Workbook for MEMT-INTERMEDIATE TEXTBOOK for the 1999 National Standard Curriculum

Workbook for Mosby's EMT-INTERMEDIATE TEXTBOOK for the 1999 National Standard Curriculum

Third Edition

Bruce R. Shade, EMT-P, EMS-I, AAS
Assistant Director of Public Safety, *Retired*
City of Cleveland, Cleveland, Ohio
Adjunct Faculty, Cuyahoga Community College, Cleveland, Ohio
Part-Time Firefighter/Paramedic, Willoughby, Ohio
Past President, National Association of Emergency Medical Technicians

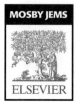

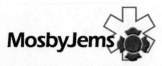

An Affiliate of Elsevier Science

11830 Westline Industrial Drive
St. Louis, Missouri 63146

Workbook for Mosby's EMT-Intermediate ISBN 13: 978-0-323-04515-5
Textbook for the 1999 National Standard Curriculum ISBN 10: 0-323-04515-4

Copyright © 2007, 2002, 1997 by Mosby, Inc., an affiliate of Elsevier Inc.

All rights reserved. No part of this publication may be reproduced or transmitted in any form or by any means, electronic or mechanical, including photocopying, recording, or any information storage and retrieval system, without permission in writing from the publisher.
Permissions may be sought directly from Elsevier's Health Sciences Rights Department in Philadelphia, PA, USA: phone: (+1) 215 239 3804, fax: (+1) 215 239 3805, e-mail: healthpermissions@elsevier.com. You may also complete your request on-line via the Elsevier homepage (http://www.elsevier.com), by selecting 'Customer Support' and then 'Obtaining Permissions'.

Notice

Knowledge and best practice in this field are constantly changing. As new research and experience broaden our knowledge, changes in practice, treatment and drug therapy may become necessary or appropriate. Readers are advised to check the most current information provided (i) on procedures featured or (ii) by the manufacturer of each product to be administered, to verify the recommended dose or formula, the method and duration of administration, and contraindications. It is the responsibility of the practitioner, relying on their own experience and knowledge of the patient, to make diagnoses, to determine dosages and the best treatment for each individual patient, and to take all appropriate safety precautions. To the fullest extent of the law, neither the Publisher nor the Authors assume any liability for any injury and/or damage to persons or property arising out or related to any use of the material contained in this book.

The Publisher

ISBN 13: 978-0-323-04515-5
ISBN 10: 0-323-04515-4

Publishing Director: Andrew Allen
Executive Editor: Linda Honeycutt
Developmental Editor: Kathleen Sartori
Publishing Services Manager: Pat Joiner
Project Manager: David Stein

Printed in the United States.

Last digit is the print number: 9 8 7 6 5 4 3 2 1

Dedication

This book is dedicated to my wife Cheri and our children Katie and Christopher. Their sacrifice allowed me to spend the countless hours needed to bring this book to print. Throughout the years, their love and support have allowed me to continue my efforts to make learning easier and more complete for out-of-hospital providers, who in turn are able to provide better patient care to those in need. My thanks and love also go to my mother, Lucille Shade, who was an aspiring author; she encouraged me to put pen to paper. Also to my father, Elmer Shade, Jr., who taught me to value a hard day's work and to continually strive for what I believe.

    This workbook is also dedicated to all my students, who over the years taught me the importance of making the learning experience interesting and challenging. It is because they become prehospital care providers and work in the field to help others that we have been able to greatly improve the quality of care provided to those in need. Lastly, I want to dedicate this book to the officers and firefighters of the Willoughby Fire Department in Ohio. They provide an outstanding, high-quality service to the community in which my family and I live.

Bruce Shade

Preface

This workbook provides a comprehensive review of the information an EMT-Intermediate (EMT-I) should know in preparation for state and national examinations as well as for working in the prehospital care setting. It includes both basic and advanced-level content.

Questions are included for each learning objective found in the textbook. Readers can use their ability to answer the questions as a gauge for determining whether they have achieved the learning objectives for the EMT-I course. The questions in this workbook were written with the intent of providing ample reinforcement of the EMT-I course content in a stimulating and challenging manner. To give readers immediate feedback, answers with rationales can be found in the back of the book. Selections to matching questions (i.e., information preceded by a letter) are bold-faced when there is a match to the selection. When there is no matching information, the selection is in italics.

To get the most from this workbook, the reader should select the most correct answer for the multiple choice and true/false questions. For the matching questions, the best corresponding answer for each item should be selected. Some matching questions have more items than corresponding answers, so some items will not be used. Other matching questions allow certain answers to be used more than one time. Writing the correct response next to each item identified by a line and letter completes labeling questions. Some labeling questions also include a coloring exercise. Colored pencils or felt tip pens can be used to complete these exercises. Some questions require short answers. It is best if readers use their own words to answer the questions rather than copying directly from the textbook. Crossword puzzles are included to make the learning more interesting. Fill-in-the-blank exercises provide blank space for the correct answer to each of these questions. Sequencing exercises are another type of questioning that is used in the workbook. With these, the reader reviews a series of skill or performance steps and identifies, by numbering, the order in which they should be performed. These exercises are meant to facilitate the mental part of learning skills—that is, what goes when.

Plentiful case histories offer readers a chance to see how well they can apply what they have learned. While reading the case, students should try to "imagine themselves responding to the emergency and actually seeing a patient in front of them." This prepares readers for the encounters they are likely to experience once they start working in the field. Several of the case histories require readers to problem solve, or in other words, to fix something that goes wrong. This, too, provides readers with a chance to develop skills they will be expected to perform each day in an often challenging and uncontrolled environment.

Readers should make every effort to answer the questions themselves before reviewing the correct answer and rationale found in the back of the textbook. This enhances learning and increases the chances for successful completion of the EMT-I course.

To provide our readers with the best possible tools for learning, we wholeheartedly encourage you to contact us with any points you feel need to be improved or changed. We want to provide the best tools available to prepare EMT-Is for working in a prehospital care setting.

Acknowledgments

As with many of these projects, a lot of work goes into making words and pictures go from the authors' minds to printed pages. A number of key people helped make this project a success. Linda Honeycutt provided resources and direction to get the project done. Her frequent phone calls and steady hand kept the project from going astray. Linda also has tremendous insight into what it takes to make these products more valuable to the learner and then has figured out a way to achieve this goal. The third editions of this textbook and workbook include several new assets that are extremely beneficial to the learner.

Our hard-working editor, Judy Ahlers, was great to work with and extremely helpful. Even though I gave her lots of stress, particularly when she had to tell Linda we were behind schedule, she hung in there and delivered an outstanding workbook to production. Furthermore, she and Linda provided emotional support along the way, helping me feel like I really could finish the project.

Contents

1 Foundations of EMT-Intermediate   1
2 Your Well-Being   11
3 Medical-Legal Aspects   19
4 Overview of Human Systems   35
5 Emergency Pharmacology   77
6 Venous Access   99
7 Medication Math   119
8 Medication Administration   125
9 Airway Management   137
10 History Taking   177
11 Techniques of Physical Examination   185
12 Patient Assessment   211
13 Clinical Decision Making   221
14 Communications   227
15 Documentation   239
16 Trauma Systems and Mechanism of Injury   249
17 Hemorrhage and Shock   259
18 Burns   277
19 Thoracic Trauma   281
20 Head and Spinal Trauma   289
21 Abdominal and Extremity Trauma   299
22 Respiratory Emergencies   307
23 Cardiovascular Anatomy and Physiology and ECG Interpretation   319
24 Cardiovascular Emergencies   359
25 Diabetic Emergencies   381
26 Allergic Reactions   387
27 Poisoning and Overdose Emergencies   391
28 Neurological Emergencies   399
29 Nontraumatic Abdominal Emergencies   407
30 Environmental Emergencies   413
31 Behavioral Emergencies and Substance Abuse   423
32 Gynecological Emergencies   429
33 Obstetrical Emergencies   435
34 Neonatal Resuscitation   445
35 Pediatric Emergencies   453
36 Geriatrics   467
37 Patients with Special Challenges   477

38 Assessment-Based Management   481
39 First Responder Procedures with Weapons of Mass Destruction   489
40 Incident Command   493
41 Tactical Emergency Medical Support   495

Answer Keys and Rationales   497

1 Foundations of EMT-Intermediate

CHAPTER TERMINAL OBJECTIVES

On completion of this chapter, the EMT-Intermediate will be able to:
- Understand his or her roles and responsibilities within an EMS system and how these roles and responsibilities differ from other levels of providers.
- Understand the role of medical direction in the prehospital environment.
- Be able to identify the importance of primary injury prevention activities as an effective way to reduce death, disabilities, and health care costs.
- Value the role that ethics play in decision making in the prehospital environment.

For the multiple-choice questions, select the single best answer to each question. For the matching questions, select the best corresponding answer for each item. Because there are sometimes more items than corresponding answers, some items may not be used.

1. To work as an EMT-I in most states, one must do all of the following *except:*
   a. attend a recognized EMT-Intermediate course
   b. become nationally registered
   c. become certified or licensed
   d. successfully complete a written and practical examination

2. The EMT-I:
   a. uses a limited amount of equipment to perform early assessment and intervention
   b. does not require on-line medical direction to make treatment decisions
   c. receives 110 hours of training
   d. employs additional skills including advanced airway adjuncts, intravenous therapy, and defibrillation

3. Certification:
   a. is the action by which an agency or association grants recognition to an individual who has met its qualifications
   b. gives the EMT-I the right to function as an EMT-I or be selected for employment
   c. is the process that allows the transfer of an EMT-I's licensure from one state to another
   d. is the process by which a governmental agency grants permission to an individual to engage in a given occupation

4. Describe the process you must follow to become certified or licensed in your state on completion of your EMT-I course.

_____

_____

_____

_____

_____

5. The process that allows the transfer of an EMT-I's licensure from one state to another is referred to as:
   a. ethics
   b. reciprocity
   c. professionalism
   d. certification

6. T F Body substance isolation is a concept that regards all body tissues and fluids as potentially infected.

7. T F To become recertified, EMT-Is are required to participate in a refresher course.

8. List three reasons why continuing education is important to an EMT-I.

   _____

   _____

   _____

9. One- or 2-day training programs such as PreHospital Trauma Life Support (PHTLS) or Basic Trauma Life Support (BTLS):
   a. can be conveniently reviewed while at home or on the job
   b. are all that are required in most states to be recertified as an EMT-I
   c. allow the EMT-I to hear a wide range of nationally recognized experts in EMS relaying the most recent information all in one location
   d. offer the benefit of requiring modest time commitment on the part of the EMT-I while providing enormous knowledge, skill learning, and remediation

10. Benefits of subscribing to professional journals include all of the following *except:*
    a. keeping the EMT-I aware of the latest changes in a constantly evolving industry
    b. highlighting tips that can be used by the EMT-I on the job
    c. typically meeting all of the requirements for state recertification
    d. providing excellent sources of continuing education to sharpen knowledge and skills

11. List two benefits an EMT-I derives from serving as an instructor in CPR, first aid, or EMT course.

    _____

    _____

12. A professional:
    a. has an advanced degree in prehospital care
    b. is a prehospital provider who is paid for his or her work
    c. is a person who has certain special skills and knowledge in a specific area and conforms to the standards of conduct and performance in that area
    d. is an individual who has permission from a governmental agency to engage in a given occupation

13. Match each of the following behaviors with professional or unprofessional conduct.

    Conduct
    a. Professional
    b. Unprofessional

    Behavior
    _____ Smoking while treating patients

    _____ Being well-groomed, wearing a clean, pressed, and well-fitting uniform

    _____ Addressing patients by their proper names

    _____ Having outbursts when persons call for EMS unnecessarily

    _____ Attending continuing education, practicing skills, reading EMS-related literature, and participating in quality improvement activities

    _____ Referring to your place of employment as being a "terrible place to work"

    _____ Working well as a member of the prehospital team, sharing equally in the workload

    _____ Not keeping the ambulance and equipment clean

    _____ Falsifying run reports

    _____ Arguing with nurses at a hospital where a patient has been transported

14. Which of the following are responsibilities of the EMT-I?
    1. interacting with first responders who are already on the scene providing care
    2. rapidly assessing and managing life-threatening illnesses and injuries
    3. a careful patient assessment, diagnosing the nature of illnesses or injuries, and prescribing emergency medical care
    4. recognizing when the limits of field care have been reached and when prompt transportation is needed
    5. administering primary and secondary cardiac medications

    Select the correct answer.
    a. 1 and 2
    b. 4 only
    c. 3, 4, and 5
    d. 1, 2, and 4

15. Ethics:
    a. relate to the willingness of the EMT-I to maintain an appropriate appearance
    b. are laws governing one's conduct as an EMT-I
    c. set standards for human morals
    d. deal with the EMT-I's relationship with his or her peers, patients, the patient's family, and society in general

16. Place a checkmark next to those behaviors listed below that are considered unethical:

    _____ Making a statement to a patient about a fellow health care worker's perceived qualities

    _____ Gently rebuffing an attractive patient's advances

    _____ Giving an attorney's business card to a victim who has fallen on icy steps in front of a public building

    _____ Discouraging a patient from going to the hospital because he or she cannot pay

    _____ Failing to maintain patient confidentiality

17. Which of the following statements regarding ethical decision making is true?
    a. These decisions should be based on what other people think is right or wrong.
    b. Employing emotion is useful when dealing with ethical questions.
    c. Maintaining a personal code of ethics that is consistent with the professional code of ethics will help an EMT-I arrive at appropriate conclusions.
    d. Sometimes making an ethical decision requires you to do something that is considered morally wrong.

18. What is one of the *first* things you should ask yourself when making an ethical decision?
    a. What does the patient really want?
    b. What does the family want?
    c. What do your protocols say?
    d. What is morally correct?

19. Patient confidentiality:
    a. is a right of all patients provided they are adults and considered competent
    b. is still considered intact if the EMT-I limits discussion of the patient's condition to what he or she knows to be fact
    c. is not breeched if the EMT-I discusses information with only his or her family
    d. is both ethically and legally required

20. T F Each person has a right to accept or decline care.

21. You are called to the home of a 50-year-old male who is apneic and pulseless. As you enter the patient's bedroom, the family presents you with a DNR order written on a prescription form and tells you not to resuscitate the patient. Your state allows EMT-Is to honor DNR orders. You should:
    a. immediately initiate CPR and continue it until you arrive at the hospital because DNR orders are not valid unless they are typewritten on a notarized document
    b. initiate CPR and advise the family to contact the patient's physician so you can speak with him or her directly
    c. honor the family's request
    d. immediately transport the patient to the hospital while providing both basic and advanced life support

22. An Emergency Medical Service (EMS) system is an _____ approach to providing _____ _____ to the _____ and _____ .

23. List the primary responsibilities of an EMS system.

    _____
    _____
    _____
    _____

24. Components of today's EMS systems may include all of the following *except:*
    a. resource management
    b. definitive trauma care
    c. transportation
    d. communications

25. Medical direction:
    a. is typically delivered via telephone to EMT-Is in the field
    b. has the responsibility of overseeing the operational aspects of EMS systems
    c. ensures that EMT-Is are providing appropriate high-quality care
    d. is usually the responsibility of nurses working in the emergency department

26. T F On-line medical direction is delivered when the EMT-I renders patient care and contacts the receiving hospital.

27. T F Protocols are a set of written instructions.

28. T F Typically, EMS managers are responsible for developing patient care protocols.

29. Portions of protocols that are completed before the EMT-I is required to contact medical direction are referred to as:
    a. direct medical orders
    b. patient care directives
    c. standing orders
    d. on-line instructions

30. List 10 duties of an EMS physician in providing medical direction.

    _____
    _____
    _____
    _____
    _____
    _____
    _____
    _____
    _____
    _____

31. Continuous quality improvement (CQI):
    a. is defined as scientific study used to establish facts and determine their significance
    b. is the evaluation of an EMS system's public image
    c. compares the care delivered with the accepted standard of care
    d. can prove that prehospital care makes a difference and is valuable

32. CQI activities are most often completed by:
    a. nurses who work in local hospital CQI departments
    b. management personnel and physicians responsible for system oversight
    c. emergency department nurses and physician assistants
    d. physicians who work in local emergency departments

33. List four benefits of the quality improvement process.

   _____

   _____

   _____

   _____

34. List four things that are checked for on patient care reports.

   _____

   _____

   _____

   _____

   _____

35. The observational phase of quality assurance involves:
    a. riding with EMT-Is as they respond to emergency calls and provide patient care
    b. conducting prehospital research on patient survival
    c. having EMT-Is demonstrate their skills on training manikins
    d. watching EMT-Is while they perform skills in the emergency department

36. Briefly explain why research is important to EMS.

   _____

   _____

   _____

   _____

   _____

37. List three benefits of conducting prehospital research.

   _____

   _____

   _____

   _____

38. Describe some reporting mechanisms and preventative measures for the following scenario.

Scenario	Reporting Mechanism	Preventative Measure
Hot summer; several deaths have occurred because children are being left unattended in cars		

39. List four reasons why EMS providers can play an important role in education and prevention activities.

_____

_____

_____

_____

40. Define the term *epidemiology*.

_____

_____

_____

41. Define the term *injury*.

_____

_____

_____

_____

42. T F Trauma is the leading cause of death in persons aged 15 to 65.

43. T F Nearly 60 million persons are injured annually in the United States.

44. T F Falls from great heights are the most common cause of fatal injuries.

45. Describe the role of the EMT-I in reducing injury.

_____

_____

_____

_____

46. Accidental injuries:
    a. are referred to as unintentional
    b. occur because of purposeful actions
    c. account for approximately one third of all injury deaths
    d. b and c

47. Determine the lost productive years of life for each of the following:

Case	Lost Productive Years of Life
33-year-old female who was killed in a head-on collision	
41-year-old male who was shot to death	
19-year-old male who was killed in an explosion	
61-year-old female who was burned to death in a house fire	

48. Match the following terms with the correct definitions. Definitions may be used more than once.

   Term
   a. Injury risk
   b. Injury
   c. Primary injury prevention
   d. Secondary and tertiary
   e. Teachable moment

   Definition
   _____ Ongoing systematic collection, analysis, and interpretation of injury data

   _____ Care and rehabilitation activities (respectively) that prevent further problems from an event that has already occurred

   _____ Real or potentially hazardous situations that put individuals in danger of sustaining injury

   _____ Essential to the planning, implementation, and evaluation of public health practice

   _____ Keeping an injury from ever occurring

   _____ An example is using power tools without wearing eye protection

   _____ Time after an injury has occurred when the patient remains acutely aware of what has happened and may be receptive to instruction about how the event or illness could be prevented

49. Fill in the missing information below regarding elements of injury risk identification and surveillance.

   EMT-Is identify injury causes
   ↓
   _____
   ↓
   These data are disseminated to those who need to know in a timely manner
   ↓
   _____

CROSSWORD PUZZLE EXERCISE

50. Complete the following crossword puzzle.

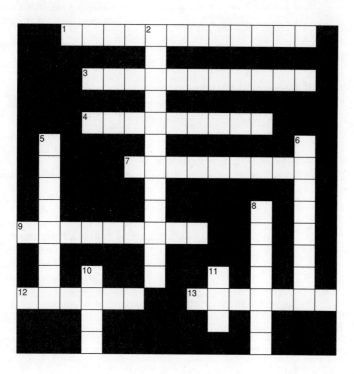

ACROSS

1. Has special skills and knowledge in a specific area and conforms to standards.
3. Process that allows the transfer of certification or licensure from one state to another.
4. Single most important behavior as an EMT-I.
7. Process by which a governmental agency grants permission to engage in a given occupation.
9. Set of written policies and procedures.
12. Derived from the Greek word meaning "character."
13. Involves identifying with and understanding the feelings, situations, and motives of others.

DOWN

2. Study of elements influencing frequency, distribution, and causes of injury and disease.
5. Type of medical direction that includes development of written instructions.
6. Scientific study conducted to establish facts and determine their significance.
8. Type of injury prevention used to keep an injury from ever occurring.
10. An injury _____ is a real or potentially hazardous situation.
11. Abbreviation for an organized approach to providing emergency care to the sick and injured.

2 Your Well-Being

CHAPTER TERMINAL OBJECTIVES

On completion of this chapter, the EMT-Intermediate will be able to understand and value the importance of personal wellness in EMS and serve as a healthy role model for peers.

For the multiple-choice questions, select the single best answer to each question. For the matching questions, select the best corresponding answer for each item. Because there are sometimes more items than corresponding answers, some items may not be used.

1. Infectious diseases are caused by:
    a. pollutants
    b. bacteria and viruses
    c. toxic substances
    d. a breakdown in the body's autoimmune system

2. Define the term *contagious disease*.

   _____

   _____

   _____

   _____

3. T F Someone who has an infectious disease will almost always exhibit signs of the illness.

4. T F EMT-Is face little risk for exposure to infectious disease.

5. T F Body substance isolation is a concept that regards all body tissues and fluids as potentially infected.

6. List four ways you may be exposed to an infectious disease during the normal course of your duties as an EMT-I.

   _____

   _____

   _____

   _____

7. List five things the EMT-I can do to reduce the risk of being exposed to or infected by an infectious disease.

___

___

___

___

___

8. The *first* rule to remember with respect to body substance isolation is:
   a. treat all blood and body fluids as though they are infectious
   b. start IVs and administer medications only to patients who absolutely need them
   c. always wear eye protection whenever conducting a patient assessment
   d. the EMT-I will likely become infected if he or she comes in contact with blood and/or body fluids

9. The most effective way to prevent disease transmission is to:
   a. always wear protective gloves when there is contact with a patient
   b. wear a gown or protective barrier during airway management procedures
   c. sterilize all equipment that comes into contact with a patient's blood and/or body fluids
   d. wash your hands as soon as possible after every patient contact or after completing a decontamination procedure

10. T F Hand washing is unnecessary as long as gloves are worn.

11. T F Latex, vinyl, or nitrile gloves can be reused as long as they are not obviously contaminated with blood or body fluids.

12. T F A safe way to remove gloves is to turn them inside out while pulling them off so as to avoid touching any contaminated areas.

13. Describe how the EMT-I can clean his or her hands when there is no access to running water.

___

___

___

___

___

14. PPE stands for:

___

___

___

15. There are three basic types of gloves: _____, _____, and _____. _____ or _____ gloves should be used if you are allergic to latex. An indication that you may be allergic is if you experience a _____ after wearing latex gloves.

16. Describe what should be done if your gloves become contaminated with blood while caring for a patient.

   _____

   _____

   _____

17. Which of the following is true regarding the use of eye protection?
    a. Eye protection should be worn whenever there is a risk of body fluids splashing into your eyes.
    b. Regular prescription glasses with side shields offer the best protection.
    c. Eye protection is required when performing airway procedures such as ventilation with a bag-mask device and insertion of an oropharyngeal airway.
    d. Rubbing your eyes while wearing contaminated gloves poses little risk of contamination.

18. Basic surgical masks:
    a. can protect the EMT-I against airborne pathogens such as those that cause tuberculosis (TB)
    b. are reusable and held in place by elastic bands or ties that fit around your head
    c. that have an attached eye shield offer little more protection than the standard mask
    d. are designed to prevent splashed or aerosolized blood and body fluids from coming into contact with your mouth and nose

19. List four signs and symptoms associated with active TB.

   _____

   _____

   _____

20. List five groups that are considered at high risk for TB.

   _____

   _____

   _____

   _____

21. Describe a precaution the EMT-I can take when treating a patient who has TB.

    _____

    _____

    _____

    _____

22. T F Disposable medical devices that become contaminated with blood or other body fluids can be placed in a wastepaper basket for disposal with normal trash.

23. T F Needles and other sharp objects must be disposed of in a puncture-proof container, often referred to as a "sharps" container.

24. Sterilizing medical equipment means:
    a. washing an item with soap and water
    b. cleaning and using a disinfectant to kill microorganisms that may be on equipment
    c. using chemical or physical methods to kill all the microorganisms on an object
    d. using heat to destroy microorganisms

25. List five actions you should take if you are exposed to blood or any other body fluid, or stuck by a needle.

    _____

    _____

    _____

    _____

    _____

26. Define the term *immunization*.

    _____

    _____

    _____

27. T F All emergency care providers should maintain immunizations for tetanus, diphtheria, polio, hepatitis B, MMR (measles, mumps, and rubella), and influenza.

28. List four factors that play a major role in maintaining physical health.

___

29. Describe a poor nutritional habit EMT-Is can easily develop because of the fast-paced environment in which they work.

___

30. List six categories of nutrients.

___

31. T F Food groups include sugar, fats, vitamins, dairy products, vegetables, fruits, and minerals.

32. T F Meat, poultry, fish, fats, eggs, and nuts are the most nutritional.

33. T F Nutrition has little to do with a person's well-being.

34. T F A healthy diet includes plenty of grain products, vegetables, and fruit and a variety of foods that are low in fat, saturated fat, and cholesterol.

35. T F Consumption of alcoholic beverages is part of a healthy diet.

36. Describe why physical fitness and weight control are important to the EMT-I.

_____

_____

_____

_____

37. Physical fitness is a condition that helps one to:
    a. work less
    b. decrease the amount of sleep necessary to feel rested
    c. look, feel, and do his or her best
    d. increase the resting heart rate and blood pressure

38. Describe why the job of the EMT-I can be extremely challenging for persons who are overweight.

_____

_____

_____

_____

39. The average adult needs _____ hours of sleep each day.
    a. 3 to 4
    b. 5 to 6
    c. 7 to 8
    d. 9 to 10

40. Which of the following will reduce the risk of *both* heart disease and cancer?
    a. using sunscreen
    b. maintaining a good total cholesterol/HDL ratio
    c. controlling high blood pressure
    d. eliminating smoking

41. Anxiety is defined as:
    a. uneasiness or dread about future uncertainties
    b. body or mental tension brought about by physical, chemical, or emotional factors
    c. good stress
    d. a negative response to an environmental stimulus

42. Likely causes of stress include all of the following *except:*
    a. a death in the family
    b. patient demands
    c. paperwork
    d. regular exercise

43. List five signs of stress.

    _____

    _____

    _____

    _____

    _____

44. Which of the following is true regarding critical incident stress management (CISM)?
    a. It is an organized, but highly informal, peer and mental health support network.
    b. It is limited to preincident stress training and on-scene support of distressed personnel.
    c. CISM services are available only to emergency responders.
    d. Two key parts of the process are the defusing and the debriefing.

CROSSWORD PUZZLE EXERCISE

45. Complete the following crossword puzzle.

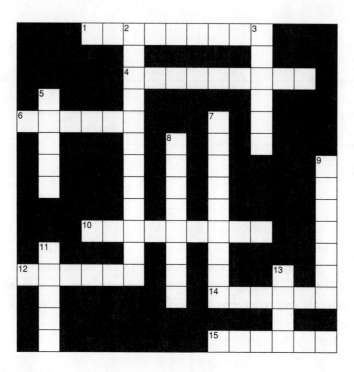

ACROSS

1. Microorganisms capable of causing disease in a suitable host.
4. Type of waste that should be placed in a red bag.
6. Caused by a change or mutation in the nucleus of a cell.
10. Cleaning and using a liquid chemical to kill microorganisms that may be on equipment.
12. Should be used whenever you come into contact with a patient.
14. Bodily or mental tension brought about by physical, chemical, or emotional factors.
15. An effective substitute to commercial disinfectants.

DOWN

2. Condition that can produce airborne pathogens.
3. Name of container in which needles and other sharp objects must be disposed.
5. Type of protective gloves that can cause allergic reaction.
7. Foods that contain the elements necessary for the body to function.
8. Washing of an item with soap and water.
9. Offer the best eye protection.
11. Helps to rejuvenate a tired body.
13. One type of respirator approved by NIOSH for use when treating patients with TB.

3 Medical-Legal Aspects

CHAPTER TERMINAL OBJECTIVES

On completion of this chapter, the EMT-Intermediate will be able to understand the legal issues that affect decisions made in the prehospital environment.

For the multiple-choice questions, select the single best answer to each question. For the matching questions, select the best corresponding answer for each item. Because there are sometimes more items than corresponding answers, some items may not be used.

1. To reduce the chances of being named in a lawsuit, EMT-Is should:
    a. adhere to state and local guidelines concerning prehospital care
    b. employ any procedure necessary to save a patient's life, even those that exceed the EMT-I's certification level
    c. reserve the use of on-line medical control for only when it is required
    d. deliver CPR to all patients in cardiac arrest, even those who have a DNR order

2. Which of the following EMT-Is is *not* demonstrating ethical behavior?
    a. Joe regularly attends continuing education classes, even those not required for recertification.
    b. Jason frequently asks attractive patients to go out for drinks after work.
    c. Mark regularly assists the hospital staff with caring for patients after delivering them to the hospital.
    d. Jill comforts patients who are experiencing serious illnesses.

3. Your local legislator initiates a law designed to clarify and expand the role and responsibilities of the EMT-I. If passed, this law will be a/an _____ law.
    a. administrative
    b. common
    c. legislative
    d. civil

4. Match each of the following types of law with the appropriate characteristics.

    Type of Law
    a. Criminal
    b. Tort

    Characteristic
    _____ Prohibits the performance of any act that is considered damaging to the public

    _____ Covers a private or public wrong or injury that occurs because of a breach, or break, of a legal duty or obligation

    _____ Covers offenses such as robbery, assault, and murder

    _____ When the plaintiff successfully proves that the defendant caused him or her harm by violating a legal duty, the plaintiff may collect damages

    _____ Also called civil law

    _____ The plaintiff files a lawsuit or legal action against the defendant

    _____ When a person is found guilty, a fine, imprisonment, or both may result

5. Place a checkmark next to those examples that are related to *civil law*.

    _____ An EMT-I is called as a witness in a drive-by shooting.

    _____ An EMT-I is charged with taking an unconscious patient's money.

    _____ A paramedic is sued for failing to intubate a patient who was in cardiac arrest.

    _____ An ambulance company fails to live up to its contract.

    _____ An EMT-I makes untrue and malicious remarks about a patient.

    _____ Two EMT-Is assault an intoxicated patient.

    _____ An EMT-I practices medicine without a license.

6. Medical Practice Acts:
    a. require EMT-Is to possess a chauffeur's license to drive an emergency vehicle
    b. outline the limits for how much a plaintiff can be awarded in a lawsuit against an EMT-I
    c. define the limits for the scope of practice of the EMT-I
    d. are laws developed by nongovernmental agencies

7. Certification:
    a. authorizes an EMT-I to deliver advanced life support
    b. is a process of occupational regulation
    c. is usually issued to the EMT-I by a state medical board
    d. grants recognition to an individual who has met predetermined qualifications

8. The EMT-I may have an obligation to report all of the following *except:*
    a. a 32-year-old who was assaulted by her husband
    b. a 16-year-old who is pregnant and unmarried
    c. a 16-year-old who was stabbed during an argument with his neighbor
    d. a 19-year-old who was allegedly raped by an acquaintance

9. The standard of care:
    a. is the degree of medical care and skill that is expected of a reasonably competent EMT-I acting in the same or similar circumstances
    b. is measured by matching the EMT-I's performance to others with lesser training and experience
    c. is based exclusively on scientific literature and EMS system standards
    d. is seldom the basis for determining whether an EMT-I is negligent in providing needed care to a given patient

CROSSWORD PUZZLE EXERCISE

10. Complete the following crossword puzzle.

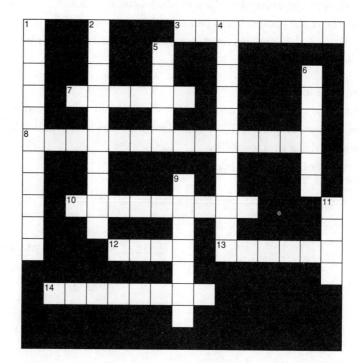

ACROSS

3. Protection against charge of negligence.
7. Judge-made law.
8. Regulations developed by a governmental agency.
10. States the reasons for the charge of negligence and asks for damages.
12. Breach of a legal duty or obligation resulting in a physical, mental, or financial injury.
13. Individual who has special knowledge and serves as a witness in a civil case.
14. Type of negligence that includes acts of omission that occur in an attempt to deliver proper care.

DOWN

1. Performing a wrongful or unlawful act.
2. Sworn statement, usually taken in an attorney's office.
4. Performing a legal act in a way that is harmful.
5. Type of negligence that is considered willful and wanton.
6. Type of damages called compensatory.
9. Unlawful touching of another person without consent.
11. Obligation to provide care.

11. The scope of practice for the EMT-I:
    a. includes such skills as placing IV lines, administering various medications, and performing nasotracheal intubation
    b. is established solely through guidelines developed by the federal government
    c. is the duties and skills he or she is expected to perform when necessary
    d. involves exercising the care, skill, and judgment that would be expected under like or similar circumstances by a similarly trained, reasonable EMT-I

12. All of the following are true *except:*
    a. on-line medical direction is care rendered under direct orders, usually over the radio or telephone
    b. each state's Medical Practice Act protects EMS system medical directors from liability
    c. medical direction is a physician's responsibility
    d. standing orders are part of off-line medical direction

13. Match each of the following terms with the correct definition.

    Term
    a. Negligence
    b. Duty to act
    c. Proximate cause
    d. Injury

    Definition
    _____ Obligation to provide care
    _____ Something that is directly responsible for damage
    _____ Conduct that falls below the standard of care

14. Describe the difference between ordinary and gross negligence.

    _____
    _____
    _____
    _____
    _____

15. List the four requirements that must be met for the EMT-I to be found negligent.

    _____
    _____
    _____
    _____

16. What is the EMT-I's best protection against being named as a defendant in a negligence case?
    a. avoiding undue risks
    b. obtaining malpractice insurance
    c. participating in high-quality training
    d. providing care only at a basic level

CASE 1 REVIEW AND DISCUSSION

REVIEW THE FOLLOWING CASES AND ANSWER THE DISCUSSION QUESTIONS POSED.

EMT-Is Jones and Landford are working for a local fire department rescue squad when they are called to the home of a 60-year-old man who is complaining of chest pain. The fire department is the agency responsible for providing emergency medical service to this community. The patient, Mr. Alfonzo, is sitting in a recliner in the living room. His wife is standing next to him; she appears worried. EMT-I Jones begins assessing the patient's vital signs while Landford obtains the present and past medical histories. According to the patient, who is alert and oriented, his chest pain started about 1 hour before the squad was called. It is described as a dull, aching pain that does not radiate and is unaffected by position or breathing. The patient tells EMT-I Landford that he has a history of diabetes for which he takes daily insulin. Mr. Alfonzo's vital signs are as follows: the pulse is 120 beats per minute (BPM) and regular; respirations are 16; blood pressure is 160/100; and his skin is pale and moist. His lung sounds are clear bilaterally. The physical exam is unremarkable. The ECG rhythm shows a pronounced elevation in the ST segment, indicating the patient is experiencing myocardial ischemia and/or infarction.

After obtaining this information, EMT-I Jones instructs Mr. Alfonzo to stand up and walk out to the ambulance, which is parked outside on the street. Mr. Alfonzo tells Jones that he feels a bit unsteady and would prefer they carry him out on the cot. "Mr. Alfonzo, you are a bit too heavy for the two of us to carry you to the ambulance," says Landford. "If we have to wait for another crew to respond here to help us move you, it will be a while before we get you to the hospital." EMT-I Jones then adds, "You really need to be seen right away, so the quickest thing to do is to go ahead and have you walk out to the ambulance." With that, Mr. Alfonzo agrees to their direction and stands up. He slowly walks from the house to the outside, assisted by EMT-I Jones. Landford follows them, carrying the jump kit, ECG monitor, and oxygen unit they brought in with them. As Mr. Alfonzo steps down off his porch onto the sidewalk that leads to the apron of his driveway, he grasps his chest and collapses to the ground. Both Landford and Jones assess him and determine he is in cardiac arrest. They start CPR right away and call for a backup unit to assist. Despite both basic and advanced life support provided to Mr. Alfonzo, he is pronounced dead at the hospital.

Two weeks after Mr. Alfonzo's funeral, Mrs. Alfonzo decides to meet with her attorney, Mr. Schaffer. As she describes the circumstances surrounding her husband's death she keeps saying, "If only they had carried him to the ambulance he would be alive today." Following a public records request, Attorney Schaffer obtains a copy of the run report that was completed for the call in question and the fire department's patient care protocol for chest pain.

The following are the relevant portions of the protocol:

a. Position the patient in the most comfortable position that satisfies his or her physiological needs.
b. Administer high-flow oxygen, 10 to 15 L (85% to 100%) by nonrebreather mask if acute myocardial infarction or ischemia is suspected and the patient is breathing adequately and has a patent airway.
c. Identify priority patients and make transport/ALS backup decision.
d. Assess and record vital signs. Be sure to note breath sounds because rales and rhonchi may indicate heart failure.
e. Apply ECG monitoring electrodes and provide continuous monitoring. Follow the appropriate protocol if dysrhythmias are seen.
f. Conduct focused history and physical examination (be sure to check the extremities for edema and presence of equal pulses, and check the abdomen for swelling).
g. Question the patient to gather present history (OPQRST and SAMPLE).
h. Determine whether there is a history of cardiac problems or other significant medical conditions.
i. Identify current medications the patient is taking.
j. Identify any allergies (particularly to medications).
k. Start an IV with normal saline and a microdrip administration set at a keep-open rate.

l. Check patient's blood pressure and administer nitroglycerin, 0.3 to 0.4 mg, sublingually if the patient is not hypotensive (blood pressure <90 mm Hg systolic or <120 mm Hg systolic in patients older than 70).
m. Contact medical command for further instruction.
n. Check patient's blood pressure and report it to medical command. The medical command physician may order repeat administration of nitroglycerin, 0.3 to 0.4 mg, sublingually every 5 minutes until chest pain is relieved or a total of 1.2 mg has been given (if the patient is not hypotensive).
o. Recheck the patient's blood pressure. If the chest pain persists and the patient is not hypotensive, the medical command physician may direct the administration of morphine sulfate, 2 to 4 mg, slow IV push (if the patient is not hypotensive).
p. Move patient to the ambulance or squad on a stair chair or cot. *Do not walk the patient to the vehicle.* Place the patient in a position of comfort based on his or her physiological needs.
q. Continue to reassess the patient's vital signs and response to treatment.
r. Unless otherwise directed by an on-duty supervisor, the patient should be transported to the nearest *appropriate* hospital.
s. Transport to hospital quietly and promptly without lights or siren.

Attorney Schaffer then obtains a copy of the autopsy report from the local coroner in which she rules Mr. Alfonzo died of "cardiac arrest suffered as a result of an acute myocardial infarction."

17. Attorney Schaffer concludes the following. Assume you are a potential expert witness. Indicate whether you agree or disagree with his conclusions. Justify your answers.

Conclusion	Agree or Disagree	Justify Your Answer
EMT-Is Landford and Jones had a duty to act.		
The care the EMT-Is provided fell below the standard of care.		
Mr. Alfonzo suffered a myocardial infarction that led to cardiac arrest and his subsequent death because of the actions of Landford and Jones.		

18. List those things EMT-Is Jones and Landford did wrong and indicate whether that action or lack of action would be considered misfeasance, malfeasance, or nonfeasance.

Action	Type of Breach of Duty

19. Attorney Schaffer alleges that the actions of these EMT-Is is grossly negligent. Briefly argue, in writing, the following:

Why he is not correct	
Why he is correct	

20. Which of the following would likely be the best expert witness for this case?
    a. an EMT-I who works for a neighboring EMS agency
    b. an emergency physician who provides medical direction of a large urban EMS system
    c. a nurse who works in the coronary care unit of a local hospital
    d. a fire chief of a suburban community

CASE 2 REVIEW AND DISCUSSION

EMT-Is Smith and Lukas are called to the home of an 80-year-old man, Mr. Taylor, who is experiencing severe shortness of breath. Mr. Taylor is sitting in a chair in the kitchen. EMT-I Smith solicits the present and past medical histories from the patient while Lukas obtains the vital signs. Speaking in short sentences, Mr. Taylor says, "I was having trouble catching my breath last night, and it got worse today, so I thought I better call." He says the shortness of breath gets worse when he lies down or exerts himself. He tells EMT-I Smith that he has a history of hypertension for which he takes daily diuretics and antihypertensives. Mr. Taylor's vital signs are as follows: he is alert and oriented; the pulse is 132 BPM and regular; respirations are 22; the blood pressure is 186/106; and his skin is pale and diaphoretic. Auscultation of his lung sounds reveals bilateral rales. The physical exam reveals swelling of both lower legs. The ECG rhythm shows a sinus tachycardia without ectopy.

Following their assessment, EMT-I Lukas tells the patient, "We need to start some treatments and take you to the hospital; is that okay with you Mr. Taylor?" The patient refuses, instead saying he wants to wait for his daughter to return from a shopping trip sometime later in the day. Despite EMT-I Lukas informing Mr. Taylor of the seriousness of his condition and that he may experience serious consequences unless treated at the hospital, he still refuses. EMT-I Smith then has Mr. Taylor talk to their on-line medical direction physician. Mr. Taylor says, "I appreciate your concern but I really want to wait for my daughter to get home." EMT-I Lukas completes the run report and then fills out a patient refusal form that he has Mr. Taylor sign. A neighbor who came over to check on Mr. Taylor signs the form as a witness to Mr. Taylor's refusal to be treated or transported to the hospital.

About 4 hours after EMT-Is Smith and Lukas leave and return to their base station they receive a call back to Mr. Taylor's home. Mr. Taylor's daughter returned home to find her father collapsed on the floor. A quick assessment suggests Mr. Taylor has been dead for at least a couple of hours.

21. You are the medical director for the EMS system where EMT-Is Lukas and Smith work. The quality assurance officer reviewed the case and made the following conclusions. Indicate whether you agree or disagree with each. Justify your answers.

Conclusion	Agree or Disagree	Justify Your Answer
EMT-Is Lukas and Smith fulfilled their duty to act.		
The care the EMT-Is provided met the standard of care.		
Mr. Taylor experienced cardiac arrest, but his death was not because of the actions of Lukas and Smith.		

22. Good Samaritan laws:
    a. provide immunity from prosecution for medical personnel who violate criminal laws at emergency scenes
    b. are in place in most states to protect persons who provide assistance at emergency scenes
    c. provide protection universally limited to laypersons
    d. typically provide funds for the defense of persons who are sued as a result of helping someone

23. T F Good Samaritan laws prevent the EMT-I from being sued.

24. T F Good Samaritan laws are largely consistent from state to state in the scope of their coverage or requirements.

25. T F Civil immunity means that an EMS service may be protected from a charge of negligence because it is a designated government agency.

26. Which of the following are likely to be protected by Good Samaritan laws?
    a. a physician who is treating a patient and charging a fee for service
    b. an EMT-I who is charged with ordinary negligence
    c. an EMT-I who performs a paramedic level intervention to treat a patient experiencing a life-threatening emergency
    d. a layperson who performs a cricothyrotomy on a patient who has an obstructed airway

27. Individual malpractice insurance is recommended for:
    a. those whose EMS systems have adequate insurance
    b. volunteer EMT-Is
    c. career EMT-Is
    d. laypersons

28. Describe the areas of responsibility in which physicians may face liability for providing medical direction.

_____
_____
_____
_____
_____

29. As an EMT-I, you:
    a. are not responsible for the actions of an EMT-Basic (EMT-B)
    b. are responsible only for you
    c. can provide medical direction to an EMT-B
    d. may be liable for the actions of an EMT-B

30. The patient's right to confidentiality:
    a. applies only to minors
    b. means that the EMT-I cannot share information with anyone other than those who are authorized to receive it
    c. applies only to the patient's history, assessment findings, and treatments rendered
    d. ends once the patient–EMT-I contact has been terminated

31. You falsely tell your partner that your patient is a felon who has a history of drug abuse. This is termed:
    a. libel
    b. malfeasance
    c. slander
    d. battery

32. Which of the following may be construed as a libelous statement?
    a. "The patient was uncooperative, refusing to allow us to assess his vital signs or provide needed treatment. . ."
    b. "The patient had one episode of emesis during transportation. . ."
    c. "The patient was falling-down drunk. . ."
    d. "The patient's gait was unsteady. . ."

33. List three ways you can avoid being sued for slander or libel.

_____
_____
_____

34. T F Hospitals are not obligated to treat persons who arrive at an emergency department and are unable to pay or who are uninsured.

35. T F Once a patient is within a hospital-owned ambulance, they must be transported to that hospital.

36. T F Patients in active labor may be transferred to another hospital if the appropriate treatment facilities are not available at the initial institution.

37. T F Consent means agreement or approval.

38. T F Conscious and mentally competent adult patients have the right to accept or refuse care or transportation as long as their condition is stable.

39. T F The EMT-I who performs assessment, care, or transport without appropriate patient consent is protected by Good Samaritan laws.

40. Expressed consent:
    a. involves the patient who is unconscious or in a condition in which he or she is unable to respond to the EMT-I
    b. is in effect only with stable patients
    c. may be withdrawn at any time by the patient
    d. means that the EMT-I assumes that a patient who is severely ill or injured would want care if the patient were able to respond

41. You respond to a baseball stadium where an 18-year-old male fell from the stands. You find him sitting on the ground. As you reach the patient he holds his up arm (which is deformed at the wrist) for you to see. This constitutes _____ consent.
    a. informed
    b. implied
    c. assumed
    d. expressed

42. After returning home from the grocery store a friend finds a 65-year-old female unconscious on her kitchen floor. EMT-Is are called to the home. They can provide treatment to this patient under _____ consent.
    a. expressed
    b. implied
    c. informed
    d. validated

43. Describe what is meant by the term *informed consent*.

_____

_____

_____

_____

44. List the information that should be presented to a patient so that he or she can make an informed decision whether to accept examination, treatment, or transport.

_____

_____

_____

_____

45. You are called to a local shopping mall where a 14-year-old male has been stabbed in the neck with a knife. You have attempted to reach his parents with no success. Which of the following are true regarding minors?
    a. Minors can legally consent to or refuse medical care.
    b. If the parent or legal guardian cannot be contacted for consent, then emergency care can be provided under the implied consent standard.
    c. Persons are no longer considered minors once they reach 16 years of age.
    d. Minors should receive only basic level care when consent cannot be obtained from a parent.

46. You are called to the home of a 16-year-old married female who is complaining of shortness of breath after escaping from a burning building. She is asking for your help. You may treat her under which of the following types of consent?
    a. valid consent by a parent
    b. expressed consent by an emancipated minor
    c. implied consent by an adult
    d. voluntary consent by a minor

47. T F A patient who has been legally determined mentally incompetent can consent to care.

48. T F If the legally responsible party is not available, a mentally incompetent patient can be cared for under the expressed consent standard.

49. T F Patients experiencing alcohol or substance intoxication can be cared for under the implied consent standard.

50. The EMT-I should do which of the following when a patient refuses examination, treatment, and/or transport to the hospital?
    1. attempt to convince the patient to allow examination, treatment, and/or transport
    2. explain the consequences of the refusal
    3. thoroughly document the refusal and have the patient sign a release
    4. force the patient to go to the hospital
    5. attempt to convince the patient that his or her beliefs are incorrect

    Select the correct answer.
    a. 1, 3, and 5
    b. 2 and 5
    c. 1, 2, and 3
    d. 4 only

51. You are called to the home of a 71-year-old female. You are informed that she is to be transported to a local hospital for admission by her physician because he believes she is suffering from cerebrovascular accident. She refuses to go and claims her son and family are just trying to move her into a nursing home. Your conversation with her reveals that she is disoriented. You should:
    a. have her sign a refusal and return to service
    b. have her son take her to the hospital in his car
    c. threaten to have her arrested if she does not cooperate
    d. provide assessment, treatment, and transport against her will

52. Match each of the following terms with the correct definition.

    Term
    a. Assault
    b. Battery
    c. False imprisonment
    d. Abandonment
    e. Libel

    Definition
    _____ When the EMT-I–patient relationship is terminated by the EMT-I without ensuring continuity of care

    _____ Intentional and unjustifiable detention of a person against his or her will

    _____ Creation of the fear of immediate bodily harm in a person, without his or her consent

53. Which of the following is considered abandonment?
    a. While driving to work, an EMT-I stops at an accident scene and provides care until a paramedic unit arrives and takes over care; he then continues on his way to work.
    b. A patient, suffering from respiratory distress, refuses care and transport despite being told of the consequences; she then signs a refusal statement, and the EMT-Is return to service.
    c. An EMT-I delivers a patient to the emergency department and leaves him or her there waiting in the triage room for the nurse to return while the EMT-I responds to another emergency call.
    d. An EMT leaves a patient with an EMT-I.

54. An advance directive:
    a. may be either a living will or a DNR order
    b. tells rescuers the wishes of a patient's family
    c. is usually communicated orally
    d. is used only in cases in which the patient has a terminal illness

55. A 68-year-old female cancer patient appears to be in cardiac arrest on your arrival. Her daughter says her mother's living will requests no extreme measures be taken to save her life and shows you a DNR order. Other family members present want you to start care. Your safest step is to:
    a. deliver all care normally provided to patients experiencing cardiac arrest because that is your responsibility when you are dispatched to an emergency call
    b. load the patient and perform a "slow code"
    c. consult medical direction if the issues cannot be quickly resolved among the involved parties
    d. start CPR and continue until you are out of sight of family members

56. The EMT-I can use force to:
   a. treat patients who are uncooperative because of a medical condition
   b. punish patients who are abusive toward the EMS team
   c. treat patients who refuse competent care
   d. assess persons who are under 18 years of age

57. Describe how a case involving a patient who is in cardiac arrest but is a potential organ donor should be handled.

_____

_____

_____

_____

_____

58. You are called to the scene of a 49-year-old man who has been shot in the stomach by his wife during a heated argument. As you arrive at the scene, one of the children runs outside yelling, "Hurry, hurry, she is going to shoot him again." Police are not at the scene yet. You should:
   a. apply your protective body armor and enter the scene
   b. wait outside the scene until police arrive and secure it
   c. position yourself and your equipment immediately outside the entranceway to the house so you can quickly reach the patient once police have secured the scene
   d. enter the scene and disarm the wife

59. Once you are in the house you should handle the crime scene by:
   1. providing good patient care and, at the same time, preserving evidence
   2. wrapping evidence in plastic bags
   3. making mental notes of what you see
   4. assisting the police in questioning witnesses
   5. asking bystanders to enter the scene to assist you in providing care

   Select the correct answer.
   a. 1 and 3
   b. 3 only
   c. 4 and 5
   d. 1, 2, and 3

60. Which of the following is true regarding child abuse?
    a. Care of the sick or injured child should be delayed until after the child abuse is reported.
    b. You should document and report any suspicious findings to the appropriate authorities.
    c. Only Florida and California have laws that protect health care professionals from liability for reporting, in good faith, suspected child abuse.
    d. EMT-Is have no legal mandate to report suspected child abuse, and if you fail to do so, you could be subject to fines, imprisonment, and loss of state certification to practice.

61. You are providing care to a 55-year-old man who was struck by a fast-moving car, when a man approaches you. He informs you that he is an emergency physician and wants to help the patient. You should:
    a. contact medical direction and allow him to speak with the on-line physician
    b. thank him for his interest and ask him politely to leave the scene
    c. ask for verification of licensure and yield to his expertise on receipt of such confirmation
    d. inform him that only the EMS medical director can give EMS providers an order

62. The *most* important legal defense measure against medical negligence claims is to always:
    a. look professional
    b. transport the patient to the hospital
    c. accurately and thoroughly document each case
    d. provide all treatments listed in the patient care protocol

63. The ambulance run report should include which of the following?
    a. accurate and thorough documentation
    b. clear and concise opinions
    c. legible handwriting
    d. a and c

CROSSWORD PUZZLE EXERCISE

64. Complete the following crossword puzzle.

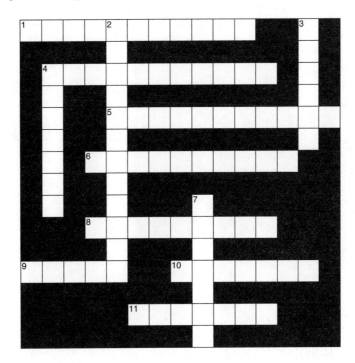

ACROSS

1. Minors who have been legally freed of the need for parental consent.
4. Means stopping care when it is still needed and desired by the patient.
5. Type of consent that involves patients held for mental health evaluation.
6. Making an untrue statement about someone's character or reputation.
8. Process of occupational regulation done by a governmental agency, such as the state medical board.
9. Injury of a person's character, name, or reputation by false and malicious writings.
10. Unlawful touching of another person without consent.
11. Type of consent that allows an EMT-I to treat a patient who is severely ill or injured.

DOWN

2. This is how all patient information must be regarded.
3. Persons younger than 18 years of age.
4. Directives indicating a patient's preference for future medical treatment.
7. Involves threatening, attempting, or causing fear of offensive physical contact with a patient

4 Overview of Human Systems

CHAPTER TERMINAL OBJECTIVES

On completion of this chapter, the EMT-Intermediate will understand basic anatomy and physiology and how it relates to the foundations of medicine.

For the multiple-choice questions, select the single best answer to each question. For the matching questions, select the best corresponding answer for each item. Because there are sometimes more items than corresponding answers, some items may not be used.

1. Define the following terms.
   Anatomy:
   _____
   _____

   Physiology:
   _____
   _____

   Pathophysiology:
   _____
   _____

2. T F The human body consists of three organizational levels.

3. Match each of the following organizational levels with the correct description.

   Organizational Level   **Description**
   a. System   _____ Groups of similar cells working together for a common function
   b. Cells
                                     _____ Carry out the processes necessary for life within each cell
   c. Tissue
   d. Organelles   _____ Composed of different types of tissues
   e. Organs   _____ The basic building blocks of all life

4. Define the term *homeostasis*.
   _____
   _____
   _____

35

Copyright © 2007 Elsevier, Inc. All rights reserved.   Chapter 4 Overview of Human Systems

5. Match each of the following anatomical and directional terms with the appropriate definition.

   Term **Definition**
   a. Prone   _____ Pertaining to the lower part of the spinal column
   b. Frontal   _____ Farthest from point of attachment
   c. Caudal   _____ The plane that vertically divides the body into a front and back portion
   d. Lateral   _____ Lying on your stomach with your face down
   e. Dorsal   _____ Above or in a higher position
   f. Distal   _____ Farther away from the midline or toward the side
   g. Superior

6. A patient has a gunshot wound to the chest, just below the sternum. This wound is on the _____ surface of the body and is _____ to the sternum.
   a. anterior; inferior
   b. posterior; lateral
   c. dorsal; caudal
   d. ventral; cranial

7. The brain is _____ to the heart.
   a. superior
   b. lateral
   c. anterior
   d. proximal

8. Label the following illustration.

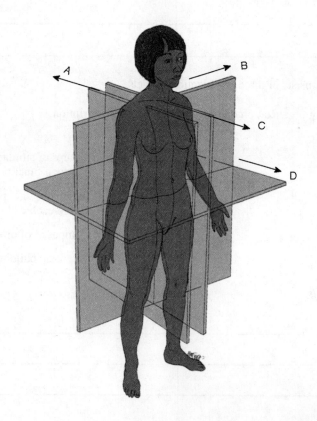

36

Chapter 4 Overview of Human Systems

9. The anatomical position means a person is:
   a. on the back with palms facing forward
   b. sitting with palms facing down
   c. on the stomach with palms facing down
   d. upright with palms facing forward

10. The knee is the _____ portion of the lower leg, whereas the ankle is the _____ portion.

11. You are called to the scene where a 31-year-old man was struck by a car as he tried to cross the street. You find him lying on his back. This patient is in a/an _____ position.
    a. supine
    b. prone
    c. lateral recumbent
    d. erect

12. Body cavities are _____ areas within the body that contain _____ and _____.

13. Match each of the following cavities with the correct characteristics.

    Cavity
    a. Thoracic
    b. Spinal
    c. Cranial
    d. Abdominal
    e. Pelvic

    Characteristic
    _____ Has a domed top and a base composed of several bones; it houses the brain

    _____ Is a single large cavity that extends from the diaphragm to the pelvic bones

    _____ Between the base of the neck and the diaphragm; is formed by the roughly circular boundary of the rib cage

    _____ Travels through the vertebral column, and contains the spinal cord

    _____ Contains the organs of digestion and excretion, which comprise the gastrointestinal and urinary systems

    _____ Comprises the lower portion of the abdominal cavity and is bounded by the ilium, ischium, pubis, sacrum, and coccyx

    _____ Major structures belong to the cardiovascular and respiratory systems—the heart, major blood vessels, and lungs

    _____ Includes organs of the gastrointestinal, reproductive, and urinary systems

14. Organs found within the cranial and spinal cavities are part of the _____ system(s).
    a. respiratory
    b. endocrine and cardiovascular
    c. reproductive
    d. nervous

15. Label the cavities in the following illustration.

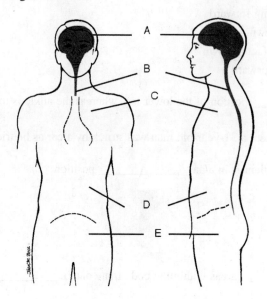

16. The mediastinum contains:
    1. bronchioles
    2. heart
    3. trachea
    4. part of the esophagus
    5. diaphragm

    Select the correct answer.
    a. 3 only
    b. 1 and 2
    c. 2, 3, and 4
    d. 3, 4, and 5

17. The digestive organs are surrounded by the:
    a. peritoneum
    b. pleural space
    c. pericardium
    d. dura mater

18. The kidneys and some of the major blood vessels of the abdominal cavity are located in an area known as the:
    a. mediastinum
    b. retroperitoneal space
    c. pleural cavity
    d. cranium

19. On the illustration below, draw two perpendicular lines that show how the abdomen is divided into four quadrants. Then list the organs that are found in each quadrant.

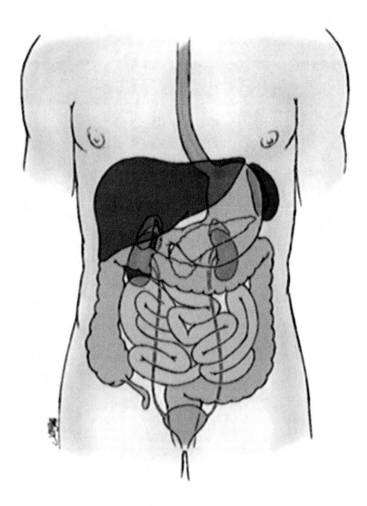

CROSSWORD PUZZLE EXERCISE

20. Complete the following crossword puzzle.

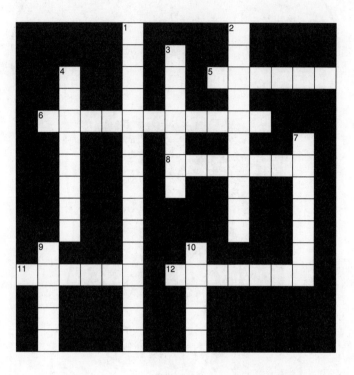

ACROSS

5. Most complex organizational level of the body
6. Normal state of balance between all of the body's systems.
8. Divides the body into equal right and left halves.
11. Toward the midline of the body.
12. Means in or near the head.

DOWN

1. Study of disease mechanisms.
2. Study of an organism's normal body functions.
3. Study of the structure of an organism and its parts.
4. Nearest to the origin of a structure.
7. Toward the front surface of the body.
9. Basic building blocks of the body.
10. Standing in an upright position.

21. The permeability of the cellular membrane refers to:
    a. the rate at which substances pass through it
    b. the makeup of its outermost layer
    c. its thickness
    d. its permanency

22. Which of the following is true regarding molecules passing through the cellular membrane?
    a. Protein molecules diffuse more easily than do water molecules.
    b. Mechanisms such as ion pumps (e.g., Na^+, K^+, H^+) act to regulate what substances pass through the cell membrane.
    c. Glucose is the one molecule that is allowed to pass freely back and forth across the cell membrane.
    d. Electrolytes easily pass through the membrane because of their electrical charge.

23. Match each of the following processes with the appropriate description.

    Process
    a. Diffusion
    b. Facilitated diffusion
    c. Osmosis
    d. Active transport

    Description
    _____ Occurs when water moves from an area of lesser solute concentration to an area of higher solute concentration

    _____ Movement of particles from an area of higher concentration to one of lower concentration until the substances scatter themselves evenly throughout an available space

    _____ Requires the assistance of a helper protein

24. On the illustration below, show the direction that particles will move during diffusion.

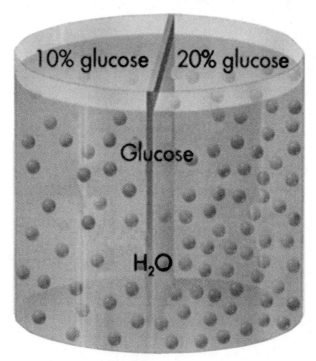

25. Which of the following requires the expenditure of energy for it to occur?
    a. facilitated diffusion
    b. diffusion
    c. osmosis
    d. active transport

26. The process that moves glucose across the cell membrane is:
    a. facilitated diffusion
    b. diffusion
    c. osmosis
    d. active transport

27. Label each portion of the illustration below as isotonic, hypotonic, or hypertonic.

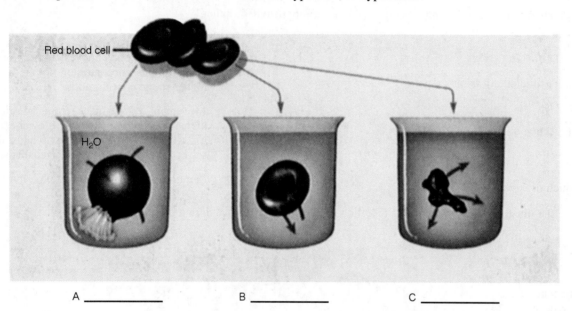

A _____   B _____   C _____

28. An isotonic IV solution has an osmotic pressure:
    a. less than that within the cell
    b. twice that of body cells
    c. greater than that within the cell
    d. equal to that within the cell

29. A hypotonic solution:
    a. has an osmotic pressure less than that of normal body fluids
    b. will draw water out of the cells and into the vascular space when administered intravenously
    c. is often used in the treatment of hypovolemia
    d. has more solutes than solvent

30. Which of the following solutions causes cells to swell by osmosis?
    a. isotonic
    b. hypotonic
    c. hypertonic
    d. hydrostatic

31. On the illustration below, use arrows to show the direction water will move across a semipermeable membrane. Use dotted lines to show how the volume of water will change on each side of the semipermeable membrane.

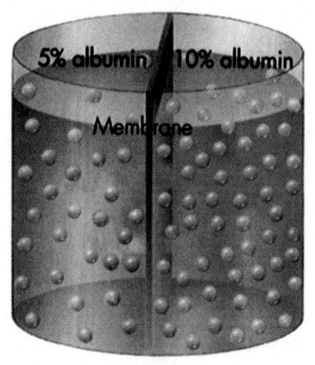

32. Which of the following is considered a hypertonic solution?
    a. normal saline (0.9%)
    b. albumin
    c. lactated Ringer's
    d. 5% dextrose in water

33. The main energy sources for the cells are:
    a. fats, calcium, sodium
    b. protein, water, ATP
    c. oxygen, nitrogen, fats
    d. glucose, amino acids, fats

34. Define the term *metabolism*.

   _____

   _____

   _____

   _____

35. T F   Glycolysis yields more ATP stores than does the Krebs cycle.

36. Cellular respiration:
    a. occurs in the same manner as respiration that occurs in the lungs
    b. produces CO_2, O_2, and chloride
    c. produces energy in the form of ATP molecules
    d. relies primarily on anaerobic metabolism

37. Anaerobic metabolism:
    a. is the primary source of energy production in the body
    b. occurs when the presence of oxygen is lowered
    c. yields a large amount of energy
    d. produces the least amount of acids

38. Cellular respiration takes place in the _____ of the cells.

CROSSWORD PUZZLE EXERCISE

39. Complete the following crossword puzzle.

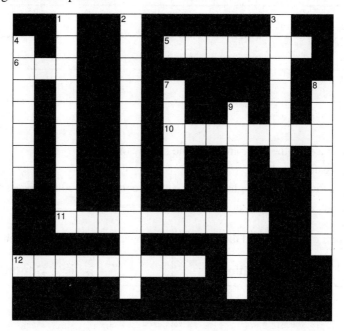

ACROSS

5. Are also referred to as particles.
6. Abbreviation for type of energy molecules produced during cellular respiration.
10. The number of particles of solutes per unit volume.
11. Breakdown phase of metabolism.
12. Constructive phase of metabolism.

DOWN

1. Has an osmotic pressure greater than that of normal body fluids.
2. Cell membrane that allows some substances to enter or leave while restricting passage of others.
3. Type of metabolism that occurs in the presence of oxygen.
4. Non–energy-requiring transport processes.
7. Only substance that passes freely back and forth across the cell membrane.
8. Some glucose is stored in this form in the liver.
9. Movement of particles from an area of higher concentration to one of lower concentration.

40. List the four types of tissue.

   _____

   _____

   _____

   _____

41. Epithelial tissue:
    a. covers all external surfaces of the body and lines the hollow organs
    b. binds other types of tissues together
    c. generates and transmits impulses throughout the body that control all bodily processes
    d. includes bone, cartilage, and adipose (fat) tissue

42. List the three major layers of the skin and then fill in the following table regarding their characteristics.

Layer	Location	Contains

43. The dermis:
    a. is the outermost layer of skin
    b. contains no blood vessels
    c. attaches the skin to the underlying bone or muscle
    d. contains connective tissue, hair follicles, glands, and nerve endings

44. The skeletal system is composed of _____ bones.
    a. 58
    b. 110
    c. 206
    d. 350

45. List four functions of the skeletal system.

_____

_____

_____

_____

46. Most of the red and white blood cells are manufactured in the:
    a. bone marrow
    b. epiphysis
    c. periosteum
    d. compact bone

47. Examples of long bones include:
    a. carpals, metacarpals
    b. vertebra
    c. femur, humerus
    d. sternum, skull

48. Label the following illustration of the skeletal system. Then use a blue highlighter to color the bones of the axial skeletal system and a yellow highlighter to color the bones of the appendicular skeleton.

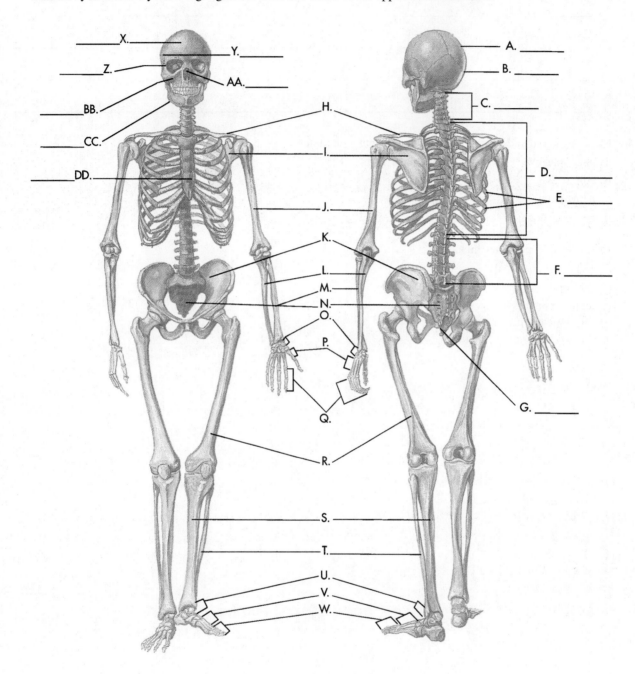

49. The brain connects with the spinal cord through a large opening at the base of the skull called the:
    a. foramen magnum
    b. styloid process
    c. squamous suture
    d. occipital bone

50. There are _____ cervical vertebrae.
    a. 4
    b. 5
    c. 7
    d. 12

51. T F The first vertebra that lies directly beneath the skull is called the axis (C1) and supports the head.

52. T F The 12 pairs of ribs that form the rib cage are attached directly to the sternum anteriorly and the thoracic vertebrae posteriorly.

53. Which of the following is located in the upper arm?
    a. scapula
    b. humerus
    c. femur
    d. radius

54. The superior portion of the ilium is called the:
    a. sacroiliac joint
    b. pelvic girdle
    c. coxa
    d. iliac crest

55. The acetabulum is the:
    a. knee cap
    b. inferior/posterior portion of the pelvis
    c. superior bone of the pelvis that contains the iliac crest
    d. socket of the hip bone

56. Match each of the following terms with the correct description.

    Term
    a. Cartilages
    b. Tendons
    c. Joints
    d. Ligaments

    Description
    _____ Where two or more bones articulate
    _____ Plates of shiny connective tissue that aid movement
    _____ Tough white bands of tissue that connect bone and cartilage

57. Describe each of the following types of joints.

    Immovable: _____

    _____

    Slightly movable: _____

    _____

    Freely movable: _____

    _____

58. Smooth muscle:
    a. is involuntary and not under conscious control
    b. has the ability to generate its own stimulus to contract if necessary
    c. includes the heart muscle
    d. has a property called *intrinsic automaticity*

59. List three types of muscle tissue.

    _____

    _____

    _____

    _____

CROSSWORD PUZZLE EXERCISE

60. Complete the following crossword puzzle.

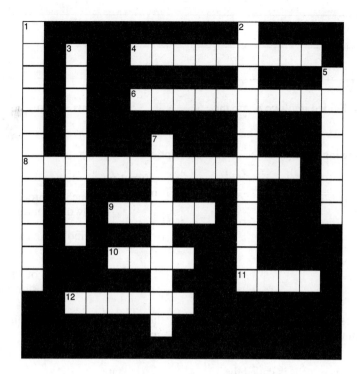

ACROSS

4. Bones that have no well-defined geometric shape.
6. Type of tissue that binds other types of tissues together.
8. Body's external surface; includes the skin, nails, hair, and sweat and oil glands.
9. Smaller bones that make up the hands and feet.
10. An example of this type of bone is the ribs.
11. Epidermis and dermis collectively are called this.
12. An example of this type of movable joint includes the knees.

DOWN

1. Component of the skeletal systems that consists of the extremities and the girdles.
2. Layer of skin that lies below the dermis.
3. Type of muscle that is under conscious control.
5. Type of tissue that includes the brain, spinal cord, and all the nerves.
7. Examples of this type of joint are those connecting the bones of the skull.

61. Describe the function of the nervous system.

_____

_____

_____

_____

62. The nervous system is divided into two parts: the _____ nervous system and the _____ nervous system.

63. Match each of the following terms with the correct description.

    Nerve Component
    a. Cell body
    b. Synapse
    c. Axon
    d. Dendrite

    Function
    _____ Branching process that extends from the cell body of a neuron
    _____ Cylinder-like extension of a neuron that carries impulses away from the cell body
    _____ Main part of the neuron containing the nucleus and surrounding tissues

64. _____ nerves transmit nerve impulses toward the spinal cord and the brain. _____ nerves transmit impulses from the brain and the spinal cord to the muscles and glands.

65. The resting state of the nerve cells is called the _____ state.
    a. depolarized
    b. repolarized
    c. activated
    d. polarized

66. Describe how depolarization occurs.

_____

_____

_____

_____

67. Match each of the following structures of the brain with its location and the functions it performs.

    Structure
    a. Cerebrum
    b. Cerebellum
    c. Medulla

    Characteristic
    _____ Top portion of the brain; consists of the left and right hemispheres
    _____ Most inferior portion of the brain
    _____ Its primary function is to control the body's coordination
    _____ Controls thinking, sensation, and voluntary movement
    _____ Is part of the brainstem
    _____ Contains important centers that control involuntary respiration, heart, and blood vessel function

68. T F The spinal cord extends from the brain to the level of the second lumbar vertebra, where it divides into individual nerves known as *cauda equina*.

69. T F The spinal cord generates nerve impulses and transmits them to the body, causing muscles to contract and movement to occur.

70. T F The brain and spinal cord are covered by three layers of cartilage.

71. The outer meningeal layer is called the:
    a. dura mater
    b. arachnoid membrane
    c. pia mater
    d. subarachnoid space

72. Cerebrospinal fluid (CSF):
    a. circulates between the pia mater and the arachnoid in the subarachnoid space
    b. is normally translucent
    c. is produced by the brain
    d. is thick and gel-like

73. The _____ _____ _____ is a specialized subdivision of the peripheral nervous system that regulates involuntary functions of the body.

74. There are _____ divisions of the autonomic nervous system—the _____ and the _____ nervous systems.

75. Stimulation of the parasympathetic nervous system causes:
    a. constriction of blood vessels
    b. elevated blood pressure
    c. a feeling of nervousness
    d. a slowing of the heart rate

CROSSWORD PUZZLE EXERCISE

76. Complete the following crossword puzzle.

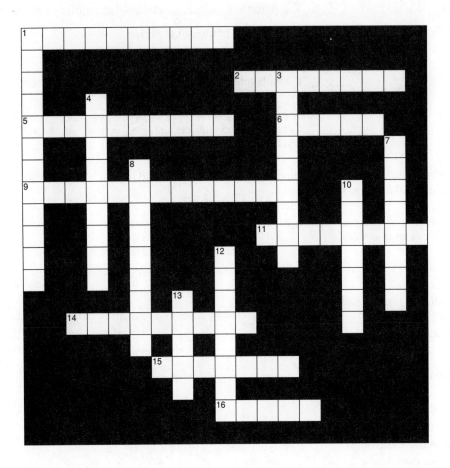

ACROSS

1. When the nerve impulse "hits" the next cell, it causes it to _____.
2. Hematoma with bleeding in the space between the dura and the arachnoid membrane.
5. Located behind and below the cerebrum.
6. Cylinder-like extension of a neuron that carries impulses away from the cell body.
9. Excess fluid accumulation in the brain with associated swelling.
11. Three layers of membranes that cover the brain and spinal cord.
14. The resting state of a nerve cell is called the _____ state.
15. Nerve cells are called this.
16. Nerves that transmit impulses from the brain and the spinal cord to the muscles and glands.

DOWN

1. Part of brain between the brainstem and the cerebrum.
3. Consists of the medulla, pons, and midbrain.
4. Branching process that extends from the cell body of a neuron.
7. Lobe that is the major site for most sensory information except smell, hearing, and vision.
8. Lobe of brain that processes visual information.
10. Region surrounding point of contact between two neurons or between a neuron and its effector organ.
12. Top portion of the brain, consisting of the left and right hemispheres.
13. Nerves that carry both sensory and motor messages.

77. Match each of the following endocrine glands with the correct facts.

    Endocrine Gland   **Fact**
    a. Pituitary   _____ Regulates sexual function, characteristics, and reproduction
    b. Adrenal   _____ Regulates glucose metabolism and other functions
    c. Pancreas   _____ Located in base of the skull
    d. Ovary   _____ Regulates all other endocrine glands
                                _____ Hormones produced include insulin
                                _____ Located in the female pelvis
                                _____ Hormones produced include adrenaline

78. These endocrine glands secrete _____, called _____, directly into the blood.

79. Describe an example of a negative feedback mechanism that acts to regulate hormonal secretion.

    _____
    _____
    _____
    _____
    _____

80. Describe the functions of hormones.

    _____
    _____
    _____
    _____
    _____
    _____

81. Which of the following is a hormone of the pancreas, along with its correct functions?
    a. insulin—increases the blood sugar by blocking its entry into the cells
    b. digestive enzyme—stimulates the small intestinal walls, preventing absorption of glucose
    c. glucagon—causes adrenergic stimulation, leading to an increase in the blood glucose level
    d. glycogen—causes the release of glucose stores from the liver

82. Describe the function of epinephrine and norepinephrine on the sympathetic nervous system.

_____

_____

_____

_____

_____

83. The adult male has about _____ L of blood.
    a. 3 to 4
    b. 5 to 6
    c. 8 to 9
    d. 10

84. Match each of the following elements of blood with the correct descriptions.

    Element
    a. Plasma
    b. Platelets
    c. White blood cells
    d. Red blood cells

    Description
    _____ Also called *erythrocytes*

    _____ Small cells that, when ruptured, release chemical factors needed to form blood clots

    _____ Carry oxygen to the tissues

    _____ Also called *leukocytes*

    _____ Pale, straw-colored fluid

    _____ Involved in destroying germs and producing substances called *antibodies* that help the body resist infection

85. A protein that bonds the oxygen to the red cells is called:
    a. prothrombin
    b. plasma
    c. insulin
    d. hemoglobin

86. Match each of the following types of white blood cells with what it does.

    Type
    a. Eosinophils and basophils
    b. Neutrophils
    c. Lymphocytes and monocytes

    Role
    _____ Fight bacterial infections
    _____ Help eliminate viruses and fungal infections
    _____ Important in allergic reactions

87. Describe what occurs if the body's blood clotting mechanisms fail.

    _____
    _____
    _____
    _____

88. List the three primary components of the cardiovascular system.

    _____
    _____
    _____

89. The heart is:
    a. a muscular, round organ
    b. about the size of grapefruit
    c. located behind the sternum
    d. completely situated in the left side of the chest

90. The pericardial sac:
    a. lines the four chambers of the heart and its valves and allows frictionless blood flow through the heart
    b. is the muscular layer of the heart that propels blood throughout the pulmonary and systemic circulations
    c. contains approximately 10 mL of serous fluid
    d. allows the heart to contract smoothly within the chest cavity

91. For this illustration of the heart, label all of the identified structures.

Use colored pencils or felt-tip pens to color this illustration according to the following: A-purple, B-green, C-blue, D-violet, E-blue, F-yellow, G-purple, H-violet, I-red, J-green, K-red, L-dark red, M-purple, and N-dark red.

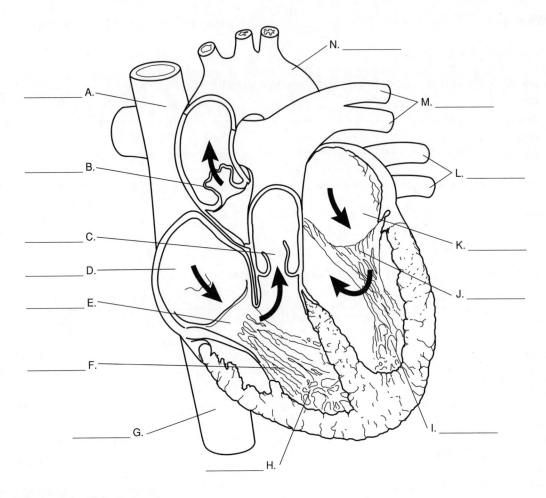

92. The left ventricle of the heart:
    a. pumps oxygen-rich blood to the cells
    b. pumps oxygen-poor blood to the lungs
    c. is the smaller of the two ventricles
    d. receives blood directly from the veins of the systemic circulation

93. The atria and ventricles are separated by valves that:
    a. prevent backward flow of blood
    b. propel the blood forward
    c. cause the blood flow to slow so as to allow proper filling of the ventricles
    d. direct blood into the proper areas of the heart

94. Blood moving from the right atrium to the right ventricle passes through the _____ valve. As the blood moves from the right ventricle to the pulmonary artery, it passes through the _____ valve. Blood moving from the left atrium to the left ventricle passes through the _____ valve. As the blood moves from the left ventricle into the aorta, it passes through the _____ valve.

95. Blood vessels that supply the heart muscle with oxygen and nutrients are the _____ arteries.
    a. coronary
    b. cerebral
    c. renal
    d. hepatic

96. Place a checkmark beside the parts of the heart that the right main coronary artery supplies.
    _____ Lateral left ventricular wall
    _____ Anterior wall of the left ventricle
    _____ Sinoatrial (SA) node
    _____ Posterior heart wall
    _____ Anterior right ventricle

97. Deoxygenated venous blood from the heart drains into _____ different coronary veins that empty into the right atrium via the _____ _____.

98. Describe the term *cardiac cycle*.

    _____
    _____
    _____
    _____
    _____

99. Cardiac output:
    a. is the amount of blood pumped through the circulatory system in 1 minute
    b. is expressed in beats per minute (BPM)
    c. is the amount of blood (volume) pumped with each heartbeat
    d. seldom fluctuates

100. The first heart sound:
    a. results from closure of both the aortic and pulmonic valves
    b. is referred to as the "lub"
    c. represents rapid ventricular filling
    d. occurs because of increased pressure in the atria

101. Bruits:
    a. are abnormal "whooshing" sounds indicating turbulent blood flow within a blood vessel
    b. are abnormal "wheezing" sounds indicating turbulent blood flow within the heart
    c. indicate abnormal cardiac valve function
    d. suggest increased pressure in the atria

102. For this illustration of the heart's conduction system, label all of the identified structures.

    Use colored pencils or felt-tip pens to color this illustration according to the following: A-yellow, B-green, C-red, D-violet, E-blue, F-purple, and G-orange.

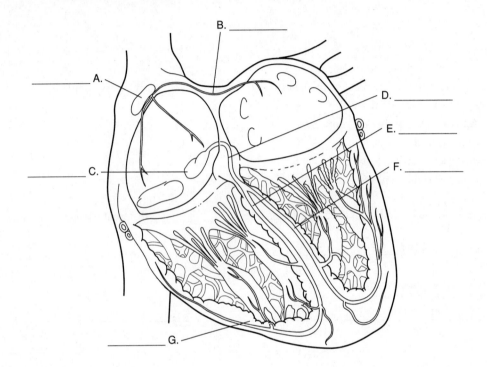

103. Identify, by numbering, the order an electrical impulse travels through the heart's conduction system.
    _____ Bundle of His
    _____ Atrioventricular node (AV node)
    _____ Sinoatrial node (SA node)
    _____ Right bundle branch and left bundle branch
    _____ Intraatrial pathways
    _____ Purkinje fibers

104. Fill in the two missing elements in the illustration shown below.

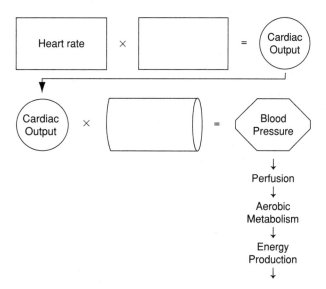

105. Control of the heart's rate and strength of contraction come from:
    a. the respiratory system
    b. the brain via the peripheral nervous system
    c. hormones of the endocrine system
    d. the bloodstream

106. Receptors in the blood vessels, kidneys, brain, and heart constantly monitor body homeostasis. _____ respond to changes in pressure, usually within the heart or the main arteries. _____ sense changes in the chemical composition of the blood.

107. If the heart is stretched, the muscle contracts _____.

108. The increase in the force of myocardial contraction caused by stretching of myocardial muscles is referred to as:
    a. cardiac output
    b. afterload
    c. stroke volume
    d. Starling's law

109. Match each of the following types of blood vessels with the correct description.

    Type   **Description**
    a. Arteries   _____ Transport blood from the body back to the heart
    b. Veins   _____ Microscopic thin-walled vessels
    c. Arterioles   _____ Blood vessels that carry blood away from the heart to the body
    d. Capillaries

110. Describe what takes place in the capillaries.

_____

_____

_____

_____

_____

111. Deoxygenated blood is returned to the right atrium via the:
    a. pulmonary veins
    b. aorta
    c. superior and inferior venae cavae
    d. iliac artery

112. Blood is pumped from the right ventricle through the _____ into the _____.
    a. aortic valve; aorta
    b. mitral valve; right atrium
    c. pulmonary vein; lungs
    d. pulmonary valve; pulmonary artery

113. Describe what occurs when blood that is being transported through the pulmonary vasculature reaches the lungs.

_____

_____

_____

_____

_____

114. The _____ deliver(s) blood to the left atrium.
    a. aorta
    b. internal jugular veins
    c. pulmonary veins
    d. superior and inferior venae cavae

115. The left ventricle pumps blood to the body via the:
    a. aorta
    b. pulmonary artery
    c. carotid artery
    d. brachial artery

116. Which of the following veins are located in the neck?
    a. external jugular
    b. radial
    c. cephalic
    d. ulnar

117. Define the term *blood pressure*.

    _____

    _____

    _____

118. The systolic phase of the blood pressure is:
    a. when ventricular relaxation and filling occur
    b. the difference between the higher blood pressure and the lower blood pressure
    c. the higher blood pressure noted during ventricular contraction
    d. when the majority of coronary artery filling occurs

119. T F The body tissues are bathed in a plasmalike fluid called *albumin*.

120. T F Lymph comes from excess cellular fluid and circulates through the body in thin-walled lymph vessels that travel close to the major arteries.

121. T F Lymphatic fluid is filtered in lymph nodes and returns to the main circulatory system via the thoracic duct, which empties into the superior vena cava.

122. Describe the role of the immune system.

    _____

    _____

    _____

    _____

    _____

123. Chemicals such as histamine, which are part of the body's immune system, work by:
    a. preventing the entry of bacteria
    b. buffering toxic substances that are released from the cells
    c. ingesting and destroying bacterial invaders and foreign matter
    d. promoting inflammation in response to foreign invaders in the body

124. Specific immunity occurs via:
    a. mechanical barriers such as the skin
    b. chemicals such as histamine
    c. white blood cells (leukocytes)
    d. antibodies that are formed in response to antigens

CROSSWORD PUZZLE EXERCISE

125. Complete the following crossword puzzle.

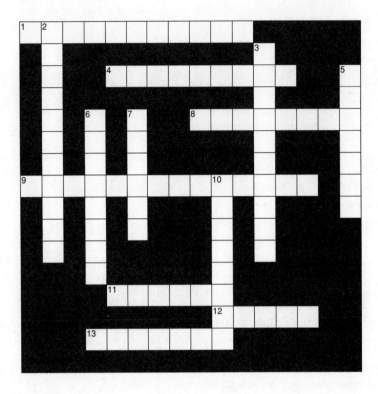

ACROSS

1. Fight bacterial infections.
4. Help eliminate viruses and fungal infections.
8. Heart receives most of its blood supply directly from this circulation.
9. Sense changes in the chemical composition of the blood.
11. System that defends the body against bacteria, viruses, and other foreign matter.
12. Two upper chambers of the heart.
13. Abnormal "whooshing-like" sound indicating turbulent blood flow within the heart.

DOWN

2. Important leukocytes in allergic reactions.
3. The protein that gives the red blood cells their reddish color.
5. Large gland situated at the base of the neck.
6. Regulate many body functions, such as growth, reproduction, temperature, metabolism, and blood pressure.
7. Valve situated between the left atrium and the left ventricle.
10. Considered an organ of both the digestive and the endocrine systems.

126. Describe the function of the respiratory system.

_____

_____

_____

_____

_____

127. Match each of the following anatomical structures with the correct description.

 Structure
 a. Oropharynx
 b. Nasopharynx
 c. Epiglottis
 d. Larynx
 e. Trachea

 Description
 _____ Tube in the front of the throat that carries air into the lungs
 _____ Inside of the mouth posterior to the tongue leading to the throat
 _____ Voice box that holds the vocal cords and the glottic opening to the trachea
 _____ Area between the nasal passages and the oropharynx
 _____ Flap of tissue that covers the glottic opening of the trachea when swallowing or gagging takes place

128. For this illustration of the respiratory system, label all of the identified structures.

Use colored pencils or felt-tip pens to color this illustration according to the following: A-orange, B-yellow, C-red, D-tan, E-yellow, F-yellow, G-yellow, H-green, I-purple, and J-red.

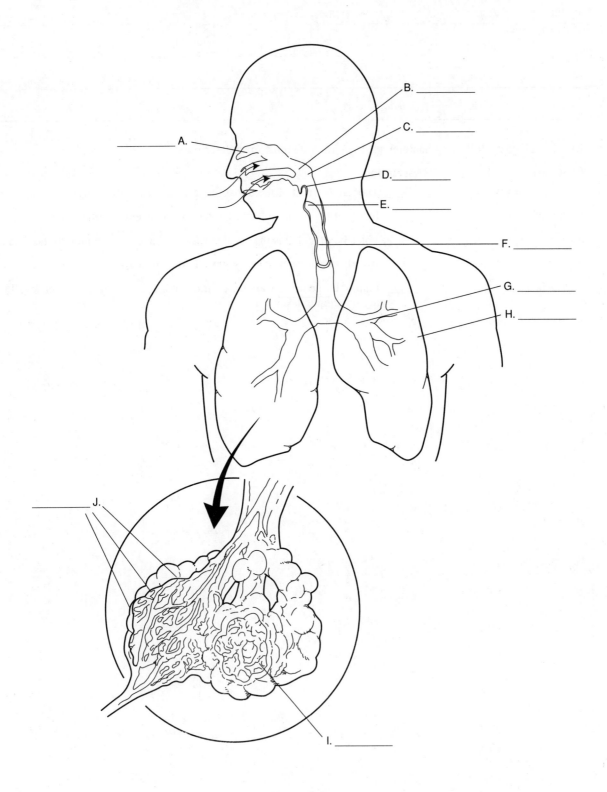

129. The alveoli are:
    a. each about 5 mm in diameter
    b. surrounded by the pulmonary venules
    c. tiny sacs of lung tissue where gas exchange takes place
    d. the most proximal portion of the respiratory tree

130. The membrane that lines the thoracic cavity is called the:
    a. diaphragm
    b. parietal pleura
    c. visceral pleura
    d. surfactant

131. The right lung consists of _____ lobes, whereas the left lung has _____ lobes.

132. Describe how inhalation occurs.

_____

_____

_____

_____

_____

133. During exhalation the:
    a. active muscular part of breathing occurs
    b. dimensions of the thorax increase
    c. diaphragm and intercostal muscles relax
    d. intercostal muscles lift the ribs

134. Ventilation refers to the:
    a. act of breathing
    b. exchange of gases at the alveolar-capillary membrane
    c. amount of oxygen being carried in the bloodstream
    d. movement of carbon dioxide in and out of the lungs

135. Inspired air contains about _____% oxygen, whereas expired air contains about _____% oxygen.

136. On the illustration below, use arrows to show the direction oxygen and carbon dioxide diffuse across the alveolar-capillary membrane following the inspiration of fresh air into the alveoli.

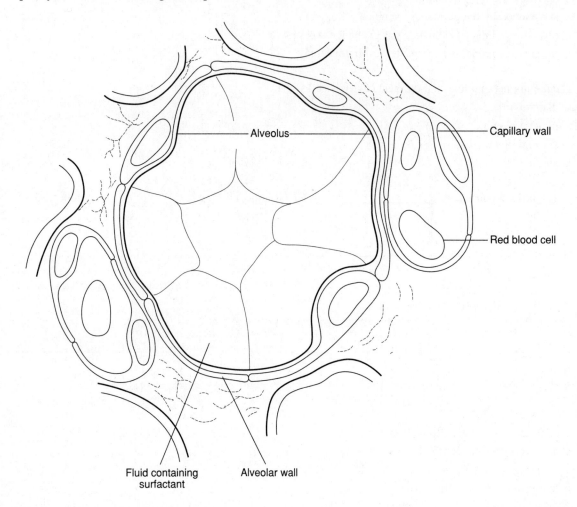

137. Oxygen is transported in the arterial blood by:
    a. bicarbonate ions
    b. hemoglobin
    c. albumin
    d. chloride

138. The majority of carbon dioxide is transported in the blood:
    a. bound to fibrinogen
    b. as free molecules
    c. combined with electrolytes
    d. in the form of bicarbonate ions

139. The primary stimulus to breathe is:
    a. excess levels of carbon dioxide
    b. low levels of oxygen
    c. fluctuations in the heart rate
    d. an elevated pH

CROSSWORD PUZZLE EXERCISE

140. Complete the following crossword puzzle.

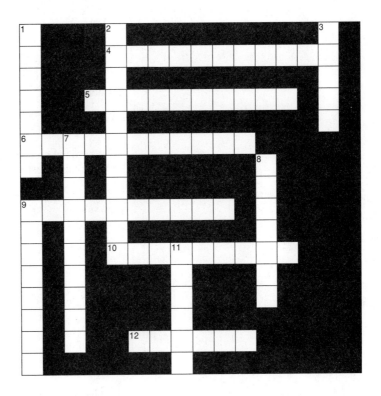

ACROSS

4. System consists of the organs and structures associated with breathing and gas exchange in the body.
5. Form the basis of antibody-mediated immunity.
6. Cell-mediated immunity is achieved by the actions of _____.
9. Passive process of respiration that normally requires no muscular effort.
10. Mainstem bronchi divide into _____ bronchi.
12. Two connective tissue membranes that surround the lungs.

DOWN

1. Tiny sacs of lung tissue where gas exchange takes place.
2. Bronchi divide into progressively smaller branches called _____.
3. Plasmalike liquid of the lymphatic system.
7. Barriers, such as the skin, that prevent the entry of many bacteria.
8. This air contains carbon dioxide and approximately 16% oxygen.
9. Abnormal collection of fluid is called a pleural _____.
11. Essential for the function of body processes.

141. Match each of the following digestive tract organs with the correct information.

    Digestive Organ

    a. Small intestine
    b. Appendix
    c. Large intestine
    d. Gallbladder
    e. Stomach

    Information

    _____ Hollow fingerlike projection situated at the beginning of the large intestine

    _____ Pear-shaped reservoir for bile, located on the posterior undersurface of the liver

    _____ Where the initial chemical breakdown of food begins, producing a semisolid substance called *chyme*

    _____ Where chemical digestion is completed and absorption of foods takes place

    _____ Where the collection and removal of wastes from the digestive system occur

142. Hollow abdominal organs include the:
    a. spleen
    b. pancreas
    c. kidneys
    d. esophagus

143. Match each of the following urinary system organs with its function.

    Organ

    a. Kidneys
    b. Ureters
    c. Urethra
    d. Urinary bladder

    Function

    _____ Thick-walled, hollow tubes that carry urine from the kidneys to the urinary bladder

    _____ Hollow, muscular sac in the midline of the lower abdominal area that stores urine until it is excreted

    _____ Filter blood, excrete body wastes in the form of urine, and are important in the regulation of the body's fluid balance and blood pressure

    _____ Hollow, tubular structure that drains urine from the bladder, passing it to the outside

144. For the illustration of the female reproductive system below, label all of the identified structures.

Use colored pencils or felt-tip pens to color this illustration according to the following: A-green, B-blue, C-yellow, D-orange, and E-red.

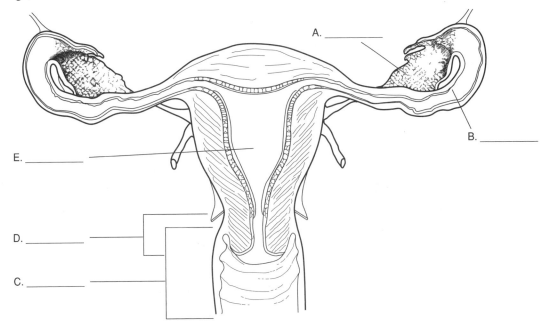

145. T F   Water makes up approximately one third of the human body.

146. T F   Water plays an important role in the maintenance of a constant internal environment of the body.

147. T F   Water functions as a universal solvent for a variety of solutes.

148. Color the following water compartments of the body: red for intravascular, blue for interstitial, and green for intracellular.

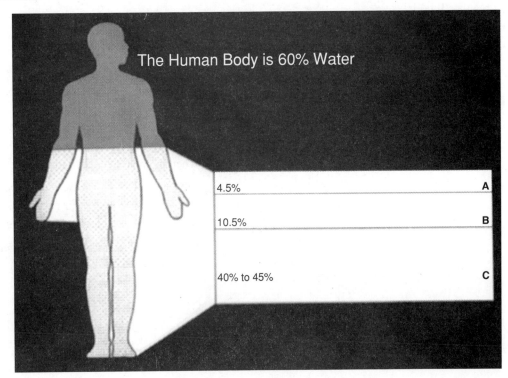

Chapter **4** **Overview of Human Systems**

149. The intracellular fluid accounts for _____ of the body weight.
    a. 4.5% to 5.5%
    b. 60% to 70%
    c. 40% to 45%
    d. 10.5% to 12%

150. Extracellular fluid:
    a. is divided into the intracellular and intravascular compartments
    b. makes up 25% of the body weight
    c. makes up approximately 50% of the body fluids
    d. is the fluid found outside the cells

151. The body's water:
    a. intake usually exceeds its output
    b. distribution in the three body compartments remains relatively constant
    c. output is increased with the secretion of antidiuretic hormone (ADH)
    d. is removed mostly through the digestive tract

152. Explain how ADH acts to reduce output of water.

    _____
    _____
    _____
    _____

153. Thirst:
    a. occurs when body fluids become increased
    b. helps regulate fluid intake
    c. stimulates the kidneys to excrete more water
    d. has little to no influence on water balance in the body

154. Match each of the following components of acid-base with the correct characteristics.

    Component
    a. Acid
    b. Base
    c. pH

    Characteristic
    _____ Substance that decreases the concentration of hydrogen ions
    _____ When in greater concentration, lowers the pH
    _____ Substance that increases the concentration of hydrogen ions in a water solution
    _____ When in greater concentration, increases the pH
    _____ Mathematical expression of hydrogen ion concentration

155. The body's three mechanisms for the regulation of acid-base balance from fastest to slowest are:
    a. lungs, buffer system, kidneys
    b. buffer system, lungs, kidneys
    c. kidneys, buffer system, lungs
    d. buffer system, kidneys, lungs

156. Match each of the following elements with the correct characteristics.

    Component
    a. Buffer system
    b. Respiratory system
    c. Renal system

    Characteristic
    _____ Provides almost immediate protection against changes in the hydrogen ion concentration of the extracellular fluid
    _____ Regulates the concentration of carbon dioxide and subsequently the amount of carbonic acid (H_2CO_3) in the body
    _____ Acts as a chemical sponge, absorbing H^+ ions when they are in excess and donating H^+ ions when they are depleted
    _____ Excretes hydrogen ions and forms bicarbonate ions in specific amounts as indicated by the pH of the blood

157. The buffer used to convert strong metabolic acids into "weak acids" is:
    a. chloride
    b. bicarbonate
    c. water
    d. carbonic acid

158. Which of the following is produced in the metabolic acid–buffering process?
    a. HCO_3
    b. H_2O
    c. H_2CO_3
    d. CO_2

159. Fill in the missing elements in the illustration of the buffering of a strong acid shown below.

    H^+(strong acid) + _____ ↔ H_2CO_3 (weak acid) ↔ H_2O (water) + _____

160. Fill in the equation below with arrows to show the changes that occur with increased breathing.

    ↑ breathing → _____ CO_2 → ↓H_2CO_3 → _____ H^+ → _____ pH

161. Fill in the equation below with arrows to show the changes that occur with decreased breathing.

    ↓ breathing → _____ CO_2 → ↑H_2CO_3 → _____ H^+ → _____ pH

162. The kidneys help in maintaining acid-base balance by:
    a. excreting or retaining hydrogen ions and bicarbonate
    b. removing carbon dioxide
    c. buffering metabolic acids
    d. all of the above

163. Which of the following is a normal pH of the human body?
    a. 7.38
    b. 7.46
    c. 7.18
    d. 7.52

164. A pH of the body fluid greater than _____ is considered *alkalosis*.
    a. 7.25
    b. 7.30
    c. 7.35
    d. 7.45

165. Respiratory acidosis:
    a. is brought on by hyperventilation
    b. occurs when exhalation of carbon dioxide is inhibited
    c. leads to an increase in the body's blood pH
    d. is treated by calming the patient and slowing his or her breathing

166. Metabolic acidosis includes:
    a. increased Pa_{CO_2}
    b. increased Pa_{O_2}
    c. depletion of bicarbonate
    d. increased pH

167. Match each of the following conditions with the appropriate case.

    Condition
    a. Respiratory acidosis
    b. Respiratory alkalosis
    c. Metabolic acidosis
    d. Metabolic alkalosis

    Description
    _____ A 19-year-old who has taken an overdose of sleeping pills and is breathing six breaths per minute

    _____ A 39-year-old diabetic patient who is suffering from diabetic ketoacidosis

    _____ A 53-year-old who has been ingesting excessive baking soda to relieve indigestion

    _____ A 30-year-old who is experiencing "hyperventilation syndrome" brought on by an argument

CROSSWORD PUZZLE EXERCISE

168. Complete the following crossword puzzle.

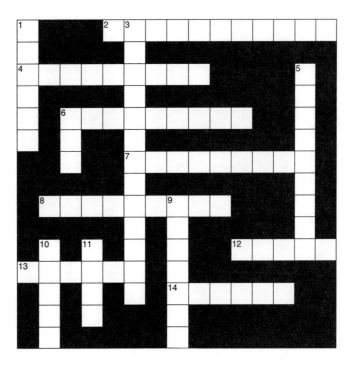

ACROSS

2. Major buffer of the body.
4. System composed of structures and organs involved in consumption, digestion, and elimination of food.
6. pH values higher than 7.45 in the arterial blood.
7. The swallowing tube.
8. Serves as the central reference point for dividing the abdomen into quadrants.
12. Semiliquid mass resulting from food being churned and mixed with digestive juices in the stomach.
13. Secreted by salivary glands.
14. Water coming into the body.

DOWN

1. Responsible for maintaining fluid balance in the body.
3. Fluid is found within individual cells.
5. Required for growth and important in the conduction of nerve impulses and muscle contraction.
6. Causes kidney tubules to reabsorb more water into the blood and excrete less urine.
9. Most abundant cation in the body.
10. Portion of the intestines where water and electrolytes are absorbed and secreted.
11. An important digestive enzyme produced by the liver and stored in the gallbladder.

5 Emergency Pharmacology

CHAPTER TERMINAL OBJECTIVES

On completion of this chapter, the EMT-Intermediate will be able to understand the basic principles of pharmacology and develop a drug profile for common emergency medications.

For the multiple-choice questions, select the single best answer to each question. For the matching questions, select the best corresponding answer for each item. Because there are sometimes more items than corresponding answers, some items may not be used.

1. Define the following terms.

    Drug: _____

    _____

    _____

    Pharmacology: _____

    _____

    _____

    _____

2. Match each of the following drug names with the appropriate description.

    Name
    a. Trade
    b. Chemical
    c. Official
    d. Generic

    Description
    _____ Name listed in the *United States Pharmacopoeia (USP)*
    _____ Compound makeup
    _____ Name assigned to a drug before it becomes officially listed
    _____ Name registered by the U.S. Patent Office and has the office mark of the patent office after its name (symbol ®)

3. Fill in the trade names for the following drugs.

Generic Name	Trade Name
Lidocaine	
Nitroglycerin	
Diazepam	

4. Furosemide is a/an _____ name.
   a. official
   b. chemical
   c. generic
   d. trade

5. Match each of the following acts with the correct description.

   Act
   a. Pure Food and Drug Act of 1906
   b. Harrison Narcotic Act of 1914
   c. Controlled Substances Act of 1970
   d. Federal Food, Drug, and Cosmetic Act of 1938

   Description
   _____ Requires that labels be used to list the possible habit-forming properties and side effects of drugs
   _____ The first federal legislation designed to stop drug addiction or dependence
   _____ Enacted to prevent the manufacture and trafficking of mislabeled, poisonous, or harmful food and drugs

6. The act that requires anyone who manufactures, prescribes, administers, or dispenses such controlled substances to register annually with the U.S. Attorney General under the Drug Enforcement Administration is the:
   a. Controlled Substances Act of 1970
   b. Narcotic Control Act of 1956
   c. Harrison Narcotic Act of 1914
   d. Federal Food, Drug, and Cosmetic Act of 1938

7. Provide a description for the following schedules, and list examples of each.

Schedule	Description	Example
I		
II		
III		
IV		
V		

8. The agency that was established to oversee the needs and controls for dangerous drugs is the:
    a. Bureau of Narcotic and Dangerous Drugs (BNDD)
    b. Drug Enforcement Administration (DEA)
    c. Federal Communications Commission (FCC)
    d. Food and Drug Administration (FDA)

9. The agency that reviews drug applications and petitions for food additives; inspects factories where drugs, cosmetics, and foods are made; and removes unsafe drugs from the market is the:
    a. Bureau of Narcotic and Dangerous Drugs (BNDD)
    b. Drug Enforcement Administration (DEA)
    c. Food and Drug Administration (FDA)
    d. Public Health Service (PHS)

10. Synthetic drugs are produced:
    a. from the pancreas of cows and pigs
    b. from medicinal plants
    c. in a pharmaceutical laboratory
    d. using inorganic sources

11. _____ are a large group of nitrogenous substances found in plants that are usually bitter, and many are pharmacologically active.
    a. Alkaloids
    b. Glycosides
    c. Gums
    d. Oils

12. Match each of the following sources with the correct drugs. Some sources may be used more than once.

    Source
    a. Plant
    b. Animal
    c. Mineral
    d. Synthetic

    Drug
    _____ Atropine
    _____ Lidocaine
    _____ Digitalis
    _____ Morphine
    _____ Insulin
    _____ Iodine
    _____ Oxytocin
    _____ Calcium

13. List two drugs that are derived from microorganisms.

    _____

    _____

14. List the three categories of drugs.

    _____

    _____

    _____

15. List four references for drug information available to the EMT-I.

    _____

    _____

    _____

    _____

16. When preparing to administer drug treatments:
    a. it is not necessary to determine whether a woman of childbearing age is pregnant
    b. drug dosage is based on a child's weight or body surface area rather than age
    c. a history of an elderly patient's specific drug use from family, friends, pharmacy, and doctors offers little information
    d. dosages must be increased in elderly patients to achieve the same therapeutic effect as in middle-aged persons

17. T F When administering drug treatments to patients who are pregnant, the expected benefits should be considered against the possible risks to the fetus.

18. T F During pregnancy the metabolism in the liver is accelerated, and the rate of drug excretion may be reduced because of the increased cardiac output that occurs.

19. T F Elderly patients may take more medications, have more illnesses, and have more adverse effects from drugs than younger patients.

20. Drugs that are _____, _____, or absorbed by the mother have the potential to harm the fetus by crossing the _____ or through _____.

21. The Food and Drug Administration has established a scale, with categories _____, _____, _____, _____, and _____ to indicate drugs that may have documented problems in animals or humans during pregnancy.

22. Usually the quickest and most reliable method for determining a child's body weight is to:
    a. ask the parents
    b. multiply their age by 4
    c. approximate it by carefully looking at the child
    d. determine the size of their little finger in centimeters, and multiply that by 2

23. Describe why doses of some medications must be altered to avoid adverse or toxic reactions in the very young.

    _____
    _____
    _____
    _____
    _____

24. Describe how changes in body composition in elderly patients affect how drugs are distributed.

    _____
    _____
    _____
    _____
    _____

25. Describe how changes in kidneys and liver in elderly patients affect how drugs are metabolized and eliminated.

    _____
    _____
    _____
    _____
    _____

26. List nine proper procedures that should be used when using drug therapy.

_____
_____
_____
_____
_____
_____
_____
_____
_____

27. Fill in the following chart regarding the autonomic nervous system.

Feature	Parasympathetic	Sympathetic
Other name		
Neurotransmitter		
Primary nerve(s)		
Stimulating drug(s)		
Blocking drug(s)		

28. Stimulation of the beta-1 receptors will cause:
    a. decreased contractility
    b. increased heart rate
    c. bronchodilation
    d. vasodilation

29. Effects of beta-2 receptor stimulation include:
    a. peripheral vasoconstriction
    b. bronchodilation
    c. increased afterload
    d. decreased heart rate

30. Alpha receptor sites are mostly located in the:
    a. lungs
    b. heart
    c. kidneys
    d. blood vessels

31. Stimulation of the parasympathetic nervous system results in:
    a. decreased heart rate
    b. increased myocardial contractility
    c. increased AV conduction velocity
    d. bronchodilation

32. A beta blocker acts by:
    a. directly absorbing epinephrine at the receptor sites
    b. preventing the movement of acetylcholine from the nerve endings
    c. blocking the release of norepinephrine from the receptor sites
    d. binding to the receptor sites, thus blocking the attachment of epinephrine

33. Their effects on bodily _____ commonly categorize drugs.

34. All drugs cause cellular change, which is their _____ _____, and a degree of physiological change, which is their _____ _____.

35. T   F   Drug actions are achieved by a physiochemical interaction between the drug and certain tissue components in the body.

36. T   F   Drugs generally exert a single effect rather than multiple actions.

37. T   F   Drugs often cause a tissue or organ to produce new functions.

38. Drugs that attach to a receptor and prevent a response are called:
    a. agonists
    b. antagonists
    c. partial agonists
    d. mimetic

39. A powdered drug that has been compressed into a hard, small disk is referred to as a:
    a. suppository
    b. tablet
    c. capsule
    d. pill

CROSSWORD PUZZLE EXERCISE

40. Complete the following crossword puzzle.

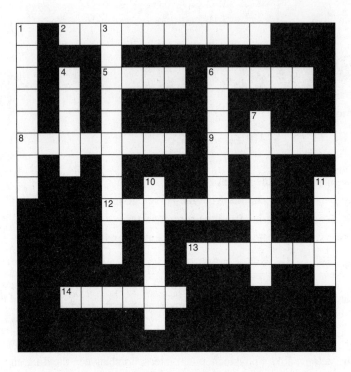

ACROSS

2. Finely ground drugs that are dissolved in a liquid, such as water.
5. One or more drugs mixed with a cohesive material in oval, round, or flattened shapes.
6. Nongreasy, semisolid preparation used on the skin.
8. Drug combined with water and oil.
9. Concentrated alcohol solution of a volatile substance.
12. Semisolid preparation of one or more drugs for prolonged contact with the skin.
13. A very concentrated form of drug made from vegetables or animals.
14. Drug dissolved in alcohol and added flavoring.

DOWN

1. Oily liquid used on the skin.
3. One or more drugs mixed in a firm base that dissolves gradually at body temperature.
4. Very sweet form of medication, resulting from high sugar content.
6. Powdered or granulated drug enclosed in a gelatin capsule.
7. An alcohol or water and alcohol solution prepared from drugs derived from plants.
10. Compressed dry form of a drug coated to withstand the stomach acidity.
11. Drug suspended in a thin gelatin base.

41. All of the following are parenteral drug administration routes *except:*
    a. IV
    b. SQ
    c. PO
    d. IM

42. Match each of the following administration routes with the appropriate characteristic.

    Route
    a. Intradermal
    b. Transdermal
    c. Intravenous
    d. Pulmonary
    e. Intramuscular
    f. Subcutaneous
    g. Sublingual

    Characteristic
    _____ Medication is injected into the fatty tissue underneath the skin that overlies the muscle
    _____ Medication is placed on the skin, where it is absorbed
    _____ Medication is absorbed into the vast capillary network immediately under the tongue
    _____ Medication is absorbed through the pulmonary capillaries of the lungs
    _____ Medication is injected into the dermal layer of the skin
    _____ Medication is administered directly into a vein
    _____ Medication is injected into the muscle tissue

43. Which of the following routes of medication administration yields a faster absorption rate and has the most potential for causing adverse reactions?
    a. PO
    b. IV
    c. IM
    d. SQ

44. List five reasons why certain drugs must be administered through a particular route and not all the available routes.

    _____
    _____
    _____
    _____
    _____

45. A systemic effect refers to:
    a. the degree of physiological change achieved
    b. a drug being absorbed into the blood and then carried to the organ or tissue on which it will act
    c. a drug's action that is limited to the area where it is administered
    d. a drug's desired effect and the reason it is prescribed

46. The movement of drugs in the body as they are absorbed, distributed, metabolized, and excreted is referred to as:
    a. pharmacodynamics
    b. the mechanism of action
    c. pharmacokinetics
    d. biotransformation

47. Match each of the following terms with the correct definition.

    Term
    a. Distribution
    b. Biotransformation
    c. Excretion
    d. Absorption

    Definition
    _____ The process involved in transferring drug molecules from the place where they are deposited in the body through the capillary walls and into the bloodstream
    _____ Refers to the manner in which a drug is transported by the bloodstream to various areas of the body
    _____ The physical and chemical alterations that a drug undergoes within the blood
    _____ The process in which drugs are removed from the body in either their original form or as metabolites

48. List eight principal factors that affect absorption of a drug.

    _____
    _____
    _____
    _____
    _____
    _____
    _____
    _____

49. Describe the three mechanisms involved in absorption of a drug.
    Diffusion:

    _____
    _____
    _____

Osmosis:

_____

_____

_____

Filtration:

_____

_____

_____

50. The blood-brain barrier:
    a. is a physical obstacle located between the capillaries and the brain tissue
    b. prevents almost all drugs from crossing it
    c. is active only in pediatric patients
    d. prevents many drugs from leaving the blood and crossing the cerebrospinal fluid into the brain

51. T F All drugs are capable of crossing the placenta from the mother to the fetus.

52. T F The most vulnerable time for drug-induced birth defects is the third trimester.

53. T F At birth, toxic reactions to drugs that remain in the newborn's system can occur because the newborn has a decreased ability to metabolize and excrete them.

54. Drug tolerance has to do with:
    a. the accelerated removal of the drug from the body
    b. a cumulative effect that leads to a dangerous and toxic level of a drug
    c. an improved ability of the liver to metabolize a given drug
    d. an increased number of receptors available to react to a drug

55. The biological half-life of a drug is:
    a. time required for the plasma level to decrease to half of a certain measured level
    b. the minimum amount of drug needed in the bloodstream to cause a therapeutic effect
    c. a profile given to determine its effectiveness
    d. a quantitative measure of the relative safety of a drug

56. Age influences the actions of drugs on the body because:
    a. elderly people have faster metabolic processes that extend the drug's breakdown and excretion times
    b. infants have immature livers and kidneys, so it is difficult for them to metabolize and eliminate the same dosages of drugs as adults
    c. a child's body and chemistry are affected by adolescence and body proportion
    d. b and c

57. Describe how the differences between men and women affect the actions of drugs on the body.

_____

_____

_____

_____

_____

58. Match each of the following terms with the correct definition.

Term
- a. Side effect
- b. Drug allergy
- c. Idiosyncratic reactions
- d. Synergism
- e. Cross-tolerance
- f. Iatrogenic responses
- g. Drug dependence
- h. Drug toxicity
- i. Cumulative effect

Definition

_____ Occurs when a repeat dose of drug is administered before the initial dose(s) are excreted. It is caused by a buildup of the drug in the blood

_____ One drug helps the action of another drug to produce an effect that neither produces alone

_____ Results from overdosage, ingestion of a drug intended for external use, or buildup of the drug in the blood caused by impaired metabolism or excretion

_____ Physical state in which withdrawal symptoms occur when a person discontinues the use of drugs

_____ Administration of many drugs can lead to symptoms that mimic naturally occurring disease states

_____ An abnormal or unexpected reaction to a drug peculiar to a certain patient

_____ An effect that is unintended

_____ Occurs in a person who has been previously exposed to the drug and has developed antibodies

CROSSWORD PUZZLE EXERCISE

59. Complete the following crossword puzzle.

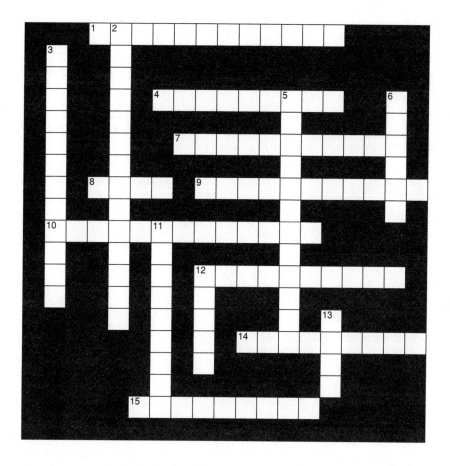

ACROSS

1. Administration route where medication is given directly into the bone marrow of a long bone.
4. One of a large group of nitrogenous substances found in plants that are usually bitter.
7. Sometimes called the adrenergic division.
8. Stimulation of these receptors results in increased heart rate.
9. Route where a drug is injected within the dermis.
10. Rapid development of tolerance.
12. A drug that prevents receptor stimulation.
14. An individual's capacity to endure medications.
15. Drugs manufactured in a pharmaceutical laboratory.

DOWN

2. Chemical neurotransmitter of the sympathetic nervous system.
3. One drug prolongs or multiplies the effects of another drug.
5. Administration route where a drug is injected within the tongue.
6. Administration route where a drug is dissolved between the cheek and the gum.
11. Administration route where a patient breathes an aerosol form of a drug.
12. Stimulation of these receptors leads to vasoconstriction.
13. Administration route where drug is swallowed and is absorbed from the stomach or small intestine.

60. Describe what is meant by the term *drug interactions*.

61. Describe what the EMT-I should keep in mind when storing drugs.

62. Describe procedures that should be used to ensure security of controlled substances stored in the ambulance.

63. List the 10 components of a drug profile.

64. In prehospital care, aspirin is given:
    a. to patients experiencing headache
    b. in combination with verapamil to convert supraventricular tachycardia
    c. for its ability to inhibit platelet aggregation
    d. to reverse severe allergic reaction

65. Amiodarone is what class of drug?
    a. bronchodilator
    b. antidysrhythmic
    c. calcium channel blocker
    d. anticholinergic

66. To treat cardiac arrest, amiodarone is given _____ at a dose of _____.

67. Which of the following medications are used to treat bronchial asthma and reversible bronchospasm associated with chronic bronchitis and emphysema?
    a. albuterol, morphine sulfate
    b. atropine, lidocaine, nitroglycerin
    c. aminophylline, albuterol, nifedipine
    d. albuterol, isoetharine

68. Which of the following side effects may develop when treating respiratory distress with bronchodilators?
    a. acute hypoglycemia
    b. bradydysrhythmias
    c. nervousness
    d. hemiparalysis

69. Describe the mechanism for action of albuterol.

    _____

    _____

    _____

    _____

    _____

70. Acetylcholine is the neurotransmitter of the parasympathetic nervous system. The compound that deactivates acetylcholine, thus terminating its effect, is:
    a. norepinephrine
    b. propranolol
    c. deoxyribonucleic acid
    d. cholinesterase

71. Atropine is a _____ drug.
    a. beta blocker
    b. parasympatholytic
    c. cholinergic
    d. sympathomimetic

72. Atropine works by:
    a. binding to acetylcholine receptors, blocking the action of acetylcholine
    b. stimulating the release of norepinephrine from the sympathetic nerve fibers
    c. stimulating the vagus nerve
    d. directly inactivating acetylcholine

73. Atropine is used to:
    a. suppress ventricular ectopy
    b. increase myocardial contractility
    c. constrict the venous circulation
    d. increase the heart rate

74. Indications for atropine administration include _____ _____, _____, pulseless electrical activity (PEA) where there is a slow rate, and _____ _____.

75. In treating bradycardia when there is a pulse, the correct dosage for atropine administration is:
    a. 5 to 10 mg, slow IV push, every 10 minutes, up to a total of 50 mg
    b. 5 mg/kg, IV push, every 5 minutes
    c. 0.5 mg, IV push, every 3 to 5 minutes, up to a total of 3.0 mg
    d. 2 to 10 mcg/min, continuous IV infusion

76. Larger than normal doses of atropine are needed in the case of:
    a. asystole
    b. organophosphate poisoning
    c. complete AV heart block
    d. profound bradycardia

77. List three indications for the administration of 50% dextrose in water ($D_{50}W$).

    _____

    _____

    _____

78. T F $D_{50}W$ is absolutely contraindicated in patients experiencing ketoacidosis.

79. T F $D_{50}W$ is administered in a dose of 25 g (50 mL of a 50% solution) IV push.

80. T F $D_{50}W$ should be administered via a large vein.

81. You have been instructed to administer 50 g of $D_{50}W$ to a 23-year-old patient who is experiencing hypoglycemia. Your kit is supplied with 50-mL prefilled syringes, each containing 25 g. To deliver the needed dose, you should administer how many prefilled syringes?

    _____

82. Epinephrine (1:10,000):
    a. is a potent alpha and beta antagonist
    b. contains 0.1 mg of medication in 10 mL of normal saline
    c. is used to convert coarse ventricular fibrillation to fine ventricular fibrillation
    d. increases myocardial oxygen demand

83. List four indications for the use of epinephrine.

    _____

    _____

    _____

    _____

84. Epinephrine, when used in the treatment of cardiac arrest, is administered at a dose of _____.
    a. 0.2 to 0.3 mg
    b. 1 mg, repeated every 3 to 5 minutes
    c. 2 to 5 mg, repeated every 8 to 10 minutes
    d. 2 to 10 mcg/min, IV infusion

85. The amount of epinephrine used to treat an adult patient experiencing an acute bronchospasm is _____ mL (1:1000 solution).
    a. 0.01 to 0.02
    b. 0.03 to 0.05
    c. 0.1 to 0.5
    d. 2.0 to 8.0

86. You have been instructed to administer 0.3 mg of epinephrine (1:1000) SQ to a 17-year-old patient who is experiencing an anaphylactic reaction following a bee sting. The number of milliliters needed to deliver the correct dose is:

    _____

87. Antidysrhythmic agents are used to:
    a. control hypertension
    b. increase the blood pressure
    c. treat or prevent cardiac dysrhythmias
    d. manage pain and anxiety

88. Place a checkmark beside the indications for the use of lidocaine.
    _____ Cardiac arrest from VF/pulseless VT
    _____ Hemodynamically compromising bradycardia
    _____ Stable ventricular tachycardia
    _____ Acute respiratory failure
    _____ Narcotic overdose
    _____ Prophylactically, in suspected myocardial infarction
    _____ Atrial fibrillation
    _____ Ventricular ectopy

89. T F Lidocaine has little effect on the fibrillation threshold.

90. T F The correct dosage for lidocaine when used to treat refractory cardiac arrest is 1.0 to 1.5 mg/kg.

91. T F A 75- to 100-mg bolus of lidocaine will typically maintain adequate therapeutic blood levels for up to 45 minutes.

92. T F Lidocaine may be used to suppress premature ventricular complexes associated with bradycardia.

93. Adverse reactions associated with lidocaine administration include:
    a. decreased level of consciousness, irritability, decreased potassium levels
    b. drowsiness, tremor, respiratory depression
    c. muscle twitching, coma, angina
    d. bradycardia, flushing, palpitations

94. You are treating a 45-year-old, 185-pound man who is complaining of chest pain and displaying ventricular tachycardia on the ECG monitor. You have been instructed to administer 1 mg/kg of lidocaine, IV push. Your kit is supplied with 100 mg/5 mL prefilled syringes. The correct dosage and number of milliliters needed is

    _____ mg, _____ mL.

95. Following your IV push administration of lidocaine, you are instructed to place 2 g of lidocaine in 500 mL of 5% dextrose in water and administer it at 2 mg/min using a microdrip administration set. The drop rate per minute needed to administer this dose is:

    _____

96. A trade name for naloxone is:
    a. Inotropin
    b. Osmitrol
    c. Narcan
    d. Dobutrex

97. List those conditions that naloxone is used to treat.

    _____

    _____

98. Place a checkmark beside those drugs for which naloxone may be used to treat an overdose.
    _____ Talwin
    _____ cocaine
    _____ Dexedrine
    _____ heroin
    _____ phencyclidine
    _____ paregoric
    _____ morphine
    _____ Demerol

99. You have been instructed to administer 2 mg of naloxone to a 31-year-old patient who has overdosed on Nubain. Your kit is supplied with prefilled syringes containing 1 mg/mL. The correct number of milliliters that needs to be delivered is:

    _____

100. Naloxone can be administered:
    1. PO
    2. SQ
    3. IV push
    4. IM

    Select the correct answer.
    a. 2 and 3
    b. 3 only
    c. 2, 3, and 4
    d. all of the above

101. Nitroglycerin administration in patients experiencing chest pain may result in:
    1. improvement of myocardial perfusion through dilation of the coronary arteries
    2. an increase in the heart rate through direct stimulation of the SA node
    3. a slowing of the heart rate through an increase in conduction time through the AV node
    4. a reduction of myocardial workload through dilation of peripheral blood vessels, thus causing a reduction in the preload and afterload

    Select the correct answer.
    a. 3 only
    b. 1 only
    c. 1 and 4
    d. 1, 3, and 4

102. T F In addition to its use in angina pectoris and acute myocardial infarction, nitroglycerin may be used in congestive heart failure.

103. T F Nitroglycerin is contraindicated in patients who have increased intracranial pressure.

104. A common side effect of nitroglycerin is:
    a. throbbing headache
    b. bradycardia
    c. dehydration
    d. seizures

105. You have been instructed to administer 0.6 mg of nitroglycerin SL to a 42-year-old patient who is complaining of chest pain following an argument with a family member. Your kit is supplied with a bottle of 0.3-mg tablets. How many tablets are needed to deliver the correct dosage?

    _____

106. Furosemide is:
    a. a loop diuretic
    b. used to treat chest pain
    c. contraindicated in pulmonary edema
    d. given rapid IV push

107. The dosage for furosemide used to treat congestive heart failure is:
    a. 0.5 to 1.0 mg/kg, IV push
    b. 75 to 100 mg, IV push
    c. 2 to 4 mg, continuous IV infusion
    d. 3 to 5 mg, IV push

108. List four adverse reactions of furosemide.

_____

_____

_____

_____

109. A trade name for furosemide is _____.

110. Morphine sulfate:
    a. is a benzodiazepine
    b. elevates the pain threshold
    c. is used to treat cardiac dysrhythmias
    d. decreases venous capacitance

111. T F Morphine sulfate is contraindicated in respiratory depression and should be used with caution in patients with emphysema.

112. T F Morphine is usually given IM in the field.

113. _____ should be used to reverse respiratory depression that follows morphine sulfate administration.

114. _____ is a brand name for adenosine.

115. Adenosine is used to treat _____ _____.

116. Adenosine is not effective in conversion of _____ _____, _____, or _____ _____.

117. Adenosine may cause _____ in asthmatic patients.

118. Describe adenosine's mechanism of action.

_____

_____

_____

_____

_____

119. The dosage for adenosine in the adult patient is:

CROSSWORD PUZZLE EXERCISE

120. Complete the following crossword puzzle.

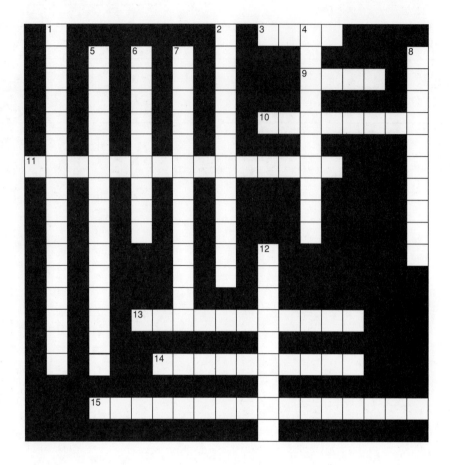

ACROSS

3. Helpful mnemonic to remember the drugs that can be given by the endotracheal route.
9. Effect of a drug that is unintended.
10. Commonly used drug that is an acetylcholine antagonist or blocker.
11. Refers to the fraction of drug administered that reaches the central circulation.
13. Drug's desired effect and the reason the drug is prescribed.
14. Drug response that mimics naturally occurring disease states.
15. Also known as drug allergy.

DOWN

1. Condition or instance for which a drug should not be used.
2. Involves the transport of an absorbed drug to its target site.
4. The process by which medications enter the body.
5. Study of the effects of drugs on the body.
6. An individual's capacity to endure medications.
7. Primary neurotransmitter of the parasympathetic nervous system.
8. Physical state where withdrawal symptoms occur when a person discontinues the use of drugs.
12. Means two drugs working together.

6 Venous Access

CHAPTER TERMINAL OBJECTIVES

On completion of this chapter, the EMT-Intermediate will understand the basic principles of intravenous therapy.

For the multiple-choice questions, select the single best answer to each question. For the matching questions, select the best corresponding answer for each item. Because there are sometimes more items than corresponding answers in some questions, some items may not be used.

1. Intravenous (IV) cannulation is defined as the:
   a. insertion of a tube into the bladder
   b. placement of a catheter into a vein
   c. placement of a needle into an artery
   d. removal of blood from a vein

2. Primary reasons for IV cannulation in the prehospital setting include:
   a. adding oxygen directly into the circulatory system
   b. sampling arterial blood
   c. monitoring the oxygen saturation levels of the venous circulation
   d. administering medications

3. T F The EMT-I can administer IV fluids without permission of on-line medical direction or standing orders.

4. T F IV therapy is an important adjunct in the management of the seriously ill or injured patient.

5. List four common conditions in which IV therapy is indicated.

   _____

   _____

   _____

   _____

6. In hypovolemic shock, IVs are used to:
   a. administer medications to restore myocardial contractility
   b. restore the body's fluid and electrolytes
   c. counter blood loss by introducing fluid into the circulatory system
   d. increase the amount of glucose in the body

7. Describe why the IV route is preferred for administering medications in the prehospital setting.

___

8. Contraindications of IV cannulation in a particular site include:
   a. small veins
   b. burned extremities
   c. veins far from joints
   d. veins close to the surface

9. T F   Transporting a critically ill or injured patient to the hospital can be delayed to initiate IV therapy.

10. T F   All blood and body substances should be regarded as potentially infected with HBV or HIV.

11. Whenever IV cannulation is performed:
    a. used needles must be placed in a puncture-resistant (sharps) container
    b. gown, mask, and eye protection should be worn
    c. used needles are recapped by hand
    d. the EMT-I should wash his or her hands after performing the procedure

12. Describe how needlestick injuries can be avoided.

___

13. Define the abbreviation HBV.

___

14. List the supplies that are needed to perform IV cannulation.

_____

_____

_____

_____

_____

_____

_____

_____

_____

_____

_____

_____

_____

15. Label the following illustration of an IV administration set.

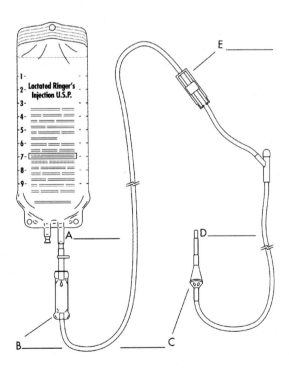

16. Containers for IV solutions used in the prehospital setting:
    a. are typically clear glass bottles
    b. come in a 250-mL size that is used for trauma emergencies, and a 1000-mL size that is used for drug administration
    c. have a port with a rubber stopper where medications can be injected into the solution
    d. have a port with a plastic tab that is removed to insert the blunt end of an IV administration set

17. The usual IV fluid replacement for hypovolemia in the prehospital setting is a:
    a. colloid solution
    b. crystalloid solution
    c. dextrose solution
    d. salt/sugar solution

18. Which of the following is true regarding crystalloid solutions?
    a. Dextran and whole blood are crystalloid solutions.
    b. Two thirds of a crystalloid solution is lost to the interstitial space within 1 hour when administered intravenously.
    c. Generally, no more than 1 L of a crystalloid solution should be administered in the field setting.
    d. Crystalloid solutions contain proteins and other large molecules.

19. It is necessary to administer _____ of IV crystalloid solution for every liter of blood lost when treating patients who have experienced hypovolemic shock.
    a. 1 L
    b. ⅔ L
    c. 0.5 L
    d. 3 L

20. Describe what is meant by the term *colloid solution*, and indicate why it is not used in the prehospital setting.

    _____

    _____

    _____

    _____

    _____

21. All of the following are examples of colloids *except:*
    a. whole blood
    b. plasma
    c. 0.45% NaCl
    d. plasma substitutes

22. T F Dextran provides immediate volume expansion, but its use may cause clotting problems and interfere with type and crossmatching of blood.

23. T F Ringer's lactate solution is an isotonic solution that contributes a buffer when metabolized.

24. T F Five percent dextrose in water is an isotonic solution that remains in the intravascular space for long periods.

25. Five percent dextrose in water (D_5W) may be used in which of the following patients?
    a. 39-year-old man who is in cardiac arrest
    b. 93-year-old woman who is suffering from a stroke
    c. 15-year-old boy who has been shot in the head with a high-powered rifle
    d. 45-year-old woman who has experienced third-degree burns over 50% of her body

26. Complete the following table regarding IV solutions.

IV Solution	1 L Contains
0.9% Sodium chloride solution (normal saline)	
Lactated Ringer's solution (LR)	

27. Match each of the following components with the correct description.

    Component
    a. Piercing spiked end
    b. Drip chamber
    c. Flow clamp
    d. Drug administration port
    e. Connector end
    f. IV administration set

    Description
    _____ Consists of a rubber stopper and a Y-shaped inlet
    _____ Portion of the administration set that is inserted into the tubing insertion port of the IV bag
    _____ Clear, cylindrical portion of the tubing where the drops passing through the administration set can be viewed and counted
    _____ Part of the IV administration set that is inserted into the hub of the IV catheter
    _____ Clear plastic tubing that connects the IV bag to the catheter
    _____ Plastic housing with a roller-type clamp that is used to control the amount of fluid the patient receives

28. Complete the following table regarding different types of administration sets.

	Also Referred to As	Drops Equal to 1 mL	Used for What Situation
Microdrip			
Macrodrip			

29. The component of the IV administration set that is used to control how much fluid the patient receives is referred to as the:
   a. infusion port
   b. extension set
   c. flow clamp
   d. drip chamber

30. Describe what is meant by the term *TKO rate*.

   _____

   _____

   _____

   _____

31. In trauma or other situations in which IV fluids are being used to replace circulatory volume, the flow rate is based on the patient's response to the IV infusion, including in the:
   a. pulse
   b. blood pressure
   c. cerebral function
   d. all of the above

32. Describe why using large amounts of IV fluids when there is uncontrolled bleeding (such as in penetrating trauma) may increase internal bleeding and lead to death.

   _____

   _____

   _____

   _____

   _____

33. The _____ is a plastic guard that prevents the piercing spike from being touched and contaminated during its insertion into the tubing insertion port of the IV bag:
   a. protective cap
   b. sheath
   c. flow clamp
   d. flange

34. Describe how the spiked piercing and connector ends of the IV administration set are protected from contamination before use.

___

35. "Volutrol chamber" IV tubing is used when:
    a. specific amounts of fluid are to be administered
    b. large amounts of fluid are to be given quickly
    c. the patient has a susceptibility to infection
    d. medications are likely to be administered

36. List two problems associated with use of an extension set.

___

37. List three types of IV catheters.

___

38. The catheter-over-needle:
    a. consists of a plastic inner catheter and an outer needle
    b. can be better anchored than most other cannulation devices
    c. permits very little movement of the extremity in which it is placed
    d. is smaller than the puncture site created by the needle

39. The outside diameter of the shaft of an IV needle is referred to as the:
    a. hub
    b. bevel
    c. lumen
    d. gauge

40. Which of the following is a larger IV catheter?
    a. 22 gauge
    b. 14 gauge
    c. 18 gauge
    d. 20 gauge

41. T F When placing an IV in a trauma patient, a 14- to 16-gauge catheter is preferred.

42. The portion of the catheter-over-needle device that the IV tubing is attached to is referred to as the:
    a. hub
    b. bevel
    c. needle
    d. flashback chamber

43. Match each of the following catheters used for prehospital care with the correct characteristics. Some items may be used more than once.

    Gauge
    a. 14 to 16
    b. 20
    c. 22

    Characteristic
    _____ Used in older children, adolescents, average-sized adult patients, suitable for most IV infusions
    _____ Used for fragile and/or small veins and when lower rates must be maintained but is more difficult to insert through tough skin
    _____ Used in adolescents and adults, for volume replacement such as in trauma, and when viscous medications such as 50% dextrose are to be administered
    _____ Painful insertion, requires large vein

44. Smaller catheters:
    a. are not well tolerated in elderly patients
    b. cause more trauma to the vein
    c. allow greater blood flow around the tip, reducing the risk of clotting
    d. are used in trauma patients

45. Which of the following can increase the IV flow rate?
    a. an IV catheter that is longer
    b. a larger-gauge IV catheter
    c. a large vein
    d. a vein that is located more distally

46. A 20-gauge catheter-over-needle should be used in which of the following?
    a. 16-year-old boy who is experiencing hypoglycemia, BP 156/96
    b. 85-year-old woman who is suffering from a stroke, BP 200/110
    c. 24-year-old man who has been shot in the chest, BP 100/78
    d. 40-year-old man who is suffering from heat stroke, BP 90/60

47. Match each of the following types of blood vessels with the correct characteristics. Each item may be used more than once.

    Blood Vessel
    a. Arteries
    b. Veins

    Characteristic
    _____ Color of blood is dark red because of decreased oxygen concentration
    _____ Run deep and are usually surrounded by muscle, which provides them the protection they need
    _____ Lie just under the skin, and drain the skin and superficial fascia
    _____ Have valves that keep blood flowing toward the heart; otherwise, muscular pressure would cause backing up of blood supply
    _____ Direction of blood flow is toward the heart
    _____ Pulsation is present

48. You have decided to place an IV line. Which of the following are preferred characteristics of any vein that you may cannulate?
    a. It is the most proximal vein available.
    b. It should be straight.
    c. It should be rolling.
    d. It is located over a joint.

49. The most suitable vein for cannulation while chest compressions are in progress is:
    a. the subclavian vein
    b. the internal jugular vein
    c. a peripheral arm vein in the antecubital space
    d. the femoral vein

50. Which of the following veins is located in the forearm?
    a. digital
    b. metacarpal
    c. cephalic
    d. saphenous

51. Which of the following veins is located in the neck?
    a. saphenous
    b. external jugular
    c. basilic
    d. cephalic

52. Label the following illustration of the veins of the arm:

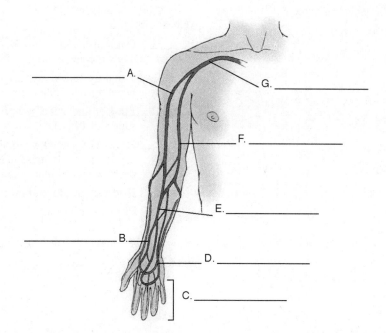

53. Match each of the following veins with the appropriate characteristics. Some items may be used more than once.

    Vein
    a. Digital vein
    b. Metacarpal vein
    c. Accessory cephalic vein
    d. Antecubital vein

    Characteristic

    _____ May be uncomfortable for patient because the arm must be kept straight; otherwise, the catheter could kink or slide in and out of the vein and damage it

    _____ Wrist movement is limited unless a short catheter is used

    _____ Readily accepts large-bore needles and its position on the forearm creates a natural splint for the needle and adapter

    _____ Cannot be used if dorsal hand veins are already being used

    _____ Insertion is more painful because of increased nerve endings in hands

    _____ Is sometimes difficult to position catheter flush with skin

    _____ Often visible or palpable in children when other veins will not dilate

54. List four things that should be explained to the patient before IV cannulation is attempted.

    _____

    _____

    _____

    _____

55. T   F   An IV bag that is leaking can be used as long as it is not cloudy.

56. To prepare an IV administration set, the EMT-I should:
    a. remove the administration set from its protective wrapping, and slide the flow control valve close to the connector end of the tubing
    b. open the flow control valve once it is in the correct location on the IV tubing
    c. using sterile technique, insert the spiked piercing end of the administration set into the tubing insertion port of the IV bag
    d. squeeze the drip chamber five or six times to fill it all the way

57. In preparation for IV cannulation, the patient should be placed into a suitable position with the selected extremity:
    a. higher than the heart
    b. lower than the heart
    c. at the patient's side
    d. above the patient's head

58. To reduce the chance of pain and discomfort while using a tourniquet:
    a. it should be tied tightly enough to impede arterial and venous blood flow
    b. release it as soon as the venipuncture device has been placed into the vein and blood samples have been drawn
    c. avoid keeping it in place for more than 1 minute
    d. keep it rolled up

59. List three ways veins can be distended for easier cannulation.

60. Describe how to cleanse the venipuncture site.

61. Describe how to stabilize the vein during venipuncture.

62. When penetrating the skin while performing venipuncture, the bevel of the needle should be pointed _____ in relation to the patient's skin.
    a. down
    b. to the side
    c. up
    d. inferiorly

63. T F An 18- to 20-gauge catheter can be used when placing an IV in patients experiencing medical conditions.

64. T F Before penetrating the skin with the needle, the tourniquet should be released.

65. T F The EMT-I can expect a great deal of resistance as the needle is advanced through the skin.

66. T F Depending on the type of venipuncture device, the needle should be held at a 15-, 30-, or 45-degree angle to the skin.

67. T F Normally, a slight "pop" or "give" is felt as the needle passes through the wall of the vein.

68. You are attempting to place an IV catheter in the forearm of a 55-year-old man who is experiencing hypoglycemia. You have penetrated the skin and are advancing the needle. The presence of dark red blood in the end of the needle is indicative of:
    a. an air embolism
    b. inadvertent arterial puncture
    c. local infiltration
    d. penetration of the vein

69. Describe why the venipuncture device is advanced another 1 to 2 cm after initial penetration of the vein.

    _____
    _____
    _____
    _____

70. After the venipuncture device has been inserted another 1 to 2 cm, the catheter is advanced into the vein until:
    a. the hub is against the skin
    b. the bevel is against the skin
    c. approximately 0.5 inch of the catheter is in the vein
    d. resistance is met

71. Describe how to prevent blood from leaking out of the catheter hub once the needle is withdrawn.

_____

_____

_____

_____

_____

72. Which of the following should be done once the IV tubing is connected to the hub of the IV catheter?
    a. A venous constricting band is applied.
    b. The flow clamp is opened, and the flow rate is adjusted accordingly.
    c. The IV site is covered with a nonsterile bandage.
    d. The time and date of insertion are written on the IV bag.

73. To ensure proper IV flow rates, the IV container must hang:
    a. below the level of the patient's heart
    b. at the same level as the patient's heart
    c. at the same level as the insertion site
    d. at least 30 to 36 inches above the insertion site

74. When infiltration occurs:
    a. the IV catheter should be kept in place until a new IV site has been established
    b. venipuncture should be attempted at another site using the same needle and catheter
    c. the tissue around the site is typically cool and swollen
    d. the IV catheter should be discarded and an occlusive dressing placed over the venipuncture site

75. Arm boards:
    a. are considered a required element of placing an IV line
    b. prevent rotation or movement of the patient's arm
    c. must be long enough to prevent flexion or extension at the tip of the venipuncture device
    d. should be covered with tape to keep them from sliding after application

---

Mathematical formula for figuring IV flow rates per minute:

volume to be infused × gtt/mL of administration set ÷ gtt/min = total time of infusion in minutes

---

76. You are instructed to administer an infusion of 1000 mL of normal saline in 4 hours, and the administration set being used provides 10 gtt/mL. The correct drip rate per minute is (round down to the nearest tenth):

77. You are instructed to administer an infusion of 750 mL of lactated Ringer's solution in 2 hours, and the administration set being used provides 10 gtt/mL. The correct drip rate per minute is (round down to the nearest tenth):

78. You are instructed to administer an infusion of 50 mL of 5% dextrose in water during your transport of a diabetic patient to the hospital. Your estimated transport time is half an hour. The administration set being used provides 60 gtt/mL. The correct drip rate per minute is (round down to the nearest tenth):

79. You are a member of a rescue team working in the Oregon wilderness. You are called in to assist with the removal and transport of a logging accident victim. You are instructed to administer an infusion of 1250 mL of lactated Ringer's solution over 2 hours. The administration set being used provides 10 gtt/mL. The correct drip rate per minute is (round down to the nearest tenth):

80. You have been called to the scene where a 38-year-old patient is believed to be experiencing an acute myocardial infarction. You have loaded the patient into the back of the ambulance when you are instructed to administer an infusion of 20 mL of 5% dextrose in water during transport to the hospital. Your estimated transport time is 20 minutes. The administration set being used provides 60 gtt/mL. The correct drip rate per minute is (round down to the nearest tenth):

81. Which of the following can be done to *slow* the IV flow rate?
    a. manually compress the IV bag
    b. raise the bag above the level of the IV site
    c. turn down the drip regulator clamp
    d. use a macrodrip administration set

82. When an IV is started, which of the following must be documented on the run report?
    1. date and time of the venipuncture
    2. type and amount of solution
    3. number of insertion attempts (if more than one)
    4. amount of blood loss by the patient during venipuncture
    5. venipuncture site

    Select the correct answer.
    a. 2 and 5
    b. 1, 3, and 5
    c. 3, 4, and 5
    d. 1, 2, 3, and 5

83. T   F   A felt-tip pen can be used to mark the outside of the IV bag with the date and time of IV cannulation.

84. Which of the following will result in the IV fluid not flowing through the administration set?
    a. a venous constricting band that has been left in place
    b. an IV bag that is too low
    c. infiltration into the tissues
    d. all of the above

85. To fix a drip chamber that is completely filled with IV solution, the EMT-I should:
    a. invert the bag, and squeeze the drip chamber to return some of the fluid into the bag
    b. move the flow regulator to a wide-open position
    c. penetrate the drip chamber with a needle attached to a 10-mL syringe, and withdraw 1 to 2 mL
    d. pinch off the IV bag above the spiked piercing end of the administration set, and squeeze the drip chamber two or three times

86. List eight complications of IV therapy.

_____

_____

_____

_____

_____

_____

_____

_____

87. Describe how catheter shear can be avoided.

_____

_____

_____

_____

88. You have established an IV line in a 51-year-old patient who is complaining of chest pain. Which of the following would be indicative of circulatory overload?
    a. acute decrease in the blood pressure
    b. absence of blood backflow when the IV bag is lowered
    c. chills and shaking
    d. shortness of breath, rales

89. When placing an IV line, the *best* indication of accidental arterial puncture is:
    a. swelling and intense pain around the puncture site
    b. an absence of a distal pulse
    c. air bubbles at the proximal end of the needle
    d. bright red blood spurting from the cannula

90. An air embolism can occur if the:
    a. IV fluid is administered too quickly
    b. IV bag is inverted anytime after the flow regulator is in an open position
    c. IV tubing becomes dislodged from the hub of the catheter
    d. patient suddenly becomes hypotensive during the course of IV cannulation

91. Pyrogenic reaction:
    a. occurs when foreign proteins, capable of producing fever, are present in the administration set or IV solution
    b. is characterized by the slow onset of fever (100 to 106° F)
    c. is managed by increasing the IV flow rate to wide open
    d. usually occurs within 2 hours of IV therapy being initiated

92. Which of the following statements regarding the drawing of venous blood samples (venipuncture) is true?
    a. Obtaining venous blood samples is rarely necessary in the comatose patient.
    b. When drawing blood, each tube should be filled completely.
    c. A 10-mL syringe is adequate for routine venous sampling.
    d. The digital veins are preferred for venipuncture.

93. Identify, by numbering, the correct sequence for performing IV cannulation.

___ While holding the needle stable between the first/middle fingers and thumb, use the first finger and thumb of the other hand to slide the catheter into the vein until the hub is against the skin.

___ Note when blood fills the flashback chamber of the needle, and lower the venipuncture device; then advance it another 1 to 2 cm until the tip of the catheter is well within the vein.

___ Apply a venous tourniquet, and select a suitable vein by palpation and sight.

___ Penetrate the skin with the bevel of the needle pointed up, and enter the vein with the needle from either the top or side.

___ Tell the patient there will be a small poke or pinch as the needle enters the skin.

___ Cleanse the site thoroughly with an alcohol wipe (or povidone-iodine).

___ Stabilize the vein by anchoring it with your thumb and stretching the skin downward.

___ Disconnect the syringe or Vacutainer device from the hub of the catheter by holding the hub between the first finger and thumb and pulling the device free with the other hand.

___ Hold the end of venipuncture device between the thumb and index/middle fingers.

___ Once the needle tip is within the catheter, apply pressure to the vein beyond the catheter tip with the little finger to prevent blood from leaking out of the catheter hub once the needle is completely withdrawn.

___ Draw a blood sample, and release the tourniquet from the patient's arm.

___ Reapply pressure to the vein beyond the catheter tip with the little finger to prevent blood from leaking out of the catheter hub once the blood-drawing device is disconnected.

___ Connect the IV tubing to the catheter hub, being careful not to contaminate either the hub or connector before insertion, and open the IV flow control valve.

___ Depending on the type of venipuncture device and the manufacturer's recommendations, hold the needle at a 15-, 30-, or 45-degree angle to the skin.

___ Cover the IV site with povidone-iodine ointment (if called for by local protocol) and a sterile dressing or an adhesive bandage, and secure the catheter, administration set tubing, and sterile dressing in place.

___ Adjust the flow rate as is appropriate for the patient's condition, and dispose of the needle(s) in a proper biomedical waste container.

94. You are attempting to place an IV line in a 41-year-old patient who is experiencing a drug overdose. Your first attempt in the dorsal aspect of his right hand was unsuccessful. You should now:
    a. select a more distal site on the dorsal aspect of the right hand
    b. proceed to the external jugular vein on the right side of the patient's neck
    c. select a site on the dorsal aspect of the patient's left hand
    d. select a site that is proximal to the first venipuncture site

95. Which of the following is done as part of discontinuing an IV line?
    a. apply a venous constricting band
    b. stop the IV fluid flow completely by closing the flow clamp
    c. lower the IV site below the level of the heart
    d. disconnect the IV administration set from the catheter hub, and then remove the catheter from the vein

96. The external jugular vein:
    a. is easy to cannulate
    b. is considered a central vein
    c. provides direct access to the superior vena cava
    d. lies superficially along the anterior portion of the neck

97. You are attempting to place an IV line in a 61-year-old female patient who is unconscious. You are unable to identify an adequate vein on either arm and decide to cannulate the patient's external jugular vein. When cannulating the external jugular vein, the:
    a. cannula should be aligned in the direction of the vein with the point aimed at the ear
    b. vein should be penetrated at a 15-degree angle
    c. puncture is made at the point where the vein pierces the deep fascia of the neck
    d. patient's head should be turned away from you.

98. You are preparing to establish an IV line in an 80-year-old woman who is experiencing heart failure. The preferred IV solution, administration set, and IV catheter for this patient is:
    a. 5% dextrose in water, microdrip, 20 gauge
    b. normal saline (0.9%), macrodrip, 18 gauge
    c. lactated Ringer's solution, microdrip, 22 gauge
    d. 5% dextrose in water, macrodrip, 22 gauge

99. You are called to the scene where a 17-year-old girl has been stabbed in the abdomen during a fight at school. Your assessment reveals she is alert and oriented, has a respiratory rate of 18, a pulse rate of 130, a blood pressure of 100/82, and cool, diaphoretic skin. Which of the following statements is true regarding initiating IV therapy in this case?
    a. Eighteen- to 20-gauge needles should be used.
    b. The IV should be started while en route to the hospital.
    c. Five percent dextrose in water should be used.
    d. Microdrip administration sets are preferred.

100. IV lines used in the management of cardiac arrest should:
    a. be placed in a forearm vein just above the wrist
    b. consist of a 5% dextrose in water solution
    c. be run wide open when overhydration is suspected
    d. be elevated above the level of the heart

CROSSWORD PUZZLE EXERCISE

101. Complete the following crossword puzzle.

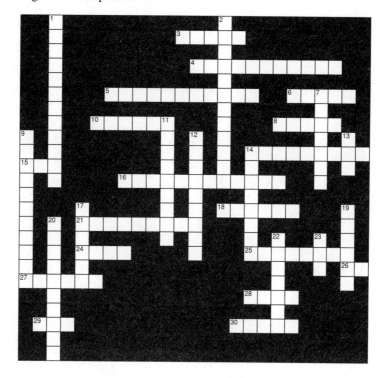

ACROSS

3. 10, 15, or 20 drops equals 1 mL of IV solution.
4. On same side of body.
5. Hand that should be used.
6. Rate that IV fluids are administered in hypovolemia.
8. Can occur when catheter is withdrawn back over or through needle.
10. Structures found only in veins.
14. Can develop if appropriate cleansing techniques are not used.
15. Abbreviation for a "to keep open" rate.
16. Within or into a bone.
18. Should be worn when establishing an IV.
21. Extra length of IV tubing.
24. Clear chamber where drops can be viewed and counted.
25. Solutions that contain proteins.
26. Direction needle bevel should be pointed when starting IV.
27. Type of catheter that slows IV flow rate.
28. Clamp used to increase or slow IV infusion rate.
29. Location on the catheter where the IV tubing connects.
30. Number of liters of IV solution administered with every liter of blood loss.

DOWN

1. Leakage and accumulation of IV fluid into tissues.
2. Dissolved crystals in water.
7. Type of catheters preferred in field setting.
9. Area where IV is placed when treating cardiac arrest.
11. Hardening or thickening of tissues.
12. Reaction that occurs when foreign proteins are present in IV solution.
13. Feeling that may be noted when needle penetrates vein.
14. Solution having same osmotic pressure as body.
17. Used to facilitate passage through skin and vein.
19. Back of hand.
20. Device used to distend distal veins.
22. Type of solution that contains sugar.
23. Abbreviation for human immunodeficiency virus.

7 Medication Math

CHAPTER TERMINAL OBJECTIVES

On completion of this chapter, the EMT-Intermediate will understand the basic math used to calculate drug dosages and volumes to be delivered for medications used in the prehospital care setting.

For the multiple-choice questions, select the single best answer to each question. For the matching questions, select the best corresponding answer for each item. Because there are sometimes more items than corresponding answers, some items may not be used.

1. A fraction is a number that expresses _____ of a group.

2. If you were told to administer ½ of a prefilled syringe containing 10 mL, how many milliliters would you deliver?
    a. 2.5
    b. 3
    c. 5
    d. 7.5

3. If you were told to administer ⅕ of a prefilled syringe containing 5 mL, how many milliliters would you deliver?
    a. 1
    b. 2.5
    c. 3
    d. 5

4. Practice exercise for decimals

0.75 + 0.25 = _____	0.66 − 0.2 = _____	12.5 × 10 = _____	14.8 ÷ 2 = _____
1.24 + 0.33 = _____	1.65 − 0.94 = _____	1.23 × 0.75 = _____	0.48 ÷ 0.6 = _____
8.76 + 1.28 = _____	44.32 − 1.16 = _____	7.52 × 1.23 = _____	12.6 ÷ 4.2 = _____
7.2 + 3.82 = _____	9.13 − 0.71 = _____	0.55 × 16.53 = _____	198.4 ÷ 12.8 = _____

5. There are two systems of measuring drug dosage: the _____ system and the _____ system.

6. The metric system is based on multiples of _____.

7. Match each of the following metric system terms with the correct abbreviation.

Term	Abbreviation
a. gram	_____ g
b. liter	_____ cc
c. kilogram	_____ mcg
d. milliliter	_____ L
e. milligram	_____ kg
f. cubic centimeter	_____ mg
g. microgram	_____ mL

8. Complete the following conversions between metric system units.

Unit	Conversion
5 mL	_____ L
3 L	_____ mL
1 g	_____ mg
4 mg	_____ mcg
1 cc	_____ mL
8 mcg	_____ mg
100 mg	_____ g

9. One kilogram is equal to _____ pound(s).
   a. 1.5
   b. 2.0
   c. 2.2
   d. 5.0

10. Convert the following patient weights in pounds to kilograms. (Round off to the nearest whole number.)

Pounds	Kilograms
100	_____
85	_____
220	_____
170	_____
150	_____

11. Complete the following table with the correct conversions.

Grams (g)	Milligrams (mg)	Micrograms (mcg)
1		
	400	
		1000
2		
	50	
		4
25		
	800	

12. With a microdrip administration set, _____ gtt is equal to 1 mL.
    a. 10
    b. 15
    c. 30
    d. 60

Mathematics Used to Determine Medication Dosages

The EMT-I may be required to make one of three calculations in order to administer medications. This includes:

- Determining the number of milliliters needed to deliver a specific medication dose
- Calculating the necessary dose of medication based on the patient's weight and then determining the number of milliliters needed to deliver the dose
- Calculating the drop rate per minute needed to deliver a specific dose of medication

To determine the number of milliliters needed to deliver a specific dose of medication, the following steps are employed.

Step 1: Multiply the desired dosage by the "volume on hand."

Step 2: Divide the answer obtained in Step 1 by the "dose on hand."

Example:

(desired dosage) × (volume on hand)
           (dose on hand)

You have been instructed to administer 80 mg of furosemide to a 67-year-old congestive heart failure patient. Furosemide is supplied in 40 mg/4 mL prefilled syringes. The following shows how to determine the number of mL needed to deliver the appropriate dosage.

Step 1: 80 mg (dose desired) × 4 mL (volume of medication on hand) = 320 mg/mL

Step 2: 320 mg/mL ÷ 40 mg (dose of medication on hand) = 8 mL (amount to be administered)

Note: When you multiply two different units of measurement (e.g., mg and mL), you show it as mg/mL. Then when you divide that number by one of the units of measurement, the one crosses out the other (shown in Step 2). The remaining unit of measurement then follows the number (shown in Step 2).

For the following cases, write the answers in the spaces provided.

13. You have been instructed to administer 0.5 mg of epinephrine (1:1000), SQ, to a 42-year-old patient who is experiencing anaphylaxis. Epinephrine is supplied in 1 mg/1 mL ampules. Indicate how many milliliters are needed to deliver the appropriate dosage.

14. You have been instructed to administer 5 mg of diazepam to a 49-year-old seizure patient. Diazepam is supplied in 10 mg/2 mL prefilled syringes. Indicate how many milliliters are needed to deliver the appropriate dosage.

15. You have been instructed to administer 3 mg of morphine sulfate to a 53-year-old female patient who is complaining of substernal chest pain. Morphine is supplied in a 1-mL syringe containing 10 mg. Indicate how many milliliters are needed to deliver the appropriate dosage.

The following steps are used to determine the amount of medication to be given based on a patient's weight.

Step 1: Divide the weight (in pounds) by 2.2 to determine the patient's weight in kilograms.

Step 2: Multiply the weight in kilograms by the drug prescribed dosage (e.g., 1 mg × ___ kg).

Step 3: Multiply the desired dosage by the "volume on hand."

Step 4: Divide the answer obtained in Step 3 by the "dose on hand."

Example:

Lidocaine is used to suppress cardiac dysrhythmias originating from the ventricles. It is generally administered at an initial dose of 1 to 1.5 mg/kg. To determine how many milliliters of the medication are needed to deliver the appropriate dose, use the four steps described above. For this exercise, lidocaine is supplied in 100 mg/5 mL (20 mg/mL) prefilled syringes.

Patient weight: 160 lb

Step 1: 160 (lb) ÷ 2.2 = 73 kg

Step 2: mg × 73 kg = 73 mg (dose desired)

Step 3: 73 mg (dose desired) × 5 mL (volume on hand) = 365 mg/mL

Step 4: 365 mg/mL ÷ 100 mg (dose on hand) = 3.65 mL (amount to be administered)

---

16. For the following patient weights, complete the four steps described above to determine the number of milliliters of lidocaine needed to deliver the appropriate dose. For this exercise, lidocaine is supplied in a 5-mL prefilled syringe containing 100 mg.

    Patient Weight in Pounds

    230

    128

    94

    198

17. Furosemide is a diuretic agent that is used to treat congestive heart failure. It may be administered at a dose of 0.5 mg/kg. To determine how many milliliters of the medication are needed to deliver the appropriate dose, complete the four steps (described earlier) for each of the patient weights listed below. For this exercise, furosemide is supplied in 40 mg/4 mL prefilled syringes.

Patient Weight in Pounds

254

112

76

172

To calculate the drop rate needed per minute to deliver a specific dose of medication, the following steps are employed.

Step 1: Multiply the "volume" (of the infusion bag) times the "desired dosage" per minute.

Step 2: Convert the concentration of the medication into a lower unit (e.g., 1 g = 1000 mg).

Step 3: Divide the answer determined in Step 2 by the dose of the drug (after it has been converted to a lower metric unit).

Step 4: Multiply the answer (determined in Step 3) times the drop rate per minute (volume of IV bag) × (dose desired)

_____ × drops/mL = _____ drops per minute (dose added to IV bag)

Example:

You have been instructed to administer 2 mg of lidocaine via continuous IV infusion to the patient described in the previous example. By protocol, you are to place 1 g of lidocaine in 250 mL of 5% dextrose in water and administer it with a microdrip administration set.

Step 1: 250 mL (volume of IV bag) × 2 mg per minute (dose desired) = 500 mL/mg/min

Step 2: 1 g (dose added to IV bag) = 1000 mg

Step 3: 500 mL/mg/min ÷ 1000 mg = 0.5 mL/min

Step 4: 0.5 mL/min × 60 drops per mL = 30 drops per minute (rate to be administered)

---

18. You have been instructed to administer 3 mg of lidocaine via continuous IV infusion to a patient who is displaying ventricular ectopy. By protocol, you are to place 2 g of lidocaine in 500 mL of 5% dextrose in water and administer it with a microdrip administration set. To determine the correct drip rate, complete the steps described earlier. Write the answer below.

19. Fill in the chart below to show how many drops per minute would be required to deliver the number of milligrams listed in the column to the left. For this exercise, assume you are delivering a premixed lidocaine solution of 1 g/250 mL or 2 g/500 mL, which provides a concentration of 4 mg/mL.

Dose	Infusion Rate
1 mg/min	
2 mg/min	
3 mg/min	
4 mg/min	

20. When converting Fahrenheit to centigrade, first _____ 32, then _____ by ⅝. When converting centigrade to Fahrenheit, first multiply by _____, then add _____.

8 Medication Administration

CHAPTER TERMINAL OBJECTIVES

On completion of this chapter, the EMT-Intermediate will be able to prepare and administer medications through the various routes used in the prehospital setting.

For the multiple-choice questions, select the single best answer to each question. For the matching questions, select the best corresponding answer for each item. Because there are sometimes more items than corresponding answers, some items may not be used.

1. You are administering a medication to a patient subcutaneously. The minimum BSI that should be used is/are:
    a. protective eyewear, gloves, and gown
    b. hand washing and the wearing of gloves
    c. hand washing and the wearing of protective mask and gloves
    d. hand washing

2. T F A gown should be worn anytime a medication is to be administered.

3. T F Hand washing is unnecessary after performing medication administration and removing your protective gloves because the gloves are a 100% effective barrier against bacteria and viruses.

4. T F Medical asepsis describes an environment free of living disease-causing microorganisms.

5. Describe what "medical asepsis" practices accomplish.

___

___

___

___

___

6. Sterilization refers to:
    a. substances that destroy or stop the growth of germs on living tissue
    b. chemicals that destroy germs on nonliving objects
    c. the complete destruction of all living organisms
    d. the topical removal of bacteria and viruses

7. T F You should strive for a sterile environment whenever administering a medication.

8. List 10 medically clean procedures and techniques used to reduce the patient's risk of infection in the prehospital setting.

   _____

   _____

   _____

   _____

   _____

   _____

   _____

   _____

   _____

   _____

9. Describe the difference between an antiseptic and a disinfectant.

   _____

   _____

   _____

   _____

10. Extreme _____ should be taken when handling needles, scalpels, lancets, and other sharp instruments or devices; when handling sharp instruments after procedures; when cleaning used instruments; and when disposing of _____ needles.

11. Disposable syringes and needles should be _____ right after their use.
    a. recapped and disposed of
    b. cleaned in a disinfectant
    c. bent or cut in half
    d. placed in a puncture-resistant container

12. T F The EMT-I has little responsibility when dispensing drugs by standing orders or by a direct order from a physician.

13. T F The EMS run report should include the type, dosage, and time each medication was administered.

14. List the six "rights" of drug administration.

15. The EMT-I should do all of the following when administering a drug *except:*
    a. read the label carefully, making sure the drug and concentration are correct
    b. confirm the order with medical direction while drawing up and administering the drug
    c. ask about any allergies that the patient may have to the drug
    d. stay with the patient while the drug is being delivered, watching for any reaction

16. Explain why it is important to check the strength of the medication and the route of administration before delivering a drug.

17. List four causes of common medication errors.

18. List six things the EMT-I should do if an incident involving a medication error occurs.

   _____

   _____

   _____

   _____

   _____

   _____

19. Label the syringe used for medication administration shown below.

20. The other types of syringes used for parenteral administration besides the hypodermic syringe are the

    _____ and _____.

21. Needle gauge varies from _____ to 27; the _____ the number, the _____ the gauge.

22. T F Most companies prepackage hypodermic syringes in color-coded envelopes with the needle attached.

23. T F When administering medications SQ, a 1- to 2-inch-long, 21-gauge needle should be used.

24. For IM medication administration, a _____-inch-long, _____-gauge needle should be used.
    a. 2; 22
    b. 5/8; 25
    c. 1; 20 to 25
    d. 1.5 to 3; 18 to 20

25. Hypodermic syringes are marked with _____ calibrations per milliliter on one side of the syringe.

    Each small line represents _____ mL.
    a. 5; 1
    b. 100; 0.01
    c. 10; 0.1
    d. 20; 0.5

CROSSWORD PUZZLE EXERCISE

26. Complete the following crossword puzzle.

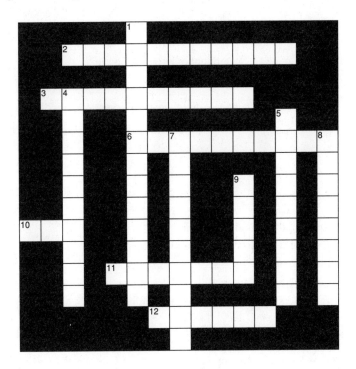

ACROSS

2. Substances that destroy or stop the growth of germs on living tissue.
3. Scale where zero is the freezing point of water, and plus 100 is its boiling point.
6. Scale where the freezing point of water is plus 32° F and its boiling point is 212° F.
10. Abbreviation for drops.
11. Means "free from all living organisms."
12. The other side of a hypodermic syringe is marked in _____.

DOWN

1. Chemicals that destroy germs on nonliving objects.
4. Date the EMT-I should check on a drug label.
5. Procedure that often results in needlestick injuries.
7. Type of syringe that is the most commonly used for injections.
8. One of these is equal to 60 drops.
9. Refers to the outside diameter of the needle lumen.

27. The tuberculin syringe is narrow and has a total capacity of _____ mL. There are _____ calibration lines marking the capacity. Each line represents _____ mL. Every tenth line is longer than the others to indicate _____ mL.

28. Prefilled syringes contain a _____ amount of a medication in a _____ cartridge with a needle attached.

29. A small sterile glass container that contains a single dose of injectable medication and is drawn up by use of a syringe and needle is referred to as a/an:
    a. ampule
    b. vial
    c. prefilled syringe
    d. Tubex syringe

30. Before being broken open, an ampule should be:
    a. shaken down to force the liquid to the lower portion of the ampule
    b. wiped off with an alcohol wipe
    c. inverted to force all the air bubbles to the top
    d. heated with a cigarette lighter to soften the neck of the container

31. T F To snap the neck of an ampule, it should be held between the forefinger and thumb of the right hand and struck against a hard, vertical surface.

32. Label the following medication container tag with the correct terms.

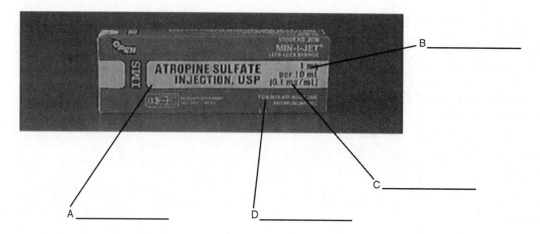

33. To prepare a prefilled medication, you would do all of the following *except:*
    a. remove the protective caps from the medication container and from the needle housing
    b. engage the medication container into the needle housing, and rotate it clockwise until it is securely fastened
    c. point the needle upward, and tap the medication container portion of the syringe until the air bubbles rise to the top
    d. uncap the needle and with the syringe needle pointed downward, expel the excess air until only the medication remains in the syringe

34. To draw up medication from a vial, you should:
    a. clean the rubber stopper with sterile water
    b. determine the amount to be withdrawn, and draw half that volume of air into the syringe
    c. invert the vial, insert the needle through the rubber stopper, and immediately pull back on the plunger
    d. insert the needle through the rubber stopper, inject air into the vial, and then withdraw the desired amount of solution

35. Two methods of enteral administration of medications are:
    a. oral, rectal
    b. endotracheal, aerosol
    c. IV, IM
    d. SL, oral

36. Match each of the following administration routes with the correct description.

    Route
    a. Oral
    b. Rectal
    c. Endotracheal
    d. Intramuscular
    e. Intravenous push
    f. Sublingual
    g. Aerosol
    h. Subcutaneous

    Description
    _____ Have a local or systemic action and are usually in the form of suppositories or solutions instilled through the enema procedure
    _____ Medications are placed in the mouth, under the tongue
    _____ Allow drugs to act directly on the structures of the lung or be absorbed into the systemic circulation
    _____ Involves the injection of a drug into the fatty tissue beneath the skin
    _____ Generally the most popular method of drug administration for nonemergency situations

37. List three reasons why the oral route is considered a popular method for medication administration for nonemergency situations.

38. List two problems that can occur with administering medications orally.

39. Describe how you can assist a patient in swallowing a tablet or pill.

40. The rectal route of drug administration:
    a. has the fastest absorption rate of all the medication administration routes
    b. has more predictable absorption than the oral route
    c. is most commonly used in the prehospital care setting
    d. can be used for delivery of pills and tablets

41. To administer a drug rectally:
    a. open the suppository package, and drop it onto a sterile gauze
    b. use one hand to separate the buttocks, exposing the internal rectum
    c. insert the suppository about 1 to 1.5 inches until it passes through the internal anal sphincter
    d. have the patient bear down once the suppository is properly positioned

42. T F Nitroglycerin is a medication that is commonly delivered sublingually.

43. T F When administering a medication sublingually, the patient should be directed to place the tablet on the tip of his or her tongue.

44. To facilitate absorption of drugs administered endotracheally, you should:
    a. inject the drug closer to the proximal end of the endotracheal tube
    b. resume assisted breathing with several large ventilations after injecting the drug
    c. allow several seconds to pass before restarting assisted breathing after injecting the drug
    d. inject half the contents of the syringe, resume assisted breathing, and then pause briefly to inject the second half of the syringe

45. For patients _____ a mouthpiece is more effective than a mask when administering an aerosolized drug.
    a. less than 5 feet tall
    b. weighing more than 120 pounds
    c. older than 5 years of age
    d. who have shallow breathing

46. To administer an aerosolized drug, you should:
    a. pour the prescribed drug into the T-piece using aseptic technique
    b. adjust the oxygen flow meter to 4 to 6 L/min to produce a steady, visible mist
    c. instruct the patient to breathe normally
    d. continue administering the treatment until there is approximately one quarter of the drug remaining in the nebulizer canister

47. Describe what should happen if changes in heart rate or dysrhythmias are noted during delivery of an aerosolized medication.

    _____
    _____
    _____
    _____

48. T F A volume of drug administered via the SQ route is usually limited to less than 1 mL.

49. T F When preparing to insert the needle during SQ medication administration, the skin should be pulled taut.

50. T F For SQ medication administration, the needle should be directed into the skin at a 45-degree angle.

51. T F As part of SQ medication administration, once the skin has been entered, the plunger should be pulled back slightly to aspirate for a blood return.

52. On the figure below, shade in the common sites for SQ injection.

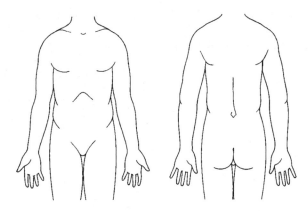

53. A medication commonly administered SQ is:
    a. atropine
    b. lidocaine
    c. dextrose
    d. 1:1000 epinephrine

54. When administering medications IM, the needle should be directed at a _____-degree angle into the skin.
    a. 15
    b. 28
    c. 45
    d. 90

55. T F Before needle insertion for IM medication administration, a venous constricting band should be applied to the arm above the injection site.

56. T F Up to 10 mL of medication can be administered into the deltoid muscle.

57. T F Once the medication has been administered, the needle is removed, and circular pressure is applied to the area to diffuse the medication into the tissue.

58. On the figure below, shade in the common sites for IM injection.

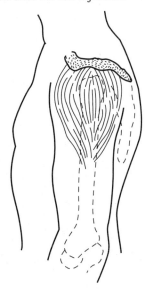

59. T F When administering IV push medications, an injection port that is closer to the patient should be selected.

60. T F Before injecting the IV medication, stop the IV flow by pinching the IV tubing below the injection site.

61. T F Following injection of the IV medication, the needle and syringe should be disposed of in a trash receptacle.

62. Describe how the IV tubing can be "flushed" after administering an IV medication.

___

63. Describe how administering a drug via the intraosseous route differs from administering an IV push medication.

___

CROSSWORD PUZZLE EXERCISE

64. Complete the following crossword puzzle.

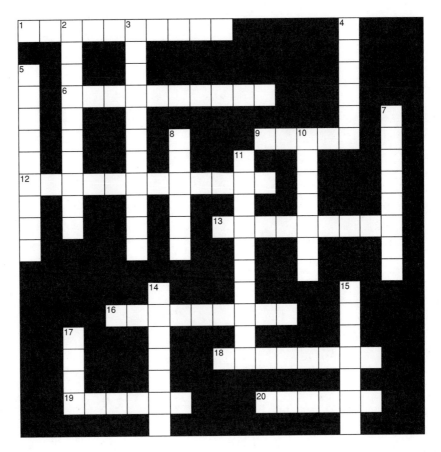

ACROSS

1. Pulling back on syringe plunger to check for blood before administering an SQ medication.
6. Date checked on the medication syringe.
9. Glass or plastic containers that have a self-sealing rubber stopper in the top.
12. Routes for drug administration that are absorbed through the mucous membranes or skin.
13. Type of mask used to administer an aerosol medication.
16. Type of syringe commonly used for administering IV drugs.
18. The syringe should be positioned in this direction to expel any excess air.
19. Measurement system that is based on multiples of 10.
20. Antiemetics and local analgesics are commonly administered using this route.

DOWN

2. Administration of any drug by the nongastrointestinal route.
3. Drugs for control of nausea and vomiting.
4. Type of container for disposing of used needles and syringes.
5. This should not be done when disposing of a used needle.
7. Equal to 2.2 lb.
8. Angle used to insert needle when delivering a medication intramuscularly.
10. Breakable glass containers from which drugs must be drawn with a syringe.
11. Syringe that is narrow and has a total capacity of 1 mL.
14. Muscle in the shoulder used to administer medications intramuscularly.
15. Refers to drugs that are absorbed through the gastrointestinal tract.
17. Equal to 1000 mg.

9 Airway Management

CHAPTER TERMINAL OBJECTIVES

On completion of this chapter, the EMT-Intermediate will be able to establish and/or maintain a patent airway, oxygenate, and ventilate a patient.

For the multiple-choice questions, select the single best answer to each question. For the matching questions, select the best corresponding answer for each item. Because there are sometimes more items than corresponding answers, some items may not be used.

1. Describe the primary objective in airway maintenance.

    _____

    _____

    _____

    _____

    _____

2. Commonly neglected airway skills in prehospital care include all of the following *except:*
    a. inserting an oropharyngeal airway too deeply
    b. failing to create an effective seal with a bag-mask device
    c. improper positioning of the patient's head and neck
    d. not reassessing the patient's condition

3. Structures of the upper airway include the:
    1. nose
    2. mouth
    3. pharynx
    4. right mainstem bronchi
    5. trachea

    Select the correct answer.
    a. 1 and 4
    b. 2, 3, and 5
    c. 2 and 3
    d. 1, 2, and 3

4. When inspired air reaches the distal passageways it is:
    a. slightly cooler than the body temperature
    b. 100% humidified
    c. 85% sterile
    d. free of carbon dioxide

5. The nose:
   a. is the inferior-most aspect of the airway
   b. has a part that protrudes from the face that is made up of skin
   c. is surrounded by the mandible along the sides and below at its base
   d. has two openings to the outside of the body that are referred to as nostrils

6. The bones located in the nasal cavity that create turbulent airflow are called the:
   a. palates
   b. turbinates
   c. alveolar ducts
   d. cricoid cartilages

7. T F Air enters the nose through the posterior nares.

8. T F The nose is lined with a mucous membrane that has a rich blood supply.

9. T F The maxillary sinus is a cartilaginous structure that separates the right and left cavities of the nose.

10. Which of the following is considered part of the nasopharynx?
    a. arytenoid folds
    b. nares
    c. soft palate
    d. mandible

11. Match each of the following structures of the upper airway with the appropriate description.

    Structure
    a. Laryngopharynx
    b. Vallecula
    c. Soft palate
    d. Nasopharynx
    e. Mouth
    f. Oropharynx
    g. Nose

    Description
    _____ Separated into right and left cavities by a cartilaginous structure
    _____ Consists of the lips, cheeks, gums, teeth, and the hard and soft palates
    _____ Extends from the soft palate in the back of the mouth to the hyoid bone below the mandible
    _____ Extends from the hyoid bone at the base of the tongue to the esophagus, posteriorly, and to the trachea, anteriorly

12. The tongue attaches to the _____ and _____ bone.

13. The three regions of the pharynx are the _____, _____, and _____.

14. Describe the function of the following structures of the upper airway.
    Trachea:

    _____
    _____
    _____
    _____

Pharynx:

Vocal cords:

Nose:

Larynx:

Tongue:

15. The hyoid bone:
    a. is shaped like a T
    b. is located superior to the chin
    c. is suspended from the temporal bone by ligaments
    d. articulates with the mandible

16. The thin, leaf-shaped structure that closes over the opening of the trachea during swallowing to prevent substances from entering is called the:
    a. epiglottis
    b. vallecula
    c. glottis
    d. cricoid membrane

17. The epiglottis lies _____ to the larynx.

18. The space between the base of the tongue and the epiglottis is referred to as the _____.

19. On either side of the epiglottis is a recess called the _____ _____.

20. T F The epiglottis is connected to the posterior pharyngeal wall by the inguinal muscle.

21. T F The larynx is a triangular-shaped structure that connects the pharynx with the trachea.

22. The "Adam's apple" is also referred to as the:
    a. hyoid
    b. carina
    c. thyroid cartilage
    d. trachea

23. The cricoid cartilage is:
    a. found superior to the thyroid cartilage
    b. attached to the first ring of tracheal cartilage
    c. open on its posterior surface
    d. the narrowest part of the upper airway in adults

24. Which of the following lies on the rear surface of the cricoid cartilage?
    a. false vocal cords
    b. hyoid bone
    c. thyroid cartilage
    d. arytenoid cartilages

25. The esophagus:
    a. is the passageway leading to the lungs
    b. is distensible
    c. is supported by C-shaped cartilage that extends throughout its length
    d. is lined with a mucous membrane, which acts to humidify and sterilize the food coming into the stomach

26. For this illustration, list the name of each anatomical structure shown.

Using colored pencils or pens, color the illustration according to the following: A-green, B-orange, C-green, D-red, E-tan, F-tan, G-blue, H-gray, I-purple, J-yellow, K-green, L-green, M-tan, N-green, O-green, and P-blue.

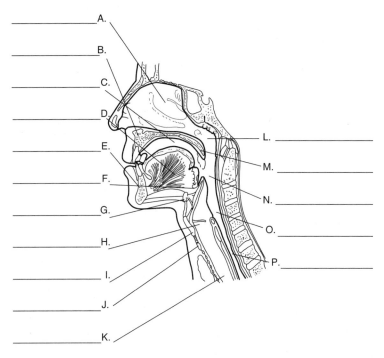

_____ A.
_____ B.
_____ C.
_____ D.
_____ E.
_____ F.
_____ G.
_____ H.
_____ I.
_____ J.
_____ K.
L. _____
M. _____
N. _____
O. _____
P. _____

27. The _____ _____ are fibrous bands that control the passage of air through the _____ and the production of sound.

28. Match each of the following structures with the most correct function or anatomical location. Letters may be used more than once.

    Structure
    a. Esophagus
    b. Pharynx
    c. Tongue
    d. Cricoid cartilage
    e. False vocal cords

    Function/Location
    _____ Slightly superior to the true vocal cords
    _____ Superior to the larynx
    _____ Superior and anterior to the larynx
    _____ Swallowing tube
    _____ A complete ring of cartilage shaped like a signet ring with the bulky portion located posteriorly
    _____ Below the thyroid cartilage
    _____ Carries food and liquid from the pharynx to the stomach

29. The true vocal cords:
    a. consist of elastic connective tissue covered by folds of mucous membrane
    b. are referred to as vestibular folds
    c. lie superior to the false vocal cords
    d. can vibrate to produce sound as expired air passes over them

30. The space between the true vocal cords is referred to as the:
    a. cricoid membrane
    b. vallecula
    c. glottic opening
    d. laryngeal inlet

31. T F The upper airway is innervated by both the parasympathetic and sympathetic nervous systems.

32. The lower airway consists of the:
    1. epiglottis
    2. larynx
    3. trachea
    4. bronchi
    5. alveoli

    Select the correct answer.
    a. 3 only
    b. 3, 4, and 5
    c. 1, 2, and 4
    d. 2 and 5

33. The trachea:
    a. lies posterior to the esophagus
    b. attaches to the larynx at the cricoid cartilage
    c. is supported by V-shaped cartilaginous rings that act to maintain its open position
    d. is a rigid, nonflexible tubular structure that divides at the septum into the right and left mainstem bronchi

34. T F The right mainstem bronchus is shorter, wider, and more in line with the trachea than the left mainstem bronchus.

35. T F At the distal end of the bronchioles, the cartilaginous rings disappear and the structures are mostly smooth muscle.

36. The alveoli:
    a. are considered the most important functional units of the respiratory system
    b. contain smooth muscle that can contract and reduce the diameter of the airway
    c. are hollow, thick-walled sacs
    d. interface with capillaries formed by terminal branches of the coronary artery

37. T F The left lung is composed of the upper, middle, and lower lobes.

38. T F The visceral pleura line the inside of the thoracic cavity.

39. T F The space between the visceral pleura and parietal pleura is called the *thoracic space*.

40. Collapse of the alveoli is referred to as:
    a. embolism
    b. pneumothorax
    c. atelectasis
    d. pleural effusion

41. Anatomical differences between adult and pediatric airways include the:
    a. overall size of the adult's airway is smaller than that of the child
    b. child's larynx lies more inferior and is oval shaped because of narrow, undeveloped cricoid cartilage
    c. child has a large, floppy, omega-shaped epiglottis
    d. cords of a child sit more posterior on the cervical spine than those of an adult

42. Describe why the upper airway of a child can become obstructed more easily than an adult's.

_____

_____

_____

_____

_____

43. The airway of a child younger than 10 years of age is narrowest at the:
    a. cricoid cartilage
    b. glottic opening
    c. false vocal cords
    d. oropharynx

44. Retching or striving to vomit is called:
    a. coughing
    b. the gag reflex
    c. atelectasis
    d. hiccoughing

45. The exchange of gases between a living organism and its environment is referred to as:
    a. respiration
    b. pulmonary ventilation
    c. inspiration
    d. diffusion

46. The respiratory cycle involves all of the following *except* the:
    a. central nervous system
    b. respiratory system
    c. endocrine system
    d. musculoskeletal system

47. The major inspiratory muscle(s) accounting for 70% of the airflow in and out the lungs is/are the:
    a. diaphragm
    b. intercostal muscles
    c. accessory muscles
    d. subclavian muscles

48. The intrapulmonic pressure after normal contraction of the diaphragm and intercostal muscles is _____ atmospheric pressure.
    a. slightly greater than
    b. equal to
    c. less than
    d. two times greater than

49. Match each of the following phases of breathing with the correct physiological processes. Items may be used more than once.

    Phase of Breathing
    a. Inspiration
    b. Expiration

    Process
    _____ Is a passive act (unless forced)
    _____ The respiratory center in the medulla of the brain signals the muscles of respiration to increase the size of the chest cavity
    _____ The diaphragm and intercostal muscles are stimulated to contract
    _____ The diaphragm and respiratory muscles relax and the chest cavity decreases in size
    _____ The intercostal muscles lift the rib cage upward and outward, thus increasing the horizontal and transverse dimensions of the thoracic cavity
    _____ The decreasing thoracic volume increases the intrathoracic pressure, and air is forced out of the lungs
    _____ A potential vacuum draws air into the enlarged lungs, filling them

50. The respiratory minute volume equals the respiratory _____ times the _____ _____.

51. Air reaching the alveoli for gas exchange equals _____ mL.

52. The tidal volume is the amount of air:
    a. exchanged by the lungs in 1 minute
    b. that actually reaches the alveoli
    c. in the inspired and expired air with each breath
    d. that interfaces with the capillaries of the pulmonary circulation

53. The maximum expiratory flow rate in liters per minute a person can deliver is called the:
    a. peak expiratory flow rate (PEFR)
    b. expiratory reserve
    c. Hering-Breuer reflex
    d. minute volume

54. Field use of the PEFR allows the EMT-I to evaluate the:
    a. percentage of oxygen saturation in the arterial blood
    b. inspiratory capacity of the lungs following maximal inspiration
    c. removal of carbon dioxide during expiration
    d. effectiveness of treatments such as bronchodilators

55. When inspired air reaches the alveoli:
    a. oxygen has a partial pressure of 160 mm Hg
    b. it is met by gas pressures that are equal on both sides of the alveolar-capillary membrane
    c. it contains more carbon dioxide and less oxygen
    d. it interfaces with capillary venous blood oxygen that has a Po_2 of 40 mm Hg

56. Which of the following is true regarding oxygen transport in the arterial blood?
    a. While blood is in the alveolar capillary, it absorbs enough oxygen to increase its partial pressure to 160 mm Hg.
    b. A small portion (3%) of oxygen is carried by hemoglobin.
    c. Oxygen carried by plasma is reflected in the blood saturation (Sao_2).
    d. Each gram of saturated hemoglobin is considered saturated to its fullest extent when carrying 1.34 mL of oxygen.

57. Hemoglobin reaches full saturation at a P_{O_2} of _____ mm Hg.
    a. 75 to 85
    b. 60 to 80
    c. 75 to 95
    d. 80 to 100

58. Once blood that is pumped through the systemic circulation reaches the capillaries:
    a. it comes into contact with tissues having a P_{O_2} of close to 100 mm Hg
    b. oxygen diffuses from the bloodstream into the tissues
    c. nitrogen moves from the bloodstream to the cells
    d. it turns bright red

59. The movement of oxygen from an area of greater concentration to an area of lesser concentration is called:
    a. diffusion
    b. osmosis
    c. active transport
    d. filtration

60. Carbon dioxide is carried in the blood in all of the following ways *except:*
    a. combined with blood proteins
    b. dissolved in plasma
    c. coupled with hemoglobin
    d. combined with water as carbonic acid and its component ions

61. The amount of carbon dioxide in the body is dependent on _____ _____ . Under normal conditions, if ventilations are increased, the carbon dioxide will _____ . If ventilations are decreased, the carbon dioxide will _____ .

62. The main nervous centers for controlling the rate and depth of breathing:
    a. are located in the medulla oblongata and the pons of the brainstem
    b. are sensitive to slight changes in the concentration of oxygen in the blood plasma
    c. increase respirations when the carbon dioxide concentration in the blood is lowered
    d. allow a person to voluntarily speed up or slow down the respiratory rate

63. The peripheral chemoreceptors:
    a. are located in the subclavian artery
    b. directly control the heart rate and stroke volume
    c. sense changes in the blood pressure (BP)
    d. sense changes in the CO_2 and O_2 concentrations and pH of the arterial blood

64. List seven factors that increase or decrease respiration.

___

65. Match each of the following modified forms of respiration with the correct description.

   Modified Forms of Respiration
   a. Cough
   b. Sneeze
   c. Sigh
   d. Hiccough
   e. Gag reflex

   Description
   _____ Sudden forceful exhalation from the nose that clears the nasopharynx
   _____ Sudden inspiration caused by spasmodic contraction of the diaphragm and intermittent spastic closure of the glottis
   _____ Forceful, spastic exhalation of a large volume of air from the lungs
   _____ Involuntary slow, deep breath followed by prolonged expiration

66. Sighing does which of the following?
   a. hyperinflates the lungs and opens atelectatic alveoli
   b. aids in clearing the bronchi and bronchioles of foreign material
   c. may bring about nausea and vomiting
   d. clears the nasopharynx

67. Which of the following should be used when performing airway assessment and management when there is little or no likelihood of body fluids splashing?
   a. protective nitrile, vinyl, or latex gloves and protective eyewear
   b. protective gown or overalls and vinyl or latex gloves
   c. heavy-duty gloves for cleaning and high-efficiency particulate air (HEPA) respirator
   d. HEPA respirator and protective eyewear

68. Describe the level of body substance isolation that should be used if there is a chance that body fluids may be splashed or aerosolized.

___

69. You have been called to a wedding reception where a 60-year-old woman collapsed while dancing with her husband. Reportedly, she just slumped to the floor. Your initial impression is that she is unresponsive, apneic, and becoming cyanotic. The first thing you should do is:
   a. check for a pulse
   b. assess respiratory effectiveness
   c. determine whether an open airway is present
   d. assist the patient's breathing

> Just a reminder: When the possibility of spinal injury exists, airway patency must be assessed and ensured in conjunction with in-line cervical spine stabilization.

70. List five indicators of respiratory function.

71. Snoring is associated with upper airway obstruction caused by:
   a. the tongue falling back against the posterior oropharynx
   b. laryngeal edema or constriction
   c. croup
   d. the presence of fluids

72. List three signs found on the neck that indicate a likely respiratory problem.

73. Pulsus paradoxus is:
   a. an indicator of circulatory failure
   b. present when the systolic BP increases greater than 10 mm Hg during inspiration
   c. seen in pulmonary embolism
   d. indicative of an increase in the intrathoracic pressure

74. Pulse oximetry:
   a. is an invasive procedure used to determine the effectiveness of patient oxygenation
   b. detects trends in a patient's oxygenation status within 6 seconds
   c. works by measuring transmission of red and near-infrared light through venous capillary beds
   d. provides valuable information in carbon monoxide poisoning and states of hypoperfusion

75. Disposable colorimetric end-tidal CO_2 detectors:
    a. can be used only in spontaneously breathing patients
    b. detect the presence of carbon dioxide in an intubated patient's expired air
    c. indicate proper placement of the endotracheal tube in the trachea by turning purple with patient expiration
    d. are 100% reliable in cardiac arrest

76. Esophageal intubation detectors:
    a. are inserted into the esophagus
    b. resemble a large syringe or flexible bulb
    c. measure the amount of carbon dioxide in the exhaled air
    d. are attached to the endotracheal tube after the initial ventilations are delivered

77. Describe how an esophageal intubation detector identifies improper placement of the endotracheal tube into the esophagus.

    _____
    _____
    _____
    _____
    _____

78. List four factors that can produce false readings when using the esophageal intubation detector.

    _____
    _____
    _____
    _____

79. List four things that should be quickly inspected for that can indicate a likely respiratory problem.

    _____
    _____
    _____
    _____

80. Auscultation of the epigastrium should:
    a. follow assessment of breath sounds
    b. be silent, with no sounds heard during ventilation
    c. be done during expiration
    d. be done only if the patient is cyanotic

81. Indicate the locations for auscultating a patient's anterior chest for breath sounds by placing X's on the illustration below.

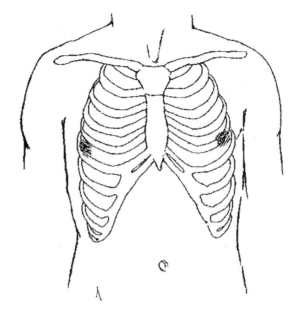

82. T F When auscultating the chest, first listen to one entire side of the chest and then the other.

83. T F Breath sounds should be equal on both sides of the chest.

84. T F The presence of airflow with auscultation over the sternal notch reveals incorrect placement of the endotracheal tube into the esophagus.

85. T F In some cases, such as with obese or barrel-chested patients, air movement into the stomach may mimic lung sounds.

86. List three things of which gastric distention is suggestive.

_____

_____

_____

87. Cyanosis:
    a. occurs early in respiratory compromise
    b. results when the sympathetic nervous system is stimulated
    c. is usually seen at the lips, fingernails, and/or skin
    d. is a reliable sign

88. Tachycardia usually accompanies hypoxemia, whereas _____ suggests anoxia with imminent cardiac arrest.

89. Hypoxia:
    a. can be recognized only when the patient becomes short of breath
    b. is defined as a decreased or inadequate supply of oxygen
    c. leads to aerobic metabolism
    d. decreases myocardial and respiratory workloads

90. List five causes of hypoxia.

___

91. Describe how to clear an oxygen supply cylinder of dust or dirt.

___

92. The _____ in a full oxygen cylinder is approximately _____ psi. This pressure is too _____ to be _____ delivered to a patient. Therefore a pressure _____ is attached to the _____ to deliver a safe working pressure of _____ to _____ psi.

93. The safe residual pressure of an oxygen cylinder is _____ psi.
    a. 50
    b. 100
    c. 200
    d. 500

94. Describe why the EMT-I must avoid allowing petroleum-based substances or adhesive tape to come into contact with the valve stem of the oxygen cylinder or the oxygen regulator.

___

95. List the volumes for the common sizes of cylinders used in the prehospital setting.
    D: _____
    E: _____
    M: _____

96. The constant flow selector valve:
    a. is the type of regulator commonly used on portable units
    b. has a gauge
    c. controls the liter flow per minute through a precision dial
    d. is more fragile than the other types of regulators and must be operated in an upright position

97. Identify, by numbering, the correct order for attaching a regulator to an oxygen cylinder and connecting an oxygen delivery device.
    _____ Crack the valve for 1 second to clear any dust or dirt.
    _____ Tighten the regulator to the cylinder valve.
    _____ Place the cylinder in an upright position and stand to one side.
    _____ Attach oxygen tubing and the delivery device.
    _____ Line up the pins in the regulator yoke to the corresponding holes in the cylinder valve (smaller tanks) or the threads of the regulator to the oxygen cylinder outlet (larger tanks).
    _____ If present, remove the plastic wrapper or cap protecting the cylinder outlet.
    _____ Select an oxygen cylinder.

98. You are using a nonrebreather mask to deliver 15 L of oxygen per minute to a dyspneic patient. Your D tank contains 1500 psi. How many minutes can you deliver oxygen to your patient before you will have to change the oxygen cylinder?

    _____
    _____
    _____
    _____
    _____

99. T F A humidifier works by running dry oxygen through a nonbreakable jar of water that is attached to the flow meter. This moisturizes the oxygen.

100. T F Even in short-term use, oxygen humidifiers can produce an adverse effect.

101. T F The water in the reservoir must be replaced with sterile fresh water as often as each shift and the reservoir cleaned according to manufacturer's instructions.

102. Describe the benefit of using humidified oxygen.

    _____
    _____
    _____
    _____
    _____

103. Match each of the following oxygen delivery devices with the concentration they can provide. Not all concentrations will be used.

    Delivered % Oxygen
    a. 17 to 22
    b. 80 to 100
    c. 40 to 50
    d. 24 to 44
    e. 35 to 60

    Oxygen Device/Liter Flow
    _____ Nasal cannula, 2 to 6 L/min
    _____ Simple face mask, 6 to 10 L/min
    _____ Nonrebreather mask, 10 to 15 L/min

104. Which of the following is the best device for delivering oxygen to a patient with chronic obstructive pulmonary disease (COPD) who is not in respiratory failure?
    a. simple face mask
    b. nonrebreather mask
    c. bag-mask
    d. Venturi mask

105. A _____ is an oxygen delivery device that has a one-way valve on each side that allows exhaled air to escape but prevents room air from being inspired.
    a. simple face mask
    b. nasal cannula
    c. Venturi mask
    d. nonrebreather mask

106. Which of the following devices is capable of delivering the highest oxygen concentration?
    a. simple face mask
    b. nonrebreather mask
    c. nasal cannula
    d. Venturi mask

107. Match each of the following oxygen delivery devices with the correct characteristics. Items may be used more than once.

Device
a. Nasal cannula
b. Simple face mask
c. Nonrebreather mask
d. Venturi mask

Characteristic

_____ At least 10 L of oxygen is needed to move sufficient oxygen into the reservoir bag and remove exhaled carbon dioxide

_____ Flow rate should be limited to 6 L/min

_____ Should be used when the patient is frightened or feels suffocated with other delivery devices

_____ No less than 6 L should be administered through the device because expired carbon dioxide can accumulate, resulting in hypercarbia

_____ Has holes in the side of the mask that allow air to be drawn into the mask during inspiration and expired air to be passed to the outside

_____ With this device the same amount of ambient air is always entrained regardless of the rate or depth of respirations

_____ Recommended for the treatment of severely hypoxic patients

_____ Offers the benefit of not interfering with assessment because the patient's response to questions can be more easily heard

_____ The reservoir bag should not be allowed to totally deflate because the patient can suffocate

_____ The device delivers oxygen concentrations of 24%, 28%, 35%, or 40%

108. Identify, by numbering, the correct order for applying the nonrebreather mask.
_____ Continuously monitor the oxygen level in the tank.
_____ Tighten the mask by adjusting the elastic strap on both sides simultaneously until the mask is secure.
_____ Adjust the flow meter to deliver 10 to 15 L/min.
_____ Apply the mask by placing it over the patient's nose, mouth, and chin.
_____ Make sure the one-way flaps are secure and functioning, and observe the reservoir bag as the patient breathes (if it collapses more than slightly during inspiration, increase the flow rate). Keep the reservoir from kinking or twisting.
_____ Press the flexible metal nosepiece so that it fits the bridge of the nose.
_____ Attach tubing of the nonrebreather mask to the oxygen flow meter nipple, and prefill the reservoir by using your finger to cover the exhaust portal (the connection between the mask and reservoir).

109. Acute hypoventilation will result in an increase in:
a. carbon dioxide
b. pH
c. oxygen saturation
d. Pao_2

110. Patients with decreased levels of consciousness and respiratory rates of less than _____ or greater than _____ breaths/min should receive ventilatory assistance.

111. When ventilating a nonbreathing adult patient, a tidal volume of approximately _____ is given over _____ second(s).
    a. 500 mL; 3 to 5
    b. 6 to 7 mL/kg or 500 to 600 mL; 1
    c. 1000 mL; 2 to 5
    d. 10 mL/kg or 700 to 1000; 2

112. Which of the following patients requires ventilatory assistance?
    a. 37-year-old woman who has overdosed on heroin, has a respiratory rate of 8, a pulse rate of 58, and a BP of 94/62
    b. 22-year-old man who is experiencing diabetic ketoacidosis (DKA), is breathing deeply at a rate of 20 breaths/min, has a pulse rate of 124, and a BP of 100/76
    c. 70-year-old man who is unconscious following a stroke, has a respiratory rate of 18, a pulse rate of 100, and a BP of 190/114
    d. 29-year-old woman who is in shock following a car crash, has normal respirations at a rate of 20 breaths/min, a pulse rate of 116, and a BP of 94/50

113. When providing mouth-to-mouth ventilation you:
    a. should deliver each breath as quickly as possible
    b. are able to deliver more oxygen than when using a bag-mask device
    c. may be exposed to communicable disease
    d. should deliver as much volume as you can with each breath

114. When providing mouth-to-mask ventilation and using supplemental oxygen, each breath should take _____ second(s) to deliver.
    a. 0.25 to 0.75
    b. 1
    c. 2.5 to 3.0
    d. 5.0 to 6.0

115. The pocket mask:
    a. delivers smaller tidal volumes than a bag-mask device
    b. eliminates exposure to the patient's exhaled air
    c. provides a higher concentration of oxygen than can be achieved with a bag-mask device
    d. does not eliminate direct contact with the patient's nose and mouth

116. Label the following components of the bag-mask device.

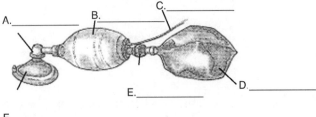

117. Bag-mask devices:
    a. convey a sense of compliance of a patient's lungs to the rescuer
    b. deliver 100% oxygen when supplied with 8 to 10 L of oxygen
    c. are equipped with a standard 30-mm adapter
    d. can be used by untrained individuals

118. When assisting a patient's breathing with a bag-mask device, the:
    a. patient's neck should be placed into a neutral position
    b. bag should be squeezed until the patient's abdomen rises
    c. use of a mask is preferred over connecting the device to an endotracheal tube
    d. mask must be held firmly to the patient's face to prevent air from leaking

119. Identify, by numbering, the correct sequence for ventilating a patient with a bag-mask device. The patient's airway has already been opened, and an oropharyngeal airway has been inserted.
    _____ Connect reservoir and oxygen tubing to the oxygen inlet of the bag-mask device, and deliver oxygen at 12 to 15 L/min.
    _____ Obtain a tight seal by applying firm downward pressure over the mask with your thumb on the dome and index and middle fingers on the base.
    _____ Select the appropriate size mask, and place it on the patient's face with the narrow end (apex) over the bridge of the nose and wide end (base) in the groove between the lower lip and chin.
    _____ Watch for the patient's chest to rise during ventilation and collapse during passive exhalation.
    _____ Hook the last two or three fingers under the jaw, and then pull the chin backward to maintain the head-tilt position.
    _____ Ventilate the patient with a tidal volume of approximately 6 to 7 mL/kg or 500 to 600 mL over 1 second (until the chest rises) in cardiac arrest.
    _____ Auscultate the chest to make sure that appropriate ventilation is occurring.
    _____ Squeeze the bag between one hand and your arm, chest, or thigh (if kneeling).

120. Fill in the volumes for the three sizes of bag-mask devices.
    Adult: _____
    Child: _____
    Infant: _____

121. You are using a bag-mask device to provide ventilatory assistance to a 50-year-old man who suffered a stroke and stopped breathing. After several minutes you notice that his abdomen appears distended, and it is becoming increasingly difficult to provide assisted ventilations. Which of the following should be done to relieve this problem?
    a. insert an esophageal obturator airway, and inflate its distal cuff
    b. straddle the patient, and deliver four quick abdominal thrusts
    c. turn the patient onto his side, place one hand over the epigastrium, between the umbilicus and the rib cage, and exert moderate pressure
    d. turn the patient onto his side, and deliver 6 to 10 back blows

122. Two- or three-person bag-mask ventilation:
    a. is especially useful for patients suffering from flail chest
    b. should be used only when you are having difficulty obtaining or maintaining an adequate mask seal
    c. offers the advantage of maintaining a superior mask seal and volume delivery
    d. has no significant disadvantages

123. Describe the procedure for ventilating a patient with a bag-mask device using two people.

___

124. The flow-restricted, oxygen-powered ventilation device:
    a. is an automatically triggered, oxygen-powered ventilatory device that delivers 100% oxygen at 60 to 100 L/min
    b. creates low airway pressures
    c. can be used with an endotracheal tube in place
    d. depends on an oxygen power source

125. Automatic transport ventilators used in the prehospital setting are:
    a. time-cycled, intermittent-flow, gas-powered devices
    b. lightweight, compact, and easy to use
    c. not effective in temperature extremes from 0 to –30° F or 110 to 125° F
    d. best used for short-term ventilation of patients

126. T F Contraindications to automatic transport ventilations are in patients who are awake, in patients who have an obstructed airway, or in patients who have increased airway resistance such as pneumothorax, asthma, and pulmonary edema.

127. T F Automatic transport ventilators are equipped with a 28-mm inside diameter/35-mm outside diameter adapter that allows them to be attached to various airway devices and masks.

128. T F Automatic transport ventilators are usually equipped with one primary control that regulates the ventilatory rate. The tidal volume is regulated automatically.

129. T F Automatic transport ventilators are typically supplied with a pop-off valve that vents a portion of the tidal volume to the atmosphere when the preset level of airway pressure is exceeded.

130. List four conditions in which pop-off valves on automatic transport ventilators may be detrimental.

___

131. List four advantages of an automatic transport ventilator.

___

132. List four disadvantages of an automatic transport ventilator.

_____

_____

_____

_____

133. Cricoid pressure is used to:
    a. insert an oropharyngeal airway
    b. relieve an obstructed airway
    c. remove fluids from the oropharynx
    d. prevent regurgitation

134. Describe how cricoid pressure works.

_____

_____

_____

_____

135. Describe how cricoid pressure can facilitate endotracheal intubation.

_____

_____

_____

_____

136. Cricoid pressure is performed by:
    a. locating and applying pressure to the depression just below the thyroid cartilage
    b. applying pressure with the index and middle fingers of one hand to the front of the cartilage just to the sides of the midline, directing it downward
    c. directing the cricoid cartilage backward and downward
    d. avoiding the application of too much pressure

137. When applying the mask of a ventilatory device to the pediatric patient's face:
    a. it is easier to achieve an adequate mask seal than in the adult
    b. apply extra-firm pressure to compress the mask against the face
    c. avoid pushing too hard on the soft tissue under the chin
    d. it is easier to obtain an adequate seal by inverting the mask

138. When ventilating infants and toddlers with a bag-mask device:
    a. their head should be maintained in a hyperextended position
    b. it is best to use a bag-mask device that provides approximately 250 cc of volume and is equipped with a pop-off valve
    c. the ventilation rate is at least 12 breaths/min
    d. a folded towel can be placed under the patient's shoulders to help maintain the sniffing position

139. Describe how to provide ventilatory assistance to the patient with a stoma.

_____

_____

_____

_____

_____

CROSSWORD PUZZLE EXERCISE

140. Complete the following crossword puzzle.

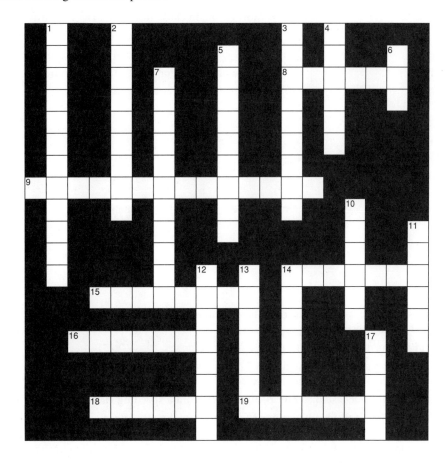

ACROSS

8. Encloses each lung.
9. Lateral curvature of the spine; can interfere with normal breathing.
14. Harsh, high-pitched sound heard on inhalation.
15. Breathing with deep, gasping respirations.
16. Airway of a child younger than 10 years of age is narrowest at this cartilage.
18. Breathing where there is a pattern of slow, shallow, irregular respirations.
19. Hyperinflates the lungs and opens atelectic alveoli.

DOWN

1. Membrane that is site for surgical and alternative airway placement.
2. Attached to an oxygen cylinder to deliver a safe working pressure of 30 to 70 psi.
3. Insufficient oxygenation of the blood.
4. Sudden forceful exhalation from the nose that clears the nasopharynx.
5. The tissues of the lungs are perfused via these arteries.
6. Retching or striving to vomit reflex that is triggered by touching soft palate or throat.
7. Collapse of the alveoli.
10. Point at which the trachea divides.
11. Triangular-shaped structure that connects the pharynx with the trachea.
12. The large bone forming the lower jaw.
13. The slitlike opening between the vocal cords.
14. Sound created by tongue obstructing the airway.
17. A forceful exhalation of a large volume of air.

141. Match each of the following types of airway obstruction with the correct description.

    Type
    a. Tongue
    b. Laryngeal edema
    c. Trauma
    d. Foreign body

    Description
    _____ Most common cause of upper airway obstruction, occurs when muscle tone is depressed or absent in the supine patient
    _____ "Café coronary," foreign body, loose teeth, dentures, toys
    _____ Clotted blood, facial bones, teeth, fractured larynx

142. Lifting the mandible forward:
    a. displaces the hyoid inferiorly
    b. pulls the tongue forward
    c. lifts the epiglottis over the glottic opening
    d. all of the above

143. The preferred procedure for opening the airway is the _____ maneuver.
    a. jaw-thrust
    b. jaw-lift
    c. Sellick
    d. head-tilt/chin-lift

144. The head-tilt/chin-lift maneuver is considered the *treatment of choice* in which of the following patients experiencing upper airway obstruction?
    a. 17-year-old girl who is unconscious following a drug overdose
    b. 3-year-old girl who is playing with an uninflated balloon when she suddenly becomes cyanotic, unable to speak, and is only able to generate a weak, ineffective cough
    c. 41-year-old man who is unconscious after being thrown from a speeding car
    d. 33-year-old woman who is displaying stridor and respiratory distress after being stung by a bee

145. Which of the following is *one of the steps* used to perform the head-tilt/chin-lift maneuver?
    a. place one hand under the neck
    b. use the thumb and index finger of one hand to apply firm downward pressure to the anterior chin
    c. place one hand on the patient's forehead and apply firm backward pressure with the palm to tip the head back
    d. grasp the angles of the patient's lower jaw with both hands, one on each side, and lift the mandible forward while tilting the head back

146. You are called to a scene where a 17-year-old girl hit her head on a diving board while jumping into the water. She is unresponsive and apneic. The preferred procedure for opening the airway of this patient is the:
    a. head tilt/chin lift
    b. sniffing position
    c. head tilt/neck lift
    d. jaw thrust without head tilt

147. An unconscious stroke patient has snoring-type breathing. If the sounds persist after repositioning the patient's head and neck you should:
    a. ventilate every 5 seconds
    b. suction vigorously
    c. perform the Sellick maneuver
    d. insert an oropharyngeal or nasopharyngeal airway

148. T F The oropharyngeal airway may be used to maintain an airway in a semiconscious patient.

149. T F A properly inserted oropharyngeal airway prevents regurgitation of stomach contents.

150. T F   The oropharyngeal airway comes in one size designed to fit all adult patients.

151. T F   When properly inserted, the flange of the oropharyngeal airway will rest against the patient's lips.

152. Describe the problems that can develop if an oropharyngeal airway is:

   Too short: _____

   Too long: _____

153. An oropharyngeal airway is indicated for a:
   a. 6-year-old boy experiencing epiglottitis
   b. 16-year-old boy who is unconscious from a drug overdose
   c. 33-year-old unconscious trauma patient who has sustained severe trauma to the mouth and neck
   d. 69-year-old tracheal stoma patient who experienced cardiac arrest

154. The nasopharyngeal airway:
   1. is an uncuffed soft plastic tube
   2. extends from the nostril to the posterior pharynx just below the base of the tongue
   3. may be used as a bite block to prevent patients from biting down on and occluding an endotracheal tube
   4. cannot be inserted when the patient's teeth are clenched
   5. should not be used when basilar skull fracture is likely present
   Select the correct answer.
   a. 2 only
   b. 3 and 5
   c. 1, 2, and 5
   d. 1, 3, 4, and 5

155. The proper size nasopharyngeal airway extends from the:
   a. eyebrow to the tip of the earlobe
   b. tip of the nose to the tip of the earlobe
   c. corner of the mouth to the inner ear
   d. lips to the tip of the earlobe

156. Describe the problems that can develop if a nasopharyngeal airway is:

   Too short: _____

   Too long: _____

157. Add a prefix to the word below to create a term that means *within the trachea*.

   _____ tracheal

158. Endotracheal intubation means:
   a. inserting a blunt-end tube into the esophagus
   b. passing a catheter through the cricoid membrane
   c. insertion of an open-ended tube into the trachea
   d. occluding the trachea with a close-ended tube

159. List seven indications for endotracheal intubation.

___

160. Endotracheal intubation:
    a. seals the trachea, thereby reducing the risk of aspirating blood, vomitus, and other foreign materials into the lungs
    b. requires a tight seal between a mask and the patient's face
    c. is usually performed "blindly"
    d. has no significant risks or complications

161. Which of the following can be administered through the endotracheal tube?
    a. atropine, 50% dextrose, epinephrine
    b. lidocaine, atropine, epinephrine, naloxone, vasopressin
    c. epinephrine, diazepam, atropine, adenosine
    d. naloxone, atropine, verapamil

162. Contraindications for endotracheal intubation include patients:
    a. in deep coma
    b. who have sustained respiratory burns
    c. under the age of 16 years
    d. with epiglottitis

163. Describe the purpose of a laryngoscope.

___

164. Label the following illustration of the laryngoscope, and describe the function of each component.

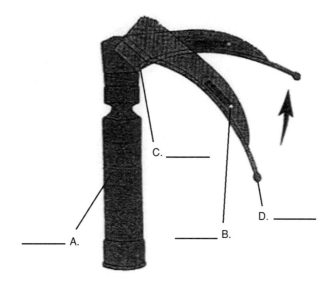

Function
A.
B.
C.
D.

165. The straight laryngoscope blade is inserted:
    a. anterior to the epiglottis
    b. posterior to the epiglottis
    c. into the esophagus
    d. between the vocal cords

166. Match each of the following types of laryngoscope blades with the correct characteristics. Answers can be used more than once.

    Type of Blade
    a. Curved
    b. Straight

    Characteristic
    _____ Also referred to as a Miller, Wisconsin, or Flagg blade
    _____ Its tip is inserted into the vallecula
    _____ Also referred to as a MacIntosh blade
    _____ Is preferred in infants
    _____ Permits more room for visualization of the glottic opening and tube insertion
    _____ Is associated with less trauma and reflex stimulation

167. The correct size for a curved laryngoscope blade in a large adult is:
    a. 1
    b. 2
    c. 3
    d. 4

168. Label the following illustration of the endotracheal tube, and describe the function of each component.

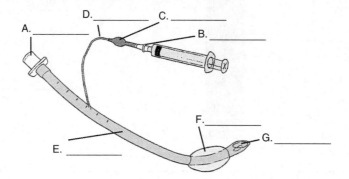

Function
A.
B.
C.
D.
E.
F.
G.

169. The abbreviation ID means _____ .

170. A(n) _____ ID endotracheal tube is recommended for the average size adult male.
    a. 6.0 to 6.5
    b. 7.0 to 7.5
    c. 8.0 to 8.5
    d. 9.0

171. Describe the problems that can develop if an endotracheal tube is:

    Too small: _____

    Too large: _____

172. Describe when an uncuffed endotracheal tube may be used.

    _____

    _____

    _____

    _____

173. The distal cuff of an endotracheal tube should be inflated with _____ mL of air.
    a. 1 to 3
    b. 5 to 10
    c. 20 to 25
    d. 30 to 35

174. Explain why it is important to keep the end of a stylet from extending beyond the distal end of an endotracheal tube while attempting to intubate a patient.

    _____

    _____

    _____

    _____

175. Magill forceps are used to:
    a. insert oropharyngeal airways in neonates
    b. extract foreign objects from the bronchi
    c. guide endotracheal tubes into place during nasotracheal intubation
    d. control hemorrhage by compressing the bleeding vessel

176. T F It is necessary to examine the distal cuff of the endotracheal tube for leaks before placement only if the protective envelope is damaged.

177. T F A laryngoscope blade that has a yellow flickering light provides insufficient illumination of the upper airway.

178. Each attempt at endotracheal intubation should not take longer than _____ seconds.
    a. 8
    b. 15
    c. 30
    d. 45

179. For this illustration, label the name of each anatomical structure shown.

    Use colored pencils or felt-tip pens to color the illustration according to the following: A-pink, B-red, C-orange, D-gray, E-brown, F-green, G-tan, and H-yellow.

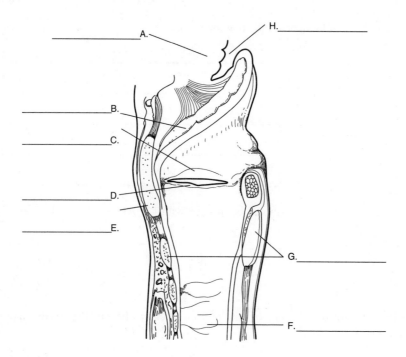

180. Describe how cricoid pressure is performed during intubation.

    _____
    _____
    _____
    _____
    _____

181. Add a prefix to the word below to create a term that means *through the mouth*.

    _____ tracheal

182. Describe the advantage the orotracheal route has over the nasotracheal route for intubation.

_____

_____

_____

_____

_____

183. Unless trauma is suspected, the patient's head should be placed in a _____ position when performing endotracheal intubation.
    a. sniffing
    b. flexed
    c. neutral
    d. hyperextended

184. Identify, by numbering, the correct order for performing endotracheal intubation.

    _____ Using the left hand, grasp the laryngoscope by its handle, and insert the blade into the right side of the patient's mouth. Using a sweeping motion, displace the tongue to the left.

    _____ Grasp the endotracheal tube in the right hand, holding it the same way a pencil is grasped. Advance it through the right corner of the patient's mouth, directing the distal end of the tube up or down to pass it into the larynx.

    _____ Move the blade slightly toward the midline, and advance it until the distal end is positioned at the base of the tongue. Visualize the tip of the epiglottis, and then place the laryngoscope blade into the proper position.

    _____ Place the patient's head and neck into an appropriate position.

    _____ Inflate the distal cuff with between 5 and 10 cc of air. Use only the minimum amount of air necessary to create an effective seal.

    _____ Keeping the left wrist straight, use the shoulder and arm to continue lifting the mandible and tongue at a 45-degree angle to the ground until the glottis is exposed.

    _____ Lift the laryngoscope slightly upward and forward to displace the jaw and airway structures without allowing the blade to touch the teeth. Suction any vomitus or secretions lying in the posterior pharynx.

    _____ Insert the endotracheal tube into the glottic opening, and advance it until the distal cuff disappears slightly (0.5 to 1.0 inch) past the vocal cords. Observe the tube as it enters the glottic opening. Hold it in place with the left hand. Do not release the endotracheal tube before it is secured in place.

    _____ Auscultate the chest for the presence of equal bilateral lung sounds.

    _____ Secure the endotracheal tube in place with umbilical tape or a commercial device while continuing ventilatory support.

    _____ Listen over the epigastrium to ensure there are no sounds when ventilations are delivered.

    _____ Attach a ventilatory device to the 15/22-mm adapter of the tube, and deliver several breaths.

    _____ Ventilate the patient with 100% oxygen, and insert an oropharyngeal airway to serve as a bite block.

185. You are having trouble intubating an unconscious stroke patient. Apparently, the patient's larynx lies anteriorly. You should:
    a. have a partner or first responder apply firm downward pressure on the patient's neck in the region of the cricoid cartilage
    b. place the patient's head into a neutral or flexed position
    c. slide the laryngoscope blade to the right, and advance it deep into the laryngeal opening
    d. have your partner grasp the tongue and lift it anteriorly

186. T F If a tube is inserted between the vocal cords sound can still be generated.

187. T F If the skin on either side of the Adam's apple "tents up" during attempts to place an endotracheal tube, the tip is likely hung up in the piriform sinus.

188. After correctly positioning the endotracheal tube, the cuff is inflated. The primary reason for inflating the distal cuff is to:
   a. stabilize the position of the tube
   b. decrease the incidence of gastric distention
   c. allow direct ventilation with 100% oxygen
   d. prevent aspiration of foreign material

189. You are attempting to place an endotracheal tube in a 53-year-old female patient who is in cardiac arrest. Signs that indicate accidental esophageal intubation include:
   a. auscultation of the chest reveals bilateral breath sounds
   b. the patient's color improves
   c. gurgling sounds are heard over the epigastric area
   d. subcutaneous emphysema quickly develops

190. As part of your management of a patient who has attempted suicide by leaving his car running in a closed garage, you have placed an endotracheal tube. On auscultating the chest, you hear breath sounds on the right side only. You most likely have:
   a. inserted the endotracheal tube too far
   b. intubated the esophagus
   c. ruptured the trachea
   d. inflated the cuff of the endotracheal tube with too much air

191. Match each of the following complications with the appropriate cause and/or how to avoid it. Some items may be used more than once.

   Complication
   a. Hypoxia
   b. Injury to teeth and tissue
   c. Vallecula misplacement
   d. Endobronchial misplacement
   e. Esophageal intubation

   Cause/How to Avoid It
   _____ Occurs when the endotracheal tube is misplaced posteriorly
   _____ Occurs when the tube is allowed to slip too far anteriorly and becomes lodged in the space between the epiglottis and base of the tongue
   _____ Occurs when intubation attempts are longer than appropriate or the EMT-I fails to provide ventilatory support between procedures
   _____ Slightly withdraw and redirect the tube posteriorly
   _____ Occurs when the endotracheal tube is inserted too far
   _____ Withdraw the tube until lung sounds are heard equally on both sides of the chest
   _____ When manipulating the jaw anteriorly, use upward traction rather than following the natural inclination to rotate and flex the wrist

192. T F Generally, the only reason to field extubate is when the patient is unreasonably intolerant of the tube.

193. T F Field extubation seldom is a problem unless the patient is elderly or overweight.

194. T F Field extubation is contraindicated if there is any risk of recurrence of respiratory failure.

195. List four indications for intubation of a child.

_____

_____

_____

_____

196. For intubation of infants and toddlers:
    a. a curved blade is preferred because it provides better visualization
    b. a No. 2 size laryngoscope blade is used
    c. uncuffed endotracheal tubes are used
    d. a 2.5 to 3.0 size endotracheal tube is indicated

197. List four ways of confirming proper endotracheal tube placement in the pediatric patient.

_____

_____

_____

_____

198. Describe three factors that make performing endotracheal intubation more challenging in children.

_____

_____

_____

199. On the illustration of the upper airway below, use a yellow highlighter to shade in the location where the cream-colored cuff of an esophageal tracheal Combitube (ETC) will rest and a green highlighter to shade in the locations where the longer tube can be inserted.

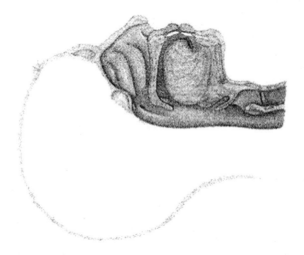

Chapter 9 Airway Management

200. The ETC airway is different from the pharyngotracheal lumen (PTL) airway in that the ETC:
    a. is a triple lumen tube having two balloon cuffs
    b. does not allow for immediate suctioning of gastric contents
    c. prevents the patient from breathing when there is undiagnosed tracheal placement
    d. has a self-adjusting, self-positioning posterior pharyngeal balloon

201. Identify, by numbering, the correct order for performing the steps used to insert the ETC.
    _____ Ventilate the patient through the blue tube.
    _____ Tell the rescuer who is providing ventilatory support to move to the side of the patient's head while you assume a position above the patient. Insert the thumb of the right hand deep into the patient's mouth, grasping the tongue and lower jaw between the thumb and index finger. Lift the tongue and lower jaw anteriorly, away from the posterior pharynx.
    _____ If a spinal injury is not likely, open the airway by hyperextending the patient's head and neck.
    _____ Hold the ETC so that it curves in the same direction as the natural curvature of the pharynx. Insert the tip into the mouth along the midline, and advance it carefully along the tongue. Gently guide the ETC along the base of the tongue and into the airway. When the ETC is at the proper depth, the teeth or alveolar ridge will be between the heavy black lines.
    _____ Connect the blue-tipped syringe (drawn up with at least 100 mL of air) to the blue one-way valve marked tube "No. 1." Then connect the white-tipped syringe (drawn up with at least 15 mL of air) to the white one-way valve marked tube "No. 2."
    _____ Observe the patient's chest and listen for lung sounds. If the chest rises and falls and breath sounds are heard, the ETC is in the esophagus. Thus the patient is being ventilated as with an esophageal obturator airway (EOA)/esophageal gastric tube airway (EGTA). When this is the case, continue to ventilate through the blue tube.
    _____ Once that cuff is inflated and the pilot balloon is tense, immediately inflate the white pilot balloon (and the distal cuff) with the smaller predrawn 15-mL syringe.
    _____ Inflate the blue pilot balloon (and cream-colored cuff) with the predrawn 100-mL blue-tipped syringe.
    _____ Continue ventilating the patient with a bag-mask device or other ventilatory device.
    _____ If the chest does not rise and breath sounds are not heard, the ETC is in the trachea. In this case, attach the bag-mask device or other ventilatory device to the shorter clear tube, and ventilate the patient through it. Again, listen for breath sounds in all lung fields and in both axillae.

202. Pharyngotracheal airways:
    a. are designed to be inserted into the trachea
    b. include the PTL and the ETC
    c. are inserted using a laryngoscope
    d. can be used only by paramedics

203. On the illustration of the upper airway below, use a yellow highlighter to shade in the location where the *short, wide tube* is inserted and a green highlighter to shade in the locations where the *longer tube* is inserted.

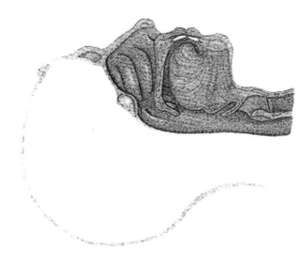

204. The PTL airway:
    a. has a longer tube that acts like an EOA when it is inserted into the esophagus
    b. has 15/22-mm connectors at its distal ends for attachment of a standard ventilatory device
    c. requires the use of a face mask to maintain a seal at the proximal end
    d. can protect the trachea from upper airway bleeding or secretions when the longer tube is in the esophagus

205. Describe the procedure for checking the cuffs of the PTL airway before insertion of the device.

_____

_____

_____

_____

_____

206. Identify, by numbering, the correct order for performing the steps for inserting the PTL airway.
    _____ Insert the device into the patient's mouth along the midline. Advance the tube until the flange rests against the patient's teeth.
    _____ Loop the white strap around the patient's head, and secure it in place.
    _____ Tell the rescuer who is providing ventilatory support to move to the side of the patient's head while you assume a position above the patient.
    _____ Use the tongue-jaw lift to move the tongue out of the way.
    _____ Once in place, inflate both distal cuffs simultaneously by taking a deep breath and blowing into the inflation valve.
    _____ Connect a ventilatory device to the green tube (oropharyngeal tube), and deliver a breath. If the chest rises, the longer tube is in the esophagus, and ventilations should be continued through the green tube.
    _____ Place the patient's head into a hyperextended position if there is no suspected spinal injury.
    _____ If the chest does not rise, the longer tube is in the trachea. The stylet must then be removed from the longer tube and assisted breathing provided through it
    _____ Continue delivering ventilatory support, and reassess for proper placement on an ongoing basis.

207. The proximal end of the laryngeal mask airway (LMA) consists of a:
    a. silicone rubber "mask" with an inflatable outer rim
    b. tube that looks like an endotracheal tube
    c. triple lumen tube having two balloon cuffs
    d. face mask that serves as a housing for the tube and face cushion

208. The role of the "grille" that covers the opening of the tube into the LMA mask is to:
    a. prevent the tongue from occluding the opening
    b. hold the vocal cords open
    c. support the epiglottis and keep it from falling into the opening of the tube
    d. seal the larynx

209. Describe how the LMA provides an open, secure airway.

    _____

    _____

    _____

    _____

    _____

210. T F The LMA provides ventilation that is equivalent to an endotracheal tube.

211. T F The LMA provides absolute protection against aspiration.

212. For various-sized patients below, fill in the correct LMA sizes.

Size of Patient	Size of LMA
Neonates/infants up to 6.5 kg	
Babies and children up to 20 kg	
Children between 20 and 30 kg	
Children and small adults more than 30 kg	
Average-sized and large adults	

213. For various-sized LMAs, fill in the correct cuff inflation volumes.

LMA Size	Cuff Inflation Volume
Size 1	
Size 2	
Size 2½	
Size 3	
Size 4	

214. The source of upper airway obstruction caused by a foreign body in the adult is usually:
    a. food
    b. bubble gum
    c. a balloon
    d. a coin

215. _____ in the spontaneously breathing patient is indicative of partial upper airway obstruction.
    a. Tracheal deviation
    b. Flushed skin
    c. Rales
    d. Stridor

216. While eating, a restaurant patron suddenly cannot speak, has ineffective breathing, and grabs at his throat. Your initial efforts at abdominal thrusts are unsuccessful, but the patient remains conscious. You should:
    a. insert an oropharyngeal airway
    b. attempt finger sweeps
    c. continue delivering abdominal thrusts
    d. deliver four back blows

217. Describe the use of direct laryngoscopy to remove a foreign body.

_____

_____

_____

_____

_____

218. Describe what the vomitus that is regurgitated into the oropharynx during states of decreased consciousness can do to the lungs.

_____

_____

_____

_____

_____

219. Gurgling sounds heard on inspiration and/or expiration indicate:
    a. the accumulation of fluids or vomitus in the upper airway
    b. swelling of the upper airway
    c. obstruction of the airway by the tongue falling back against the oropharynx
    d. spasm of the bronchial airways

220. All of the following are true regarding suctioning *except:*
    a. suctioning is used to remove vomitus, blood, fluids, and secretions from the airway
    b. each attempt at suctioning should be limited to 15 seconds
    c. the suction unit should provide a vacuum in excess of 30 mm Hg when the tube is clamped
    d. after inserting the catheter into the oropharynx, suction is applied while rotating the catheter as it is removed

221. Match each of the following suction catheters with the appropriate descriptions/characteristics. Answers may be used more than once.

    Type
    a. Tonsil tip
    b. Whistle tip

    Description/Characteristic
    _____ Is ineffective in removing large volumes of secretions rapidly
    _____ Also referred to as the Yankauer suction
    _____ Can be inserted through the nares, into the oropharynx or nasopharynx, through a nasopharyngeal airway, along an oropharyngeal airway, or through an endotracheal tube
    _____ Is a rigid tube that has a ball-like tip with multiple holes at its distal end
    _____ Is designed to remove larger particles and voluminous secretions
    _____ Is a small, easy to use flexible tube that is long enough to extend into the lower respiratory tract
    _____ Vigorous insertion can cause lacerations or other injuries

222. When fluids in the upper airway are so voluminous or thick that the tonsil-tip or whistle-tip suction catheters cannot provide adequate suctioning, the EMT-I should:
    a. insert the catheter deeper into the oropharynx than normal
    b. remove the catheter and use the thick-walled, wide-bore suction tubing alone
    c. alternately squeeze and release the tubing at its proximal end
    d. suction isoproterenol alcohol through the tubing between suctioning attempts

CROSSWORD PUZZLE EXERCISE

223. Complete the following crossword puzzle.

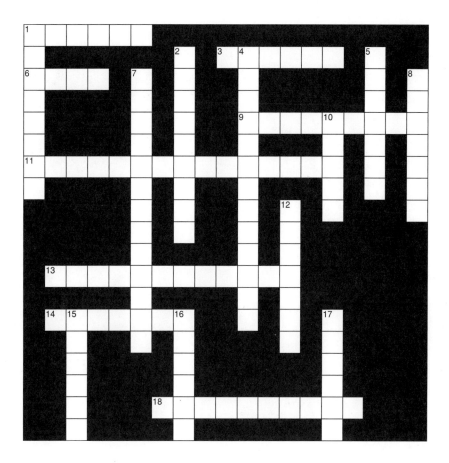

ACROSS

1. This face mask can deliver a concentration of 40% to 60% oxygen.
3. Clear plastic mask that covers the patient's mouth and nose.
6. Fracture of these may lead to hypoxia.
9. Process of generating sounds or speech with the vocal cords.
11. Reduced rate of depth of breathing.
13. Within or through the trachea.
14. Environmental or room air.
18. Oxygen is moisturized.

DOWN

1. Laryngoscope blade that is positioned posterior to the epiglottis.
2. Double lumen tube with two balloon cuffs.
4. Plastic J-shaped airway that conforms to the curvature of the palate.
5. Posterior portion of the head.
7. This mask is capable of delivering a 60% to 100% concentration of oxygen.
8. Mask is a high-flow oxygen delivery device.
10. Absence of breathing.
12. Maneuver is quick, effective way of preventing gastric distention and/or regurgitation.
15. Forceps that resemble a bent pair of scissors with circle-shaped tips.
16. Most common cause of upper airway obstruction in the unresponsive patient.
17. Semirigid, bendable plastic-coated wire.

10 History Taking

CHAPTER TERMINAL OBJECTIVES

On completion of this chapter, the EMT-Intermediate will be able to use the appropriate techniques to obtain a medical history from a patient.

For the multiple-choice questions, select the single best answer to each question. For the matching questions, select the best corresponding answer for each item. Because there are sometimes more items than corresponding answers, some items may not be used.

1. T F When doing assessments, historical information is usually gathered from only one source, the patient; otherwise, the data tend to be unreliable.

2. T F You must weigh the reliability of the history in a nonjudgmental manner at the end of the evaluation, not the beginning.

3. T F At a minimum, when determining the patient's current health status, you should always strive to find a history of allergies, use of medications, and use of drugs, alcohol, or tobacco.

4. List four factors that affect the quality of the historical data obtained during patient assessment.

   _____

   _____

   _____

   _____

5. Match each of the following history-taking terms with the correct description.

   Term
   a. Chief complaint
   b. History of the present illness
   c. Past medical history
   d. Current health status

   Description
   _____ Focuses on the patient's present state of health
   _____ Includes any significant past injuries, hospitalizations, operations, or diseases
   _____ Identifies, in the patient's own words, the symptoms for which the patient is seeking medical care
   _____ Should include a full, clear, and chronological account of the patient's symptoms

6. List at least 10 factors of interest that should be assessed as part of determining a patient's current health status.

___

7. The best place to conduct history taking is:
   a. in the back of the ambulance
   b. in the patient's home
   c. at the hospital
   d. dependent on each situation

8. During history taking you should respect the other person's personal space by:
   a. standing to the person's side
   b. not getting closer than 2 to 3 feet
   c. kneeling next to the person
   d. using frequent hand gestures to emphasize the points you are making

9. Studies have shown that the majority of our interpersonal communication occurs by:
   a. words
   b. actions
   c. voice inflection
   d. body language

10. When addressing patients you should refer to them:
    a. in an endearing term such as "dear," "sweetie," or "honey"
    b. respectfully by using terms such as "sir" or "madam"
    c. by their name
    d. by their favorite nickname

11. Describe what you should do if a patient expresses concern over your taking notes while conducting the history taking.

12. Open-ended questions:
    a. require a simple answer
    b. tend to yield far more helpful information than closed-ended questions
    c. can cause patients to say only what they think you want to hear
    d. often lead to frustration by the patient

13. Place a checkmark beside those questions that are open ended.
    _____ "How long have you been feeling ill?"
    _____ "Can you describe your pain?"
    _____ "Do you feel nauseated?"
    _____ "Does sitting up make it easier for you to breathe?"
    _____ "Did your chest pain subside after you took the nitroglycerin tablets?"
    _____ "How did you feel earlier today?"

14. Give an example of when closed-ended questions may be better.

    _____
    _____
    _____
    _____

15. Match each of the following history-taking terms with the correct description.

    Term
    a. Facilitation
    b. Reflection
    c. Clarification
    d. Empathetic responses
    e. Confrontation
    f. Interpretation

    Description
    _____ More direct but potentially disruptive to your relationship with the patient
    _____ Repeating the patient's words (or your summary of them) back to make certain you both are communicating
    _____ Combination of verbal and nonverbal actions that are used to encourage the patient to say more
    _____ Requires you to synthesize what the patient has told you (verbally and body language) with your own knowledge and "gut feelings"
    _____ Interrupting or asking additional questions to clarify points
    _____ Identifying with one's feelings or symptoms

16. During history taking an EMT-I says, "Tell me more . . . I am listening." This is an example of:
    a. reflection
    b. confrontation
    c. empathy
    d. facilitation

17. After listening to a patient describe his shortness of breath an EMT-I says, "What I understand you to have said is you haven't been able to catch your breath since last night and that you were treated for the same thing about a month ago—is that correct?" This is an example of:
    a. reflection
    b. empathy
    c. confrontation
    d. interpretation

18. "We are trying to help you—if you don't lie still on the backboard you can worsen your injuries!" is an example of:
    a. reflection
    b. empathy
    c. confrontation
    d. interpretation

19. T F While conducting the history taking avoid saying, "I am listening" when you are obviously doing something else, such as taking a blood pressure.

20. T F Done properly, reflection does not bias the story or interrupt the patient's train of thought.

21. T F Empathy is the same thing as sympathy.

22. T F Generally, you should share your interpretation of the patient's condition with him or her.

23. Describe an easy way to quantify the severity of a symptom.

    _____

    _____

    _____

24. List the meaning for each letter of the mnemonic SAMPLE.

    S: _____

    A: _____

    M: _____

    P: _____

    L: _____

    E: _____

25. List the meaning for each letter of the mnemonic OPQRST.

    O: _____

    P: _____

    Q: _____

    R: _____

    S: _____

    T: _____

26. While conducting history taking, the best way to deal with a silent patient is to:
    a. pressure him or her to immediately respond following your question
    b. accept a less comprehensive history
    c. show patience and remain alert for nonverbal clues of distress
    d. ask direct questions

27. List five things you can do to cope with the talkative patient during history taking.

28. Describe the most important thing that must be done when dealing with a patient who has multiple complaints.

29. You are assessing a patient who has multiple complaints. You have ruled out any immediate life threats. You should next have the patient:
    a. identify the least bothersome
    b. focus on the past medical history
    c. use a numerical rating scale to convey to you the severity of each complaint
    d. help you rank the complaints, starting with the most bothersome, then second worst, and so on

30. T F For the most part, persons who are anxious as a result of being sick or injured talk fast as a response.

31. T F Reassurance is the best tool for gathering information from persons who are anxious.

32. T F In cases in which a patient's behavioral response seems out of proportion to the apparent degree of illness or injury, the EMT-I should remain objective and empathetic.

33. T F Sometimes the best way to deal with a crying patient is simply to offer tissues.

34. T F Depression is confusing or unusual behavior resulting from a potentially serious medical problem.

35. List six signs of depression.

_____
_____
_____
_____
_____
_____

36. Angry and hostile patients:
    a. often purposely displace anger toward the EMT-I
    b. are best managed by redirecting the hostility and anger back to them
    c. should be left for police to handle
    d. are best handled when the EMT-I remains calm in response to the patient

37. When dealing with intoxicated patients the EMT-I should:
    a. use it as an opportunity to point out the adverse effects of alcoholism
    b. direct them to keep their voice down
    c. talk calmly and avoid sudden moves
    d. move closer to them and occasionally gently touch their shoulder or hand

38. Describe how the EMT-I should deal with a seductive patient.

_____
_____
_____
_____

39. Describe why the EMT-I should consider confusing or unusual behavior to be caused by a potentially serious medical problem until proven otherwise.

_____
_____
_____
_____

40. Match each of the following special challenges with the correct way to manage them.

    Challenge
    a. Patient with limited intelligence
    b. EMT-I/patient language barrier
    c. Patient with a hearing problem
    d. Blind patient

    Method for Managing

    _____ Try to find a translator, including the dial-up services for language translation offered by several telephone companies. Be aware of your local resources.

    _____ Find a translator if the patient can sign. Ask patients if they read lips by looking them in the eyes, pointing to your mouth, and saying, "Do you read lips?" If the answer is yes, speak slowly and avoid unusual terms and idiomatic language.

    _____ Speak clearly, but normally; although it may not be the case, expect more time than usual for the patient to respond to your question. Getting additional information from family or friends is always helpful. If patients are capable of communicating, direct your interview toward them first. Remember to be patient and professional.

41. T F The patient who has a hearing problem will be able to communicate with you even when you turn your head out of the patient's line of vision.

42. T F One way to communicate with the patient who has a hearing problem is by writing notes, if the patient is able.

43. T F Often, family members and friends are excellent collateral sources of data.

44. T F When soliciting information from a patient's family and friends, any medical information is not considered confidential.

CROSSWORD PUZZLE EXERCISE

45. Complete the following crossword puzzle.

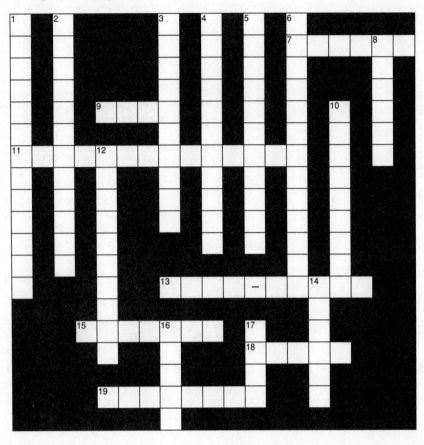

ACROSS

7. Mnemonic that helps you remember what you need to know about the patient's chief complaint.
9. Medical history that includes any significant previous hospitalizations, operations, or diseases.
11. Questioning techniques that require you to synthesize what the patient has told you.
13. Questions that require more than a simple, often one-word answer.
15. From where historical information often comes.
18. "When did the problem begin?" refers to what part of assessing the chief complaint?
19. "On a scale of 0 to 10, how bad is the pain?" refers to what part of assessing the chief complaint?

DOWN

1. Technique of interrupting or asking additional questions to clarify points.
2. Combination of verbal and nonverbal actions that we use to encourage the patient to say more.
3. Type of responses that identify with a person's feelings or symptoms.
4. "What makes the problem worse?" refers to what part of assessing the chief complaint?
5. In a nonjudgmental fashion, you must weigh the _____ of the history gathered from sources.
6. Questioning technique that is more direct but potentially disruptive to relationship with patient.
8. A mnemonic that helps you remember what to ask in the present history.
10. This patient is the opposite of the silent patient.
12. Repeating patient's words back to make certain you both are communicating.
14. Type of questions that require a simple answer, such as "yes" or "no."
16. The _____ complaint is the symptom for which the patient is seeking medical care.
17. The majority of our interpersonal communication occurs by this language.

11 Techniques of Physical Examination

CHAPTER TERMINAL OBJECTIVES

On completion of this chapter, the EMT-Intermediate will be able to explain the significance of physical examination findings commonly found in emergencies.

For the multiple-choice questions, select the single best answer to each question. For the matching questions, select the best corresponding answer for each item. Because there are sometimes more items than corresponding answers, some items may not be used.

1. Match each of the following physical examination procedures with the correct description.

   Procedure
   a. Inspection
   b. Auscultation
   c. Percussion
   d. Palpation

   Description
   _____ Process in which the examiner feels the texture, size, consistency, and location of certain parts of the body with the hands

   _____ Technique involving gently striking or tapping a part of the body to evaluate the size, borders, and consistency of the internal organs and to discover the presence of fluid in body cavities

   _____ Act of listening for sounds within the body to evaluate the condition of the heart, lungs, pleura, intestines, or other organs or to detect fetal heart sounds

2. Which procedure involves the use of a stethoscope?
   a. inspection
   b. palpation
   c. percussion
   d. auscultation

3. List the four vital signs.

   _____

   _____

   _____

   _____

4. T F Recheck vital signs every 1 to 3 minutes, sooner if the patient's condition changes.

5. T F Normal vital signs can vary within large ranges and differ considerably by age.

6. T F In the prehospital setting, especially during an acute situation, exact determination of the patient's weight is not usually necessary—an estimate will do.

7. Give the correct description for each item of examination equipment.

Examination Equipment	Description
ECG monitor	
Pulse oximeter	
Peak flow meter	
Capnometer	
Glucose meter	

8. One of the best indicators of a person's condition is the:
   a. blood pressure
   b. mental status
   c. pulse oximetry
   d. respirations

9. The V in the mnemonic AVPU stands for:
   a. unresponsive
   b. responsive to painful stimuli
   c. alert
   d. responsive to verbal stimuli

10. Describe what is meant by *normal mentation*.

   _____
   _____
   _____
   _____
   _____

11. Match each of the following levels of consciousness with the correct description.

    Level of Consciousness
    a. Stupor
    b. Obtundation
    c. Coma
    d. Drowsy
    e. Lethargic

    Description
    _____ Patients are drowsy but open their eyes to look at you, respond, then fall back to sleep
    _____ State of profound unconsciousness; the patient cannot be aroused by any stimulation
    _____ State of lethargy and unresponsiveness in which a person seems unaware of the surroundings
    _____ Reduced level of consciousness resulting in insensitivity to unpleasant or painful stimuli; often caused by an anesthetic or analgesic (pain) medication
    _____ Sleepy, but otherwise normal

12. Label the illustrations below with the type of posturing each is displaying.

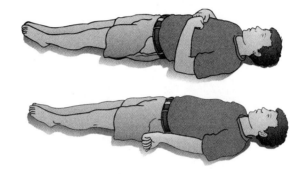

13. Acute arching of the back with the head bent back on the neck, the heels bent back on the legs, and the arms and hands flexed rigidly at the joints describes which of the following types of posturing?
    a. decerebrate
    b. decorticate
    c. opisthotonic
    d. anatomical

14. Match each of the following posture and motor behaviors with the correct description.

    Posture and Motor Behavior
    a. Opisthotonic posturing
    b. Motor tics
    c. Decerebrate posturing
    d. Rigidity
    e. Tremor

    Description
    _____ Spasmodic muscular contractions most commonly involving the face, mouth, eyes, head, neck, or shoulders
    _____ Involuntary alternating contraction and relaxation of opposing groups of skeletal muscles
    _____ Results from severe muscle spasms, such as during a seizure or from tetanus
    _____ A severe injury to the brain at the level of the brainstem is the usual cause
    _____ Hardness, stiffness, or inflexibility, usually of the extremities; a sign of neurological disease, such as Parkinson's disease

15. T F Restlessness or agitation may indicate a serious underlying medical condition, such as hypoxia (lack of oxygen).

16. T F Patients with altered mental status are usually well groomed.

17. Patients who do not smile or show other facial expressions, are quiet, and provide simple answers with no variation in voice tone are said to have:

    a. tremors
    b. a low Glasgow Coma Scale score
    c. a flat affect
    d. obtundation

18. List four things related to a person's ability to speak (that are part of the mental status evaluation) that the EMT-I should assess.

    _____
    _____
    _____
    _____

19. Impaired speech caused by dysfunction of the tongue or other muscles essential to speech is called:

    a. dysarthria
    b. aphasia
    c. apnea
    d. dysphonia

20. List the three things the standard evaluation of a person's orientation centers around.

    _____
    _____
    _____

21. Describe what is meant by the phrase "A & O × 3."

    _____
    _____
    _____
    _____

CROSSWORD PUZZLE EXERCISE

22. Complete the following crossword puzzle.

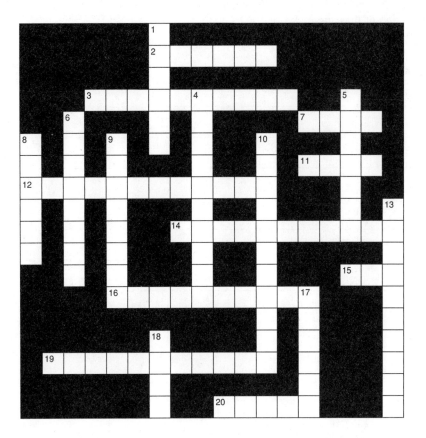

ACROSS

2. Rhythmic, purposeless, quivering movements.
3. Act of visually evaluating the patient.
7. Mnemonic for determining patient's level of consciousness.
11. Affect in which the patient appears emotionally unresponsive.
12. Posturing that results from severe muscle spasms, such as during a seizure or from tetanus.
14. Posturing where upper extremities are flexed at the elbows and at the wrists.
15. Refers to how much awareness people have regarding their immediate surroundings.
16. Impaired speech caused by dysfunction of the tongue or other muscles essential to speech.
19. Instrument consisting of two earpieces connected by means of flexible tubing to a diaphragm.
20. Abbreviation for head, eyes, ears, nose, and throat.

DOWN

1. State of lethargy and unresponsiveness where a person seems unaware of the surroundings.
4. Electronic device that measures how much carbon dioxide is exhaled during breathing.
5. Abnormal neurologic condition in which language function is defective or absent.
6. Hardness, stiffness, or inflexibility, usually of the extremities.
8. Sleepy, but otherwise normal.
9. Patients open their eyes and look at you, but respond slowly and are confused.
10. Posturing where arms are extended and internally rotated while feet are extended and in forced plantar flexion.
13. Technique involving gently striking or tapping a part of the body.
17. A person's outward manifestations of emotion.
18. State of profound unconsciousness.

23. The general survey is a:
    a. rapid assessment of priority conditions
    b. universal overview of the patient's general condition
    c. detailed examination of the patient
    d. combination of the physical examination and history taking

24. List the 11 components of the general survey.

    _____
    _____
    _____
    _____
    _____
    _____
    _____
    _____
    _____
    _____
    _____

25. List the things you should do during examination of the skin.

    _____
    _____
    _____
    _____
    _____

26. List the six things you should pay particular attention to as you evaluate the skin and the fingernails.

_____

_____

_____

_____

_____

_____

27. Skin that stays up when it is pinched:
    a. indicates overhydration
    b. is called decreased skin turgor
    c. indicates hypoxia
    d. is associated with fever

28. Cyanosis is caused by:
    a. an excess of deoxygenated hemoglobin in the blood
    b. greater than normal amounts of bilirubin in the blood
    c. the leakage of blood into the subcutaneous tissues because of trauma to the underlying blood vessels
    d. vasodilatation of the peripheral blood vessels

29. Describe the assessment of the head.

_____

_____

_____

_____

_____

30. List three things you should do when checking the eyes.

_____

_____

_____

31. The term *conjugate gaze* means:
    a. the pupils are round and reactive to light
    b. each pupil moves separate from the other
    c. the eyes move in the same direction
    d. the patient is staring straight forward

32. To check for proper conjugate gaze you would:
    a. have the patient follow your light or finger in the six cardinal directions
    b. shine a light into the patient's eyes while watching each pupil react
    c. have the patient look straight ahead while you shine a light into the side of the eye
    d. have the patient look up and down while you follow the movement with a penlight

33. Describe how an injury to the muscles or nerves of the eye can be detected.

    _____
    _____
    _____
    _____

34. Label the figure of the pupils below as either normal, dilated, small, or unequal.

35. Describe what the figure of the pupils above may indicate.

    _____
    _____
    _____
    _____

36. List the steps for checking a patient's pupils.

    _____
    _____
    _____
    _____

37. The condition in which the pupils are normally unequal is called:
    a. aphasia
    b. anisocoria
    c. ataxia
    d. consensual reaction

38. Causes of constricted pupils include:
    a. direct trauma to the eye
    b. shock
    c. poisoning
    d. cardiac arrest

39. You can perform a visual acuity exam by:
    a. shining a light into the patient's eyes
    b. having the patient view an eye chart
    c. having the patient follow a pen or light with the eyes as you move it from one side to the other and back again
    d. asking the patient to count your fingers that you hold in front of him or her

40. Describe what things you should check for when examining a patient's ears.

    _____

    _____

    _____

    _____

41. Which of the following may indicate a basilar skull fracture?
    a. blood or cerebrospinal fluid (CSF) in the ear canal
    b. bruising in front of the ears
    c. laceration of the outer ear
    d. a and b

42. Referring to the picture of the unresponsive patient below, describe the procedures used to assess the mouth.

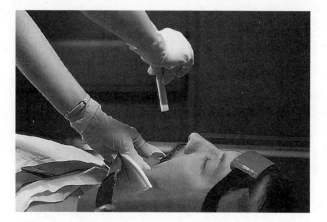

43. Which of the following is true regarding assessing the airway?
    a. Bleeding into the mouth can obstruct the upper airway.
    b. Dentures should be routinely removed.
    c. Airway compromise leads to the patient being reclassified to "priority" status only if accompanied by circulatory compromise.
    d. Alcohol ingestion usually is difficult to detect.

44. Nuchal rigidity:
    a. is defined as an increased range of motion of the neck
    b. may indicate infection, such as meningitis, or may be caused by muscle spasm from a whiplash type of injury
    c. is usually associated with minor conditions
    d. should prompt the EMT-I to apply cervical immobilization

45. T F You palpate the anterior neck of a patient who was shot in the chest and note that the trachea is deviated to the left. This is considered normal.

46. T F Never palpate both sides of the neck simultaneously.

47. T F The extrication collar is removed during assessment of the neck to give the EMT-I needed access.

48. T F Ecchymosis in the neck region may signify trauma and impending airway obstruction.

49. T F Jugular vein distention (JVD) evaluation is best done with the patient sitting at a 15-degree angle.

50. T F Minor open wounds to the anterior neck are typically insignificant.

51. Neck vein distention:
    a. is normal in elderly patients
    b. is said to be present when the veins are distended and pulsating
    c. indicates conditions such as congestive heart failure and cardiac tamponade
    d. may be seen with hypovolemic shock and dehydration

52. Subcutaneous emphysema:
    a. feels like jelly when pressed
    b. occurs when air leaks into the subcutaneous tissue
    c. is indicative of tension pneumothorax
    d. occurs only in pediatric patients

CROSSWORD PUZZLE EXERCISE

53. Complete the following crossword puzzle.

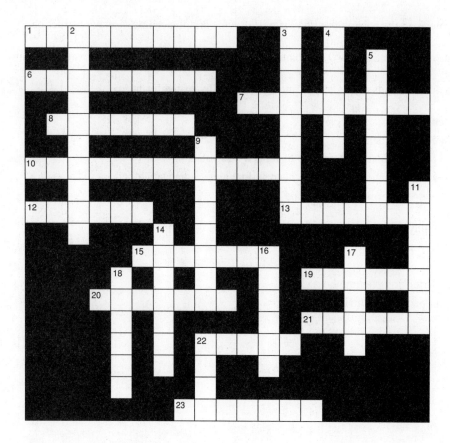

ACROSS

1. Discoloration of an area of skin or mucous membrane caused by leakage of blood into tissues.
6. Gaze in which the eyes move in the same direction.
7. _____ reactivity means how quickly the patient's pupils constrict when exposed to bright light.
8. Type of cyanosis best seen in the lips, oral mucosa, and tongue.
10. Abnormal tone or color.
12. Unable to coordinate movements.
13. An abnormal neurologic condition in which language function is defective or absent.
15. Scars, moles, birthmarks, wounds, bruises.
19. _____ rigidity is defined as stiffness of the neck with decreased range of motion.
20. This sign is a discoloration behind the ears.
21. Elasticity ("snapability") of the skin.
22. Stands for Pupils are Equal, Round, and React to Light.
23. This age group's normal rate of breathing is 40 breaths/min.

DOWN

2. Reaction where when a light is shined in one eye and it constricts so does the other.
3. Difficulty in speaking.
4. Unnatural paleness or absence of color in the skin.
5. Bluish discoloration of skin, mucous membranes, and sclera of the eyes.
9. Yellowish discoloration of skin, mucous membranes, and sclera of the eyes.
11. Blood or clear watery fluid, CSF, in ear may indicate _____ skull fracture.
14. When skin stays up when it is pinched.
16. White part of the eye.
17. Mark left in the skin or an internal organ by the healing of a wound, sore, or injury.
18. General term for any type of abnormal skin eruption.
22. This color of the lower eyelid when retracted indicates poor perfusion.

54. Referring to the picture of the patient below, pretend you are an EMT-I who is conducting a patient examination. Your partner is maintaining cervical stabilization. Describe the procedures used to assess the chest.

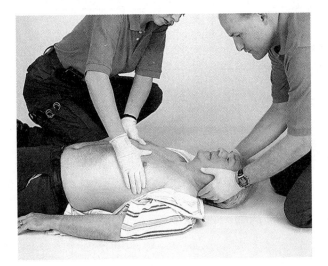

_____

_____

_____

_____

_____

55. List the average respiratory rates for the following:

   Newborn: _____

   Infant (less than 1 year): _____

   Toddler: _____

   Preschooler: _____

   School age: _____

   Adolescent: _____

   Adult: _____

56. _____ is a respiratory rate that is too slow, and _____ is a respiratory rate that is too fast.

57. List seven indicators of respiratory distress.

_____
_____
_____
_____
_____
_____
_____

58. Match each of the following breathing patterns with the correct description.

    Breathing Pattern
    a. Bradypnea
    b. Cheyne-Stokes
    c. Tachypnea
    d. Kussmaul
    e. Apnea

    Description
    _____ Absence of breathing
    _____ Rapid and deep respirations usually found in diabetic patients or others with imbalances of the acid content in their bodies
    _____ Slow respirations
    _____ Series of rapid then slow respirations, followed by periods of apnea
    _____ Rapid and usually shallow respirations

59. To palpate a patient's chest, begin with the _____, and then palpate the _____ _____. Note pain, _____, possible fractures, or _____ _____. After palpation, _____ the chest to verify _____ _____.

60. List three things for which to inspect the chest.

_____
_____
_____

61. T F Percussion of the chest helps the EMT-I identify whether the underlying tissues are air filled, fluid filled, or solid.

62. T F Percussion involves striking one finger against a wrist of the other hand, which is held against the chest.

63. T F The thorax should be percussed symmetrically, from top to bottom.

64. Dullness heard with percussion:
    a. is relatively loud, low pitched, and of long duration
    b. often occurs in the face of pneumothorax or chronic obstructive pulmonary disease (COPD)
    c. occurs if the pleural space becomes filled with fluid such as with pleural effusion
    d. is normal

65. Hyperresonance is:
    a. detected with the use of a stethoscope
    b. the sound heard over solid organs such as the liver
    c. commonly heard when assessing the thorax
    d. heard when the chest contains more air than usual

66. Auscultation of the chest:
    a. is used to assess whether the tissues are air filled, fluid filled, or solid
    b. involves listening to the sounds generated by breathing and checking for symmetry
    c. cannot determine whether additional adventitious sounds are present; this requires more precise listening devices
    d. is done in at least 12 different areas

67. On the figure below, draw circles to show the locations where the chest is auscultated.

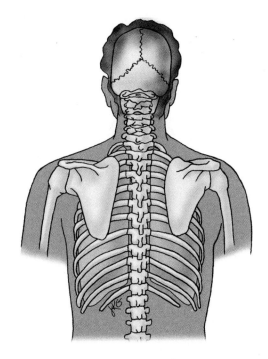

68. Match each of the following types of sounds with the correct description.

    Sound Heard
    a. Tracheal
    b. Vesicular
    c. Bronchial
    d. Bronchovesicular

    Description
    _____ Normal sound of rustling or swishing heard with the stethoscope over the lung periphery; usually higher pitched during inspiration, fading rapidly during expiration

    _____ Normal if heard over the anterior sternum; otherwise, an abnormal sound heard with a stethoscope over the lungs, indicating consolidation or compression of normal lung

    _____ Sounds intermediate between tracheal sounds and vesicular sounds. These may be normal in the first and second interspaces anteriorly and between the scapulae, but otherwise suggest fluid in the lungs

69. "Discontinuous" adventitious lung sounds include:
    a. rales
    b. rhonchi
    c. wheezing
    d. absent

70. Rhonchi:
    a. are crackling or bubbling sounds that represent fluid in the alveoli and are present in heart failure or pneumonia
    b. are squeaking, high-pitched sounds that may occur on either inspiration, expiration, or both
    c. represent spasms in the airways and are present in patients with asthma, COPD, or heart failure
    d. are coarser gurgling-like sounds that are often present over the larger airways only and may be heard on both inspiration and expiration

71. Describe what diminished lung sounds indicate.

    _____

    _____

    _____

    _____

72. A heart rate that is greater than 100 BPM is called _____, whereas a heart rate less than 60 BPM is referred to as _____.

73. The average pulse rate for the preschooler (aged 4 to 5 years old) is _____ BPM.
    a. 60 to 105
    b. 70 to 150
    c. 80 to 140
    d. 120 to 160

74. List the four pulses that are most commonly used to assess vital signs.

    _____

    _____

    _____

    _____

75. Describe why the radial pulse is not the preferred pulse to check in the presence of shock or poor circulation.

_____

_____

_____

_____

_____

76. List the three important characteristics to evaluate when checking the pulse.

_____

_____

_____

77. List the average pulse ranges for the following:

    Newly born (birth to 4 wk): _____

    Infant (1-12 mo): _____

    Toddler (1-3 yr): _____

    Preschool (4-5 yr): _____

    School age (6-12 yr): _____

    Adolescent (12-18 yr): _____

    Adult (>18 yr): _____

78. Cardiac dysrhythmias:
    a. may produce an irregular pulse
    b. usually go unnoticed by the patient
    c. have no effect on cardiac output
    d. are described as a bounding pulse

79. List three factors that affect a person's blood pressure.

_____

_____

_____

80. Errors that occur in the measurement of blood pressures include:
    a. a cuff that is too small, which acts as a tourniquet and can lead to falsely low readings
    b. a cuff that is placed too loosely, which can lead to readings that are almost always too high
    c. sounds that may be incorrectly heard
    d. a cuff that is too large, which produces falsely high readings

81. Orthostatic hypotension:
    a. is a condition in which the blood pressure suddenly increases when a person stands up
    b. is more common in smaller female patients, elderly persons, and those who are dehydrated or bleeding internally
    c. is said to be present when there is an increase in the pulse rate of 30 to 40 BPM or greater, along with a decrease in the systolic blood pressure of 10 to 20 mm Hg or greater
    d. is said to be present only if the patient's blood pressure decreases

82. The pulse pressure:
    a. is the difference between systolic blood pressure and diastolic blood pressure
    b. is normally 20 mm Hg
    c. increases when there is a loss of blood volume
    d. increases in the presence of early cardiac tamponade or tension pneumothorax

83. Which of the following would be regarded as a narrowed pulse pressure?
    a. 100/62
    b. 210/140
    c. 90/70
    d. 144/88

84. You are called to the home of a 60-year-old woman who is complaining of a headache. You determine that her blood pressure is 190/110. This patient is experiencing:
    a. normotension
    b. hypotension
    c. orthostatic hypotension
    d. hypertension

85. Venous pulsations:
    a. can usually be felt
    b. are eliminated by light pressure on the vein just above the sternal end of the clavicle
    c. increase in intensity as the patient becomes more upright
    d. can be easily seen

86. On the illustration of the chest below, insert an arrow pointing to the area that represents the point of maximum impulse.

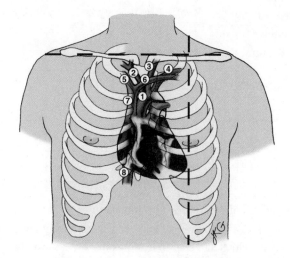

87. The point of maximum impulse (PMI) of the heart is:
    a. in the seventh intercostal space of the thorax
    b. lateral to the left midclavicular line
    c. where the apical beat of the heart is observed
    d. where the chest is percussed to identify the heart sounds

88. The first heart sound:
    a. sounds like a "dub"
    b. is called S_1
    c. normally sounds muffled
    d. sounds the same for all persons

89. T F To examine the abdomen you should place the patient into a sitting position.

90. T F When examining the abdomen begin with the most sensitive areas first.

91. The abdomen should be inspected for signs of obvious injury, _____, or _____.

92. Abdominal striae:
    a. are defined as constriction of veins
    b. may be a sign of endocrine disease
    c. indicate the presence of fluid in the abdomen
    d. are typically asymmetrical

93. Dilated veins, especially those that appear like a "bundle of worms," suggest:
    a. severe liver disease
    b. diabetes
    c. obesity
    d. cancer

94. A scaphoid abdomen is:
    a. flat
    b. bulging
    c. markedly concave
    d. common with ascites

95. Excessive pulsations well below the epigastrium may indicate:
    a. an aortic aneurysm
    b. hypertension
    c. hypovolemic shock
    d. appendicitis

96. Describe why it is preferable to auscultate the abdomen before palpating it.

_____

_____

_____

_____

97. Normally, bowel sounds in the abdomen are:
    a. absent
    b. decreased
    c. relatively noisy
    d. hyperactive

98. Absent bowel sounds:
    a. represent normal peristalsis of food through the gut
    b. occur with anxiety, diet, and hunger
    c. are referred to as borborygmi
    d. can indicate serious intraabdominal pathology such as peritonitis

99. It is important to listen to all four quadrants of the abdomen with:
    a. decreased bowel sounds
    b. hyperactive bowel sounds
    c. normal bowel sounds
    d. borborygmi

100. Bruits heard over the abdomen:
    a. sound like a low-pitched "bubbling"
    b. are more significant if they are in the upper quadrant
    c. represent turbulent blood flow in arteries
    d. are more common during diastole

101. Describe the significance of bruits found in each of the following locations.

Location	Suggests
Upper abdominal quadrant	
Lower abdomen or back	
Over the groin	

102. Using the figure below, describe how to perform light palpation of the abdomen.

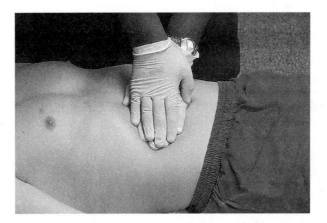

_____

_____

_____

_____

_____

103. When palpating the abdomen you note tenderness, _____, and muscular _____, and any masses or lesions. Observe the patient's face for any _____ response or _____.

104. Describe what the term *guarding* means and what it represents.

_____

_____

_____

_____

_____

105. Describe what is meant by the term *boardlike rigidity*.

_____

_____

_____

_____

_____

106. The costovertebral angle (CVA) is:
    a. located anteriorly
    b. at the junction of the 12th rib and the 12th thoracic vertebra
    c. percussed to identify kidney disorders
    d. seldom assessed in the field setting

107. To assess for rebound tenderness:
    a. begin by palpating the abdominal area with light palpation, except that you gently press a little harder and deeper—if there is an area of tenderness, slowly withdraw your hand to see whether the slow withdrawal worsens the pain
    b. apply deep, quick palpation to the tender areas of the abdomen
    c. first assess the abdominal area with gentle palpation—if there is an area of tenderness, quickly and deeply palpate the area to see whether that worsens the pain
    d. start by palpating the abdominal area with light palpation, except that you gently press a little harder and deeper—if there is an area of tenderness, quickly withdraw your hand to see whether the quick withdrawal worsens the pain

108. Rebound tenderness suggests:
    a. cancer
    b. bowel obstruction
    c. peritoneal irritation
    d. gastritis

109. Patients with abdominal discoloration, rigidity, exposed intestines (evisceration), or severe pain should be classified as _____ .

110. Describe considerations that should be given to examining patients who are a different sex than the EMT-I.

    _____
    _____
    _____
    _____
    _____

111. Describe what should be noted with examining the external genitalia.

    _____
    _____
    _____
    _____
    _____
    _____

CROSSWORD PUZZLE EXERCISE

112. Complete the following crossword puzzle.

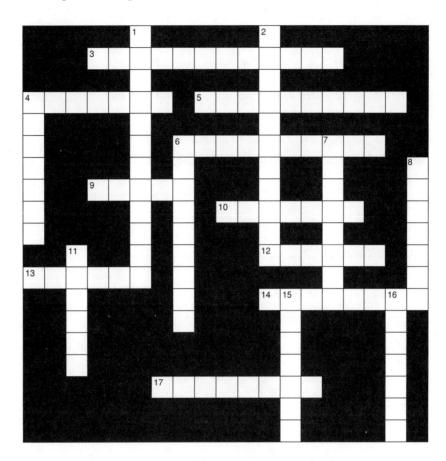

ACROSS

3. Paralysis of both arms and both legs.
4. Fluid in the abdominal cavity.
5. Paralysis of the arm and leg on one side of the body.
6. Rumbling, gurgling, and tinkling noises indicating hyperperistalsis.
9. Swelling caused by accumulation of fluid in the tissues.
10. Is said to exist when pressure over an edematous area results in depression in skin.
12. "Stretch marks."
13. High-pitched "whooshing" sounds that represent turbulent blood flow in arteries.
14. Bubbling sound from fluid in the airways.
17. Palpable or audible crunching produced by movement of a body part.

DOWN

1. Numbness or tingling sensation in the arms or legs.
2. Peritoneal irritation.
4. Loss of substance, especially muscle mass.
6. Respiratory rate that is abnormally slow.
7. Abnormal, short, and loud breaks during exhalation.
8. Widening of the nostrils during inspiration.
11. _____ rigidity is stiffness of the neck with decreased range of motion.
15. Pupils seen with head injury, bleeding in the brain, direct trauma to the eye, or cataract surgery.
16. Has a normal respiratory rate of 40 breaths/min.

113. To assess the extremities, consider the functional implications of any _____ or _____ and the underlying _____ . Assess the patient's general _____, body proportions, and ease of _____. Be certain to note any _____ in the range of motion or any unusual _____ in the _____ of a joint.

114. Decreased range of motion in the extremities is common in patients with arthritis, _____, or _____.

115. List 11 things that should be evaluated as part of examining the extremities.

_____
_____
_____
_____
_____
_____
_____
_____
_____
_____
_____

116. Match each of the following lower extremity pulses with the correct location.

Pulse
a. Dorsalis pedis
b. Femoral
c. Posterior tibial
d. Popliteal

Location
_____ In the inguinal region, about halfway between the anterior superior iliac spine and the symphysis pubis
_____ On the dorsum of the foot, lateral to the great toe extensor tendon
_____ In the back of the knee joint
_____ Posterior to the medial malleolus of the ankle

117. Pitting edema:
  a. is swelling caused by accumulation of blood in the tissues
  b. is said to be present when pressure applied to an edematous area results in a depression in the skin
  c. should be checked for over the dorsum of each foot, behind each medial malleolus, and in the popliteal recess
  d. is considered to indicate the presence of a serious condition only when it is four-plus

118. Identify how much edema is represented by each value of the four-point scale:

    One-plus: _____

    Two-plus: _____

    Three-plus: _____

    Four-plus: _____

119. T F If possible, the spine should be inspected from both the side and from behind.

120. T F From behind the patient, the EMT-I should assess that the normal cervical, thoracic, and lumbar curves are visible.

121. T F From the back, an imaginary line drawn from the spinous process of C1 should run perpendicular to the ground and between the gluteal cleft.

122. Describe how the spine should be palpated during the physical examination.

    _____
    _____
    _____
    _____
    _____

123. A patient with paresthesias:
    a. has numbness or tingling sensation in the arms or legs
    b. may have possible spinal cord damage or local circulatory problems
    c. should be treated as if he or she has possible extremity fractures
    d. a and b

12 Patient Assessment

CHAPTER TERMINAL OBJECTIVES

On completion of this chapter, the EMT-Intermediate will be able to integrate the principles of history taking and techniques of a physical exam to perform patient assessment on an emergency patient.

For the multiple-choice questions, select the single best answer to each question. For the matching questions, select the best corresponding answer for each item. Because there are sometimes more items than corresponding answers, some items may not be used.

1. _____ _____ is a structured method of evaluating a patient's physical condition.

2. A _____ is a subjective indication of a disease or condition as perceived by the patient.

3. A _____ is an objective finding detected by you, such as a rash or deformed arm.

4. List six phases of assessment.

   _____
   _____
   _____
   _____
   _____
   _____

5. List four pieces of information the emergency medical dispatcher (EMD) can typically provide to the responding emergency medical services (EMS) crew.

   _____
   _____
   _____
   _____

6. List five on-scene observations that should be made by the EMT-I.

   _____

   _____

   _____

   _____

   _____

7. The first phase of patient assessment is the:
   a. resuscitation phase
   b. initial assessment
   c. scene size-up
   d. focused trauma assessment

8. Potentially hazardous situations include calls to:
   a. high crime or drug use areas
   b. gang fights
   c. scenes involving domestic violence
   d. all of the above

9. _____ _____ _____ is a set of guidelines for prehospital care providers to follow that minimizes one's exposure to contagious diseases.

10. Latex, nitrile, or vinyl gloves:
    a. should be worn whenever the EMT-I is likely to come in contact with blood or other body fluids, mucous membranes, or nonintact skin of any patient
    b. are not needed when handling items soiled with blood or body fluids
    c. protect the EMT-I from sharp objects such as wood, metal, or glass
    d. should be worn when taking a blood pressure

11. T F Protective eyewear or masks should be worn whenever there is a potential for splashing or spraying of blood or body fluids to your eyes, nose, or mouth.

12. T F Avoid recapping of needles—always dispose of sharp objects in medical waste containers.

13. You arrive at a scene where a man was shot by his wife. He can be seen lying on the ground next to the front door. He appears unresponsive. The wife is standing beside him with weapon in hand. She pleads for you to come help him. Police are not on scene yet. You should:
    a. rush up to her, get the weapon, and handcuff her hands behind her back
    b. stay back an appropriate distance and wait until police arrive to secure the scene before entering
    c. have the wife surrender the weapon to you, then initiate care for the husband
    d. have the wife come to you with her hands raised in the air, then take the weapon from her

14. You arrive at the scene where five people have been shot. Police were there first and have secured the area. You should call for additional help:
    a. after you have triaged the patients
    b. once the patients are loaded into the ambulance
    c. after initial assessments have been done on all the patients
    d. immediately on arriving on the scene

15. You and your partner are treating a patient who overdosed on phencyclidine (PCP) and a host of other drugs. Several family members are standing around watching you provide care. Police are not at the scene. Initially, the patient is subdued and allows you to begin your assessment. Then he begins thrashing about, attempting to kick and strike you and your partner. You should:
    a. move to a safe area and wait for police to arrive
    b. have the family members sign a refusal and then leave the scene
    c. wrestle the patient to the ground and restrain him
    d. hit the patient on the head with your clipboard to subdue him

16. As part of evaluating a patient, all available information must be gathered. The force that causes an injury and how it is applied to the body is referred to as the:
    a. chief complaint
    b. mechanism of injury
    c. kinematic factor
    d. primary mechanism

17. Which of the following is part of the *initial assessment* of a patient?
    a. obtaining a general impression
    b. inspecting and palpating the patient for injuries
    c. assessing for distal pulses, and motor function and sensation in each extremity
    d. obtaining baseline vital signs

18. You are called to the scene where a 47-year-old man suddenly collapsed at work. As you come through the door you can see him lying supine on the floor next to his desk. There are several bystanders attempting to provide care. By your observation you determine that he is unresponsive. There is no indication of trauma. Which of the following assessment steps should be done first?
    a. obtain a blood pressure
    b. check for a pulse
    c. open the airway
    d. assess the breathing

19. You have opened the airway and assessed for breathing. The patient is apneic. The next thing you should do is:
    a. obtain a blood pressure
    b. check for a pulse
    c. assess the airway
    d. begin delivering ventilatory support

20. The general impression of the patient is formed by your immediate _____ assessment and the patient's _____ complaint.

21. If you suspect _____ and potential _____ to the cervical spine, stabilize the spine.

22. Place a checkmark beside those conditions regarded as life threatening.
    _____ An obstructed airway
    _____ A fractured arm
    _____ Capillary bleeding
    _____ Marked breathing difficulty
    _____ Severe bleeding

23. Fill in the meaning for each letter of the AVPU mnemonic.

    A: _____

    V: _____

    P: _____

    U: _____

24. If the patient is conscious and able to speak clearly, the:
    a. breathing is within normal levels
    b. blood pressure is normal
    c. airway is open
    d. pulse rate is adequate

25. A patient is unconscious after falling from a motorcycle that was traveling at a high rate of speed. To open his airway you should:
    a. stabilize the cervical spine and perform the jaw-thrust maneuver
    b. perform the head tilt/chin lift
    c. place a pillow under his shoulder blades and move his head into "sniffing position"
    d. logroll him onto his side and perform the head tilt/chin lift

26. List three techniques that should be used to evaluate the effectiveness of a patient's breathing.

    _____

    _____

    _____

27. A 20-year-old patient is unconscious from a drug overdose. Assessment reveals that he responds to painful stimuli by moaning and withdrawing, has shallow respirations at a rate of 8 breaths/min, a pulse rate of 46 BPM, a blood pressure of 100/74, and a pulse oximetry reading of 90%. You should:
    a. ventilate the patient by either mouth to mask or by an adjunct device supplied with high-concentration oxygen
    b. administer 15 L/min of oxygen via nonrebreather mask
    c. deliver cardiopulmonary resuscitation (CPR)
    d. place the patient's head in a neutral position

28. List five things that can be used to determine whether you are providing the patient with effective ventilatory support.

    _____

    _____

    _____

    _____

    _____

29. Describe when a patient should receive a high concentration of oxygen.

_____

_____

_____

_____

_____

30. T F The brachial pulse should be palpated when assessing circulation in the responsive adult patient.

31. T F Medical patients who are at least 1 year old, pulseless, and in ventricular fibrillation should receive CPR and defibrillation.

32. Match each of the following pulse locations with the approximate systolic blood pressure its presence represents.

   Pulse Location
   a. Carotid artery
   b. Femoral artery
   c. Radial artery

   Systolic Pressure
   _____ 80 mm Hg
   _____ 60 mm Hg
   _____ 70 mm Hg

33. Mottled red, pale, or blue skin is associated with:
    a. kidney disease
    b. cocaine ingestion
    c. anemia
    d. poor perfusion

34. Jaundiced skin is indicative of:
    a. heart attack
    b. allergic reaction
    c. liver disease
    d. high blood pressure

35. Pallor is seen with which of the following conditions?
    a. diabetic coma
    b. shock
    c. heatstroke
    d. fever

36. Capillary refill:
    a. is checked by pressing on the nail bed of the patient's finger or toe, releasing the pressure, and determining the time it takes for the nail bed to return to its initial color
    b. that is slow (greater than 2 seconds) indicates adequate tissue perfusion, whereas capillary refill that is fast (less than 2 seconds) indicates a state of poor perfusion
    c. is assessed at the time of evaluating skin color and temperature
    d. should be assessed only in the conscious patient

37. Capillary refill can be used to effectively assess circulation in which of the following?
    a. 44-year-old woman who has been shot in the head with a large-caliber gun
    b. 5-year-old boy who fell from a third-story window
    c. 19-year-old woman suffering from vaginal bleeding
    d. 70-year-old man who is experiencing heart failure

38. Priority patients:
    a. are unstable patients who require more advanced level care as soon as possible
    b. are typically transported to the nearest appropriate medical facility
    c. should be promptly transported
    d. all of the above

39. List 10 patient conditions that would be considered priorities.

    _____
    _____
    _____
    _____
    _____
    _____
    _____
    _____
    _____
    _____
    _____

40. You are called to treat a patient experiencing congestive heart failure. He is awake and talking, has labored respirations at a rate of 22, a pulse rate of 136, a blood pressure of 190/112, and cool, moist skin. The pulse oximetry reading is 84%, and auscultation of chest reveals bilateral crackles. This patient should be regarded as:
    a. unstable
    b. stable

41. The resuscitation phase of patient assessment includes all of the following *except:*
    a. splinting fractures
    b. initiating airway management
    c. controlling hemorrhage
    d. initiation of shock management

42. Match each of the letters of the mnemonic OPQRST with the question each represents.

    Letter
    a. O
    b. P
    c. Q
    d. R
    e. S
    f. T

    Description
    _____ Does the symptom come and go, or is it always there?
    _____ When did the problem begin?
    _____ Does the pain go anywhere?
    _____ On a scale of 1 to 10, how bad is the pain?
    _____ What makes the problem worse?
    _____ What is the pain like—is it sharp, crushing, or viselike?

43. Which of the following is part of the focused history and physical exam of a trauma patient who has a significant mechanism of injury?
    a. initial assessment
    b. thorough neurological evaluation
    c. detailed examination
    d. rapid trauma assessment

44. List the seven areas of the body that should be examined as part of the rapid trauma assessment.

    _____

    _____

    _____

    _____

    _____

    _____

    _____

45. List the meaning for each letter of the mnemonic DCAP-BTLS.

    D: _____

    C: _____

    A: _____

    P: _____

    B: _____

    T: _____

    L: _____

    S: _____

46. Describe what should be done as part of the focused history and physical exam if cervical spine injury is suspected.

_____

_____

_____

_____

_____

47. Place a checkmark beside those activities that are considered part of the detailed assessment.
    _____ Determining the chief complaint
    _____ Examining the neck, chest, and abdomen
    _____ Palpating the pelvis and lower extremities
    _____ Checking pupillary response
    _____ Ensuring a patent airway with regard to possible cervical spine injury
    _____ Checking the effectiveness of breathing
    _____ Having the patient grasp your hands
    _____ Palpating for a radial pulse
    _____ Obtaining the patient's history

48. T F A 30-year-old patient who has a simple cut finger should receive a detailed assessment.

49. T F A detailed assessment should be performed on "priority" patients while at the scene.

50. In a stable patient, repeat your assessment every _____ minutes. In an unstable patient, repeat the assessment every _____ minutes.
    a. 10; 5
    b. 15; 5
    c. 8; 4
    d. 5; 2

51. List those things the EMT-I should do as part of the ongoing assessment.

_____

_____

_____

_____

_____

_____

_____

52. T F Fracture stabilization, bandaging, and immobilization to the stretcher improve comfort and make it safer to transport the trauma patient to the hospital.

53. Which facility a patient is transported to depends on:
    a. available transport modes
    b. patient condition
    c. available facilities
    d. all of the above

54. Helicopter transport is appropriate:
    a. for removing patients from freeway accidents
    b. for transporting combative patients
    c. for conveying patients contaminated by hazardous materials
    d. during lightning or high wind conditions

55. List six pieces of information that should be communicated to the medical direction or the receiving hospital when transporting a patient.

    _____
    _____
    _____
    _____
    _____
    _____
    _____

56. Describe the benefits of accurate documentation.

    _____
    _____
    _____
    _____
    _____
    _____
    _____

CROSSWORD PUZZLE EXERCISE

57. Complete the following crossword puzzle.

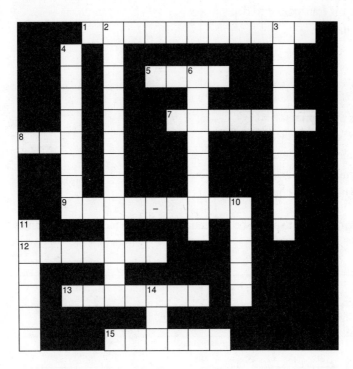

ACROSS

1. Typically, persons develop tachycardia and then _____ with respiratory compromise.
5. Mnemonic used to determine patient's level of responsiveness.
7. With a stable patient, the ongoing assessment should be repeated every _____ minutes.
8. Abbreviation that means the use of protective equipment to reduce exposure to contagious diseases.
9. Mnemonic for the rapid head-to-toe examination of a trauma patient.
12. Portion of the patient assessment that is a rapid, organized, and systematic evaluation.
13. _____ impression is based on immediate sensory assessment of environment and the chief complaint.
15. During the initial assessment if the patient is responsive, check quickly for a _____ pulse.

DOWN

2. Performed as necessary throughout assessment as soon as life-threatening problems are identified.
3. The EMT-I must immediately assist ventilation or ventilate patients with _____ breathing.
4. Portion of assessment that is an organized subjective and objective examination of the patient.
6. Also referred to as unstable patients.
10. _____ size-up is an assessment of the scene and surroundings.
11. The patient who is responsive and can speak clearly has an open _____.
14. Skin color seen with alcohol or cocaine ingestion, anaphylaxis, hyperthermia, stroke, or heart attack.

13 Clinical Decision Making

CHAPTER TERMINAL OBJECTIVES

On completion of this chapter, the EMT-Intermediate will be able to apply the decision-making process to form a field impression from information gathered during patient assessment.

For the multiple-choice questions, select the single best answer to each question. For the matching questions, select the best corresponding answer for each item. Because there are sometimes more items than corresponding answers, some items may not be used.

1. Describe the difference between the prehospital environment and the emergency department environment.

   _____

   _____

   _____

   _____

2. Place a checkmark beside those patients considered to be experiencing critical life-threatening emergencies.
   - _____ 61-year-old with a gunshot wound to the head
   - _____ 28-year-old suffering from acute gastroenteritis and experiencing frequent episodes of forceful vomiting and diarrhea
   - _____ 32-year-old who has severe wounds to his chest, abdomen, and extremities from an explosion
   - _____ 75-year-old who has a history of chronic obstructive pulmonary disorder (COPD) and is in extreme respiratory distress
   - _____ 45-year-old who has a fractured and deformed lower leg
   - _____ 81-year-old patient with cancer who is emaciated, obtunded, and has minimal respirations

3. T F Usually the mechanism of injury itself is enough to alert the provider to the potential for serious injury.

4. T F Patients with "potentially serious" injuries or illnesses require the greatest amount of scrutiny and evaluation.

5. T F Chronic medical conditions seldom affect a patient's response to new illnesses or injuries.

6. Well-defined protocols, standing orders, and patient care algorithms:
   a. eliminate the need to contact on-line medical command for orders
   b. can prepare the EMT-I for each potential patient encounter
   c. provide a standardized approach to common presentations
   d. are usually referred to while delivering patient care

7. Medical ambiguity:
   a. can cause the EMT-I to misclassify the patient
   b. puts the EMT-I on the correct course for evaluating and treating patients
   c. is a strength of patient care protocols
   d. occurs when the patient is focused on all aspects of his or her illness

8. List four disadvantages of protocols.

   _____

   _____

   _____

   _____

9. The mechanism of collecting, integrating, and synthesizing information takes part largely at the _____ level.

10. The product of critical thinking is an understanding of the patient's _____ or _____ and

    development of a _____ plan.

11. Match each of the following components of the critical thinking process with the correct definition.

    Component of Thinking Process
    a. Concept formation
    b. Data interpretation
    c. Application of principle
    d. Evaluation
    e. Reflection on action

    Definition
    _____ Comparing current information with past education and experience to draw conclusions
    _____ Formulating an initial impression of what disease processes or injuries are affecting the patient
    _____ Critiquing the actions and interventions performed on each individual call
    _____ Pattern of understanding based on initial information gathered
    _____ Constantly reassessing the patient

12. Radio alert tones suddenly pierce the air, and the dispatcher announces that an ambulance is needed at a local bakery for a female who burned her arm on an oven. From this information, the EMT-I begins to:
    a. interpret data
    b. form the first concepts
    c. evaluate the situation
    d. formulate an initial impression

13. General patient _____ can provide clues to the patient's mental status.

14. Mental status directly relates to _____ of the central nervous system (CNS), electrolyte disturbances,

    intoxication, _____ trauma, and _____ disorders.

15. Initial interventions are selected based on the _____ interpretation of all the _____ the EMT-I

    has received with the current patient, as well as _____ patients who have been cared for in the past.

16. The EMT-I should routinely reevaluate the _____ signs and physical state of the patient to determine the response to _____ or progression of the physiological insult.

17. T F Generally, new information does not change the EMT-I's working diagnosis.

18. T F Honest and in-depth reflection on the aspects of the run that were challenging will help the EMT-I prepare for the next patient with similar problems.

19. List the eight elements that form the foundation of critical thinking for the EMT-I.

_____
_____
_____
_____
_____
_____
_____
_____

20. The level of understanding the EMT-I possesses regarding how injuries and diseases affect patients is acquired through all of the following *except:*
    a. training
    b. continuing education
    c. patient encounters
    d. type of emergency medical services (EMS) system

21. One of the true attributes that separate the seasoned, veteran EMT-I from a new graduate is the:
    a. salary he or she earns
    b. ability to work under extreme pressure
    c. amount of knowledge he or she has regarding human anatomy and physiology
    d. ability to work with medical direction

22. Which of the following occurs in reaction to stressful situations?
    a. The sympathetic nervous system stimulation is blocked.
    b. Critical thinking skills are enhanced.
    c. The abilities to focus on problems and perform thorough assessments are improved.
    d. Muscle strength and reflexes are increased.

23. The _____ nervous system releases _____, which is responsible for the "fight or flight" response.

24. The useful aspects of this _____ surge are heightened senses of vision and _____ .

25. Describe strategies for effective thinking under pressure.

___

26. List five key points that are part of the EMT-I's mental checklist for effective thinking during each patient encounter.

___

27. List two questions the EMT-I should address while assessing the patient for a current acute event.

___

28. List the "six R's" the EMT-I should use during each patient encounter.

___

29. List five critical questions the EMT-I should keep in mind while approaching the patient.

___

30. The hallmark of every EMT-I is the ability to:
    a. recognize a life-threatening emergency and react quickly
    b. always form a clear working diagnosis
    c. occasionally reevaluate the condition of the patient
    d. perform all required skills perfectly

31. The initial assessment is designed to:
    a. identify the chief complaint and determine the initial treatment
    b. quickly identify critical patients and prompt the EMT-I to intervene with airway, respiratory, and cardiac support
    c. determine the patient's mental status, vital signs, and the presence of any injuries
    d. make the EMT-I aware of the environmental surroundings

CROSSWORD PUZZLE EXERCISE

32. Complete the crossword puzzle.

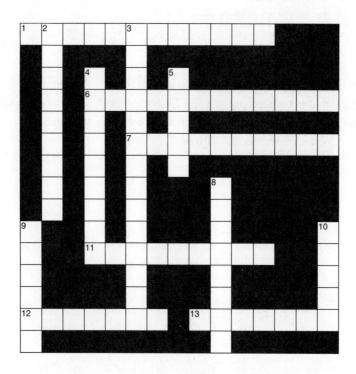

ACROSS

1. Patterns of behaviors and actions that promote efficient and appropriate patient care.
6. Ongoing assessment of the patient to determine change in condition or response to therapy.
7. Data _____ style is the divergent development of ideas versus convergent focused processing.
11. Analysis that is reflective in nature versus impulsive action.
12. Allows the EMT-I to gain further insight into the current crisis.
13. _____ formation is a pattern of understanding based on initial information gathered.

DOWN

2. Medical _____ is a vagueness in symptoms or complaints.
3. Data _____ is comparing current information with past education and experience.
4. Well-defined practice guidelines for specific patient presentations, illnesses, or injuries.
5. Type of trauma where mechanism of injury places the patient at great risk of death or disability.
8. _____ making style allows the EMT-I to prepare for additional interventions.
9. Spectrum of _____ is the wide range of patient presentations, illnesses, or injuries.
10. _____ or flight response involves activation of the sympathetic nervous system.

14 Communications

CHAPTER TERMINAL OBJECTIVES

On completion of this chapter, the EMT-Intermediate will be able to follow an accepted format for the dissemination of patient information in verbal form, either in person or over the radio.

For the multiple-choice questions, select the single best answer to each question. For the matching questions, select the best corresponding answer for each item. Because there are sometimes more items than corresponding answers, some items may not be used.

1. Effective _____ is essential to the smooth and _____ operation of the emergency medical services (EMS) team.

2. There must be a coordinated _____ system that allows information to flow internally and _____, in both routine and _____ modes.

3. Communications that take place as part of providing EMS are done verbally through _____ means or _____.

4. Identify, by numbering, the order of the basic communications model.
   _____ You select the medium for sending your message, such as speaking to someone face to face or over the radio or telephone, leaving a voice mail, writing a note or letter, or sending a fax or electronic mail.
   _____ The receiver provides feedback to you that the message has been received and understood.
   _____ You form an idea or message you wish to pass along.
   _____ Your message arrives at its destination, and the receiver decodes it.
   _____ You encode message in a language that can be understood by the person who will receive the message or in a manner that is appropriate for the situation.

5. Label the components of the basic communication model shown below.

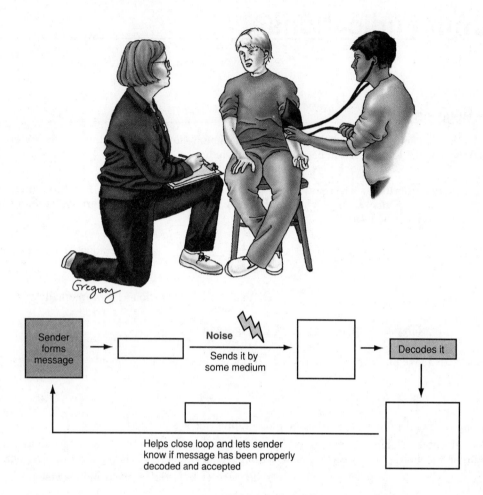

6. _____ is putting a message into words, numbers, symbols, pictures, codes, signals, and such.
   a. Forming an idea
   b. Encoding
   c. Decoding
   d. Providing feedback

7. Describe why feedback is particularly critical in emergency communications.

_____

_____

_____

_____

_____

8. T F Verbal communication is the only way to exchange system and patient information with other members of the EMS team.

9. T F Semantic factors only act to boost communications.

10. T F To improve your communications, make sure they are unambiguous, to the point, and include ample technical and semantic jargon.

11. T F Using abbreviations and acronyms commonly used by the physicians, nurses, and other health care professionals in your local hospitals can facilitate communications.

12. List the factors that lead to noise in the communication model.

_____
_____
_____
_____
_____
_____
_____

13. List two techniques that can be used to overcome noise in emergency communications.

_____
_____

14. The typical EMS communication system configuration includes all of the following *except:*
    a. telephones
    b. automatic vehicle-locating system
    c. pagers
    d. radios

15. T F Ready availability of the telephone makes it an excellent communication link for EMS systems.

16. T F The recommended telephone number for accessing EMS is 4-1-1.

17. T F The enhanced version of the recommended emergency telephone number includes a visual system that displays the caller's telephone number and address.

18. Dedicated land lines:
    a. are telephone lines with intermittent connections from one geographical location to another
    b. may be used by dispatchers to notify EMS personnel of emergency calls
    c. are not an efficient method of communicating with receiving hospitals, communication consoles, or police and fire dispatch centers
    d. require the dispatcher to go through a switchboard to reach EMS personnel

19. One problem that can occur with cellular telephones is that:
    a. EMT-Is are often not familiar with how to use the equipment
    b. they can only transmit voice communications
    c. they typically have poor reception in urban areas
    d. available cells can become tied up with public communication

20. Match each of the following radio system components with the correct characteristics.

    Component
    a. Base station
    b. Mobile radios
    c. Portable radios

    Characteristic
    _____ Typical power output of 1 to 5 W
    _____ Typical power output of 45 to 275 W
    _____ Mounted in vehicles such as ambulances, rescue units, or supervisory vehicles
    _____ Most powerful radio in the system
    _____ Typical power output of 40 to 100 W
    _____ Allow communications to take place while EMT-Is are away from the ambulance
    _____ Usually located in a dispatch center that serves as the communication network for the EMS system
    _____ Characteristic transmission range is 10 to 15 miles over the average terrain
    _____ Hand-held devices
    _____ May be controlled by a remote console
    _____ Will maximize coverage when it is held in a vertical and elevated position

21. Which of the following statements best describes a remote console?
    a. It resembles a telephone dial that causes pulsed tones to be sent out over the air when dialed.
    b. It receives a signal on one frequency and retransmits that signal on another frequency.
    c. It receives only properly coded messages.
    d. It is a control console connected to the base station by telephone lines.

22. All of the following factors will decrease the range of a mobile radio *except:*
    a. dense foliage
    b. mountainous terrain
    c. water
    d. urban areas

23. Radio frequencies are designated by cycles per second called:
    a. bands
    b. watts
    c. megahertz
    d. joules

24. Match the following MHz ranges with the correct bands.

    Range
    a. 5 to 25 MHz
    b. 30 to 50 MHz
    c. 80 to 95 MHz
    d. 450 to 470 MHz
    e. 150 to 170 MHz

    Band
    _____ VHF low band
    _____ VHF high band
    _____ UHF

25. T F UHF has a shorter range and better penetration in dense urban areas than VHF.

26. T F Medical channels 9 and 10 are used for EMT-I–to–physician communications.

27. T F VHF low band is limited to voice communications because it is against Federal Communications Commission (FCC) regulations to transmit telemetry in VHF low band frequencies.

28. T F UHF frequencies are often paired together to allow duplex operations.

29. VHF high band:
    a. is not as effective for communications in metropolitan areas as VHF low band
    b. signals are transmitted in a straight line and do not follow the curvature of the earth
    c. base station antennas are usually located on low sites to increase the area of coverage
    d. is more susceptible to electrical disturbances or skip phenomenon

30. Radios that operate on the 800-MHz frequency:
    a. permit more effective utilization of the assigned frequencies and can permit interagency communications
    b. are not effective for use in major metropolitan operations
    c. have transmissions that are able to bend and follow the curvature of the earth, allowing transmission to stations over the horizon
    d. have poor penetration of buildings

31. Maximizing the range for low-power mobile or portable radios is best achieved by the use of:
    a. repeater systems
    b. encoders
    c. decoders
    d. remote consoles

32. Describe how repeater systems work.

    _____
    _____
    _____
    _____
    _____

33. T F Repeater systems receive and retransmit on the same frequency.

34. T F Repeaters can only be located in satellite base stations.

35. The process by which the repeater station receiving the strongest incoming signal is chosen to rebroadcast that signal is referred to as:
    a. transmitting
    b. voting
    c. repeating
    d. casting

36. Match each of the following modes with the correct characteristics.

    Mode
    a. Simplex
    b. Duplex
    c. Multiplex

    Characteristic

    _____ Most complicated type of communication

    _____ The EMT-I must avoid starting any communication until all other communications have ended

    _____ Used by many base station hospitals that provide on-line medical direction

    _____ Communication can occur in only one direction at a time

    _____ Has the ability to simultaneously transmit two or more different types of information (e.g., voice and telemetry) in either or both directions over the same frequency

    _____ Two separate frequencies are paired together to allow simultaneous transmission and reception to take place

    _____ Least complicated type of communication

37. All of the following are functions of the FCC *except:*
    a. issuing frequency and license regulations
    b. conducting spot checks of base stations and their records
    c. monitoring assigned radio frequencies
    d. providing funds for biotelemetry communications

38. T F Because of federal regulations, cellular telephones cannot be used for EMS communications.

39. T F The FCC is the agency charged with dispatching ambulances across state borders.

40. Describe why proper documentation during an EMS event is important.

    _____

    _____

    _____

    _____

    _____

41. Describe the precautions that should be taken at the hospital to ensure patient confidentiality.

    _____

    _____

    _____

    _____

    _____

    _____

42. Advantages of electronic information gathering include all the following *except:*
    a. it can allow for real-time capturing of information
    b. medical diagnostic technology can be integrated into it
    c. it eliminates the burden of ensuring patient confidentiality
    d. it facilitates data collection for quality improvement, research activities, and patient billing

43. Define each of the following terms.

    Biotelemetry: _____

    _____

    Computer: _____

    _____

    Facsimile: _____

    _____

44. List five causes of interference.

    _____

    _____

    _____

    _____

    _____

45. Define what is meant by the term *encrypting,* and state why it is used in the prehospital care setting.

    _____

    _____

    _____

    _____

    _____

46. What precautions should be taken at the hospital to prevent breaching of patient confidentiality?

    _____

    _____

    _____

    _____

    _____

CROSSWORD PUZZLE EXERCISE

47. Complete the following crossword puzzle.

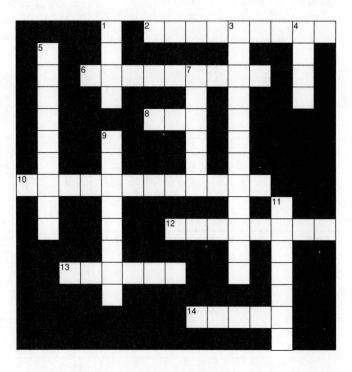

ACROSS

2. Duplex system that allows transmission of voice and data simultaneously.
6. Radio frequencies designated by cycles per second.
8. Federal agency that controls and regulates all radio communications in the United States.
10. Process of transmitting physiologic data, such as an ECG, over distance, usually by radio.
12. A pooling of frequencies.
13. Converting a message into understandable language.
14. Things that interfere with receiving a message.

DOWN

1. The intended meaning of the communication.
3. Preventing or inhibiting clear reception.
4. Means to immediately repeat back each radio transmission received.
5. Relates to the meaning of words.
7. Putting an idea or message into a language or code.
9. Confirmation from the receiver that a message has been received and understood.
11. Communication system that transmits and receives on the same frequency.

48. List the steps in the progression of a typical response to an emergency.

_____
_____
_____
_____
_____
_____

49. Responsibilities of the emergency medical dispatcher (EMD) include all of the following *except:*
    a. giving medical direction to EMT-Is working in the field
    b. directing the appropriate emergency response unit(s) to the scene
    c. monitoring and overseeing communications between EMS and other public safety personnel
    d. obtaining, in a rapid and controlled manner, as much information about the emergency from the caller as possible

50. T   F   Typically, the first information the EMD should solicit is the age and weight of the patient.

51. T   F   When gathering information from a caller, the EMD should solicit a call-back number in case of accidental telephone disconnect.

52. T   F   After an EMS unit is dispatched, many EMS systems have the EMD give the caller prearrival medical instructions over the phone.

53. List at least five reasons for medical communications.

_____
_____
_____
_____
_____
_____

54. List two reasons why a standard format should be used when transmitting the findings of a patient assessment.

_____
_____

55. All of the following information should be conveyed to medical command *except:*
    a. a description of the scene
    b. the patient's name
    c. a brief, pertinent history of the present illness
    d. an estimated time of arrival at the hospital

56. T   F   To prevent mistakes, the EMT-I should avoid repeating back orders from the medical direction physician.

57. T   F   Even when the orders from medical command seem inappropriate for the patient's condition, the EMT-I should not question the physician over the air.

58. T   F   The EMT-I should keep the physician aware of any changes in the patient's condition.

59. Using the following case presentation, organize the information into a report that can be delivered to your local medical direction.

   It is a Friday afternoon, and you receive a call to aid a "female short of breath." After a 4-minute response time, you arrive at the address given by the dispatcher. A fire engine first-responder company is already on scene. You pull the oxygen unit, jump kit, drug box, and ECG monitor out of the ambulance and carry them to the house. A firefighter meets you at the front door of the single house and says, "She's in the living room . . . looks like an allergic reaction."
   You enter to find the 21-year-old patient sitting bolt upright on the couch. One of the first responders has just taken her pulse, respiration, and blood pressure and reports, "The patient has a respiratory rate of 24, a pulse rate of 132, a blood pressure of 164/82, and cool, moist skin."
   Your partner auscultates the lung sounds while you check the pulse oximetry. The patient's mother, who is visibly upset, states, "She was mowing the lawn when she got stung by a bee. She immediately started itching all over. Then she said she couldn't catch her breath." Auscultation of the chest reveals bilateral wheezing, and the pulse oximetry shows an Sao_2 of 88%. You note that there is swelling about the patient's face, particularly around the eyes. On questioning, the mother tells you the patient is allergic to bee stings.
   Your partner sets up a 1000-cc bag of normal saline with a macrodrip administration set and clears the line of air while you attach an ECG monitor to the patient. You tell your partner, "Looks like sinus tachycardia, with no ectopy." The IV line is quickly established in the patient's right forearm and run at a TKO rate. You deliver a breathing treatment while your partner draws up and administers epinephrine subcutaneously. The patient responds favorably to the treatment. So far, she has received oxygen at 15 L/min via nonrebreather mask, an IV of normal saline delivered at a TKO rate, 0.3 cc of 1:1000 epinephrine subcutaneously, and an albuterol breathing treatment. Your reassessment reveals the patient has a respiratory rate of 18, a pulse rate of 116, a blood pressure of 130/84, and warm, dry skin. Auscultation of her chest reveals a marked decrease in the bilateral wheezing, and she appears to be moving air much better. The ECG monitor continues to show sinus tachycardia without ectopy, and the pulse oximetry reveals an Sao_2 of 94%.

60. List least three reasons for verbally communicating patient information to the receiving hospital.

61. When speaking into the radio, the EMT-I should:
    a. speak in a monotone
    b. use codes in all situations
    c. use words like "affirmative" and "negative"
    d. voice activate the system before using the frequency

62. Proper radio communication techniques include:
    a. pressing the transmit button for approximately 1 second before you begin to speak
    b. holding the microphone 10 to 12 inches away from your face
    c. speaking quickly to avoid tying up radio time
    d. conveying the patient's name over the air

63. T F Codes and abbreviations should be used routinely.

64. T F Slang and profanity should not be conveyed over the air.

65. T F Longer transmissions are preferred when communicating with the dispatch center.

66. T F Always listen to the frequency to be sure no one is transmitting before you start talking.

67. T F Before transmitting, reduce the background noise as much as possible by closing the window, turning the volume down on other radios, and so on.

68. T F Hold portable radios in a horizontal position to achieve maximum radio coverage.

69. Which of the following is considered appropriate handling and maintenance of portable radio equipment?
    a. The radio should be carried in the hip pocket.
    b. The exterior case should be cleaned with solvents.
    c. A fresh, recharged battery should be placed in the unit every day.
    d. The radio should be placed in the charging device whenever the radio is not in use.

70. EMS communication capabilities are often limited during disasters because of what four factors?

_____

_____

_____

_____

15 Documentation

CHAPTER TERMINAL OBJECTIVES

On completion of this chapter, the EMT-Intermediate will be able apply the necessary knowledge and skills to properly document various types of emergency medical services (EMS) events.

For the multiple-choice questions, select the single best answer to each question. For the matching questions, select the best corresponding answer for each item. Because there are sometimes more items than corresponding answers in the matching questions, some items may not be used.

1. List three reasons for patient care documentation.

2. Describe why EMS run reports are important to the EMS system.

3. Hand-held data entry or pen-based computers:
   a. increase the amount of information that can be managed but do little to expedite data entry
   b. allow the data to be analyzed and quality improvement activities performed more quickly and efficiently
   c. usually transfer patient information to the hospital using hard-wired telephone systems
   d. transfer the data from the field to administrative entities in about the same amount of time as when paper-based systems are used

4. Which of the following is true regarding documenting information on the run report?
   a. When the situation is unclear, it is acceptable for the EMT-I to document assumptions about what has taken place.
   b. It is better to be general rather than specific.
   c. Cursive is preferred to printing.
   d. The EMT-I must be as objective as possible.

5. A _____ should be used to record information on the run report.
   a. felt-tip pen
   b. pencil
   c. ballpoint pen
   d. highlighter pen

6. Which of the following is true regarding the use of abbreviations as part of prehospital documentation?
   a. Abbreviations allow more information to be included in narrative sections of the run report.
   b. Using abbreviations increases the amount of time it takes to document information.
   c. Abbreviations have only one meaning.
   d. Abbreviations used in the prehospital setting should be limited to two letters.

CROSSWORD PUZZLE EXERCISE

7. Complete the following crossword puzzle.

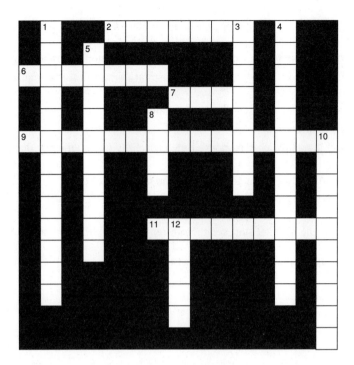

ACROSS

2. Type of writing that is often more readable than cursive writing.
6. Word that is formed by combining the first letter or letters of a name or a phrase.
7. Acronym for Subjective, Objective, Assessment, Plan.
9. An example is, "The patient was uncooperative."
11. This is a description of what you observed at the scene.

DOWN

1. Process used to record patient information.
3. First block of information on the run report.
4. Documentation that follows care of patient by identifying steps taken in the order they were performed.
5. The EMS run report is a key source for data _____.
8. The treatment you provide or that which is refused by the patient.
10. What the patient experiences and tells you about his or her condition.
12. _____ boxes or lines render a report incomplete.

8. T F   Gloves used to provide patient care may be worn while the EMT-I fills out the run report.

9. T F   To increase efficiency, the run report should be filled out close to where patient care is occurring.

10. T F   Recording of information on the run report is the first step of providing patient care to ill or injured patients.

11. Place a checkmark next to those statements considered extraneous or nonprofessional information.

    _____ "The patient stated he was already seen in the hospital five times for the same problem and they didn't do anything to help him."

    _____ "The patient has been feeling ill for the past 48 hours."

    _____ "The patient is stinking drunk."

    _____ "There was a significant delay in response time caused by the emergency department not moving patients through triage fast enough."

    _____ "The patient reports he has had a headache for the past several days."

    _____ "The patient is alert and oriented × 3."

12. T F   Only the EMT-I and the hospital staff see the run report that is filled out about a particular patient.

13. T F   The run report should be reviewed by other EMS team members before it is turned in.

14. List the meaning of the acronym SOAP.

    S: _____

    O: _____

    A: _____

    P: _____

15. Describe the difference between subjective and objective.

    _____

    _____

    _____

    _____

16. Place an "O" (for objective) or an "S" (for subjective) in front of each of the following to represent whether it is an objective or subjective narrative.

    _____ "I can't feel my toes."

    _____ "My head hurts."

    _____ "The steering wheel was bent, and the patient's chest was bruised."

    _____ The patient says he felt nauseous at the same time as his chest started to hurt and he became sweaty.

    _____ Skin is cool, pale, and diaphoretic.

    _____ Patient has decreased grip on right side.

17. Match each of the following assessment methods with the correct description.

    Method
    a. Chronological method
    b. Head-to-toe method
    c. Body systems approach

    Description

    _____ Documents the assessment the same way you performed it. Start by noting the patient's age, sex, and level of consciousness, and how the patient was initially found.

    _____ Uses a comprehensive review of the primary body systems. It includes a detailed review of the skin, skeletal, head, endocrine, respiratory, cardiac, hematological, lymph nodes, gastrointestinal, genitourinary, neurological, and psychiatric systems.

    _____ Documentation follows the care of the patient by identifying the steps taken in the order in which they were performed. It begins with the time of arrival on the scene. Each entry starts with a time notation followed by the pertinent information for that time period.

18. List 10 pieces of information that should be included on the run report.

    _____
    _____
    _____
    _____
    _____
    _____
    _____
    _____
    _____
    _____

19. The chief complaint:
    a. is the reason why the person called for EMS assistance
    b. should be stated in the EMT-I's own words
    c. is denoted as "man down" in cases where the patient is unconscious or in cardiac arrest
    d. is the first piece of information that is written on the run report

20. The past medical history includes:
    a. surgeries and hospitalizations
    b. care being provided before arrival of the EMT-I
    c. pertinent positives and negatives
    d. how the patient describes his or her complaint

21. List those elements of the patient's vital signs that should be documented on the run report.

_____

_____

_____

_____

_____

22. Repeat vital signs:
    a. should be documented on a supplemental sheet that is then attached to the run report
    b. provide important information regarding changes in the patient's condition
    c. are only necessary when medications are administered
    d. should be taken and recorded every minute

23. Documentation of treatments provided should include:

_____

_____

_____

24. Place a checkmark next to those treatments that are described in appropriate detail.
    _____ "placed an endotracheal tube"
    _____ "Proventil, 0.25 mL, by inhalation, administered at 0804 per medical command"
    _____ "applied traction splint to the patient's right leg"
    _____ "IV of D_5W, 18-gauge needle to right antecubital fossa, microdrip administration set, run TKO, established at 1805 according to standing orders"
    _____ "15 L of oxygen administered via nonrebreather mask, started at 10:15 PM."

25. Match each of the following elements of the run report with the correct examples. Elements may be used more than once.

Elements
a. Chief complaint
b. Past medical history
c. Physical assessment
d. Pertinent positives or negatives
e. Patient's response or lack of response to treatment
f. Present history
g. Treatment

Examples
_____ Patient was found sitting at kitchen table on arrival.
_____ Patient denies shortness of breath and nausea.
_____ Cyanosis subsided after oxygen administration.
_____ Chest pain subsided after the patient took a nitroglycerin tablet.
_____ BP 190/110, pulse 110 and regular, labored respirations at a rate of 20 per minute.
_____ Patient says he "is having a hard time breathing."
_____ Patient's blood pressure increased to 110/86 after infusion of 500 mL of normal saline.
_____ Patient takes Diabinese for diabetes.
_____ Patient has deformity and swelling to his left upper leg.
_____ Administered 15 L of oxygen via nonrebreather mask.

26. Which of the following is a "pertinent negative?"
    a. Patient states he feels "a heaviness in his chest."
    b. Chest pain is accompanied by nausea and vomiting.
    c. Shortness of breath is not relieved with oxygen administration.
    d. The patient experienced a syncopal episode following the nitroglycerin administration.

27. As part of documentation, the EMT-I should collect demographic information such as name, _____, sex, date of birth, _____, and _____ _____. In some systems you also may be required to obtain _____ _____, such as type of medical insurance.

28. T F   Once the run report has been completed and signed, it is too late to make corrections.

29. T F   Late entries can be added, without making any other adjustments, after a run report has been completed.

30. Mistakes on run reports should be corrected by:
    a. erasing or scratching out the inaccurate section
    b. indicating that they are errors, initialing and dating them
    c. writing the correct information on a separate sheet and attaching it to the run report
    d. covering them completely with correction fluid

31. The following is an example of information contained on a run report:
    You determine that the patient uses the medication Lopressor instead of Digitalis. Fix the mistake.

    _____

    Patient takes Lasix and Digitalis for hypertension and heart failure.

    _____

32. List three items that should be listed if the normal protocol or standard of care is not followed.

_____

_____

_____

33. List the two things that falsification of information on the run report may lead to.

_____

_____

34. You are the instructor of a continuing education session for EMT-Is. You are showing sample run reports to give the students examples of good documentation. Which of the following should be done to protect patient confidentiality?
    a. Avoid writing the patient's name on the run report.
    b. Write the patient's name in cursive.
    c. Cross out or blacken the patient's name to prevent disclosing his or her name.
    d. List only the last name of the patient.

35. When a patient refuses care:
    a. assessment findings and emergency medical care given should be documented, and the patient should be asked to sign a refusal form
    b. one of the EMT-Is handling the call should sign the form as a witness
    c. documentation should be limited to just identifying the reason for the patient refusal of care and/or transport
    d. a family member should be the first person asked to sign as a witness

36. When documenting care in multiple-casualty incidents, the EMT-I:
    a. should fill the run reports out at the same time as patient care is being delivered
    b. is expected to fill out the run report in the same way he or she would on a typical call
    c. should only complete the treatment section and leave the rest of the report blank
    d. must do the best he or she can with the limited information available

37. T F Documentation of invasive or advanced treatments should include a brief notation as to whether they were done with permission of medical direction.

38. T F Treatments that are attempted without success or problems with delivering treatment should be noted on the run report.

39. T F The only person responsible for signing the run report is the EMT-I who is completing it.

CROSSWORD PUZZLE EXERCISE

40. Complete the following crossword puzzle.

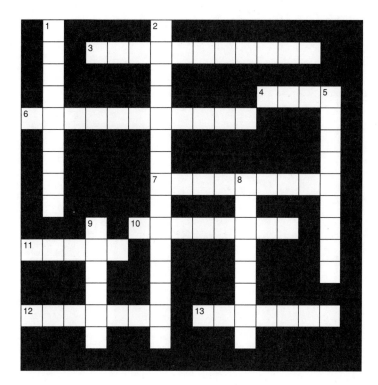

ACROSS

3. Information that includes patient's name, address, age, and telephone number.
4. Medical history of significant illnesses or traumatic injury that the patient has experienced.
6. How the emergency call for assistance is concluded.
7. Portion of the run report that is written out in longhand.
10. Times used to record the run times.
11. Complaint that prompted the patient, family member, friend, or bystander to call for EMS assistance.
12. This history relates to events or complaints associated with the patient's complaint.
13. Remember, if it was not _____ in the report, it was not done.

DOWN

1. The run report provides for a _____ of care.
2. Great care must be taken to protect the patient's right to this.
5. _____ with the run report can cause serious trouble for you.
8. Figure of a human body, with anterior and posterior views.
9. Competent adult patients have the right to _____ treatment.

16 Trauma Systems and Mechanism of Injury

CHAPTER TERMINAL OBJECTIVES

On completion of this chapter, the EMT-Intermediate will be able to apply the principles of kinematics to enhance patient assessment and predict the likelihood of injuries based on the patient's mechanism of injury.

For the multiple-choice questions, select the single best answer to each question. For the matching questions, select the best corresponding answer for each item. Because there are sometimes more items than corresponding answers in the matching questions, some items may not be used.

1. Trauma is the leading cause of death in people ages _____ to _____ years.
   a. 5, 62
   b. 21, 38
   c. 1, 44
   d. 12, 50

2. Trauma:
   a. is linked to alcohol in many fatal motor vehicle crashes
   b. results in 1 million years in lost productivity from disabilities, at a cost of $5 billion
   c. permanently disables 150,000 people each year
   d. is the leading cause of death in people who are older than age 60

3. List the top five causes of unintentional trauma deaths.

   _____

   _____

   _____

   _____

   _____

4. T F In the postincident phase, the focus is on prevention of intentional and unintentional trauma deaths.

5. T F Properly preparing the patient for transportation to an appropriate medical facility is considered part of the incident phase.

6. Describe activities that can be taken by health care providers to reduce trauma.

   _____
   _____
   _____
   _____
   _____

7. The Golden Hour refers to trauma patients receiving _____ within 1 hour of the incident.
   a. advanced life support
   b. surgical intervention
   c. aggressive oxygen therapy
   d. whole blood

8. Definitive intervention provided to the trauma patient within the Golden Hour can enhance _____ and reduce _____.

9. The EMT-I must recognize critically injured patients and ensure that prehospital _____ activities do not unnecessarily delay patient _____.

10. Describe the responsibilities of the EMT-I in the postincident phase of trauma.

    _____
    _____
    _____
    _____
    _____

11. List the eight components of a sophisticated trauma system, and underline those that involve the EMT-I.

    _____
    _____
    _____
    _____
    _____
    _____
    _____
    _____

12. The _____ has taken the lead in describing resources necessary to provide appropriate care to a trauma patient.
    a. American College of Surgeons (ACS)
    b. U.S. Department of Health and Human Services (USDHHS)
    c. U.S. Department of Justice (DOJ)
    d. American Hospital Association (AHA)

13. The document called *Resources for Optimal Care of the Injured Patient* outlines all of the following necessary for an institution to provide quality trauma care *except:*
    a. resources
    b. personnel
    c. training
    d. fees for treatment

14. Trauma centers are categorized based on the _____ and _____ available at the facility.

15. This categorization identifies those hospitals capable of handling trauma patients and enables emergency medical service (EMS) providers to _____ transport patients to the most _____ medical facilities.

16. Match each of the following levels with the correct capability.

    Level
    a. Level I
    b. Level II
    c. Level III
    d. Level IV

    Capability
    _____ May not be a hospital but rather it can be a clinic-type facility; provides initial stabilization and then transfers the patient
    _____ Usually a community hospital that provides evaluation, resuscitation, and operative intervention for stabilization
    _____ Usually provides initial definitive patient care; research is not an essential component
    _____ Provides a full spectrum of services from prevention programs to patient rehabilitation and serves as the leader in trauma care for a geographic area

17. Fill in the following chart regarding the structure of a Trauma Care System.

Environments	Components	Providers

18. Describe what factors determine the appropriate level of care and hospital destination for a given trauma patient.

_____

_____

_____

_____

_____

19. List three situations in which air transportation should be considered.

_____

_____

_____

20. Which of the following is considered an appropriate reason to delay transport of a seriously injured patient?
    a. to perform a thorough physical examination
    b. to place one or two IV lines using a large-bore cannula and lactated Ringer's solution
    c. to perform a series of diagnostic maneuvers to determine the exact nature of the injury
    d. none of the above

21. Define the term *kinematics*.

_____

_____

_____

22. Newton's first law of motion states that a body in motion will remain in motion unless acted upon by a(n) _____ _____.

23. The second principle of physics is that energy cannot be _____ or _____.

24. T F   In trauma, the weight of the patient has no effect on the amount of injury he or she will sustain.

25. T F   Sudden deceleration is likely to produce injuries, whereas gradual deceleration is usually uneventful.

26. Match each of the following terms with the correct description.

    Terms
    a. Motion
    b. Inertia
    c. Kinetic energy
    d. Acceleration
    e. Impact
    f. Mass
    g. Deceleration

    Description
    _____ Forceful contact or collision
    _____ The rate at which speed or velocity increases
    _____ The process of changing place; movement
    _____ The tendency of an object to remain at rest or to remain in motion unless acted upon by an external force
    _____ The energy an object has while it is in motion; related to the object's velocity and mass
    _____ The rate at which speed decreases
    _____ Weight

27. Blunt trauma:
    a. results from change of speed and compression
    b. usually causes a split or tear in the skin
    c. produces an injury only on the superficial layers of tissue
    d. causes contusions and lacerations of solid organs but does not lead to rupture of hollow organs

28. T F During a change in speed, the body accelerates or decelerates, which may cause shearing or tearing injuries.

29. List four types of impact seen in motor vehicle collisions.

    _____
    _____
    _____
    _____

30. Describe when the "second collision" occurs during a head-on car crash.

    _____
    _____
    _____
    _____

31. A "down-and-under" frontal impact:
    a. throws the occupant over the steering wheel and into the windshield
    b. can produce knee dislocation, patellar fracture, femur fracture, fracture or posterior dislocation of the hip, fracture of the acetabulum, vascular injury, or hemorrhage
    c. produces a shattered windshield
    d. can cause rib fracture, ruptured diaphragm, hemopneumothorax, pulmonary contusion, cardiac contusion, myocardial rupture, or vascular disruption

32. Transection of the aorta is associated with _____ collisions.
    a. rollover
    b. side impact
    c. rear impact
    d. frontal impact

33. List four injuries that are predictable when the abdomen, in forward motion, strikes the steering wheel of a vehicle.

    _____

    _____

    _____

    _____

34. All of the following indicate a frontal impact *except:*
    a. knee imprints in the dashboard
    b. bent steering wheel
    c. starring of the windshield
    d. intrusion of the vehicle into the passenger compartment

35. The anatomical region most commonly injured in the rear-end collision is the:
    a. head
    b. neck
    c. chest
    d. extremities

36. When a vehicle is struck from the side:
    a. injury patterns depend on whether the damaged automobile remains in place or moves away from the point of impact
    b. predictable injuries result from compression to the torso, pelvis, and head
    c. the kidneys, liver, and spleen are subject to vascular tears from supporting tissue, including the disruption of renal vessels from their points of attachment to the inferior vena cava and descending aorta
    d. secondary collisions with other passengers in the vehicle are unlikely

37. A person who is ejected from a vehicle:
    a. is more likely to have severe injuries and is at greater risk of death
    b. tends to have a definable injury pattern
    c. is less likely to suffer a spinal fracture than those who remain in the vehicle
    d. is always struck by the vehicle as it rolls over

38. List the four types of restraints available in the United States.

    _____

    _____

    _____

    _____

39. T F Small motorized vehicles are considered to be more dangerous than other motor vehicles because they offer minimal protection to the rider from the transfer of energy associated with collisions.

40. T F The injuries sustained in small motor vehicle crashes usually are less severe than those received from automobile crashes.

41. When a motorcycle strikes an object that stops its forward motion:
    a. the rest of the bike and the rider continue forward until acted on by an outside force
    b. the motorcycle tips backward and the rider is thrown off
    c. the rider impacts with the gas tank
    d. the driver experiences crushing-type injuries to his or her affected side

42. Describe what can happen if a rider is involved in a frontal impact collision on a motorcycle and his or her feet remain on the footrests during impact.

    _____
    _____
    _____
    _____
    _____

43. Describe three common injury mechanisms to riders of all-terrain vehicles (ATVs).

    _____
    _____
    _____

44. Adult pedestrians:
    a. threatened by an approaching vehicle attempt to protect themselves by facing toward the oncoming automobile
    b. are usually struck by the vehicle bumper in the upper legs, producing hip and femur fractures
    c. are often thrown onto the hood of the vehicle after being struck
    d. are usually pulled under the car on impact and then dragged

45. When an auto strikes a child:
    a. his or her pelvis and legs are the first to be struck by the bumper
    b. he or she is often knocked to the ground by the vehicle, then run over
    c. he or she tends to have injuries to the torso, head, neck, and arms
    d. it causes the child to be thrown up into the air

46. Which of the following causes the initial injury in a blast?
    a. the pressure wave
    b. objects in the blast wave
    c. the individual becoming a missile
    d. none of the above

47. The pressure wave:
    a. produces tertiary injuries
    b. has the same effect as any other penetrating trauma on the body
    c. causes the least significant internal injuries
    d. produces injuries that often affect the hollow, gas-containing organs of the body

48. Objects contained within the blast wave:
    a. seldom injure the victim
    b. may include flying glass, metal, falling mortar, and other items
    c. lead to numerous internal injuries
    d. produce the most serious and obvious injuries

49. Tertiary blast injuries:
    a. are produced when victims are thrown significant distances
    b. include chest and abdominal injuries more often than head, neck, and spinal injuries
    c. result from radiation exposure
    d. are caused by the victims being impaled on objects when they land

50. The pressure wave that accompanies a bullet as it travels through human tissue is called:
    a. drag
    b. cavitation
    c. trajectory
    d. ballistics

51. T F With penetrating trauma, there is a temporary cavity created, as well as a permanent cavity when the skin is broken.

52. Weapons that have a low level of energy include:
    a. handguns and some rifles
    b. hunting rifles, assault weapons
    c. knives, axes, needles, or ice picks
    d. explosive devices

53. An entrance wound:
    a. is larger than the exit wound
    b. is usually round or oval and lies against the underlying tissue
    c. usually has ragged and torn tissue
    d. always has a corresponding exit wound

54. When a firearm causes penetrating injury, it is useful to know all of the following *except:*
    a. the place where it was purchased
    b. the type of gun and the type and caliber of the bullet
    c. the distance fired
    d. the location of the shooter

CROSSWORD PUZZLE EXERCISE

55. Complete the following crossword puzzle.

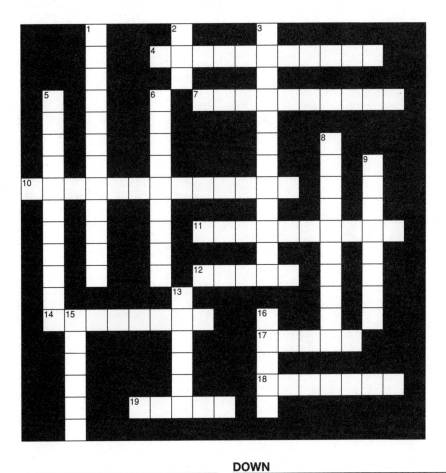

ACROSS

4. Direct _____ is most common type of force applied in blunt trauma.
7. Process of predicting injury patterns that may result from forces and motions of energy.
10. Primary blast injuries result from sudden changes in _____ pressure.
11. Opening produced by a force that pushes body tissues laterally away from the track of a projectile.
12. Injury that occurs from any type of impact.
14. Blast injuries caused by being propelled by an explosion and striking a stationary object.
17. _____ pedestrians threatened by an approaching vehicle turn away from the oncoming automobile.
18. Impact that occurs when a vehicle is struck from the side.
19. Type of injury to a patient exposed to a pressure field produced by an explosion.

DOWN

1. Phase when the EMT-I traditionally uses the skills he or she has gained.
2. Weapons with a _____ level of energy include those used by the attacker's hands.
3. Injuries that occur when body organs are put into motion after an impact.
5. During this phase of trauma care, focus is prevention of intentional and unintentional trauma deaths.
6. Blast injuries that result when bystanders are struck by flying debris.
8. Impacts that occur when an off-center portion of an automobile strikes an immovable object.
9. Speed is also known as _____.
13. Leading cause of death in people ages 1 through 44 years.
15. Conservation of _____ law states that energy cannot be created or destroyed.
16. One of the top causes of trauma deaths in 2003.

17 Hemorrhage and Shock

CHAPTER TERMINAL OBJECTIVES

On completion of this chapter, the EMT-Intermediate will be able to utilize the assessment findings to formulate a field impression and implement the treatment plan for the patient with hemorrhage or shock.

For the multiple-choice questions, select the single best answer to each question. For the matching questions, select the best corresponding answer for each item. Because there are sometimes more items than corresponding answers in the matching questions, some items may not be used.

1. Describe why perfusion is important.

    _____
    _____
    _____
    _____
    _____

2. List the four elements of the Fick principle.

    _____
    _____
    _____
    _____

3. Which of the following interferes with appropriate loading of oxygen onto the red blood cells in the lungs?
    a. a tidal volume of 500 to 800 mL of air
    b. peripheral vasoconstriction
    c. normal hemoglobin levels
    d. a lack of erythrocytes

4. List three elements necessary for off-loading of oxygen from the red blood cells at the tissue level.

    _____
    _____
    _____

5. The body's cells require a continuous supply of _____ and _____ to live.

6. The main energy source for the cells is:
   a. lipid
   b. protein
   c. oxygen
   d. glucose

7. The first step of cellular respiration yields a very small amount of energy and produces a byproduct called:
   a. lactic acid
   b. oxygen
   c. pyruvic acid
   d. carbon dioxide

8. Match each of the following types of metabolism with the correct characteristics. Items may be used more than once.

   Type of Metabolism
   a. Aerobic
   b. Anaerobic

   Characteristic
   _____ Occurs without oxygen
   _____ Produces carbon dioxide, water, and acid as waste products
   _____ Yields a very small amount of energy
   _____ Occurs in the mitochondria of the cell
   _____ Some small and primitive organisms such as certain bacteria can survive using this type of metabolism alone
   _____ Yields a great deal of energy
   _____ Is the first part of cellular metabolism
   _____ Is the primary source of energy production in the body

9. Color the following illustration of the cell and metabolism. Use blue to show the cell membrane, yellow to show the mitochondria, orange to show anaerobic metabolism, purple to show pyruvic molecules, green to show oxygen, and red to show aerobic metabolism.

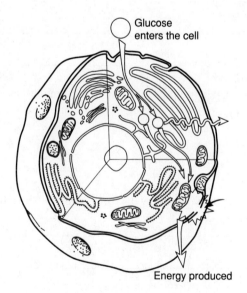

Chapter 17 **Hemorrhage and Shock**

10. Stroke volume:
    a. is the blood volume found in the capillary bed
    b. has no effect on cardiac output
    c. is defined as the amount of blood pumped through the circulatory system by the heart per minute
    d. is affected by circulatory volume, preload, afterload, and myocardial contractility

11. Match the following terms with the correct descriptions.

    Term
    a. Preload
    b. Contractility
    c. Afterload
    d. Perfusion
    e. Cardiac output

    Description
    _____ Blood passing through an organ or part of the body
    _____ Passive stretching force exerted on the ventricular muscle at the end of diastole
    _____ The resistance against which the heart must pump
    _____ Extent and velocity (quickness) of muscle fiber shortening
    _____ The amount of blood pumped through the circulatory system over 1 minute

12. Which of the following is true regarding contractility?
    a. Sodium triggers the action that produces a shortening of the muscle fibers and subsequent myocardial contraction.
    b. The ventricular walls squeeze in on the blood contained in the chamber, resulting in the same amount of blood occupying a larger space.
    c. Blood is ejected out of the heart when ventricular pressure, resulting from ventricular contraction, exceeds the pressure in the aorta and pulmonary artery.
    d. Contractility is the extent and velocity or quickness of muscle fiber lengthening.

13. The increase in the force of myocardial contraction caused by stretching of myocardial muscles is referred to as:
    a. cardiac output
    b. Starling's law
    c. stroke volume
    d. afterload

14. Below is an illustration of the heart. Show by drawing on the picture, the stretch applied to the heart muscle at end diastole.

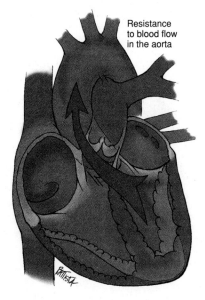

15. Preload is influenced by the _____ of blood returning to the heart. More blood returning _____ preload, whereas less blood returning _____ preload.

16. The greater the afterload, the _____ it is for the ventricles to eject blood into the arteries.

17. Factors that lead to increased afterload include:
    a. obstruction of the aortic valve
    b. hypotension
    c. myocardial depression
    d. dehydration

18. The blood pressure:
    a. is the force that blood exerts against the walls of the arteries as it passes through them
    b. is equal to cardiac output times peripheral vascular resistance
    c. affects the perfusion of the tissues
    d. all of the above

19. Blood pressure can be reduced by all of the following *except:*
    a. severe damage to the myocardium
    b. decreased heart rate
    c. increased myocardial contractility
    d. an excessive heart rate

20. T F An abnormally low or high blood pressure generally has no effect on perfusion.

21. T F When perfusion is decreased, the body cells do not receive enough oxygen and nutrients; therefore cellular function is compromised.

22. Increased blood pressure may be caused by:
    a. vasodilation
    b. increases in the heart rate
    c. decreases in myocardial contractility
    d. increased vagal tone

23. Cardiac output is the product of _____ times _____ .
    a. heart rate; blood pressure
    b. stroke volume; peripheral resistance
    c. stroke volume; heart rate
    d. tissue perfusion; contractility

24. Decrease in either the heart rate or stroke volume results in:
    a. a decrease in oxygen intake
    b. an increase in blood pressure
    c. an improvement in tissue perfusion
    d. a decrease in cardiac output

25. Which of the following is true regarding the blood vessels?
    a. They are rigid and cannot readily adjust their diameter to accommodate for blood volume changes.
    b. The vascular system size is changed by either the dilation or constriction of the blood vessels.
    c. The volume of the container has no relationship to the diameter of the blood vessels.
    d. Only large changes in the diameter of the blood vessels will change the size of the container.

26. A 5-L container and 3 L of blood are equal to a:
    a. a half-filled container
    b. partially full container
    c. full container
    d. none of the above

27. Describe two regulatory mechanisms used to control blood flow to the tissues.

    _____

    _____

28. Which of the following plasma proteins is the most abundant?
    a. albumin
    b. globulin
    c. fibrinogen
    d. thrombin

29. Match the following elements of blood with the correct descriptions. Some items may be used more than once.

    Element
    a. Plasma
    b. Platelets
    c. White blood cells
    d. Red blood cells

    Description
    _____ Also called erythrocytes
    _____ Tiny formed elements that when ruptured, release chemical factors needed to form blood clots
    _____ Are the most abundant of the blood cells; carry oxygen to the tissues and carbon dioxide away from tissues
    _____ Also called leukocytes
    _____ Watery, salty fluid that makes up more than half the volume of blood
    _____ Involved in destroying germs and producing substances called antibodies that help the body resist infection

30. Hemoglobin:
    a. is a protein that contains iron and bonds the oxygen
    b. carries carbon dioxide from the lungs to the tissues, and oxygen from the tissues to the lungs
    c. is 100% saturated with oxygen when it is returned to the heart via the pulmonary veins
    d. turns dark red when it combines with oxygen

31. The hematocrit:
    a. represents the percentage of oxygen carried in the blood
    b. on average is 42 for a woman and 45 for a man
    c. is a useful tool for determining the ratio of white blood cells to plasma in the blood
    d. can be determined only through arterial blood sampling

32. Blood:
    a. is thinner and more fluid than water
    b. flows more quickly than water
    c. viscosity has no effect on peripheral resistance
    d. viscosity is determined by the ratio of plasma cells and formed elements

33. Match each of the following types of closed wounds with the correct characteristics.

    Type of Closed Wound

    a. Contusions and hematomas
    b. Crush injuries
    c. Compartment syndrome
    d. Crush syndrome

    Characteristic

    _____ Caused by blunt trauma or compressive forces to areas with a minimal ability to stretch, it develops as bleeding and swelling increase pressure in a closed area, which compromises circulation and leads to ischemia of the tissues.

    _____ With these injuries the blood vessels are torn beneath the dermis. Bruising may result. The blood also may leak into deeper tissues and lead to swelling.

    _____ Usually involve the extremities, torso, or pelvis; can result in blood vessel injury and internal organ rupture.

    _____ Life-threatening condition caused by prolonged compression or immobilization (beyond 4 to 6 hours). This condition is rare, and the exact mechanism is unknown.

34. Fill in the following table regarding open wounds.

	Mechanism	Signs and Symptoms	Treatment
Abrasions			
Lacerations			
Punctures			
Avulsions			
Amputation			

35. Describe how hemorrhage occurs.

   _____

   _____

   _____

   _____

   _____

36. Match each of the following types of bleeding with the correct characteristics. Items may be used more than once.

    Bleeding Type
    a. Arterial
    b. Venous
    c. Capillary

    Characteristic
    _____ Blood is dark red and flows slowly and steadily.
    _____ Blood is medium red and oozes slowly.
    _____ Blood is bright red and, if the artery is exposed, the blood may escape in spurts synchronized with the pulse.
    _____ This type of bleeding is the least frequent but the most serious.
    _____ This type of bleeding is associated with minor scrapes and cuts.
    _____ This is the type of bleeding associated with deeper cuts.

37. T F For direct pressure to control external bleeding from an ordinary cut it must be followed by elevation of the extremity.

38. T F Whenever tissue is cut the body releases chemicals that constrict the blood vessels sufficiently to stop the bleeding.

39. T F Internal bleeding is usually readily apparent.

40. An adult can lose _____ of blood without any harm, but the loss of _____ may cause death in an infant.

41. Match the following types of bleeding with the correct characteristics. Items may be used more than once.

    Stage of Hemorrhage
    a. Stage 1
    b. Stage 2
    c. Stage 3
    d. Stage 4

    Characteristic

    _____ Classic signs of hypovolemic shock

    _____ Loss of greater than 35%

    _____ Up to 15% to 25% intravascular loss; cardiac output cannot be maintained by arteriolar constriction

    _____ Reflex tachycardia, increased respiratory rate, blood pressure maintained; catecholamines increase peripheral resistance; narrow pulse pressure; diaphoresis from sympathetic stimulation

    _____ Up to 25% to 35% intravascular loss

    _____ Up to 15% intravascular loss; compensated for by constriction of vascular bed

    _____ Blood pressure maintained; normal pulse pressure, respiratory rate, and renal output, skin pallor; anxiety

    _____ Extreme tachycardia; pronounced tachypnea; significantly decreased systolic blood pressure; confusion, lethargy, and unconsciousness; skin is diaphoretic, cool, and extremely pale

42. T F Serious injuries almost always bleed heavily, whereas minor injuries only have minor bleeding.

43. T F People who take blood-thinning medication can bleed easily.

44. T F Puncture wounds usually bleed heavily and carry a high risk of infection.

45. Describe hemostasis.

    _____

    _____

    _____

    _____

46. The most effective method used to control bleeding is:
    a. elevation
    b. application of a tourniquet
    c. direct pressure
    d. pressure points

47. Identify, by numbering, the correct order for applying bleeding control measures.

_____ Apply additional dressings if the wound continues to bleed.

_____ Apply direct pressure to the wound with sterile dressings and a gloved hand.

_____ If the bleeding is uncontrolled, elevate the wound (if it is on an extremity).

_____ Locate and apply pressure to the appropriate arterial pressure point if the wound continues to bleed. These pressure points are found on the main artery above the wound.

_____ Use body substance isolation precautions.

_____ If the bleeding continues, apply a pressure dressing and bandage to the wound.

48. List 15 signs of internal bleeding.

49. Describe what occurs with a lack of perfusion.

50. Shock is defined as:
    a. a low blood pressure, fast pulse rate, and shallow respirations
    b. cool and clammy skin
    c. a lack of oxygen delivered to the tissues
    d. a state of hyperperfusion

51. Add a prefix to the word below to create a word that means *deficient perfusion*.

    _____ perfusion

52. Baroreceptors:
    a. detect changes in the blood pressure
    b. are small structures found in the branch of the carotid arteries, arch of the aorta, and ventricles
    c. stimulate reflex mechanisms that allow the body to adapt to carbon dioxide changes
    d. have a direct role in retaining water in the body

53. Initially in shock, compensatory adjustments begin with the _____ detecting a decrease in arterial blood pressure. Messages are sent to a regulatory center in the brain that activates the _____ nervous system. The _____ nervous system stimulates the heart to beat _____ and more _____ in an effort to compensate for the decreased blood flow.

54. Stimulation of the sympathetic nervous system also causes a release of _____ from sympathetic nerve endings and _____ from the adrenal glands.

55. Chemoreceptors:
    a. are sensitive to changes in the osmotic pressure of the capillaries
    b. directly stimulate the precapillary and postcapillary sphincters to constrict or dilate
    c. detect changes in the blood pressure
    d. are located in the walls of the atria of the heart, vena cava, aortic arch, and carotid sinus

56. In sustained anaerobic metabolism, there is an outpouring of lactic acid that can lead to:
    a. unresolved acidosis
    b. an elevation of the pH
    c. metabolic alkalosis
    d. a decrease in hydrogen ions

57. The word *ischemia* means:
    a. insufficient blood supply
    b. tissue sloughing
    c. rapid heart rate
    d. death of tissue

58. During the precapillary relaxation phase:
    a. there is minimal blood flow to the capillaries, resulting in stagnation
    b. cardiac output increases
    c. the capillaries become engorged with fluid
    d. the red blood cells separate

59. During the washout phase:
    a. the lining of the capillary loses its ability to retain large molecular structures within its walls
    b. plasma is pushed into the interstitial spaces by hydrostatic pressure
    c. the postcapillary sphincters relax
    d. metabolic alkalosis develops

60. During compensatory shock the:
    a. signs and symptoms can be hidden by activation of the sympathetic nervous system
    b. blood pressure begins to decrease
    c. precapillary sphincters relax and the postcapillary sphincters remain closed
    d. vital organs such as the kidneys, liver, lungs, and heart begin to falter and eventually become ineffective

61. Sympathetic vasoconstriction during shock results in:
    a. tachycardia
    b. pupillary constriction
    c. pale, cool skin
    d. increased container size

62. If blood volume decreases more than _____, the shock becomes steadily worse because _____ mechanisms are no longer able to maintain _____ .

63. As the cardiovascular system progressively deteriorates, cardiac output _____ dramatically. This condition can lead to further reductions in _____ _____ and _____ _____ .

64. Which of the following occurs with decompensated (progressive) shock?
    a. The cells of the vital organs begin to die from inadequate perfusion.
    b. Clinical symptoms of shock are minimal.
    c. Adult respiratory distress syndrome (ARDS) develops.
    d. The body's compensatory mechanisms fail, and normal function cannot be maintained.

65. Add a prefix to the word below to create the word that means *low blood pressure*.

    _____ tension

66. Thirst:
    a. occurs when body fluids become increased
    b. helps regulate fluid intake
    c. stimulates the kidneys to excrete more water
    d. has little to no influence on water balance in the body

67. Children often lose _____ % of their blood supply before they experience a decrease in blood pressure.
    a. 10
    b. 30
    c. 45
    d. 60

68. With irreversible shock:
    a. the patient will recover provided prompt prehospital care is initiated
    b. the patient's mental status improves
    c. the liver, kidneys, and lungs become progressively ischemic and begin to falter, eventually becoming ineffective
    d. the patient's blood pressure is relatively normal

69. Match the following phases of shock with the appropriate characteristics. Items may be used more than once.

    Phase of Shock
    a. Compensatory
    b. Decompensated
    c. Irreversible

    Characteristic
    _____ Vital organs begin to die because of inadequate perfusion
    _____ Earliest phase of shock
    _____ Includes signs and symptoms such as sweating; cold, clammy skin; narrowing pulse pressure; hypotension; and nausea and vomiting
    _____ Body recognizes the catastrophic event that is occurring and triggers corrective action in an attempt to return cardiac output and arterial blood pressure to normal
    _____ ARDS, renal failure, liver failure, and sepsis may develop
    _____ Arteries that are deprived of their blood supply cannot remain constricted and begin to dilate, resulting in decreased venous return, which in turn decreases cardiac output
    _____ The heart deteriorates to the point that it can no longer effectively pump blood, and there are life-threatening reductions in cardiac output, blood pressure, and tissue perfusion
    _____ The cells in the tissues become hypoxic, leading to anaerobic metabolism and the production of harmful acids, eventually bringing about metabolic acidosis

70. Hypovolemic shock may be caused by:
    a. bacterial infection
    b. profuse sweating
    c. severe spinal cord injury
    d. severe left ventricular depression

71. T F Cardiogenic shock is the most common type of shock seen in the prehospital setting.

72. T F Cardiogenic shock is caused by profound failure of the heart.

73. Which of the following is regarded as relative hypovolemia?
    a. pooling of blood in the peripheral circulation caused by severe vasodilatation
    b. plasma loss from burns
    c. direct blood loss
    d. obstruction of blood flow out of the heart as a result of cardiac tamponade

74. In neurogenic shock:
    a. more epinephrine is released
    b. blood pools in the blood vessels in certain areas of the body
    c. the blood vessels constrict, cutting off blood flow to vital areas of the body
    d. venous return to the heart is abruptly increased

75. The signs and symptoms of neurogenic shock:
    a. are the same as those seen in hypovolemic shock
    b. include tachycardia, sweating, and pale skin color
    c. usually appear after the patient has been in shock for awhile
    d. usually include hypotension and an abnormal mental status

76. Which of the following may cause anaphylactic shock?
    a. severe electrolyte imbalance
    b. blood loss
    c. profound and persistent diarrhea
    d. the reaction between an antigen and antibody

77. An antibody is a:
    a. substance that enters the body and triggers the release of compounds designed to destroy it
    b. molecule made by the body to defend against bacteria, viruses, or other foreign substances such as antigens
    c. compound released during inflammation and allergic responses
    d. chemical compound that provides energy for use by body cells

78. All of the following may occur with release of histamine during anaphylaxis *except*:
    a. intense vasodilatation
    b. blood loss
    c. sudden, severe bronchoconstriction
    d. leakage of fluid from the blood vessels

79. Septic shock:
    a. is caused by an overwhelming infection
    b. leads to ineffective circulation because blood is pooled or trapped in constricted veins
    c. results in a loss of blood volume caused by internal hemorrhage
    d. is more common in pediatric patients

80. Signs and symptoms of septic shock include:
    a. a cold body and warm extremities
    b. fever
    c. hypertension
    d. bradycardia

81. In shock, anaerobic metabolism occurs as a result of:
    a. increased bicarbonate in the body
    b. hypoxia at the cellular level
    c. a decrease in carbonic acid in the arterial blood
    d. increased perfusion at the cellular level

82. Treatment of a patient experiencing hypovolemic shock includes:
    a. administering 35% to 60% oxygen
    b. establishing one IV line and running it at 40 to 60 drops/min
    c. administering one or two IVs of lactated Ringer's or normal saline solution
    d. placing the patient into a semisitting position

83. _____ is often the first sign of shock.
    a. Cold, clammy skin
    b. Rapid breathing
    c. Hypotension
    d. An altered mental status

84. Compensatory hyperventilation seen with shock:
    a. tends to occur in late shock
    b. acts to reduce the carbon dioxide content of the blood and to compensate for metabolic acidosis
    c. occurs when the respiratory center of the brain becomes depressed because of hypoperfusion
    d. produces respiratory acidosis

85. Any indication of hypoventilation should prompt the EMT-I to:
    a. perform emergency chest decompression
    b. administer bronchodilators
    c. assist the patient's breathing with a bag-mask device
    d. administer 100% oxygen using a nonrebreather mask

86. T F Compensatory mechanisms can maintain a normal pulse rate even in the presence of a 25% volume deficit.

87. T F A fast, weak, or thready pulse indicates decreased circulatory volume.

88. T F Initially in shock, the skin appears pale.

89. Capillary refill:
    a. is checked by pressing on the nail bed of the patient's finger or toe, releasing the pressure, and determining the time it takes for the nail bed to return to its initial color
    b. that is slow (greater than 2 seconds) indicates adequate tissue perfusion, whereas capillary refill that is fast (less than 2 seconds) indicates a state of poor perfusion
    c. is a reliable vital sign in both children and adults
    d. should be assessed only in the conscious patient

90. The blood pressure of a patient experiencing shock will:
    a. be high
    b. be profoundly low
    c. go from low to high
    d. usually be low but may be normal

91. In the patient experiencing hypovolemic shock, fluid replacement is generally:
    a. guided by medical direction and established protocol
    b. administered slightly faster than in the heart failure patient
    c. run wide open
    d. 10 drops/min for each 10-mm Hg decrease in the patient's blood pressure

92. T F When treating a patient experiencing shock, the IV should be started while en route to the hospital.

93. T F Normal saline (0.9%) is considered a hypotonic solution.

94. T F Lactated Ringer's solution is a hypertonic solution that contains calcium chloride and sodium lactate in water.

95. T F Five percent dextrose in water (D_5W) is used to replace fluid volume in patients experiencing shock because its administration causes an immediate expansion of the circulatory volume.

96. Which of the following IV solutions and blood preparations has oxygen-carrying capacity?
    a. plasma substitutes
    b. platelets
    c. whole blood
    d. plasma

97. Match the appropriate IV solution to be administered in each of the following conditions. Some items may be used more than once.

    Solution
    a. D_5W
    b. Lactated Ringer's or normal saline (0.9%)

    Condition
    _____ 17-year-old girl experiencing vaginal hemorrhage with a blood pressure of 80/60
    _____ 41-year-old man who has a gunshot wound to the head and a blood pressure of 240/110
    _____ 45-year-old man who is complaining of chest pain and has a blood pressure of 170/96
    _____ 33-year-old man stabbed four times in the chest with a blood pressure of 70 by palpation
    _____ 65-year-old man with severe diarrhea for the past week and a blood pressure of 100/78

98. The pneumatic antishock garment (PASG):
    a. is indicated when the systolic blood pressure is below 100 mm Hg, with or without obvious signs and symptoms of shock
    b. may be used in patients experiencing bleeding, trauma, sepsis, a ruptured aneurysm, or ectopic pregnancy
    c. can bring about an autotransfusion of 3 to 5 L of blood
    d. is contraindicated in patients suffering from pelvic fracture

99. _____ is an absolute contraindication to the use of the PASG.
    a. Spinal injury
    b. Pulmonary edema
    c. Head injury
    d. Blunt abdominal trauma

100. When applying the PASG, the EMT-I should:
    a. position it so that the garment top is just below the rib cage
    b. apply it with the inside portion facing the patient
    c. wrap the three sections of the garment around the patient loosely
    d. initially connect the foot pump to the pump connections on the legs only

101. When inflating the PASG, the EMT-I should quickly compress the foot pump until:
    a. the vents on the stopcocks stop leaking
    b. crackling sounds are heard from the Velcro
    c. the systolic blood pressure increases to 80 mm Hg
    d. the shocklike symptoms completely subside

102. The PASG should be removed:
    a. only when a physician orders the removal of the garment
    b. once an adequate blood pressure is achieved
    c. as soon as the patient is transferred over to the care of emergency department personnel
    d. if the patient's mental status improves

103. When deflating the PASG:
    a. the stopcock(s) should be opened to allow a large amount of air to escape
    b. deflation should be discontinued if the blood pressure decreases by more than 20 mm Hg systolic
    c. the legs should be deflated first
    d. the patient's vital signs should be reassessed every 5 minutes

It is a Friday afternoon when you are called to an office building where a 44-year-old man attempted to commit suicide by cutting his wrists and taking a handful of sleeping pills. You find him sitting on the restroom floor in blood-soaked clothes with dark red blood flowing from two large cuts across his wrists. Your assessment reveals that he is awake but agitated; has a respiratory rate of 18 breaths/min; a weak, thready pulse at a rate of 130 BPM; a blood pressure of 90/52; and pale, diaphoretic skin. The pulse oximetry reading is 90%. He reportedly has a past medical history of epilepsy.

104. This patient is experiencing _____ bleeding with _____ shock.
    a. arterial; hypovolemic
    b. venous; neurogenic
    c. capillary; cardiogenic
    d. venous; hypovolemic

105. Treatment for this patient includes:
    a. applying tourniquets to both arms at the elbows
    b. establishing one or two IV lines with normal saline or lactated Ringer's solution and macrodrip administration sets
    c. applying and inflating the PASG
    d. administering 2 to 3 L of oxygen via nasal cannula

It is 7:30 PM on a Friday when you are called to a restaurant where a 28-year-old woman is complaining of dyspnea. You find her sitting on the floor next to her table. Her husband states that she was eating dinner when she suddenly began itching all over. The difficulty breathing began shortly after that. Your assessment reveals that the patient is apprehensive, has a respiratory rate of 22, a pulse rate of 130, a blood pressure of 108/72, and flushed skin. The pulse oximetry reading is 90%. You note the presence of urticaria. Auscultation of the chest reveals bilateral wheezing. She has swelling about her face, particularly around the eyes and tongue. She is also complaining of abdominal cramps. You are able to determine that she is allergic to shellfish and has a history of diabetes.

106. Your patient is experiencing:
    a. anaphylactic shock
    b. food poisoning
    c. neurogenic shock
    d. diabetic ketoacidosis (DKA)

107. Treatment for this patient includes:
    a. administering 2 to 3 L of oxygen via simple face mask
    b. placing her into a supine position
    c. administering epinephrine, 1:1000 solution, subcutaneously
    d. establishing two IV lines with macrodrip administration sets and normal saline or lactated Ringer's solution and running them wide open

Your patient is an 18-year-old man who was shot during an attempted robbery. You find him lying on his back next to the cash register. He has been shot in both upper legs and the right wrist. He is alert and oriented, has a respiratory rate of 18, a pulse rate of 102, a blood pressure of 104/80, and warm, diaphoretic skin. Auscultation of the chest reveals slight bilateral wheezing. The pulse oximetry reading is 94%. You note a small entrance wound with swelling and bleeding to the wrist, and large, open wounds to both upper legs. There appears to be no deformity to either leg. You are able to establish that the patient has a previous medical history of asthma.

108. Your patient is suffering from:
    a. neurogenic shock
    b. fractured tibias
    c. respiratory acidosis
    d. hypovolemic shock

109. You begin administering oxygen at 15 L via nonrebreather mask, apply direct pressure to the wounds, place him in a supine position on a full backboard with cervical spine stabilization, and move him to the patient module of the ambulance. The *next* treatment for this patient is to:
    a. transport him to the nearest hospital
    b. establish one or two IV lines with macrodrip administration sets and normal saline or lactated Ringer's solution
    c. perform endotracheal intubation
    d. apply cold compresses to the wounds

You are called to a local hotel where a 52-year-old woman is complaining of chest pain after attending a rally and dinner. You note that she is also short of breath and nauseated. She has a history of hypertension, angina, and diabetes for which she takes furosemide, Dyazide, nitroglycerin, and insulin. According to the patient she was fine until about 20 minutes ago when she suddenly felt a crushing pain in her chest. Your assessment reveals that she is extremely anxious, has a respiratory rate of 20 breaths/min, a pulse rate of 128 BPM, a blood pressure of 80/56, and cool, sweaty skin. Auscultation of the chest reveals bilateral rales. The pulse oximetry reading is 88%.

110. This patient is experiencing:
    a. septic shock
    b. cardiogenic shock
    c. insulin shock
    d. neurogenic shock

111. Treatment of this patient includes:
    a. applying and inflating the PASG
    b. having her breathe into a paper sack
    c. administering 100% (at least 15 L) oxygen via nonrebreather mask
    d. establishing an IV line with a macrodrip administration set and normal saline and running it wide open until at least 1000 mL has been administered

You are called to the scene of a skier who has fallen while coming down a steep hill. You find the patient lying supine in a snow bank. He tells you that he is not able to move his arms or legs. Assessment reveals that the patient is awake and oriented, has shallow breathing at a rate of 24, a pulse rate of 80, a blood pressure of 114/62, and cool, moist skin. The pulse oximetry reading is 92%. The physical examination reveals bumps, bruises, and abrasions to the forehead. Auscultation of the chest reveals clear bilateral lung sounds. According to his friends, the patient has no previous medical history.

112. This patient is suffering from:
    a. cardiogenic shock
    b. anaphylactic shock
    c. neurogenic shock
    d. hypovolemic shock

113. Treatment for this patient includes:
    a. establishing two IV lines with macrodrip administration sets and normal saline and running them wide open
    b. administering 15 L of oxygen using a nonrebreather mask
    c. stabilizing him (including the cervical spine) onto a full backboard
    d. inserting an oropharyngeal airway

    You are called to the home of a 40-year-old woman who is complaining of a fever. You find her lying on her bed. Assessment reveals that the patient is well oriented, has a respiratory rate of 18 breaths/min, a pulse rate of 120 BPM, and a blood pressure of 86/54. You note that her body is warm, but her legs are cool. Auscultation of the chest reveals clear bilateral lung sounds. The patient tells you that she has been sick with a urinary tract infection for almost a week. According to her husband, she has no other past medical history.

114. This patient is suffering from:
    a. septic shock
    b. anaphylactic shock
    c. neurogenic shock
    d. hypovolemic shock

115. Treatment for this patient includes:
    a. administering 10 L of oxygen using a simple face mask
    b. placing her in a supine position with legs elevated 10 to 12 inches
    c. applying ice or cold compresses over the groin and in the armpits
    d. administering epinephrine, 1:1000 solution, subcutaneously

18 Burns

CHAPTER TERMINAL OBJECTIVES

On completion of this chapter, the EMT-Intermediate will be able to assess and manage a patient who has sustained burn injuries.

For the multiple-choice questions, select the single best answer to each question. For the matching questions, select the best corresponding answer for each item. Because there are sometimes more items than corresponding answers in the matching questions, some items may not be used.

1. Fires rank _____ among unintentional injuries.

2. Morbidity and mortality rates from burn injuries depend on _____, _____, and _____ _____.

3. Deaths from residential fires are most commonly caused by:
   a. careless use of cigarettes
   b. heating equipment malfunction
   c. electrical equipment malfunction
   d. children playing with matches or cigarette lighters

4. T F The consumption of alcohol has been shown to be the strongest independent risk factor for death after the fire begins.

5. T F Children playing with ignition sources such as matches or cigarette lighters cause about 50% of the burn fatalities.

6. T F Three fourths of all fire deaths occur in the home, with the highest incidence in lower-income households.

7. T F Direct contact with either a flame or hot liquid such as water or grease will cause thermal burns.

8. T F The length of contact with the substance or flame does not affect the extent of a burn injury.

9. List four factors that influence the body's ability to resist burn injury.

   _____

   _____

   _____

   _____

10. Major burns have _____ distinct zones of injury that usually appear in a _____ eye pattern.

11. The central area of the burn wound:
    a. is called the zone of stasis
    b. dies within 24 to 48 hours after injury if no supportive measures are taken
    c. sustains the most intense contact with the thermal source
    d. has increased blood flow as a result of the normal inflammatory response

12. Tissues in the zone of hyperemia:
    a. recover in 7 to 10 days if infection or profound shock does not develop
    b. surround the critically injured area and consist of potentially viable tissue
    c. die within 24 to 48 hours after injury if no supportive measures are taken
    d. are ischemic because of clotting and vasoconstriction

13. The zone of _____ surrounds the critically injured area and consists of potentially viable tissue despite the serious thermal injury. In this area, cells are _____ because of clotting and _____. These cells die within _____ to _____ hours after injury if no supportive measures are taken.

14. A large thermal injury can cause _____ shock with a decrease in venous return, _____ cardiac output, and _____ vascular resistance except in the hyperemic zone.

15. Match the following characteristics with the various depths of burns. Some items may be used more than once.

    Depth of Burn
    a. Superficial
    b. Partial thickness
    c. Full thickness

    Characteristic
    _____ Appears very dry and leathery or white, dark brown, or charred
    _____ There are blisters with weeping
    _____ Heals in 3 to 6 days
    _____ Skin is red
    _____ There is no sensation in the skin

16. List four elements that are used to categorize the severity of a burn.

    _____

    _____

    _____

    _____

17. Using the "rule of nines," label the following illustration of the adult with the percentage it represents, and color it according to the following: a-blue, b-red, c-yellow, d-tan, and e-green.

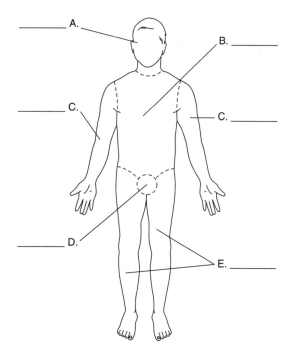

You are called to the scene where a 60-year-old man has been burned in a house fire. Apparently he fell asleep on the couch while smoking a cigarette. He has partial- and full-thickness burns to the anterior surface of his neck, chest, and abdomen. Your assessment reveals that he has a respiratory rate of 22, a pulse rate of 120, a blood pressure of 160/100, and warm, moist skin. He appears to be well oriented but is in a great deal of pain. Also, you note that he has singed nasal hairs, soot about the nostrils and mouth, and his voice seems hoarse.

18. The severity of this injury is considered:
    a. insignificant
    b. minor
    c. moderate
    d. critical

19. The approximate percentage of burn injury is _____.
    a. 1% to 5%
    b. 8% to 14%
    c. 18% to 20%
    d. 40% to 45%

20. Treatment for this patient includes all of the following *except:*
    a. administering 100% oxygen
    b. removing any smoldering clothing
    c. ensuring a patent airway
    d. applying ice to the burned area

CROSSWORD PUZZLE EXERCISE

21. Complete the following crossword puzzle.

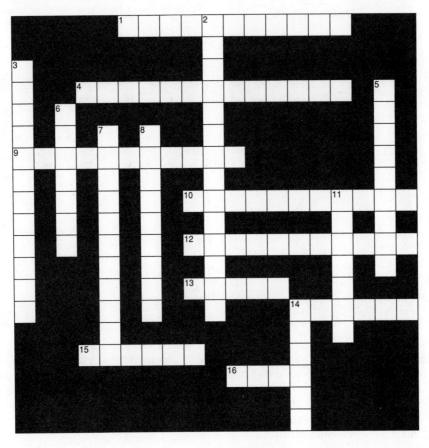

ACROSS

1. Burn that involves only the epidermis.
4. Myoglobin in the urine.
9. _____ globin is formed by the combination of carbon monoxide with the hemoglobin molecule.
10. The zone of _____ is the central area of the burn wound.
12. A large thermal injury can cause this type of shock.
13. Rule of _____ is commonly used in the prehospital setting to assess percentage of burned area.
14. The zone of _____ surrounds the critically injured area and consists of potentially viable tissue
15. Cramps, seizures, twitching of muscles, and sharp flexion of wrist and ankle joints.
16. A _____ -thickness burn is one that extends through all of the dermal layers.

DOWN

2. Breakdown of striated or skeletal muscle.
3. Discharge of fluid in the bronchi.
5. Molecular complex responsible for red color of muscle and its ability to store oxygen.
6. _____ -thickness is a burn that involves epidermis and dermis but no underlying tissue.
7. Permanent condition of a joint characterized by flexion and fixation.
8. The zone of _____ is at the periphery of the zone of stasis.
11. Type of burns caused by direct contact with either a flame or hot liquid such as water or grease.
14. The wound caused by the burn usually _____ rapidly.

19 Thoracic Trauma

CHAPTER TERMINAL OBJECTIVES

On completion of this chapter, the EMT-Intermediate will be able to assess and manage a patient who has thoracic injuries.

For the multiple-choice questions, select the single best answer to each question. For the matching questions, select the best corresponding answer for each item. Because there are sometimes more items than corresponding answers in the matching questions, some items may not be used.

1. Label the following illustration of the thorax, and color it according to the following: A-blue, B-red, C-yellow, D-tan, and E-green.

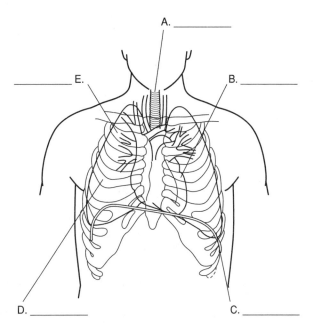

A. _____
B. _____
C. _____
D. _____
E. _____

2. Match the following components of the respiratory system with the correct description.

   Component
   a. Visceral pleura
   b. Pleural space
   c. Trachea
   d. Parietal pleura
   e. Alveoli
   f. Lobes
   g. Alveolar-capillary membrane

   Description
   _____ Microscopic chambers within the lungs where the gases of respiration are exchanged
   _____ Fine fibrous sheath covering the interior of the thorax
   _____ Regions of the lung
   _____ Provides interface between the respiratory and circulatory systems
   _____ Fine lining covering the lungs
   _____ The potential space between the parietal pleura and the visceral pleura
   _____ Windpipe, the main conduit for air passing to and from the lungs

3. Chest injuries account for about _____ deaths per year in the United States and are directly responsible for more than _____% of all traumatic deaths, regardless of the mechanism of _____.

4. The most commonly fractured bone is the:
   a. scapula
   b. clavicle
   c. sternum
   d. humerus

5. A rib is most commonly broken on the _____ aspect of ribs _____ through _____.
   a. anterior; three; five
   b. posterior; two; seven
   c. lateral-superior; one; seven
   d. lateral; three; eight

6. The mortality rate with sternal fractures is between _____% and _____%.
   a. 5; 10
   b. 20; 30
   c. 25; 45
   d. 50; 75

7. List three causes of sternal fractures.

   _____

   _____

   _____

8. List three significant injuries that can be associated with sternal fractures.

   _____

   _____

   _____

9. With a flail chest:
   a. there are at least four or more fractured ribs in two or more places
   b. the trachea will be noticeably deviated away from the affected side
   c. there is decreased ventilation because of paradoxical movement of the involved segment of the thoracic wall
   d. the lung sounds will be equal on both sides

10. Describe how a flail chest should be stabilized in the field setting:

_____
_____
_____
_____
_____

11. A pulmonary contusion:
    a. usually occurs as a result of penetrating trauma
    b. is frequently seen under a flail chest
    c. has minimal effect on respiratory effectiveness
    d. can be described as bleeding that occurs in the bronchiolar areas of the lung

12. A closed or simple pneumothorax:
    a. is present when air is introduced into the pericardial space
    b. occurs in more than 50% of patients with blunt chest trauma
    c. can cause the affected lung to collapse as the pressure in the pleural space increases
    d. is seldom associated with life-threatening complications

13. An open pneumothorax:
    a. is caused by penetrating trauma
    b. occurs when an opening is created between the alveoli and the outside of the body
    c. allows air to freely enter but not exit the pleural cavity
    d. usually seals independently and seldom progresses to a life-threatening tension pneumothorax

14. A pneumothorax may occur from all of the following *except:*
    a. rupture of bleb or cystic lesion on the lobe of a lung
    b. a fractured clavicle
    c. blunt chest trauma
    d. inhalation of carbon monoxide

15. T F With pneumothorax, there is a loss of pleural seal integrity.

16. T F With pneumothorax, auscultation of the chest will reveal equal bilateral lung sounds.

17. T F A closed pneumothorax is generally associated with penetrating trauma.

18. An open pneumothorax that has a bubbling sound is referred to as a/an _____ chest wound.

19. To treat an open pneumothorax, it should be covered with a/an _____ dressing.

20. With tension pneumothorax:
    a. there is only partial collapse of the involved lung
    b. the mediastinum is pushed to the opposite side
    c. cardiac output is increased because of the kinking of the vena cava and increased intrapleural pressure
    d. there is improved ventilation in the opposite lung

21. Place a checkmark beside those signs and symptoms that are characteristic of tension pneumothorax. Also, circle those considered to be "late signs."

    _____ tachycardia, hypotension
    _____ external jugular vein distention
    _____ muffled heart sounds
    _____ tracheal deviation, severe dyspnea
    _____ increasing cyanosis
    _____ warm, diaphoretic skin
    _____ equal bilateral lung sounds
    _____ apprehension, agitation

22. Your patient has been involved in a serious car crash and is suffering from a tension pneumothorax. Which of the following is considered a correct treatment for this condition?
    a. placing the patient into a supine position with the legs elevated 10 to 12 inches
    b. performing needle thoracentesis
    c. administering oxygen via nasal cannula
    d. performing pericardiocentesis

23. To perform needle decompression of the chest:
    a. a 16- to 18-gauge catheter-over-needle should be used
    b. a flutter valve is created by passing a catheter-over-needle device through the finger of a sterile glove and piercing the distal tip
    c. the needle is inserted on the contralateral side
    d. the needle is advanced into the pericardial space until a rush of escaping air is noted

24. On the illustration below, mark with asterisks or dots the anterior and lateral sites for needle decompression of the chest.

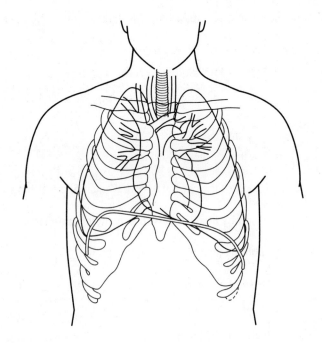

25. Severe blunt trauma to the abdomen may rupture the _____, permitting the abdominal contents to enter the thoracic cavity.

26. List four signs of diaphragmatic rupture.

   _____

   _____

   _____

   _____

27. During trauma, compression of the chest may:
    a. cause aortic rupture
    b. result in rupture of the liver and spleen
    c. burst the trachea
    d. cause traumatic asphyxia

28. List three signs of traumatic asphyxia.

   _____

   _____

   _____

29. When bleeding into the thoracic cavity occurs, it is referred to as _____.

30. The type of shock that results from hemothorax is _____.

31. T F Cardiac tamponade occurs as a result of bruising of the myocardium.

32. T F Cardiac tamponade only occurs as a result of penetrating trauma.

33. Fill in the signs of cardiac tamponade in the following table.

	Signs Seen With Cardiac Tamponade
Jugular veins	
Tracheal position	
Lung sounds	
Pulse	
Blood pressure	
Heart sounds	

34. Describe the importance of rapid transport to definitive care.

_____

_____

_____

_____

_____

A 31-year-old patient has been shot in the chest with a small-caliber pistol during a fight with his ex-wife. You find him lying supine on the kitchen floor. He is responsive to pain and questions but seems confused, has labored breathing at a rate of 20 breaths/min, and his skin is cool and diaphoretic.

35. You palpate the patient's radial pulse to find that it is weak and fast. The presence of a radial pulse indicates that this patient has a blood pressure of at least _____ mm Hg.
    a. 40
    b. 60
    c. 80
    d. 100

36. Your physical assessment reveals an entrance wound just above the patient's right nipple. You note that his neck veins are flat and the trachea is in the midline. Auscultation of the chest reveals an absence of breath sounds on the right side, but the left side is normal. This patient is most likely experiencing:
    a. cardiac tamponade
    b. pneumothorax
    c. traumatic asphyxia
    d. tension pneumothorax

37. Treatment of this patient includes:
    a. administering 8 L of oxygen via simple face mask
    b. placing him on the uninjured side
    c. applying and inflating the pneumatic antishock garment
    d. covering the wound with an occlusive dressing

38. This patient should be transported to:
    a. a trauma center
    b. an urgent care center
    c. the nearest hospital
    d. a regional cardiac center

A 25-year-old patient was stabbed in the chest during a domestic fight and is lying on the sidewalk in a pool of blood. On your arrival on scene, a police officer escorts you in. They abruptly leave to pursue the assailant, who is reportedly running down the street. As you get to the patient's side, the assailant suddenly emerges from a nearby bush. She is waving a knife, threatening to cut anyone who comes near. After several minutes, you are able to persuade her to surrender the weapon, and a police officer returns to take her into custody. Assessment reveals the patient is awake; has a respiratory rate of 30; a weak, thready pulse at a rate of 122; a blood pressure of 84/52; and cool, pale, diaphoretic skin. Exposure of the chest reveals a knife wound about 1 cm to the left of the sternum. Auscultation of the chest reveals clear bilateral lung sounds, but the heart sounds are muffled. You note that there is external jugular vein distention and the trachea is in a midline position.

39. This patient is suffering from:
    a. pericardial tamponade
    b. sucking chest wound
    c. a flail chest
    d. tension pneumothorax

40. The two treatments that should be provided to this patient first include:
    a. stabilizing the cervical spine, administering 100% oxygen
    b. stabilizing the cervical spine, ensuring a patent airway
    c. performing emergency chest decompression, establishing two IV lines using large-bore catheters (14 to 16 gauge) and normal saline solution
    d. ensuring a patent airway, covering the wound with a sterile gauze dressing

41. The next two treatments that should be provided to this patient include:
    a. administering 100% oxygen, establishing one or two IV lines using large-bore catheters (14 to 16 gauge) and lactated Ringer's or normal saline (0.9%) solution
    b. performing needle pericardiocentesis, applying and inflating the pneumatic antishock garment
    c. securing the patient to a long backboard, assisting the patient's breathing with a bag-mask device
    d. establishing two IV lines using large-bore catheters (14 to 16 gauge) and lactated Ringer's or normal saline (0.9%) solution, performing emergency chest decompression

42. While en route to the hospital with the patient, you notice that the drip chamber of one of the IV administration sets becomes completely filled. To correct this problem, the IV:
    a. should be discontinued
    b. site should be raised above the level of the patient's heart
    c. bag should be inverted and the drip chamber squeezed
    d. bag should be lowered below the level of the insertion site

It is Sunday afternoon when you are called to the home of a 42-year-old man who was hit in the chest by a baseball. You identify the scene as safe. The patient is sitting on the back porch steps. He is alert and talking as you approach.

43. The first thing you should do is:
    a. form a general impression
    b. check the airway
    c. determine the chief complaint
    d. check for a pulse

The patient is complaining of chest pain. Your assessment reveals he is alert, has a respiratory rate of 22, a pulse rate of 128, a blood pressure of 106/82, and cool, moist skin. Auscultation of the chest reveals clear bilateral lung sounds. The patient's wife states he has a history of hypertension. You note there is bruising in the midsternal area of the chest.

44. Your patient is most likely experiencing:
    a. cardiac contusion
    b. tension pneumothorax
    c. aortic disruption
    d. cardiac tamponade

45. Treatment of this patient includes:
    a. administering 6 L of oxygen via nonrebreather mask
    b. monitoring his electrocardiogram (ECG)
    c. establishing an IV line of normal saline or lactated Ringer's solution and running it wide open
    d. performing emergency chest decompression

CROSSWORD PUZZLE EXERCISE

46. Complete the following crossword puzzle.

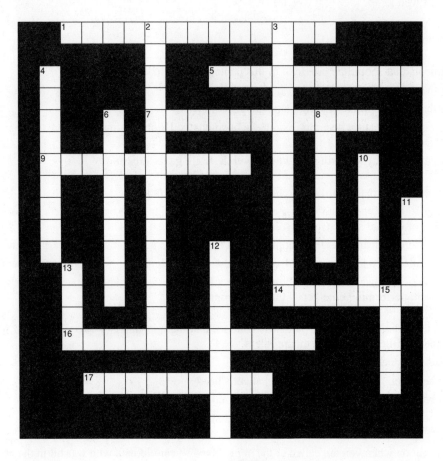

ACROSS

1. Type of rupture that may allow intraabdominal organs to enter thoracic cavity.
5. Thoracic injury in which blood collects within the pleural space.
7. Esophageal injuries are most frequently caused by _____ trauma.
9. Rupture of this refers to an acute traumatic perforation of the ventricles or atria.
14. Fracture caused by a direct blow to the chest as in a massive crush injury.
16. Air in the pleural cavity.
17. Type of contusion that usually occurs as a result of blunt trauma and is seen frequently under a flail chest.

DOWN

2. Blood in the pericardial sac.
3. A needle _____ can be used to relieve a tension pneumothorax.
4. _____ asphyxia describes a severe crushing injury to the chest and abdomen.
6. To treat an open pneumothorax, cover the open area with a/an _____ dressing.
8. These objects should be left in place and stabilized for transport.
10. This pneumothorax occurs when air enters the pleural space but does not exit and pressure builds up.
11. Chest injury that occurs when two or more ribs are broken in two or more places.
12. Sheet of voluntary muscle that separates the abdominal cavity from the thoracic cavity.
13. Abbreviation for positive end-expiratory pressure.
15. Can be ruptured or torn in accidents involving high energy.

20 Head and Spinal Trauma

CHAPTER TERMINAL OBJECTIVES

On completion of this chapter, the EMT-Intermediate should be able to utilize the assessment findings to formulate a field impression and implement the management plan for the patient with a head or neck injury.

For the multiple-choice questions, select the single best answer to each question. For the matching questions, select the best corresponding answer for each item. Because there are sometimes more items than corresponding answers in the matching questions, some items may not be used.

1. Head injuries:
    a. affect nearly 10 million people each year in the United States
    b. lead to death in about 100,000 patients before they reach the emergency department
    c. are usually isolated to one area
    d. may be difficult to treat because the patient may be unresponsive

2. The two age groups at highest risk for traumatic brain injury are _____ to _____ years of age and _____ to _____ years of age.

3. Which of the following signs is usually not associated with a skull fracture?
    a. Battle's sign
    b. blood and/or cerebrospinal fluid (CSF) draining from the ears
    c. deteriorating mental status
    d. hypotension

4. The anatomical components of the skull are the scalp, followed by the cranial vault, under which are the:
    a. pia mater, cerebellum, arachnoid
    b. meninges, CSF, dura mater
    c. dura mater, CSF, arachnoid, medulla oblongata
    d. dura mater, arachnoid layer, pia mater, brain

5. Describe how the appearance of blood and CSF occurs in the ears and/or nose of a patient with a skull fracture.

_____

_____

_____

_____

6. Black-and-blue discoloration that results from the collection of blood in the tissue around the eye sockets as a result of a head injury is referred to as:
   a. decorticate posturing
   b. Battle's sign
   c. raccoon eyes
   d. subcutaneous emphysema

7. T F   Unequal pupils are seldom associated with brain injury.

8. T F   Bleeding within and around the brain can compress brain tissue, impair neurological function, and lead to death.

9. The most important sign indicating that the intracerebral pressure (ICP) is increasing is:
   a. vomiting
   b. deterioration in the level of consciousness
   c. unequal pupils
   d. a progressive increase in the blood pressure

10. Match the following signs with the correct description.

    Sign
    a. Cheyne-Stokes
    b. Cushing reflex or triad
    c. Hemiplegia
    d. Quadriplegia
    e. Decorticate posturing
    f. Decerebrate posturing
    g. Paraplegia

    Description
    _____ Paralysis on one side of the body
    _____ Position in which the arms are extended and internally rotated and the legs are extended with the feet in forced plantar flexion
    _____ A repetitive pattern of slow, shallow breathing to rapid, deep ventilations back to slow, shallow breaths followed by a period of apnea
    _____ Position of a patient in which the upper extremities are flexed at the elbows and at the wrists
    _____ Progressive increase in the blood pressure (especially the systolic reading), an increase in the respiratory rate, and a decreasing pulse rate
    _____ Paralysis of the lower extremities
    _____ Paralysis of all four extremities

11. T F   Administration of oxygen in the presence of head injury should be delivered at 2 to 4 L/min via nasal cannula.

12. T F   Both the insertion of a nasopharyngeal airway and nasotracheal intubation are contraindicated in basilar skull fractures.

It is 2:40 AM when you are called to the scene of a street fight to find a male who has been shot in the head with a small-caliber pistol. As you approach the scene, several bystanders who are attempting to flee from the gun-wielding assailant meet you. You remain in a distant location until police arrive and arrest the assailant. Your assessment of the patient reveals that he is unconscious, has a respiratory rate of 8, a pulse rate of 50, a blood pressure of 220/138, and cold, diaphoretic skin. The entrance wound is to the forehead, just above the right eyebrow, and you are unable to locate an exit wound. You note there is CSF and blood coming from his nose and ears.

13. Treatment of this patient includes:
    a. controlling the bleeding and leakage of CSF from the nose and ears with direct pressure
    b. limiting the number of times vital signs are taken to prevent agitating him
    c. applying cervical immobilization and placing him on a long backboard
    d. establishing an IV line using a microdrip administration set and 5% dextrose in water and running it at a TKO rate

14. T F The EMT-I should assume a patient with a closed scalp injury has a cervical spine and brain injury until proven otherwise.

15. T F For individuals with long hair, the scalp can be avulsed if the hair is caught in and pulled by a mechanical device.

16. T F The EMT-I should apply direct pressure with the fingers to control bleeding in a patient with an open scalp injury in which there is significant bleeding.

17. Match the following fracture locations with the correct signs and symptoms.

    Type of Location
    a. Mandibular
    b. Orbital
    c. Zygomatic
    d. Nasal

    Sign

    _____ Periorbital edema, subconjunctival ecchymosis, double vision, recessed globe, epistaxis, and anesthesia in the region of the anterior cheek. Double vision and impaired extraocular movements may also be present.

    _____ Flatness of a usually rounded cheek area; numbness of the cheek, nose, and upper lip; and epistaxis. Altered vision may also be present.

    _____ Malocclusion, numbness in the chin, and inability to open the mouth. The patient also may have difficulty swallowing and excessive salivation.

    _____ Injuries may depress the affected body part or displace it to one side. In some instances, fractures may result only in epistaxis and swelling without apparent skeletal deformity.

18. List 16 common mechanisms of anterior neck injury.

___

You are called to a hardware store where a 50-year-old man was stabbed in the neck during a robbery. The patient is sitting on a stool in the front of the store. Several policemen are holding him to keep him from falling. There is a 3- to 4-inch-long knife impaled in the left lateral side of his neck. The entrance wound is just below the lobe of his ear, and the knife appears to be angled straight down. There is dark red blood flowing steadily from around the wound. Your assessment of the patient reveals that he is alert and oriented, has a respiratory rate of 22, a pulse rate of 126, a blood pressure of 170/100, and warm, moist skin. Auscultation of the chest reveals no lung sounds on the left side. Although there is noticeable swelling around the injury site, you note that the patient is able to speak, and there is no external jugular vein distention or tracheal deviation. You are able to determine that the patient has a history of lung cancer and had a pneumonectomy on the left side several years ago. The patient is able to move all of his extremities and denies numbness or tingling sensation.

19. This patient is experiencing:
    a. pneumothorax
    b. tracheal perforation
    c. venous bleeding
    d. laryngotracheal avulsion

20. Treatment of this patient includes all of the following *except:*
    a. removing the knife and applying a sterile dressing over the wound
    b. applying direct pressure to control the bleeding
    c. administering high-concentration oxygen
    d. stabilizing the head and neck

21. Match the mechanisms of spinal injury with the correct description.

    Mechanism
    a. Extension
    b. Flexion
    c. Rotation
    d. Vertical compression

    Description
    _____ Occurs when the spinal structures are violently bent forward such as when hitting one's head while diving
    _____ Occurs when a force is directed along the axis of the spine. The intervertebral disk is crushed into the body of the vertebra, leading to spinal cord damage
    _____ Seldom occurs as an isolated event, occurring instead as a combination with rotation of the spine that causes dislocation of the intervertebral joints
    _____ Tear of the ligaments and vertebral instability that occur with hyperextension

22. Spinal shock:
    a. is a form of hypovolemic shock that results from blood loss from the spinal cord
    b. may result in the patient becoming hypotensive because of the loss of vascular control caused by the injury
    c. is associated with the patient having an elevated pulse rate, and pink, warm, moist skin
    d. is the most common cause of shock resulting from trauma

23. List three benefits of manual stabilization of the cervical vertebrae.

    _____

    _____

    _____

24. To stabilize a supine trauma patient's cervical spine, the EMT-I should *first:*
    a. flex the neck
    b. hold traction on the neck while applying a cervical collar
    c. place his or her hands at the corner of the patient's jaw on both sides
    d. put the head into a "sniffing position"

25. T F A rigid cervical collar alone provides sufficient support to immobilize the cervical spine.

26. T F Soft cervical collars provide inadequate stabilization of the injured spine and therefore should not be used.

27. When using a short (half) spine board or vest-type device, several important rules must be followed, including:
    a. loosely secure the device to allow for easy chest expansion
    b. apply a rigid cervical collar if the head is in a neutral position
    c. secure the patient's head to the immobilization device before the device has been secured to the torso
    d. allow the patient to move while applying the device

28. When applying a short spine board, a pad should be placed:
    a. behind the head to fill any void
    b. between the cervical collar and the board
    c. between the shoulder blades and the board
    d. below the seventh cervical vertebra

29. Describe how the EMT-I should immobilize the patient's head in preparation to apply a short spine board or vest-type device:

_____

_____

_____

_____

_____

30. T F The EMT-I should assess motor, sensory, and distal circulation in only the patient's lower extremities before- and after application of a short spine board or vest-type device.

31. T F When applying a vest-type device there is no need to pad voids.

32. T F When using the KED, at least 2 to 3 inches of space should be left between the device and the patient's axillae (armpits).

33. T F When pulling the straps of the KED tight, hold the buckles to prevent the device from rotating.

34. T F Typically, when applying the KED, the groin straps are applied first and then the chest straps.

You have been called to the scene of a neighborhood swimming pool where a 20-year-old man struck his head on a diving board while jumping into the water. Your assessment reveals he is unconscious and apneic, has a pulse rate of 80 BPM, a blood pressure of 90/70, and warm, wet, flushed skin. You note that there is a large bump on the occipital area of his head. No other injuries are found during your assessment.

35. The preferred procedure for opening this patient's airway is the:
    a. jaw thrust without head tilt
    b. head tilt/chin lift
    c. sniffing position
    d. head tilt/neck lift

36. This patient is most likely suffering from:
    a. increased intracranial pressure
    b. cerebral contusion
    c. cervical spine injury
    d. hypovolemic shock

37. Treatment of this patient includes:
    a. securing him to a long backboard
    b. using the head-tilt/chin-lift procedure to open his airway
    c. administering high-concentration oxygen
    d. applying manual traction to his head and neck

38. To logroll a patient who is in a supine position onto a long backboard:
    a. four people are needed
    b. approach the patient from the side of his or her head to limit the patient's motion before you begin cervical immobilization, and then carefully move the patient's head into neutral in-line alignment
    c. straighten the patient's arms so that they are in a "palm-in" position next to the torso, direct your second partner or EMT assistant to bring the legs together into neutral alignment, and then raise the patient's arm on the side the patient will be logrolled
    d. the rescuer at the chest decides when the patient is logrolled

39. When securing a patient to a long backboard, the straps should be placed:
    a. one strap over the nipple line, one strap over the abdomen, one strap just above the knees, one strap midway between the ankles and knees
    b. one strap above the nipple line, one strap below the iliac crests, one strap just below the knees, one strap midway between the ankles and knees
    c. one strap over the nipple line, one strap over the iliac crests, one strap just above the knees, one strap midway between the ankles and knees
    d. one strap over the clavicular line, one strap over the iliac crests, one strap just below the knees, one strap midway between the ankles and knees

40. Describe how a patient's head should be immobilized to the long backboard.

    _____
    _____
    _____
    _____
    _____

41. Describe how to logroll a patient who is found in a prone position onto a long backboard.

    _____
    _____
    _____
    _____
    _____

42. Rapid extrication techniques are used in two instances: a/an _____ scene or patients with _____ injuries

43. All of the following are examples that justify rapid extrication *except:*
    a. rising water
    b. danger of explosion
    c. threat of fire
    d. a stabilized vehicle lying on its side

44. List five life-threatening injuries that may also require rapid removal.

45. List three things that would give the EMT-I reason *not to remove* a football helmet.

CROSSWORD PUZZLE EXERCISE

46. Complete the following crossword puzzle.

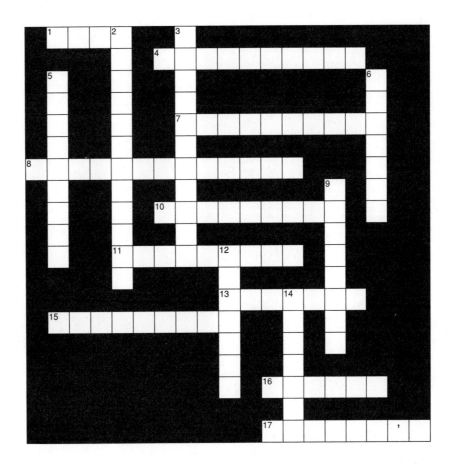

ACROSS

1. Skull fracture that involves skin that has been disrupted, exposing the central nervous system.
4. Paralysis on one side of the body.
7. Amnesia in which there is no recall of events before the injury.
8. Caused by the release of gastric contents into the thoracic cavity.
10. Occurs when an individual is exposed to great changes in barometric pressure.
11. Amnesia in which there is no recall of events immediately after recovery of consciousness.
13. This reflex or triad is a late sign of increased intracranial pressure.
15. Fractures that include flatness of normally rounded cheek area, numbness of cheek, nose, and upper lip.
16. Fracture pattern produced in the mid-face region.
17. Skin discoloration at the mastoid region behind the ear is called _____ sign.

DOWN

2. This type of intubation is contraindicated if a basilar skull fracture is suspected.
3. Posturing in which upper extremities are flexed at elbows and wrists; legs also may be flexed.
5. Skull fractures where the bony fragments have been forced inward toward the brain.
6. Head injury may produce this type of papillary change.
9. Type of IV solution that should be used in head injury.
12. _____ eyes is a black and blue discoloration caused by collection of blood in tissue around eyes.
14. Bleeding into the anterior chamber of the eye.

21 Abdominal and Extremity Trauma

CHAPTER TERMINAL OBJECTIVES

On completion of this chapter, the EMT-Intermediate will be able to integrate pathophysiological principles and the assessment findings to formulate a field impression and implement a treatment plan for the patient with abdominal trauma.

For the multiple-choice questions, select the single best answer to each question. For the matching questions, select the best corresponding answer for each item. Because there are sometimes more items than corresponding answers in the matching questions, some items may not be used.

1. T F It is easy to identify traumatic injuries in the abdomen that may require surgical repair.

2. T F There are only a few main organs in the abdomen that may be injured.

3. T F When unrecognized, abdominal injury is one of the major causes of death in the trauma patient.

4. With abdominal injuries the Emergency Medical Technician–Intermediate (EMT-I) must have a high degree of suspicion based on the _____ of injury because death usually results from continuing _____ and/or delay of _____ repair.

5. The primary cause of shock in abdominally injured patients is:
   a. release of acids, enzymes, or bacteria from the gastrointestinal tract into the peritoneal cavity
   b. loss of blood into the abdominal cavity
   c. severe, inappropriate vasodilation
   d. rupture of hollow organs

6. Define the term peritonitis, and describe how it occurs as a result of abdominal injury.

   _____
   _____
   _____
   _____
   _____
   _____

7. Blunt abdominal trauma is usually the result of:
   a. compression or shear injuries
   b. stab wounds, gunshot wounds, or impaled objects
   c. falls from great distances
   d. blows to the abdomen

8. The degree of abdominal injury caused by blunt forces is related to the:
   a. age of the patient
   b. type of abdominal structure injured
   c. quantity and duration of force applied
   d. b and c

9. T F A stab wound is more likely to produce multiple organ damage than is a gunshot wound.

10. T F The intestine is the most frequently injured organ in penetrating trauma.

11. Injury to the _____ abdominal organs usually results in rapid and significant blood loss. The two solid organs commonly injured are the _____ and _____. Both of these are primary sources of _____.

12. Injury to the _____ should be suspected in any patient with a steering wheel injury, lap belt injury, or history of epigastric trauma.

13. Patients with splenic injury may complain of pain in the left shoulder. This is referred to as:
    a. Kehr's sign
    b. rebound tenderness
    c. ascites
    d. Crone's sign

14. Describe why hollow organ injury presents with different signs and symptoms than solid abdominal organ injury.

    _____
    _____
    _____
    _____
    _____

15. T F The stomach is damaged in about 1% of blunt abdominal trauma and in about 19% of cases of penetrating trauma.

16. T F The colon and small intestine are injured less often as a result of blunt trauma cases as compared with penetrating trauma.

17. The potential space behind the "true" abdominal cavity is referred to as the:
    a. peritoneum
    b. pelvic cavity
    c. retroperitoneal space
    d. thoracic region

18. Hemorrhage within the retroperitoneal space may be massive and usually results from _____ and/or _____ fractures.

19. Injuries to the kidneys involve _____ fractures and _____, resulting in hemorrhage, urine extravasation, or both.

20. Injury to the bladder:
    a. is more likely if the bladder is empty at the time of injury
    b. can cause urine to leak into the peritoneal cavity
    c. may result in the presence of bile in the urine
    d. usually does not interfere with a person's ability to void

21. List five indicators for establishing the index of suspicion for abdominal injury signs/symptoms of abdominal trauma.

    _____

    _____

    _____

    _____

    _____

22. T F The pregnant patient should be immobilized to the long backboard in a supine position with her legs elevated 10 to 12 inches.

You are called to the scene where a 23-year-old man was injured while doing a woodworking project at his home. You arrive to find him lying on his side on the ground with his knees bent and holding his stomach. You move his hands to reveal abdominal organs protruding from a cut that extends the entire width of his abdomen. Assessment reveals that he is alert, has a respiratory rate of 20 breaths/min, a pulse rate of 126, a blood pressure of 106/90, and cool, moist skin.

23. This patient is suffering from a/an:
    a. perforation
    b. evisceration
    c. contusion
    d. laceration

24. Treatment for this patient includes:
    a. pushing the organs back into the abdominal cavity
    b. covering the organs with a dry, sterile dressing
    c. straightening his legs
    d. administering 100% oxygen via a nonrebreather mask

It is 9:30 pm on Wednesday when you are called to the scene where a 49-year-old man accidentally shot himself in the abdomen while cleaning his small-caliber pistol. You find him sitting on the living room sofa. He has a small entrance wound just above his umbilicus. Dark red blood is flowing from it. There is no exit wound. Your assessment reveals he is semiconscious; has a respiratory rate of 18; a blood pressure of 70/52; a weak, thready pulse at a rate of 130; and pale, diaphoretic skin. He has no known medical history.

25. This patient is experiencing _____ bleeding with _____ shock.
    a. venous; hypovolemic
    b. capillary; neurogenic
    c. arterial; cardiogenic
    d. arterial; hypovolemic

26. Treatment for this patient includes:
    a. administering high-concentration oxygen
    b. placing one or two IV lines with microdrip administration sets and normal saline
    c. applying the pneumatic antishock garment (PASG) but inflating only the leg sections
    d. applying an occlusive dressing over the wound

A 17-year-old patient was struck in the abdomen with a large wrench during a fight at a local repair garage. You find him lying on his side on the sidewalk in front of the garage. You begin your assessment to find that he is awake, has a respiratory rate of 20; a weak, thready pulse at a rate of 126; a blood pressure of 90/78; and cool, pale, diaphoretic skin. Auscultation of the chest reveals clear bilateral lung sounds. Your inspection and palpation reveal bruising and rigidity in the upper right abdominal quadrant. No other injuries are noted.

27. This patient is experiencing:
    a. neurogenic shock
    b. blunt abdominal trauma
    c. abdominal evisceration
    d. aortic rupture

28. The abdominal organ that is likely injured is the:
    a. spleen
    b. right kidney
    c. liver
    d. small intestine

29. Treatment of this patient includes:
    a. administering 6 L of oxygen by nonrebreather mask
    b. placing him into a sitting position on the cot
    c. placing an IV line using 5% dextrose in water
    d. promptly transporting him to a trauma center

CROSSWORD PUZZLE EXERCISE

30. Complete the following crossword puzzle.

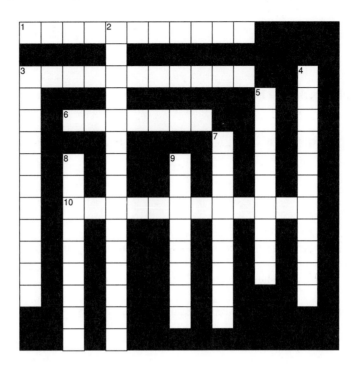

ACROSS

1. These mechanisms cause organs of the abdomen to be crushed between solid objects.
3. Trauma caused by stab wounds, gunshot wounds, or impaled objects.
6. Usually protected during blunt mechanisms because of its location in the abdomen.
10. Protrusion of an internal organ or peritoneal contents through a wound or surgical incision.

DOWN

2. Potential space behind the "true" abdominal cavity.
3. Propulsive, muscular movements of the intestines.
4. Inflammation of the peritoneum.
5. Body cavity extending from below the diaphragm to the pelvic bone.
7. Blood in the urine.
8. Causes anatomical and physiological changes to the body's system.
9. Incidents that create rupture of solid organs or rupture of blood vessels in the abdominal cavity.

31. T F Extremity trauma tends to occur with other injuries.

32. T F Fractures occur when there is a complete break in the continuity of bone or cartilage.

33. T F Fractures are seldom life threatening unless circumstances such as uncontrolled bleeding are present.

34. T F A fractured femur can produce severe internal bleeding.

35. You are called to a baseball park for a 56-year-old man who was struck several times with a baseball bat during an altercation. Assessment reveals deformity to the upper arm with the bone ends protruding through the wound.

    This type of fracture is referred to as a/an _____ fracture.
    a. simple
    b. closed
    c. impacted
    d. open

36. A _____ occurs when there is a separation of two bones at the joint. It can cause an area of

    _____ that may produce a large amount of pain.

37. List six complications that can occur from extremity trauma.

    _____

    _____

    _____

    _____

    _____

    _____

38. A grating noise heard with the movement of broken bone ends rubbing together is called:
    a. urticaria
    b. crepitus
    c. adduction
    d. ascites

39. When immobilizing a fracture, which of the rules below should be followed?
    a. Immobilize the joints above and below the injury site.
    b. Allow the patient to continue wearing rings or other pieces of jewelry.
    c. Straighten all angulated fractures of the extremities, including those that involve joints such as the shoulder and wrist.
    d. Leave all open wounds associated with fractures uncovered.

40. What major blood vessel can be found in the thigh?
    a. femoral artery
    b. common iliac artery
    c. radial vein
    d. subclavian artery

41. Provide one example of each type of splint listed below.

    Rigid splint: _____

    Formable splint: _____

    Traction splint: _____

    A 27-year-old patient has been injured in a motorcycle accident. Your assessment reveals that the patient is conscious but is obviously inebriated, has a normal respiration rate of 22, a strong pulse of 110, a blood pressure of 128/86, and warm, diaphoretic skin. Examination reveals deformity and swelling to the upper right leg, just above the knee. There are no other noticeable injuries. According to his friends, the patient has been drinking beer and snorting cocaine for the past 4 hours.

42. You have decided to apply the Hare traction splint. When applying the device:
    a. mechanical traction should be applied before securing the ischial strap in place
    b. the patient should be placed on a long backboard
    c. the ischial pad should be seated approximately 6 inches below the ischial tuberosity
    d. only one rescuer is needed

43. Which of the following pulse sites would be used to assess vascular function in the lower extremity of this patient?
    a. radial and ulnar
    b. femoral and popliteal
    c. axillary and brachiocephalic
    d. posterior tibial and dorsalis pedis

44. List three complications from splinting.

    _____

    _____

    _____

CROSSWORD PUZZLE EXERCISE

45. Complete the following crossword puzzle.

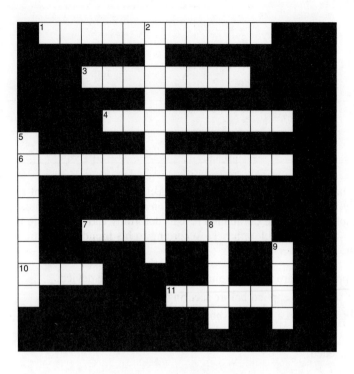

ACROSS

1. Occurs when there is a separation of two bones at the joint.
3. Splint that accommodates the shape of the injured extremity.
4. Occur when there is any break in the continuity of bone or cartilage.
6. May initially restore distal pulse in circulatory compromise seen with dislocation or fracture.
7. Traction splint should be measured against this leg.
10. Injury that occurs when there is a break in the bone, as well as a disruption of the skin.
11. Occur where two or more bones meet or articulate.

DOWN

2. _____ syndrome is ischemia and compromised circulation that occur from a vascular injury.
5. Type of splint most commonly used to stabilize femur fractures.
8. Type of splint that requires positioning of body part to fit the splint's shape.
9. Can be used for initial stabilization of pelvic fracture.

22 Respiratory Emergencies

CHAPTER TERMINAL OBJECTIVES

On completion of this chapter, the EMT-Intermediate will be able to use assessment findings to formulate a field impression and carry out a treatment plan for the patient with respiratory emergencies.

For the multiple-choice questions, select the single best answer to each question. For the matching questions, select the best corresponding answer for each item. Because there are sometimes more items than corresponding answers in the matching questions, some items may not be used.

1. The respiratory system is responsible for _____, warming, _____, and _____ more than 10,000 L of air per day in an adult.

2. Place a U next to the structures that are part of the upper respiratory system and an L next to the structures that are part of the lower airway.
   _____ Alveoli
   _____ Mouth
   _____ Trachea
   _____ Larynx
   _____ Vocal cords
   _____ Oral cavity
   _____ Bronchi
   _____ Bronchioles
   _____ Nasal cavity

3. Match the following terms with the correct description.

   Term
   a. Respiration
   b. Ventilation
   c. Oxygenation
   d. Diffusion
   e. Perfusion

   Description
   _____ The process in which oxygenated blood is pumped to the tissues, and waste products are returned to the lungs
   _____ Refers specifically to the exchange of carbon dioxide
   _____ Involves inspiring oxygen-containing air and exhaling carbon dioxide
   _____ Movement of oxygen and carbon dioxide from areas of greater concentration to areas of lesser concentration
   _____ Refers only to the exchange of oxygen

4. In the following table, list three functions that are affected by respiratory abnormalities, the respiratory abnormalities that can affect these functions, and specific conditions related to each.

Function	Respiratory Abnormality Affecting Function	Specific Conditions
Ventilation		
Diffusion		
Perfusion		

5. List eight signs of potential life-threatening respiratory distress in adults.

___

6. When the Emergency Medical Technician–Intermediate (EMT-I) sees a person suffering from respiratory distress who is in a tripod position, it means he or she:
   a. is leaning forward with arms raised over the head
   b. is experiencing moderately severe dyspnea
   c. is experiencing congestive heart failure
   d. has been in respiratory distress for at least an hour

7. T F Diaphoresis is a specific finding that indicates that the patient is in more distress than someone who is not diaphoretic.

8. T F Cyanosis is concerning to the EMT-I only when it is associated with diaphoresis and tachycardia.

9. T F Bradycardia is a sign of hypoxemia, fear, or sympathomimetic medication use.

10. A pattern of breathing marked by rapid and regular respirations at a rate of about 25 breaths/min is referred to as:
    a. eupnea
    b. tachypnea
    c. Cheyne-Stokes breathing
    d. central neurological hyperventilation

11. Jugular venous distention (JVD) may accompany:
    a. stroke
    b. right-sided heart failure
    c. shock
    d. diabetic coma

12. _____ _____ are abnormally deep, very rapid sighing respirations often caused by the presence of metabolic acidosis such as diabetic ketoacidosis.

13. _____ is a type of breathing characterized by a series of several short inspirations followed by regular or irregular periods of apnea.

14. Describe air trapping.

    _____
    _____
    _____
    _____
    _____

15. Pursed-lip breathing is often present in patients with:
    a. asthma and chronic obstructive pulmonary disorder (COPD)
    b. shock
    c. pneumothorax and flail chest
    d. pneumonia

16. T F Increasing amounts of sputum suggest infection.

17. T F Thick green or brown sputum suggests allergy or inflammation.

18. T F Pink, frothy sputum is usually associated with acute pulmonary edema.

19. Describe what barrel chest deformity suggests.

    _____
    _____
    _____
    _____
    _____

20. Describe what capnometry is used to assess.

_____
_____
_____
_____
_____

21. Match the following respiratory conditions with the correct description.

    Condition
    a. Asthma
    b. Hyperventilation
    c. Spontaneous pneumothorax
    d. Emphysema
    e. Pulmonary embolism
    f. Pulmonary edema

    Description
    _____ Sudden accumulation of air in the pleural space caused by rupture of a weak area on the lung surface; as the air enters the pleural space, the lung on the involved side collapses

    _____ Blockage of a pulmonary artery by foreign matter, most often caused by a piece of a blood clot that has broken away from a pelvic or deep leg vein

    _____ Chronic disease that involves the lower airway, beyond the level of the trachea and mainstem bronchi; it occurs when the bronchial airways narrow and make breathing difficult

    _____ Refers to filling of the lungs with fluid in the interstitial spaces, the alveoli, or both. It is not a disease in itself, but rather a pathophysiological condition resulting from many possible causes.

22. T F The major cause of COPD is industrial inhalants.

23. The underlying pathophysiology of all forms of obstructive lung disease is decreased _____ airflow and air _____ primarily caused by obstruction in the small bronchioles.

24. List three factors that may exacerbate underlying conditions in COPD.

_____
_____
_____

25. List four external stimuli that may also play a significant contributory role in exacerbating underlying conditions in COPD.

_____
_____
_____
_____

26. List four things that happen when bronchial airways of an asthma patient are irritated.

_____

_____

_____

_____

27. T F Asthma is most common in older adults.

28. T F Acute asthma is a chronic inflammatory pulmonary disorder that is characterized by reversible obstruction of the airways.

29. T F About one third of the adults who have asthma outgrow it.

30. T F With intrinsic asthma, a specific outside substance such as pollen causes the air tubes to narrow.

31. List seven groups of common asthma triggers.

_____

_____

_____

_____

_____

_____

_____

32. Signs and symptoms of an acute asthma attack include:
    a. blood-tinged sputum
    b. hypotension
    c. wheezing
    d. bradycardia

33. Status asthmaticus:
    a. is frequently precipitated by a pulmonary embolism
    b. is a true emergency that requires immediate transport
    c. is a severe prolonged asthma attack that responds to standard medications
    d. requires that the patient be intubated

34. _____ _____ _____ _____ is a progressive and irreversible disease of the airway marked by decreased inspiratory and expiratory capacity of the lungs. It may result from _____ or _____ .

35. After a period of time, the right side of the heart may develop failure because of the effort required to move blood through diseased lungs. This condition is known as chronic _____ _____ and indicates severe COPD.

36. Which of the following are characteristics of chronic lung disease patients?
    a. Their chests often take on a concave-shaped appearance.
    b. They are typically cigarette smokers.
    c. They tend to be less than 30 years old.
    d. They tend to be individuals who use birth control pills.

37. List three signs that may be present if the COPD patient also has cor pulmonale.

    _____

    _____

    _____

38. Albuterol:
    a. is used in the treatment of bronchospasm
    b. is typically supplied in a concentration of 2.5 mg/10 mL
    c. has side effects that include bradycardia, hypotension, and respiratory depression
    d. is a pure alpha stimulant

39. Treatment of a patient experiencing obstructive lung disease (acute asthma attack or COPD) includes:
    a. administering epinephrine at a dose of 0.5 to 1.0 mL of a 1:1000 solution subcutaneously
    b. placing him or her in a supine position
    c. administering 6 L/min using a nonrebreather mask if the patient can tolerate the mask
    d. administering an aerosolized bronchodilator such as albuterol (Proventil), isoetharine (Bronkosol), or metaproterenol (Alupent)

40. T F COPD patients who are carbon dioxide retainers and given high concentrations of oxygen may experience respiratory depression and arrest.

41. T F Pneumonia is an acute inflammatory condition of the lungs, usually caused by inhalation of toxic substances.

42. List five risk factors that make people more susceptible to pneumonia.

    _____

    _____

    _____

    _____

43. The "typical" picture of bacterial pneumonia is heralded by acute onset of _____ and _____. Cough productive of _____ sputum soon follows. Depending on the location of the infection, the patient may have _____ chest pain—pain that worsens with deep _____ or _____.

44. Describe the type of breath sounds heard with bacterial pneumonia.

_____

_____

_____

_____

_____

45. Treatment the EMT-I can provide the patient experiencing pneumonia includes:
    a. ensuring his or her own safety
    b. administering 2 to 3 L/min of oxygen via nasal cannula
    c. establishing an IV line of normal saline and administering it at a wide-open rate
    d. administering antibiotics

46. Match the following types of pulmonary edema with the correct characteristics. Items may be used more than once.

    Term
    a. High pressure
    b. High permeability

    Characteristic

    _____ May be caused by acute hypoxemia, near-drowning, cardiac arrest, shock, high altitude exposure, inhalation of pulmonary irritants (e.g., chlorine gas), or adult respiratory distress syndrome (ARDS)

    _____ The inability of the ventricle to pump blood adequately results in an increase in ventricular pressure. The increased ventricular pressure is back-transmitted to the left atrium, then the pulmonary vessels, causing an increase in the pulmonary venous pressure.

    _____ Most commonly results from acute myocardial ischemia but may also be caused by heart valve disease, chronic hypertension, or myocarditis

    _____ The alveolar-capillary membrane is disrupted, and fluid leaks into the interstitial space. Widening of the interstitial space by fluid impairs diffusion.

    _____ Symptoms may develop over a longer period, but an acute onset is still common.

47. The patient with pulmonary edema may complain of dyspnea that worsens when lying down. This is referred to as:
    a. paroxysmal dyspnea
    b. orthopnea
    c. agonal breathing
    d. Kussmaul breathing

48. All of the following are effects of furosemide in acute pulmonary edema *except:*
    a. it vasodilates, causing a decrease in the cardiac preload
    b. it increases lymphatic flow from the lungs back into the circulatory system, helping to drain the lungs of fluid
    c. it is a narcotic analgesic that helps alleviate the patient's fear and anxiety
    d. it causes the kidneys to eliminate excess fluid from the body

49. Treatment of pulmonary edema includes:
    a. placing the patient into a supine position
    b. placing an IV line and running it at a medium flow rate
    c. placing the patient in an upright position with the legs dangling
    d. administering 2 to 3 L of oxygen via nasal cannula

50. Risks for pulmonary embolism include all of the following *except:*
    a. thrombophlebitis
    b. oral contraceptives
    c. fracture of a long bone
    d. an acute asthma attack

51. Patients with massive pulmonary emboli often suffer cardiac _____ or _____ spell as the first symptom of the illness.
    a. sudden onset of chest pain; respiratory distress
    b. cardiac arrest; syncopal
    c. wheezing; coughing up of blood
    d. anxiety; hypotension

52. T   F   Spontaneous pneumothorax is a common cause of sudden-onset shortness of breath and chest pain in younger persons.

53. T   F   Spontaneous pneumothorax is more common in women than in men.

54. T   F   The most frequent cause of spontaneous pneumothorax is excessive pressure buildup in the chest during exercise.

55. Place a checkmark beside the signs of spontaneous pneumothorax.
    _____ Increasing respiratory distress
    _____ Bounding pulse
    _____ Cyanosis
    _____ Hypertension
    _____ Decreased breath sounds on the affected side
    _____ Flat neck veins
    _____ Subcutaneous emphysema

56. Treatment of a patient believed to be experiencing a tension pneumothorax as a result of a spontaneous pneumothorax includes:
    a. needle decompression
    b. increasing the flow rate of the IV to wide open
    c. placing the patient on the unaffected side
    d. assisting the patient's breathing with a bag-mask device

57. A 15-year-old patient is hyperventilating, apparently brought on by an argument with her father. Her respiratory rate is 24, pulse rate is 110, and blood pressure is 142/84. The increased respiratory rate will likely lead to a decreased:
    a. Pao_2
    b. pH
    c. bicarbonate level
    d. $Paco_2$

58. This patient will likely develop:
    a. metabolic acidosis
    b. respiratory alkalosis
    c. normal pH
    d. respiratory acidosis

59. List five conditions that can result in hyperventilation.

    _____

    _____

    _____

    _____

    _____

60. Carpopedal spasm is a:
    a. numbness and tingling feeling of the face, fingers, and toes
    b. violent contraction of the muscles of the bronchial walls, causing marked constriction of the bronchi
    c. contorted position of the hand in which the fingers flex in a clawlike fashion
    d. tightness or a lump in the throat that restricts airflow and creates a high-pitched sound

61. Having a hyperventilating patient breathe into a paper sack is appropriate when the patient:
    a. is younger than 21 years
    b. is breathing faster than 20 times per minute
    c. displays tachycardia
    d. none of the above

You have been called to local state university for a 19-year-old young man who is having trouble breathing. According to the school nurse, the patient was walking to class when he became dyspneic. Assessment reveals the patient is awake but agitated, has a respiratory rate of 26, a weak thready pulse, a blood pressure of 116/74, and cool, diaphoretic skin. You note the presence of cyanosis about the lips. Auscultation of the chest reveals bilateral wheezing. You are able to determine the patient has a previous medical history of respiratory trouble.

62. This patient is experiencing:
    a. hyperventilation syndrome
    b. anaphylactic shock
    c. an acute asthma attack
    d. pulmonary embolism

63. Treatment includes:
    a. administering atropine, 0.5 mg, IV push
    b. administering nonhumidified oxygen, 10 to 15 L/min, via nonrebreather mask
    c. withholding an IV line unless the patient becomes severely hypotensive
    d. administering an aerosolized bronchodilator such as albuterol (Proventil), isoetharine (Bronkosol), or metaproterenol (Alupent)

You have been called to the residence of a 75-year-old woman who is complaining of dyspnea. Your assessment reveals that she is awake but agitated, has labored respirations of 24 breaths/min, an irregular pulse of 124, a blood pressure of 174/106, and cool, diaphoretic skin. Auscultation of the chest reveals bilateral wheezes and rales. You note that she has a barrel-shaped chest and is breathing through pursed lips. Examination of her lower extremities reveals pitting bilateral edema. According to her son and daughter-in-law, the patient has a history of respiratory and heart problems, smokes two packs of cigarettes a day, and is allergic to penicillin.

64. Your patient is suffering from:
    a. a pulmonary embolus
    b. spontaneous pneumothorax
    c. hyperventilation syndrome
    d. an acute COPD episode

65. Treatment includes:
    a. assisting the patient's breathing with a bag-mask device and 100% oxygen
    b. having her rebreathe into a paper sack
    c. loosening any restrictive garments
    d. transporting the patient in a lateral recumbent position

You have been called to an international airport for a 23-year-old woman who is reportedly having chest pain and shortness of breath. The chest pain increases in intensity with a deep breath. According to the flight attendant, the patient was in midflight when she suddenly began having the problem. Assessment reveals she is awake but confused; has a respiratory rate of 26; a weak, thready, irregular pulse of 110; a blood pressure of 106/82; cool, diaphoretic skin; and a pulse oximetry reading of 75%. Auscultation of the chest reveals bilateral wheezing. You are able to determine the patient has had a recent surgery and takes birth control pills.

66. This patient is experiencing:
    a. hyperventilation syndrome
    b. anaphylactic shock
    c. an acute asthma attack
    d. pulmonary embolism

67. Treatment includes:
    a. administering atropine, 0.5 to 1.0 mg, IV push
    b. administering high-concentration oxygen, via nonrebreather mask
    c. withholding an IV line unless the patient becomes severely hypotensive
    d. administering epinephrine, 0.5 mg of a 1:10,000 solution, subcutaneously

CROSSWORD PUZZLE EXERCISE

68. Complete the following crossword puzzle.

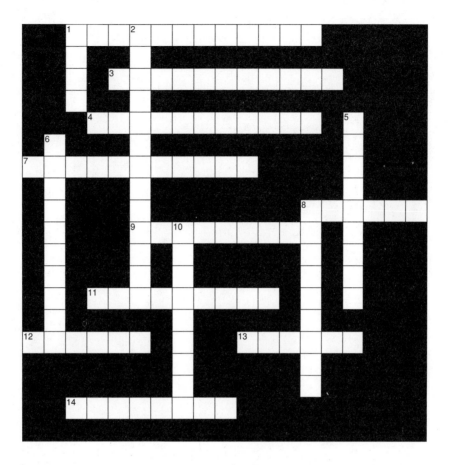

ACROSS

1. Spasm of tiny muscle layers surrounding the bronchioles.
3. Alveolar collapse.
4. Pneumothorax caused by the rupture of a weak area on the lung surface.
7. Involves moving oxygen into and carbon dioxide out of the body via the lungs.
8. Position that suggests moderately severe respiratory distress.
9. Lung tissue damage with loss of elastic recoil of the lungs.
11. Breathing characterized by a prolonged inspiratory phase followed by expiration apnea.
12. Recurring condition of completely or partially reversible acute airflow obstruction in lower airway.
13. Normal breathing rate.
14. Abnormally deep, very rapid sighing respirations.

DOWN

1. Congenital defect on the surface of the lung.
2. Cardiac drug that dilates both the veins and the arteries.
5. Asthma for which no specific substance can be identified as causing the air tubes to narrow.
6. Coughing up of blood.
8. Rapid breathing rate.
10. Acute inflammatory condition of the lungs, usually caused by either bacterial or viral infection.

23 Cardiovascular Anatomy and Physiology and ECG Interpretation

CHAPTER TERMINAL OBJECTIVES

On completion of this chapter, the EMT-Intermediate will understand the anatomy and physiology of the cardiovascular system and be able to interpret basic electrocardiography.

For the multiple-choice questions, select the single best answer to each question. For the matching questions, select the best corresponding answer for each item. Because there are sometimes more items than corresponding answers, some items may not be used.

1. The heart:
    a. is divided into right and left sides, separated by a thick wall
    b. is made up of a thick muscle called the endocardium
    c. consists of two upper chambers—the ventricles—and two lower chambers—the atria
    d. is about the size of a large grapefruit

2. The thick set of two membranes surrounding the heart is called the:
    a. epicardium
    b. myocardium
    c. pericardium
    d. endocardium

3. By numbering the correct order, trace how blood returning from the systemic venous circulation comes into contact with each of the following structures of the heart.
    _____ Blood traverses the mitral (bicuspid) valve into the left ventricle.
    _____ Blood is pumped through the aortic (semilunar) valve into the aorta.
    _____ Blood flows from the right ventricle through the pulmonary (semilunar) valve into the main pulmonary artery.
    _____ Deoxygenated blood returns to the right atrium via the superior and inferior venae cavae.
    _____ Blood that was oxygenated in the lungs is returned to the left atrium via the pulmonary veins.
    _____ Blood passes through the tricuspid valve into the right ventricle.

4. The valve that separates the right atrium from the right ventricle is the _____ valve.
    a. tricuspid
    b. mitral
    c. aortic
    d. pulmonic

5. The systolic blood pressure is:
    a. the pressure within the arteries during contraction of the atria and ventricles
    b. the pressure in the heart during its relaxation phase
    c. what forces the blood supply from the coronary arteries into the heart muscle
    d. the amount of blood pumped through the cardiovascular system

6. Cardiac output is the product of _____ × _____.
   a. heart rate; blood pressure
   b. stroke volume; peripheral resistance
   c. preload; blood pressure
   d. stroke volume; heart rate

7. Which of the following is true regarding *preload?*
   a. The greater the presystolic ventricular stretch (within limits), the lesser the subsequent ventricular contraction.
   b. If preload is decreased, ventricular contraction is unaffected.
   c. Preload is unaffected by the ventricular compliance.
   d. Preload is the pressure within the ventricle at the end of diastole.

8. The principle of "the heart pumping blood more forcefully when it is filled and the ventricles are stretched" is:
   a. Boyle's law
   b. Starling's law
   c. Hering-Breuer reflex
   d. systolic stretch principle

9. Match the following terms with the correct definition.

   Term
   a. Afterload
   b. Stroke volume
   c. Ejection fraction
   d. Cardiac output

   Definition
   _____ The amount of blood pumped by the heart in 1 minute
   _____ Resistance to blood flow out of the ventricle
   _____ The amount of blood pumped out of the ventricle during each contraction
   _____ The amount of blood returning to the right atrium, which varies somewhat from minute to minute

10. _____ are blood vessels that carry blood away from the heart to the body. _____ transport blood from the body back to the heart. _____ decrease in size as they move away from the heart, branching into many small _____. _____ then divide many times until they form _____, microscopic thin-walled vessels through which oxygen, carbon dioxide, and other nutrients and waste products are exchanged.

11. For the illustration of the coronary circulation below, label the arteries and veins.

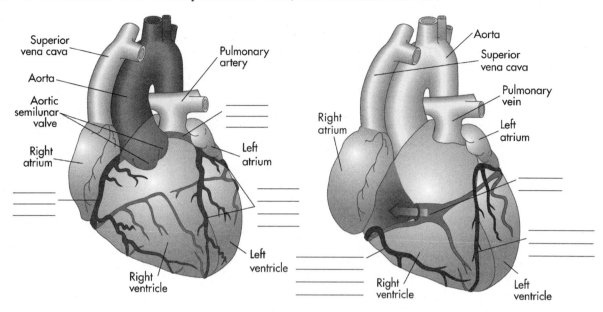

12. Briefly describe the function of the electrical conduction system of the heart.

_____

_____

_____

_____

_____

13. For the illustration of the conduction system of the heart on p. 322, label the components of the conduction system, describe the function of each, and color each structure as indicated.

Name	Function	Color of Pencil That Should Be Used
A		red
B		green
C		yellow
D		orange
E		blue

321

Copyright © 2007 Elsevier, Inc. All rights reserved. Chapter **23** **Cardiovascular Anatomy and Physiology and ECG Interpretation**

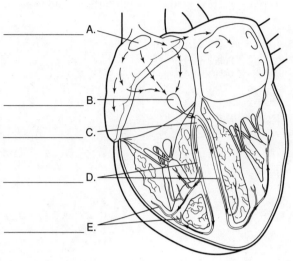

_____ A.

_____ B.

_____ C.

_____ D.

_____ E.

14. The SA node has an intrinsic rate of _____ beats per minute (BPM).

15. The AV junctional tissue has an intrinsic rate of _____ BPM.

16. The ventricles have an intrinsic rate of _____ BPM.

17. Identify, by numbering, the correct sequence in which an electrical impulse is initiated and travels through the heart.
    _____ Purkinje fibers
    _____ SA node
    _____ Bundle branches
    _____ Bundle of His
    _____ Interatrial and internodal tracts
    _____ AV node

18. The Purkinje fibers:
    a. have an inherent rate of 40 to 60 BPM
    b. serve as the primary pacemaker site of the heart
    c. are located in the superior aspect of the right atrium
    d. supply a conduction pathway to the individual cells of the ventricles

19. Match four unique characteristics of the myocardial cells with the correct description.

    Characteristic
    a. Automaticity
    b. Excitability
    c. Conductivity
    d. Contractility

    Description
    _____ The ability to respond to an appropriate electrical stimulus
    _____ The ability of the myocardial cell to contract when stimulated by an appropriate electrical stimulus
    _____ The ability to self-generate electrical activity (action potential) without the need for extraneous nerve stimulation
    _____ The ability to transmit an appropriate electrical stimulus from cell to cell throughout the myocardium

20. The interior of the heart cell (myocyte) is _____ charged during the resting phase. This is referred to as the _____ _____ _____.

21. When depolarization begins, _____, _____, and _____ ions move from their "resting" locations in and out of the cell. The net result is that the interior of the myocyte becomes more _____ charged.

22. When a certain level or _____ is reached, _____ of the entire cell occurs.

23. After a period of time, each cell returns back to the _____ state, again as a result of the movement of _____, _____, and _____, waiting for the next stimulus.

24. The electrical term for the process of depolarization and repolarization is:
    a. refractory period
    b. membrane threshold
    c. dromotropic state
    d. action potential

25. Describe the "wave of depolarization."
    _____
    _____
    _____
    _____

26. T F Pacemaker cells are capable of self-initiated depolarization.

27. T F Repolarization is the process by which cells reestablish internal negativity and are readied for stimulation.

28. During the absolute refractory period:
    a. a sufficiently strong stimulus will depolarize the myocardium
    b. the heart is less amenable to receiving new electrical stimuli
    c. no stimulus will depolarize the myocyte
    d. only ectopic stimuli will depolarize the myocardium

29. The term *dromotropic* refers to the:
    a. heart rate
    b. contractility of the heart
    c. velocity of electrical impulse conduction through the heart
    d. amount of stretch applied to the ventricle at the end of diastole

30. A medication that has positive inotropic effects:
    a. increases the heart rate
    b. decreases coronary perfusion
    c. increases myocardial contractility
    d. decreases the heart's conductivity

31. List three things that influence the chronotropic, dromotropic, and inotropic states of the heart.

_____

_____

_____

32. Stimulation of the parasympathetic nervous system:
    a. decreases the heart rate
    b. causes vasoconstriction
    c. results in bronchodilation
    d. enhances conduction velocity through the AV node

33. Which of the following is true regarding the sympathetic nervous system?
    a. Its primary receptor is the vagus nerve.
    b. Acetylcholine is its neurotransmitter.
    c. It is part of the central nervous system.
    d. It is associated with "fight or flight."

34. Stimulation of beta-1 receptors:
    a. leads to peripheral vasoconstriction
    b. increases the heart rate
    c. brings about relaxation of the bronchial smooth muscle
    d. causes dilation of the renal and mesenteric arteries

35. Stimulation of the alpha-1 receptors of the sympathetic nervous system will cause:
    a. vasoconstriction
    b. increases in the heart rate
    c. decreases in myocardial contractility
    d. increased vagal tone

36. The baroreceptors:
    a. are located in the subclavian artery
    b. directly control the heart rate and stroke volume
    c. sense changes in the blood pressure
    d. sense changes in the CO_2 and O_2 concentrations and pH of the arterial blood

37. T F The electrocardiograph (ECG) records the mechanical action of the heart.

38. The ECG is a _____ representation of the electrical activity of the heart, which is picked up by _____ that are placed on the patient's skin in at least _____ different places.

39. The electrodes are attached to the cardiac monitor by means of a _____.

40. All of the following information can be gained from a monitoring lead or rhythm strip *except:*
    a. how fast the heart is beating
    b. how long the conduction is taking to occur in different parts of the heart
    c. axis deviation and chamber enlargement
    d. how regular the heartbeat is

41. When stimulated by the electrical impulse of the conduction system, the heart muscle cell becomes

    _____ and contracts in response.

42. Match the following ECG representations with the correct cardiac event.

    ECG Representation
    a. P wave
    b. PR interval
    c. QRS complex
    d. ST segment
    e. T wave
    f. R-to-R interval

    Cardiac Event
    _____ Time between two ventricular depolarizations
    _____ Electrical depolarization of the atria
    _____ Electrical depolarization of the ventricles
    _____ Period between ventricular electrical depolarization and repolarization

43. Use the directions below to color the illustration of the ECG complex.

    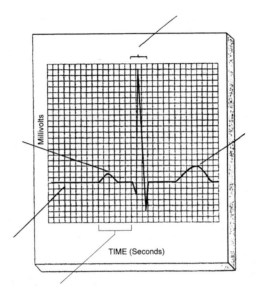

    a. Label and color the isoelectric line yellow.
    b. Label and color the P wave green.
    c. Label and color the remainder of the PR interval red.
    d. Label and color the QRS complex orange.
    e. Label and color the T wave blue.

44. Atrial repolarization is:
    a. denoted by the ST segment
    b. denoted by the P wave
    c. buried within the QRS complex
    d. represented by the first downward deflection following the P wave

45. List five elements that should be evaluated when analyzing an ECG rhythm strip.

_____

_____

_____

_____

_____

46. To count the heart rate per minute, the 3-second marks at the top of ECG paper can be used. Two complete sections represent _____ in time. The number of R waves that occur within this time are counted and the number multiplied by _____ to obtain the patient's heart rate.
    a. 3 seconds; 2
    b. 10 seconds; 5
    c. 6 seconds; 10
    d. 4 seconds; 25

47. In example A below, using the 6 second times 10 method, determine the heart rate of this dysrhythmia.

_____

_____

A

B

48. Another method for estimating the heart rate involves using a series of numbers to denote the value of each vertical bold (heavy) line beyond an R wave that falls on a bold line. In example B (above), using that method, determine the heart rate of this dysrhythmia.

49. If the distance between consecutive R waves remains constant, the ventricular rhythm is considered to be

    _____. If the interval varies, the rhythm is _____.

50. An upright, rounded P wave usually indicates an impulse originating from the _____ _____.

51. If each P wave on the ECG is followed by a _____ complex, it indicates that the impulses are being transmitted to the ventricles.

52. In the healthy adult, the PR interval is between _____ and _____ small squares, or _____ to _____ second(s) in duration.

53. Normal QRS duration is less than _____ small squares, or less than _____ second(s). A duration of _____ small squares or more indicates a delay in the conduction of the impulse through the _____ .

54. Define the term *dysrhythmia*.

_____
_____
_____
_____

55. List 10 causes of dysrhythmia.

_____
_____
_____
_____
_____
_____
_____
_____
_____
_____

56. Characteristics of sinus rhythm include:
    a. an irregular rhythm
    b. a rate of between 60 and 100 BPM
    c. an inverted P wave that precedes each QRS complex
    d. PR intervals that vary slightly

57. In sinus bradycardia, the pacemaker site is in the:
    a. SA node
    b. atrial conduction pathways
    c. AV junction
    d. bundle of His

58. Sinus bradycardia has a rate of _____ BPM.
    a. less than 80
    b. 20 to 40
    c. less than 60
    d. 60 to 100

59. Sinus tachycardia is a regular sinus rhythm with a rate greater than _____ BPM. Usually the rate does not exceed _____ BPM.

60. In sinus tachycardia, the P waves, PR intervals, and QRS intervals are _____.

61. On the following illustration, mark the location where sinus rhythm, sinus bradycardia, sinus tachycardia, and sinus dysrhythmia originate.

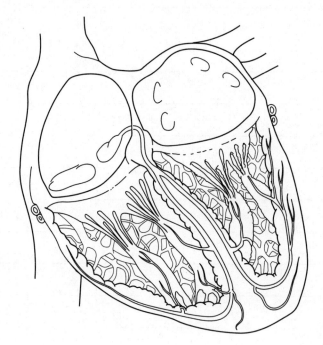

62. Fill in the following table regarding sinus rhythms.

	Rate	Rhythm	QRS Complex	P Wave	PR Interval
Sinus rhythm					
Sinus tachycardia					
Sinus bradycardia					
Sinus dysrhythmia					

63. With sinus dysrhythmia, the:
    a. P waves all appear different
    b. QRS complexes are greater than 0.12 second in duration
    c. rhythm is regularly irregular
    d. PR intervals vary

64. With sinus arrest, the:
    a. rhythm is irregular because of the pause in the rhythm
    b. rate is usually greater than 80 BPM
    c. P waves are inverted, and a QRS complex follows each
    d. QRS complexes are usually greater than 0.12 second

65. On the following illustration, indicate the area where atrial dysrhythmias originate.

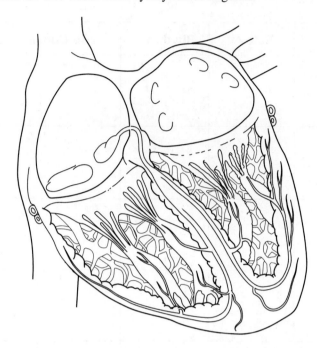

66. With atrial rhythms, the QRS complexes are typically _____ than _____ second(s) in duration.

67. Match the following atrial dysrhythmias with the correct characteristics. Letters can be used more than once.

   Dysrhythmia
   a. Wandering pacemaker
   b. Premature atrial contraction (PAC)
   c. Supraventricular tachycardia (SVT)
   d. Atrial flutter
   e. Atrial fibrillation

   Characteristic
   _____ Rhythm is totally (grossly) irregular
   _____ Atrial rate is 250 to 350 BPM
   _____ Early beat causes the underlying rhythm to be irregular
   _____ Normal P waves absent; "sawtooth" flutter waves present
   _____ Atrial and ventricular rate is 150 to 250 BPM
   _____ Morphology of P wave changes from beat to beat
   _____ The baseline is chaotic because the atrial activity is represented by "fibrillatory waves" or "f" waves
   _____ Atrial rate is between 350 and 700 BPM

68. With a wandering atrial pacemaker, the rhythm is:
   a. slightly irregular
   b. regular
   c. totally irregular
   d. a patterned irregularity

69. Atrial flutter:
   a. severely hampers cardiac output
   b. originates from the AV node
   c. has an atrial rate of greater than 350 BPM
   d. may have a varying conduction ratio

70. The P waves associated with atrial fibrillation are _____, and the PR intervals are _____.
    a. referred to as sawtoothed; variable
    b. indiscernible; nonexistent
    c. inverted; less than 0.12 second
    d. dissociated; between 0.12 and 0.20 second

71. Fill in the following table regarding atrial dysrhythmias.

	Rate	Rhythm	QRS Complex	P Wave	PR Interval
Wandering atrial pacemaker					
PAC					
SVT					
Atrial flutter					
Atrial fibrillation					

72. Describe why P waves seen with atrial dysrhythmias differ from normal.

_____

_____

_____

_____

73. On the following illustration, indicate the area where junctional dysrhythmias originate.

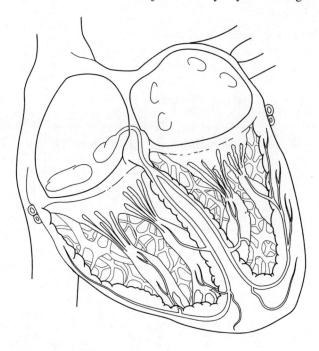

74. P waves seen with junctional rhythms will:
    a. appear upright and rounded
    b. be inverted when present and may precede, follow, or be lost in (absent) the QRS complex
    c. often have a different appearance than normal and vary from beat to beat
    d. be flattened or notched

75. PR intervals seen with junctional rhythms will appear:
    a. longer than 0.20 second in duration
    b. shorter than 0.12 second in duration
    c. within normal ranges
    d. varied

76. Describe why QRS complexes seen with junctional rhythms are usually less than 0.12 second in duration.

_____

_____

_____

_____

_____

77. Fill in the following table regarding junctional rhythms.

	Rate	Rhythm	QRS Complex	P Wave	PR Interval
Premature junctional contraction (PJC)					
Junctional escape rhythm					
Accelerated junctional rhythm					
Junctional tachycardia					

78. On the following illustration, indicate the area where ventricular ectopy originates.

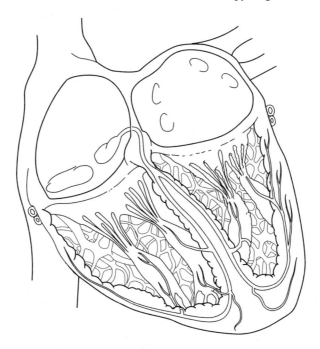

79. T F A premature ventricular complex (PVC) is a single irritable focus within the atrium that fires prematurely to initiate an ectopic complex.

80. T F Because the PVC arises from an irritable focus, the complex will come earlier in the cardiac cycle and will interrupt the regularity of the underlying rhythm.

81. A PVC:
    a. has a QRS complex that appears narrow and normal in configuration
    b. has a T wave that takes an opposite deflection of the QRS complex
    c. is preceded by an inverted P wave
    d. is seldom followed by a compensatory pause

82. List five types of PVCs that are considered malignant.

    _____

    _____

    _____

    _____

83. Match the following types of PVCs with the correct description.

    Types of PVC
    a. Trigeminal
    b. Multiformed
    c. Bigeminal
    d. Couplets
    e. Uniform
    f. R-on-T phenomenon
    g. A run of PVCs

    Description
    _____ Occurs when the PVC wave falls on the T wave
    _____ PVCs that occur every other beat
    _____ Three or more PVCs in a row
    _____ PVCs that appear different from each other
    _____ PVCs that occur every third beat
    _____ Two PVCs that occur together without a normal complex between
    _____ PVCs that have the same morphology (appearance)

84. Which of the following rhythms may result in hypotension?
    a. sinus rhythm
    b. ventricular tachycardia
    c. occasional PVCs
    d. sinus tachycardia

85. Ventricular tachycardia has:
    a. an irregular rhythm
    b. a rate of between 20 and 40 BPM
    c. P waves preceding each QRS complex
    d. wide and bizarre QRS complexes (greater than 0.12 second in duration)

86. Ventricular fibrillation appears on the ECG monitor as having:
    a. an overall pattern that appears irregularly shaped, chaotic, and lacks any regular repeating features
    b. narrow QRS complexes
    c. electrical signals that are the same height
    d. a distance between the peaks of the electrical signal that varies greatly

87. Idioventricular rhythm has a rate of _____ BPM.
    a. fewer than 40
    b. 30 to 60
    c. 50 to 75
    d. 100 to 150

88. Place a checkmark beside those dysrhythmias that are considered life threatening.
    _____ Sinus tachycardia
    _____ Occasional unifocal PVCs
    _____ Ventricular fibrillation
    _____ Sinus bradycardia
    _____ Asystole
    _____ Pulseless electrical activity (PEA)

89. Which of the following is referred to as the "ultimate bradycardia"?
    a. ventricular fibrillation
    b. sinus bradycardia
    c. asystole
    d. PEA

90. Which of the following has an organized electrical rhythm but no pulse?
    a. ventricular fibrillation
    b. PEA
    c. asystole
    d. ventricular tachycardia

91. List at least four reversible causes of PEA.

_____

_____

_____

_____

92. Fill in the following table regarding ventricular rhythms.

	Rate	Rhythm	QRS Complex	P Wave	PR Interval
PVC					
Ventricular escape rhythm					
Ventricular tachycardia					
Ventricular fibrillation					
Asystole					

93. The most common cause of sudden death in the patient experiencing acute myocardial infarction is:
    a. pump failure
    b. asystole
    c. electrical mechanical dissociation (EMD)
    d. ventricular fibrillation

94. On the following illustration, shade in the area where heart blocks occur.

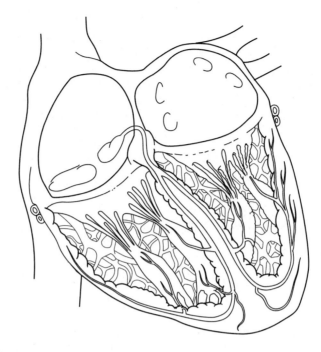

95. With first-degree heart block:
    a. the PR intervals are greater than 0.20 second in duration
    b. not all the P waves are followed by QRS complexes
    c. the P waves are inverted
    d. the underlying rhythm is slow

96. With second-degree heart block, Wenckebach:
    a. the PR intervals get progressively shorter
    b. not all the P waves are followed by a QRS complex
    c. the P waves are inverted
    d. the rhythm appears to be irregularly irregular

97. With second-degree AV heart block, Mobitz II, the:
    a. P waves are upright and uniform
    b. QRS complex follows each P wave
    c. pacemaker site is in the AV junction
    d. ventricular rate is less than 40 BPM

98. Match the following heart blocks with the correct characteristics.

    Heart Block
    a. First-degree AV block
    b. Second-degree AV block, Wenckebach
    c. Second-degree AV block, Mobitz II
    d. Third-degree AV block

    Characteristic
    _____ PR interval gets progressively longer until a P wave fails to conduct, resulting in a "dropped" QRS complex. After the blocked beat, the cycle starts all over again.
    _____ There is a complete block at or below the AV node; there is no relationship between the P waves and QRS complexes
    _____ Some beats are conducted, and others are blocked
    _____ Not a true block; there is a delay at the AV node; each impulse is eventually conducted

99. Which of the following rhythms has a constant PR interval?
    a. second-degree AV heart block, Wenckebach
    b. third-degree AV heart block
    c. second-degree AV heart block, Mobitz II
    d. all of the above

100. The difference between Wenckebach and Mobitz II is that with:
    a. Wenckebach, the PR intervals are constant
    b. Mobitz II, the ventricular rate is usually greater than 60 BPM
    c. Mobitz II, the P waves appear to march right through the QRS complexes
    d. Wenckebach, there appears to be a pattern to the irregularity

101. Which of the following dysrhythmias has P waves that seem to march through the QRS complexes?
    a. second-degree AV block, Wenckebach
    b. second-degree AV block, Mobitz II
    c. third-degree AV block
    d. first-degree AV block

102. T F With third-degree AV heart block, the ventricular rate is usually greater than 60 BPM.

103. T F With second-degree AV heart block, Mobitz II, the PR interval becomes progressively longer until a QRS complex is dropped.

104. T F With third-degree AV heart block, the R-to-R waves are irregular.

105. T F With second-degree AV heart block, Mobitz II, the rhythm is typically regular.

106. T F Atropine is not recommended in the treatment of second-degree AV block, Mobitz II, or in third-degree block with new wide QRS complexes.

107. Fill in the following table regarding heart blocks.

	Rate	Rhythm	QRS Complex	P Wave	PR Interval
First-degree AV block					
Second-degree AV block, Wenckebach					
Second-degree AV block, Mobitz II					
Third-degree AV block					

108. Which of the following originates from the SA node?
    a. wandering atrial pacemaker
    b. junctional escape rhythm
    c. premature atrial complex
    d. sinus dysrhythmia

109. In _____, each of the QRS complexes is preceded by an upright, normal P wave.
    a. atrial fibrillation
    b. junctional tachycardia
    c. sinus bradycardia
    d. idioventricular rhythm

110. Which of the following dysrhythmias is irregular?
    a. atrial tachycardia
    b. sinus bradycardia
    c. junctional escape rhythm
    d. wandering atrial pacemaker

111. Which of the following rhythms is preceded by an inverted P wave?
    a. atrial flutter
    b. junctional escape rhythm
    c. atrial tachycardia
    d. idioventricular rhythm

112. Which of the following rhythms has a longer than normal PR interval?
    a. atrial fibrillation with a controlled ventricular response
    b. ventricular tachycardia
    c. first-degree AV block
    d. accelerated junctional rhythm

113. Which of the following dysrhythmias is fast?
    a. atrial tachycardia
    b. sinus bradycardia
    c. accelerated junctional rhythm
    d. sinus dysrhythmia

114. With artificial pacemaker rhythm, the:
    a. heart rate varies according to pacer settings; usually 60 to 80/min
    b. QRS complex is normal in width and appearance
    c. QRS complex is preceded by a round and upright P wave
    d. PR intervals are within normal duration

115. T F Pacemaker failure is a true emergency.

116. T F With pacemaker failure, the EMT-I should use immediate synchronized cardioversion.

117. T F Ventricular conduction disturbances involve complete blockage in electrical conduction through either the bundle branches (right or left) or the fascicles (anterior, posterior).

118. T F The presence of R and R' waves in a wide, upright QRS complex in lead MCL1 strongly favors an ECG diagnosis of right bundle branch block.

119. The hemiblocks (LAHB, LPHB) involve a block of conduction in one of the _____ _____.

    _____ _____ hemiblock is far more common.

120. With hemiblock, the normal conduction pathway is _____. The affected myocardium receives its electrical innervation "_____" from the remaining intact parts of the _____ system.

121. Patients with any type of _____ conduction block, and especially those with a combination, are at high risk of developing _____ heart block. Consider standby _____ _____ for these individuals, especially in the face of acute myocardial ischemia.

122. Describe preexcitation syndromes.

    _____
    _____
    _____
    _____
    _____

123. List the ECG features of Wolff-Parkinson-White (WPW) syndrome.

    _____
    _____

Identify the following cardiac ECG rhythms.

124.

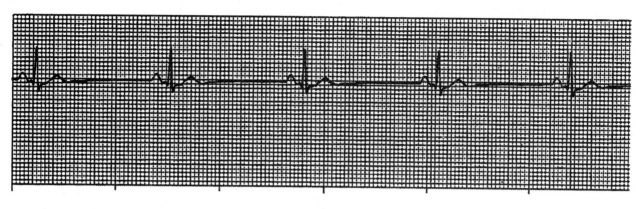

Rate: Rhythm: P waves:
QRS complexes: PR intervals: Interpretation:

125.

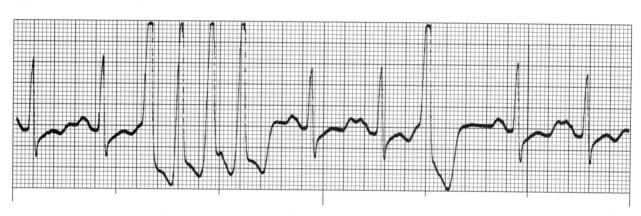

Rate: Rhythm: P waves:
QRS complexes: PR intervals: Interpretation:

126.

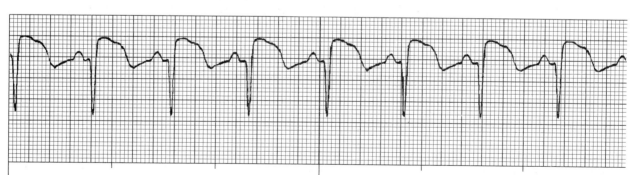

Rate: Rhythm: P waves:
QRS complexes: PR intervals: Interpretation:

127.

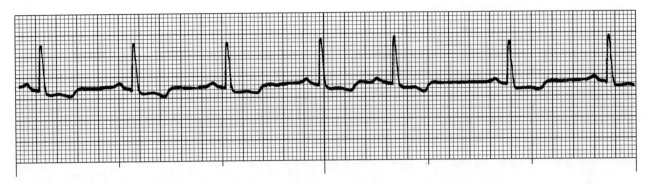

Rate: Rhythm: P waves:
QRS complexes: PR intervals: Interpretation:

128.

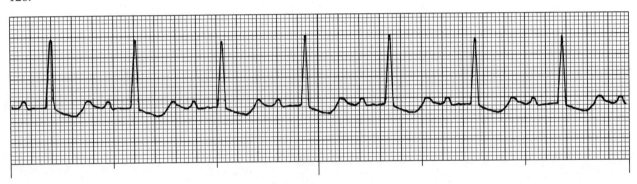

Rate: Rhythm: P waves:
QRS complexes: PR intervals: Interpretation:

129.

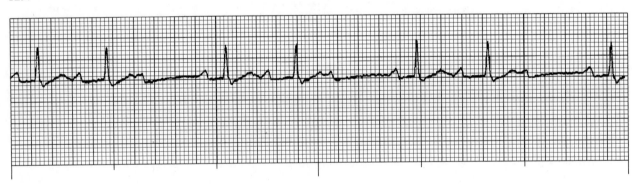

Rate: Rhythm: P waves:
QRS complexes: PR intervals: Interpretation:

130.

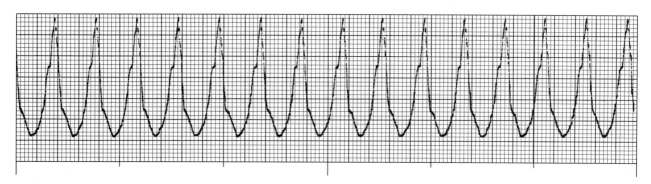

Rate: Rhythm: P waves:
QRS complexes: PR intervals: Interpretation:

131.

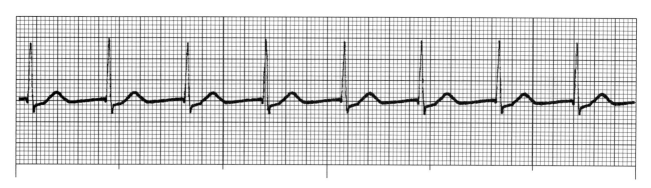

Rate: Rhythm: P waves:
QRS complexes: PR intervals: Interpretation:

132.

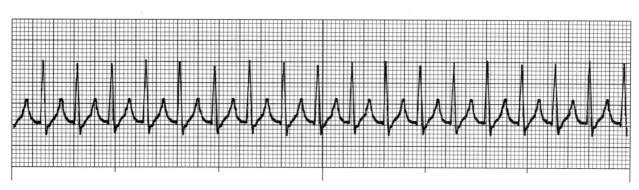

Rate: Rhythm: P waves:
QRS complexes: PR intervals: Interpretation:

133.

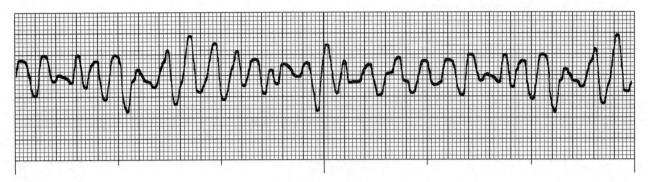

Rate: Rhythm: P waves:
QRS complexes: PR intervals: Interpretation:

134.

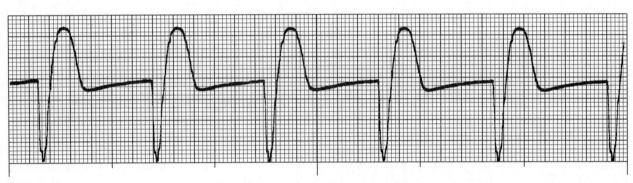

Rate: Rhythm: P waves:
QRS complexes: PR intervals: Interpretation:

135.

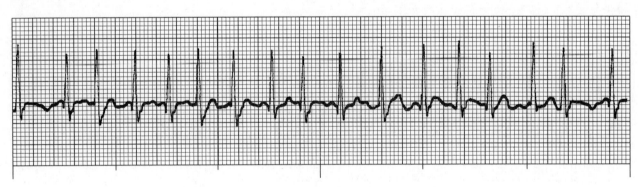

Rate: Rhythm: P waves:
QRS complexes: PR intervals: Interpretation:

136.

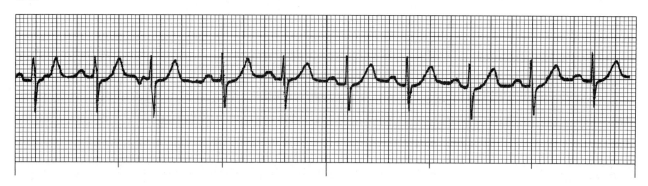

Rate: Rhythm: P waves:
QRS complexes: PR intervals: Interpretation:

137.

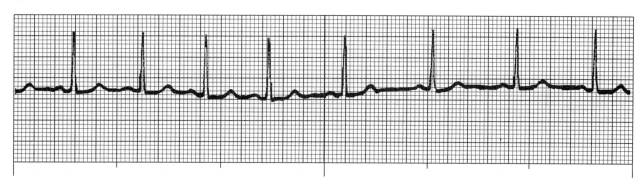

Rate: Rhythm: P waves:
QRS complexes: PR intervals: Interpretation:

138.

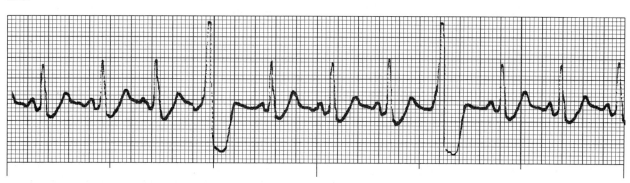

Rate: Rhythm: P waves:
QRS complexes: PR intervals: Interpretation:

139.

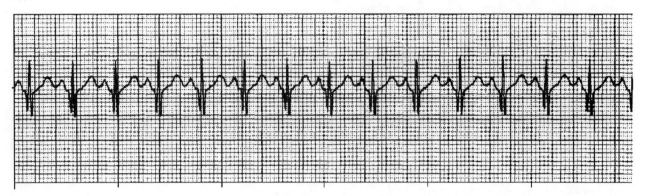

Rate: Rhythm: P waves:
QRS complexes: PR intervals: Interpretation:

140.

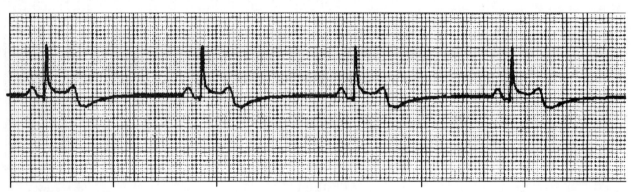

Rate: Rhythm: P waves:
QRS complexes: PR intervals: Interpretation:

141.

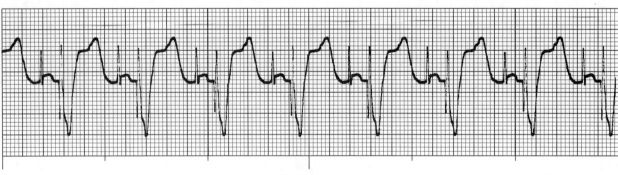

Rate: Rhythm: P waves:
QRS complexes: PR intervals: Interpretation:

142.

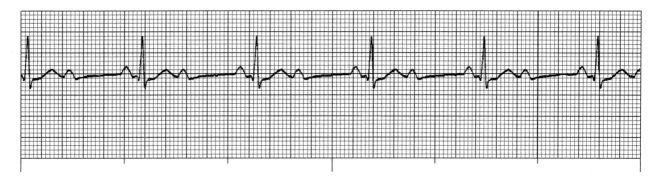

Rate: Rhythm: P waves:
QRS complexes: PR intervals: Interpretation:

143.

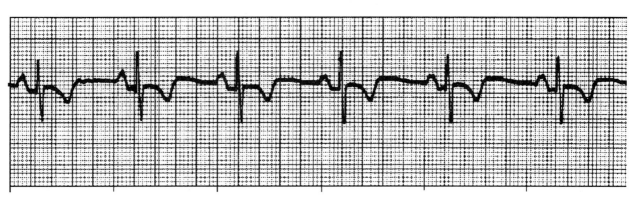

Rate: Rhythm: P waves:
QRS complexes: PR intervals: Interpretation:

144.

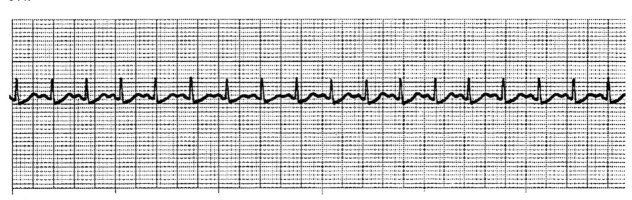

Rate: Rhythm: P waves:
QRS complexes: PR intervals: Interpretation:

145.

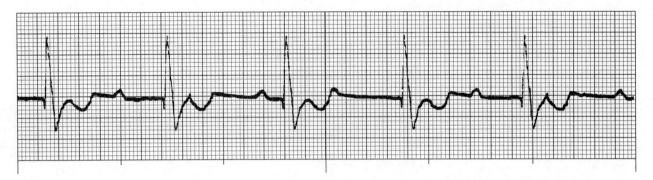

Rate: Rhythm: P waves:
QRS complexes: PR intervals: Interpretation:

146.

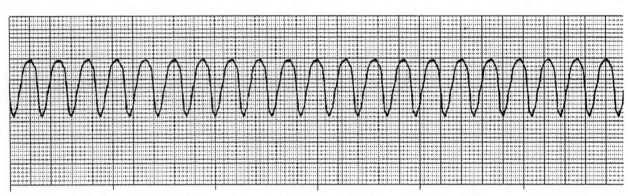

Rate: Rhythm: P waves:
QRS complexes: PR intervals: Interpretation:

147.

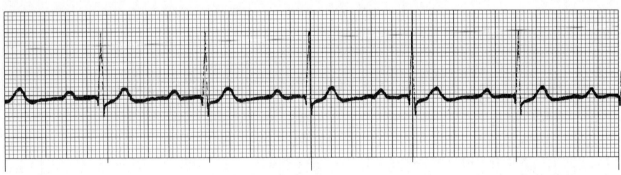

Rate: Rhythm: P waves:
QRS complexes: PR intervals: Interpretation:

148.

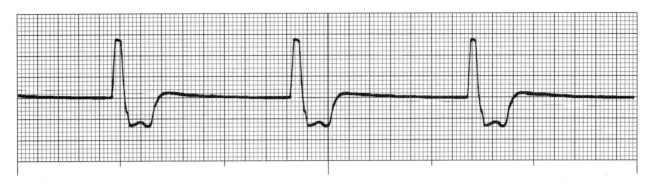

Rate: Rhythm: P waves:
QRS complexes: PR intervals: Interpretation:

149.

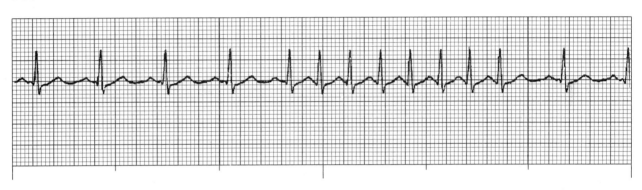

Rate: Rhythm: P waves:
QRS complexes: PR intervals: Interpretation:

150.

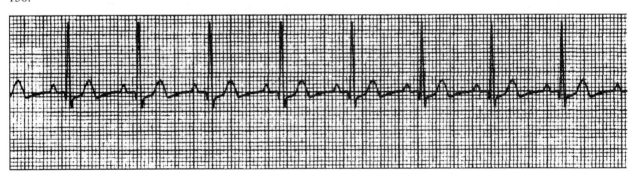

Rate: Rhythm: P waves:
QRS complexes: PR intervals: Interpretation:

151.

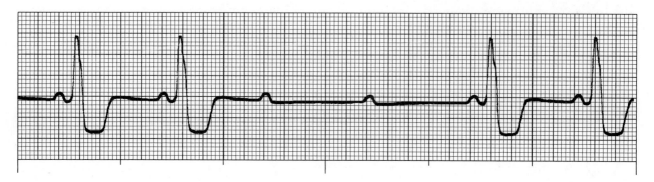

Rate: Rhythm: P waves:
QRS complexes: PR intervals: Interpretation:

152.

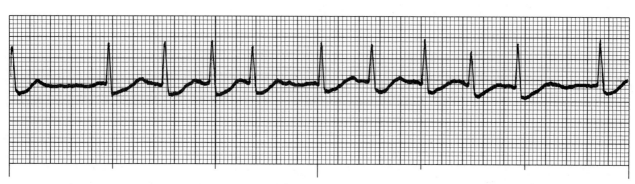

Rate: Rhythm: P waves:
QRS complexes: PR intervals: Interpretation:

153.

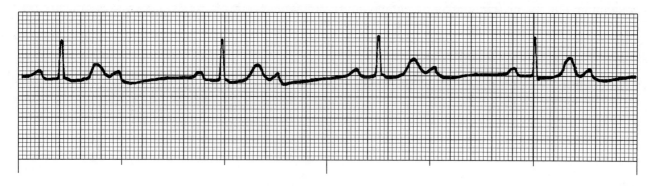

Rate: Rhythm: P waves:
QRS complexes: PR intervals: Interpretation:

154.

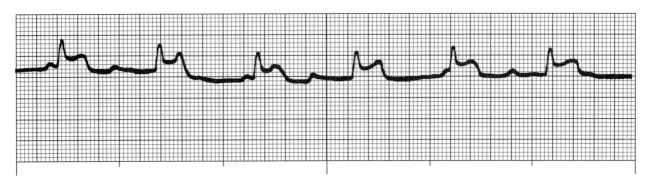

Rate: Rhythm: P waves:
QRS complexes: PR intervals: Interpretation:

155.

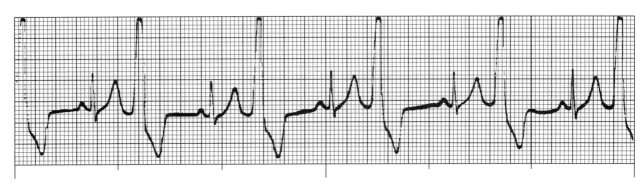

Rate: Rhythm: P waves:
QRS complexes: PR intervals: Interpretation:

156.

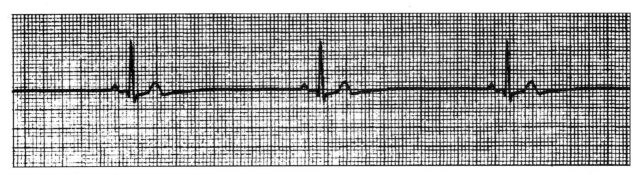

Rate: Rhythm: P waves:
QRS complexes: PR intervals: Interpretation:

157.

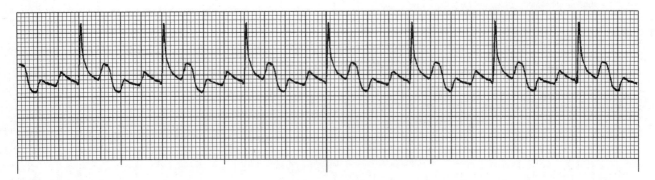

Rate: Rhythm: P waves:
QRS complexes: PR intervals: Interpretation:

158.

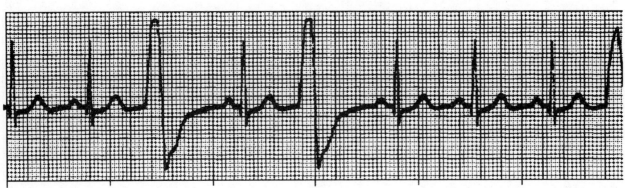

Rate: Rhythm: P waves:
QRS complexes: PR intervals: Interpretation:

159.

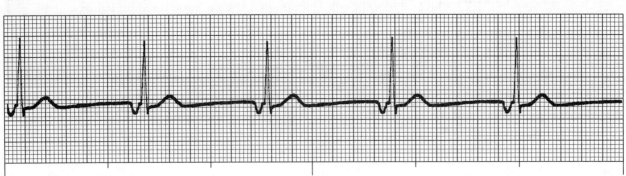

Rate: Rhythm: P waves:
QRS complexes: PR intervals: Interpretation:

160.

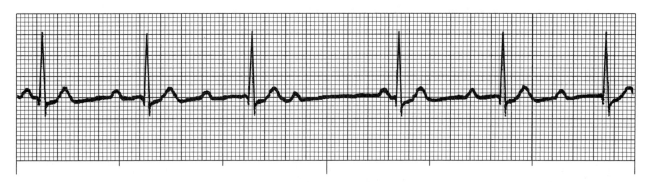

Rate: Rhythm: P waves:
QRS complexes: PR intervals: Interpretation:

161.

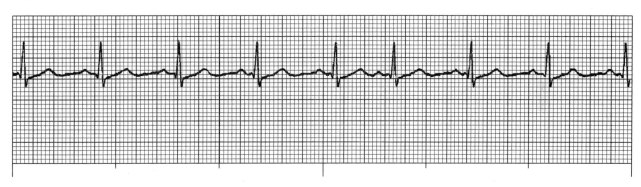

Rate: Rhythm: P waves:
QRS complexes: PR intervals: Interpretation:

162.

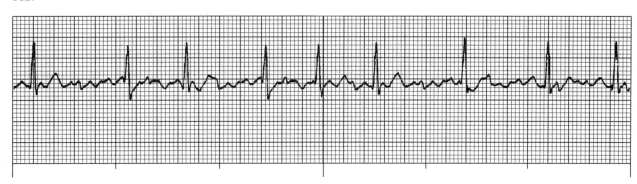

Rate: Rhythm: P waves:
QRS complexes: PR intervals: Interpretation:

163.

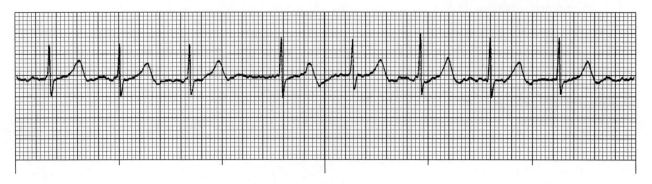

Rate: Rhythm: P waves:
QRS complexes: PR intervals: Interpretation:

164.

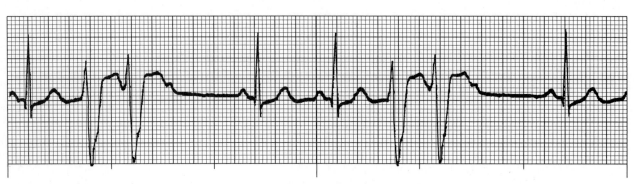

Rate: Rhythm: P waves:
QRS complexes: PR intervals: Interpretation:

165.

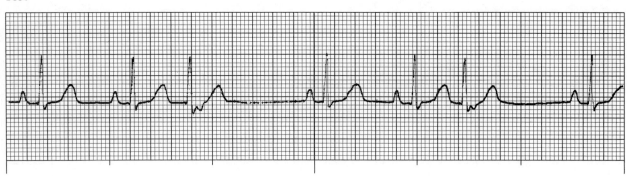

Rate: Rhythm: P waves:
QRS complexes: PR intervals: Interpretation:

166.

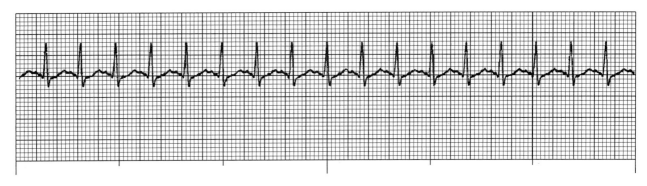

Rate: Rhythm: P waves:
QRS complexes: PR intervals: Interpretation:

167.

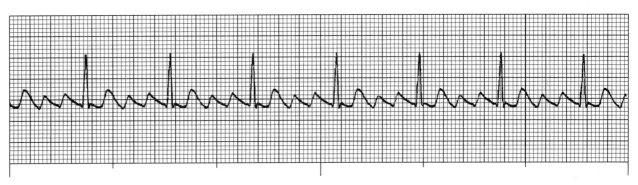

Rate: Rhythm: P waves:
QRS complexes: PR intervals: Interpretation:

168.

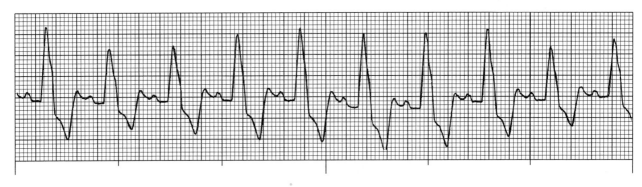

Rate: Rhythm: P waves:
QRS complexes: PR intervals: Interpretation:

169.

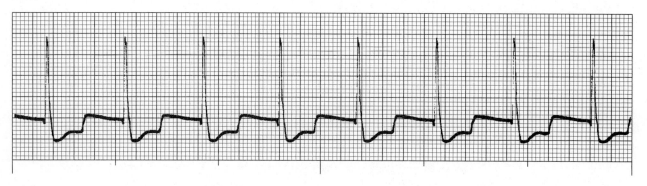

Rate: Rhythm: P waves:
QRS complexes: PR intervals: Interpretation:

170.

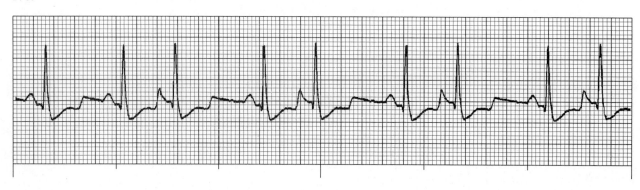

Rate: Rhythm: P waves:
QRS complexes: PR intervals: Interpretation:

171.

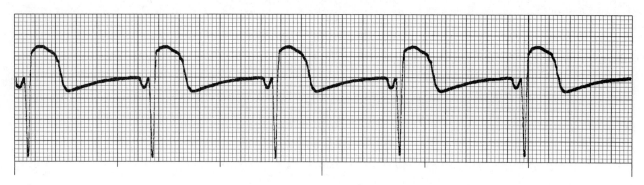

Rate: Rhythm: P waves:
QRS complexes: PR intervals: Interpretation:

172.

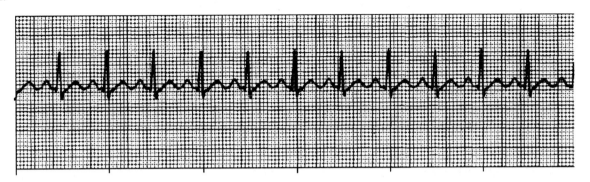

Rate: Rhythm: P waves:
QRS complexes: PR intervals: Interpretation:

24 Cardiovascular Emergencies

CHAPTER TERMINAL OBJECTIVES

On completion of this chapter, the EMT-Intermediate will be able to utilize assessment findings to formulate a field impression, and implement and evaluate a management plan for the patient experiencing a cardiac emergency.

For the multiple-choice questions, select the single best answer to each question. For the matching questions, select the best corresponding answer for each item. Because there are sometimes more items than corresponding answers, some items may not be used.

1. The number one killer in the United States is:
    a. respiratory disease
    b. cardiovascular disease
    c. endocrine disorders
    d. cancer

2. Between 1963 and 1995, there was a _____ decrease in the death rate from ischemic heart disease (IHD) in the United States.
    a. 10%
    b. 25%
    c. 50%
    d. 75%

3. IHD includes _____ _____ _____, _____ _____, _____ _____, and congestive heart failure (CHF).

4. List four reasons for the decrease in the death rate from IHD in the United States.

    _____

    _____

    _____

    _____

5. In the United States about 225,000 people a year die of IHD without being hospitalized. Many of these are sudden deaths caused by cardiac arrest, usually resulting from:
    a. ventricular fibrillation (VF)
    b. asystole
    c. idioventricular rhythm
    d. heart failure

6. List seven major risk factors that predispose to IHD.

_____

_____

_____

_____

_____

_____

_____

7. The presence of pink-tinged frothy sputum may suggest acute _____ _____.

8. The most common symptom of cardiac problems is _____ _____.

9. T F Pain associated with myocardial ischemia and infarction is not always felt in the chest.

10. T F It is quite common for persons to have a feeling of impending doom before cardiac arrest.

11. T F The sudden onset of profuse sweating is usually not associated with cardiac problems unless it accompanies chest pain.

12. T F Nausea quite commonly accompanies myocardial infarction.

13. List seven findings suggestive of acute myocardial ischemia.

_____

_____

_____

_____

_____

_____

_____

14. List 11 elements that may be seen in the past medical history of the cardiac patient.

_____

_____

_____

_____

_____

_____

_____

_____

_____

_____

_____

15. Most patients complain of "_____ _____ _____," or palpitations, rather than of a/an "_____ _____ _____."

16. Patients who are uncomfortable for any reason, especially those who are hypoxic, will feel _____.

17. A patient is hypotensive secondary to a slow heart rate. To treat this patient you would administer:
    a. lidocaine, 1 mg/kg, IV push
    b. atropine, 0.5 mg, IV push
    c. 6 L/min of oxygen via simple face mask
    d. epinephrine, 0.5 to 1.0 mg, IV push

18. Management of sinus tachycardia focuses on treating the _____ of the tachycardia.

19. Fill in the following treatment algorithm for bradycardia.

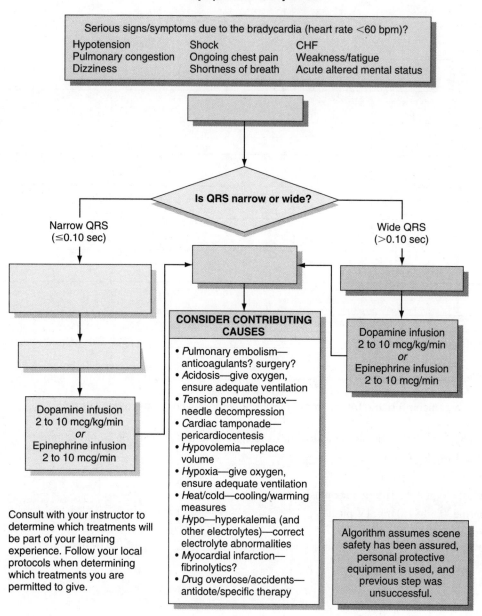

20. Fill in the following treatment algorithm for supraventricular tachycardia.

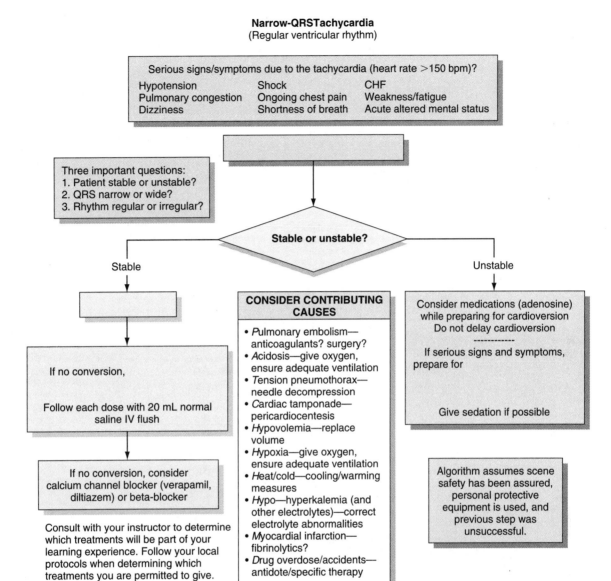

21. Treatment for stable ventricular tachycardia (VT) includes:
    a. atropine
    b. adenosine
    c. oxygen
    d. defibrillation

22. Fill in the following universal cardiac treatment algorithm.

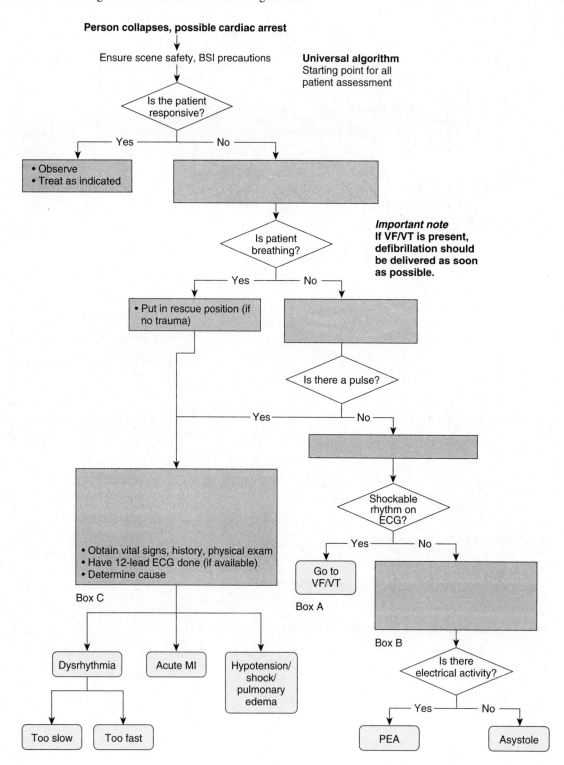

23. Which of the following is considered a treatment for pulseless VT?
    a. atropine
    b. naloxone
    c. D_{50}
    d. defibrillation

24. Which of the following drugs is used to treat VF?
    a. D_{50}
    b. epinephrine
    c. atropine
    d. nitroglycerin

25. Treatment for asystole includes:
    a. lidocaine, 1 mg/kg, IV push
    b. epinephrine, 100 mg, IV push
    c. atropine, 1 mg, IV push
    d. naloxone, 2 mg, IV push

26. Which of the following would be considered a treatment for pulseless electrical activity (PEA)?
    a. bretylium, 5 mg/kg, IV push
    b. epinephrine, 1 mg, IV push
    c. atropine, 10 to 20 mg, IV push
    d. defibrillation, 200 J

27. The most common cause of sudden death in the patient experiencing acute myocardial infarction (AMI) is:
    a. pump failure
    b. asystole
    c. electrical mechanical dissociation (EMD)
    d. VF

28. Fill in the following treatment algorithm for VF/pulseless VT.

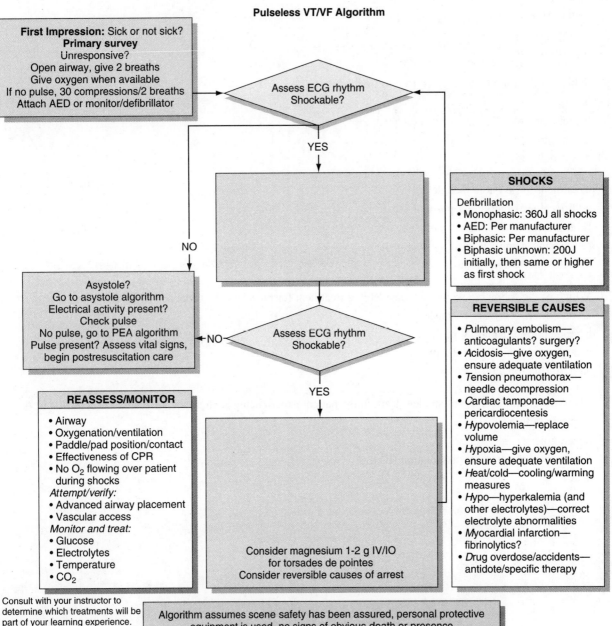

29. Fill in the following treatment algorithm for asystole.

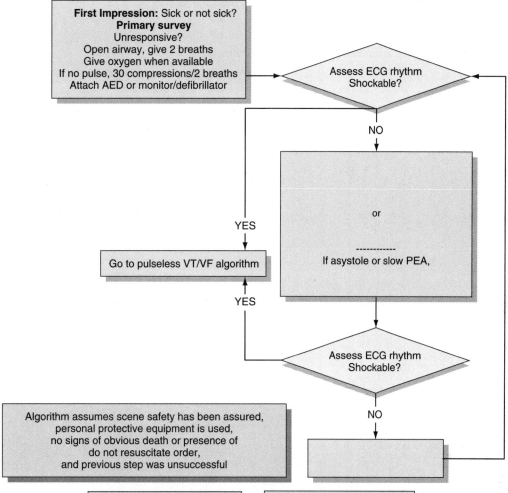

30. Vagal maneuvers:
    a. are used to stimulate the sympathetic nervous system
    b. should be used in the treatment of unstable PSVT
    c. should be preceded by the placement of an IV line and ECG monitoring
    d. are usually performed under standing orders

31. Match the following vagal maneuvers with the correct information.

    Vagal Maneuver
    a. Valsalva maneuver
    b. Ice-water maneuver
    c. Unilateral carotid sinus pressure

    Information
    _____ Should not be performed if IHD is present or suspected
    _____ Should be done only after auscultating both carotid arteries for a bruit
    _____ Involves having the patient take in a deep breath and "bear down" as if to have a bowel movement
    _____ Involves having the patient hold his or her breath and then immersing the face briefly into ice water
    _____ Is done using your index and middle fingers placed over the carotid artery on the neck, just below the angle of the jaw
    _____ Results in forced expiration against a closed glottis and vagal nerve stimulation
    _____ Stimulates the vagus nerve because of the mammalian diving reflex

32. List three contraindications to unilateral carotid sinus pressure.

    _____

    _____

    _____

33. To perform unilateral carotid sinus pressure:
    a. compress the carotid artery firmly while massaging the area
    b. maintain pressure for no longer than 15 to 20 seconds
    c. stop immediately if bradycardia or heart block develops, or if the tachycardia breaks
    d. compress both sides at the same time

34. Adenosine:
    a. may be used in the treatment of wide complex tachycardia of uncertain type
    b. enhances AV node and SA node activity
    c. is administered slowly by IV push
    d. administration should be followed immediately with a 20-mL saline flush

35. Adenosine is effective in terminating _____ .

36. The initial dose of adenosine is a _____ -mg rapid IV bolus followed by a 20-mL normal saline flush. If there is no response in _____ minutes, a _____ -mg dose should be administered in the same manner.

37. List three side effects of adenosine.

_____

_____

_____

38. Atropine _____ discharge from the _____ nervous system, leading to a/an _____ in the heart rate.

39. Indications for atropine include hemodynamically significant _____, _____, and bradycardic PEA.

40. Atropine is administered at a dose of:
    a. 5 to 10 mg IV push in symptomatic bradycardia
    b. 1 mg IV push in cardiac arrest
    c. 2 mg IV push in bradycardic PEA
    d. 1.0 to 1.5 mg when delivered endotracheally

41. Describe the repeat doses for atropine.

_____

_____

_____

42. Describe when atropine may be used as a temporizing measure.

_____

_____

_____

43. Place a checkmark beside the effects of epinephrine.
    _____ Increased aortic diastolic pressure
    _____ Peripheral vasodilation
    _____ Decreased heart rate
    _____ Increased coronary perfusion pressure
    _____ Decreased coarseness of fibrillation

44. List three types of cardiac arrest epinephrine may be used to treat.

_____

_____

_____

45. In the treatment of cardiac arrest, epinephrine can be administered at a dose of:
    a. 0.5 to 1.0 mg, IV push, repeated every 5 to 10 minutes
    b. 0.3 to 0.4 5g/kg IV infusion
    c. 1 mg, IV push, repeated every 3 to 5 minutes
    d. 1 mg/kg, IV push, repeated every 3 to 5 minutes

46. Lidocaine is:
    a. an antidysrhythmic agent
    b. contraindicated in patients who are in cardiac arrest
    c. used to suppress supraventricular ectopy
    d. generally administered intramuscularly

47. T   F   Lidocaine stabilizes the cardiac membrane and decreases the frequency of rhythm problems.

48. Lidocaine is currently considered acceptable for:
    a. VF/pulseless VT that persists after defibrillation and administration of epinephrine
    b. asystole
    c. PEA
    d. hemodynamically stable PSVT

49. In cardiac arrest, the dose of lidocaine is:
    a. 1.0 mg, IV push (2.0 to 2.5 mg ETT), every 3 to 5 minutes an unlimited number of times
    b. 1.0 to 1.5 mg/kg, IV push (3.0 to 3.5 mg/kg ETT), 0.5- to 0.75-mg/kg boluses every 5 to 10 minutes to a maximum of 3.0 mg/kg
    c. 1.0 mg, IV push (2.0 to 2.5 mg ETT), every 3 to 5 minutes until a total of 0.03 to 0.04
    d. 1.0 mg/kg, IV push every 3 to 5 minutes until a maximum dose of 3.0 mg/kg has been delivered

    Note to students: The following questions relate to medications that are not included in the most recent version of the DOT EMT-I curriculum. However, because these medications are part of the revised American Heart Association ACLS guidelines, they are included for your review. Consult with your instructor regarding your requirement to learn these medications, as well as your need to complete these questions.

50. Amiodarone is:
    a. a complex drug with very specific effects
    b. useful for both atrial and ventricular dysrhythmias
    c. used to treat cardiac arrest with persistent VT or VF and is delivered before defibrillation and epinephrine administration
    d. contraindicated in patients with severely impaired heart function

51. List four indications for amiodarone.

    _____

    _____

    _____

    _____

52. Vasopressin is the _____ occurring _____ hormone. In high doses it acts as a powerful _____ by direct stimulation of specific _____ receptors.

53. Describe how vasopressin may be used in the treatment of cardiac arrest.

54. Describe what should be done if there is no response to the administration of vasopressin in the treatment of cardiac arrest.

55. Match the following cardiac medications with the correct dosages. Some medications may be used more than once.

    Medication
    a. Vasopressin
    b. Amiodarone

    Dosage
    _____ In nonarrest situations give 150 mg IV over 10 minutes, followed by 1-mg/min infusion for 6 hours
    _____ In cardiac arrest caused by pulseless VT or VF, give 300 mg, IV push (diluted in a volume of 20 to 30 mL of saline)
    _____ Given as a one-time dose of 40 units, IV
    _____ Can repeat at dose of 150 mg (diluted in a volume of 10 to 15 mL of saline) if VF/VT recurs

56. List five mechanical interventions used to treat cardiac emergencies that require no special equipment.

57. Which of the following is considered to be an *initial* treatment for VF?
    a. atropine
    b. defibrillation
    c. epinephrine
    d. D_{50}

58. Electrical defibrillation when properly applied:
    a. revitalizes the electrical conduction system of the heart
    b. causes a depolarization of a critical mass of myocardium
    c. stimulates an impulse to be generated from the SA node
    d. results in contraction of the heart muscle

59. Successful defibrillation depends on:
    a. energy output
    b. paddle placement
    c. transthoracic resistance
    d. all of the above

60. Describe synchronized cardioversion.

    _____

    _____

    _____

    _____

61. Defibrillation precedes initiation of cardiopulmonary resuscitation (CPR) in:
    a. witnessed VF (or VT without a pulse)
    b. hemodynamically compromising bradycardia
    c. asystole
    d. electromechanical dissociation

62. T F The time it takes for defibrillation to be performed following the onset of VF does little to influence the success of the defibrillation attempt.

63. T F Resistance to passage of the countershock caused by the tissues of the chest is referred to as transthoracic resistance.

64. T F The greater the transthoracic resistance, the more energy delivered to the heart.

65. List seven factors that influence transthoracic resistance to defibrillation.

    _____

    _____

    _____

    _____

    _____

    _____

66. The first countershock administered in VF should be delivered at a dose of _____ J.
    a. 100
    b. 200
    c. 300
    d. 360

67. List the basic steps for use of any automated external defibrillator.

68. Proper defibrillation involves which of the following?
    a. placing defibrillation pads on the patient's chest or applying conductive gel to the paddles
    b. keeping at least two thirds of the paddle surface in contact with the patient's skin
    c. pushing down on the paddles with 10 to 15 lb of firm arm pressure
    d. delivering the countershock during delivery of a breath so that the patient's chest is fully inflated

69. List nine precautions the EMT-I should follow to use a defibrillator.

70. Transcutaneous pacing:
    a. is effective in treating most cases of asystole
    b. can be used for patients who are in a wet environment
    c. may be effective in resolving symptomatic bradycardia and heart block that is not responsive to atropine
    d. is generally effective in resolving PEA

71. When managing a patient in cardiac arrest, the EMT-I should:
    a. in an unwitnessed arrest, delay the start of CPR until after defibrillation has been performed
    b. place an IV line of normal saline in the dorsum of the hand
    c. in VF, insert an endotracheal tube immediately after starting CPR
    d. administer 1 mg of epinephrine in all types of arrest

72. Which of the following is true regarding atherosclerosis?
    a. Atherosclerosis is an acute disease of the medium and larger arteries.
    b. Atherosclerotic plaque consists of calcium, cholesterol, and connective tissue.
    c. Atherosclerosis does little to interfere with blood flow.
    d. The development of atherosclerosis occurs only in elderly persons.

73. Substernal chest pain that is provoked by effort and is usually relieved with rest and nitroglycerin is associated with:
    a. angina
    b. dissecting aortic aneurysm
    c. pulmonary embolism
    d. AMI

74. Which of the following is true of angina pectoris?
    a. With angina there is injury and death to the heart muscle.
    b. It results when a damaged or weakened heart cannot pump blood well enough to maintain proper circulation throughout the body.
    c. It occurs secondary to AMI.
    d. It is an intermittent attack of chest pain and related symptoms caused by a reduction in blood flow to the heart muscle.

75. Stable angina:
    a. is chest pain that occurs at rest
    b. is also called preinfarction angina
    c. is brought on by stress or exertion
    d. generally fails to respond to nitroglycerin

76. Describe what is meant by the term *unstable angina*.

    _____
    _____
    _____
    _____

77. In patients experiencing chest pain, nitroglycerin administration may result in:
    a. improvement of myocardial perfusion through constriction of the coronary arteries
    b. slowing of the heart rate by increasing conduction time through the AV node
    c. an increase of the heart rate by directly stimulating the SA node
    d. a decrease in the myocardial workload by dilating peripheral blood vessels, thus reducing preload and afterload

78. T F An AMI occurs when there is death of an area of heart muscle caused by complete blockage of coronary blood flow.

79. T F A patient experiencing AMI will have chest pain.

80. Chest pain associated with AMI:
    a. increases in severity on inspiration
    b. is sometimes described as discomfort, an aching pain, or heaviness
    c. will disappear following nitroglycerin administration
    d. is usually not noticed until 2 to 3 hours following the onset of myocardial ischemia

81. All of the following are precipitating factors of AMI *except:*
    a. coronary artery trauma
    b. coronary artery spasm
    c. inflammation of the blood vessels
    d. cerebral thrombosis

82. The most common complication that leads to death in AMI is:
    a. cardiogenic shock (pump failure)
    b. myocardial rupture
    c. cardiac dysrhythmia (sudden death)
    d. hypovolemia

83. T F Oxygen administration is of little benefit in the patient experiencing AMI.

84. Signs characteristic of an aortic dissection include:
    a. bradycardia
    b. severe tearing-like chest pain
    c. hypertension
    d. distended neck veins

85. Signs and symptoms of pulmonary emboli include:
    a. sudden, unexplained onset of chest pain that increases in intensity with a deep breath
    b. substernal pain that is often aggravated with movement
    c. cough, fever, chills
    d. all of the above

86. CHF:
    a. is characterized by tachycardia, dyspnea, elevated blood pressure, rales, and edema to the lower extremities
    b. occurs secondary to angina pectoris
    c. results in blood traveling through the pulmonary and systemic circulations faster
    d. is best treated in the field setting by placing the patient in a supine position and elevating the legs approximately 10 to 12 inches

87. The presence of cyanosis is indicative of:
    a. hypertension
    b. an irregular heartbeat
    c. increased sympathetic activity
    d. hypoxia

88. Match the following terms with the correct description.

   Term
   a. Paroxysmal nocturnal dyspnea
   b. Orthopnea
   c. Ascites
   d. Pedal edema

   Description
   _____ Abdominal swelling
   _____ Shortness of breath at night—the patient may wake up unable to breathe
   _____ Worsening of shortness of breath when lying down
   _____ Fluid collects in the feet and legs

89. With left-sided CHF:
   a. the pumping capability of the right ventricle is decreased
   b. fluid backs up into the body, causing peripheral edema
   c. the patient will often display pink, frothy sputum
   d. blood draining into the right heart backs up into the vascular system

90. T F To be classified as hypertensive crisis, the patient's systolic pressure must be greater than 250 mm Hg and the diastolic pressure greater than 120 mm Hg.

91. T F Treatment of hypertensive crisis includes the administration of nitroglycerin 1.5 to 2.5 mg, SL.

92. Place a checkmark beside those signs that are characteristic of cardiogenic shock.
   _____ Normal mental status
   _____ Systolic blood pressure of less than 80 mm Hg
   _____ An ECG reading of sinus rhythm with a bundle branch block
   _____ Cool and clammy skin
   _____ Tachypnea

93. Which of the following would be considered appropriate treatment for a patient who is hypotensive secondary to cardiogenic shock?
   a. administering nitroglycerin, 1 tablet, SL
   b. starting an IV line of normal saline at a KVO (keep vein open) rate; give a 250- to 500-cc fluid challenge
   c. administering a low concentration of oxygen
   d. defibrillating the patient with 200 J

94. All of the following medications may be administered in cardiac arrest and repeated *except:*
   a. lidocaine
   b. epinephrine
   c. atropine
   d. vasopressin

95. You are called to the scene where a 53-year-old woman collapsed while at work at her office. You arrive at the scene to find her fellow workers performing CPR. Your partner begins ventilating the patient with a bag-mask device supplied with 100% oxygen while you have one of the bystanders continue chest compressions. You attach the ECG monitor leads to see VF. Identify, by numbering, the correct sequence for treating a patient who is in VF. Assume that CPR is being provided throughout the resuscitation effort.
   _____ Defibrillation at 360 J.
   _____ Administer lidocaine or amiodarone.
   _____ Establish an IV line.
   _____ Deliver the fourth defibrillation at 360 J.
   _____ Place an endotracheal tube.
   _____ Deliver the second defibrillation at 360 J.

_____ Deliver the third defibrillation at 360 J.
_____ Deliver the fifth defibrillation at 360 J.
_____ Administer epinephrine, 1 mg, IV push.

You are called to an apartment of a 79-year-old, 114-lb woman who is complaining of shortness of breath. The patient has difficulty speaking in short sentences and has labored breathing. She states that it is getting progressively harder for her to breathe. According to her husband, the dyspnea began acutely, approximately 1 hour before you were called. On questioning, the patient acknowledges a dull aching pain in her chest but denies any radiation of the pain, dizziness, or vomiting. According to her husband, the patient has a medical history of CHF and takes Lasix, Lanoxin, Transderm, and Aldomet. Your physical assessment reveals she is oriented but seems anxious and apprehensive; has labored respirations at a rate of 22 breaths/min; a blood pressure of 176/128; cool, sweaty skin; and a pulse oximetry reading of 85%. The focused exam reveals external jugular vein distention, accessory muscle usage, and intercostal retraction but no peripheral edema. Auscultation of the chest reveals bilateral rales and wheezing in all bases. You attach the patient to the ECG monitor and see sinus tachycardia.

96. This patient is suffering from:
    a. cardiogenic shock
    b. pneumonia
    c. an acute asthma attack
    d. left-sided heart failure

97. Treatment for this patient includes:
    a. administering oxygen at 2 to 3 L/min via nasal cannula
    b. establishing an IV with lactated Ringer's solution and a macrodrip administration set
    c. placing her in a supine position
    d. administering furosemide, 20 to 80 mg, IV push

It is 12:52 AM on Sunday when you are called to the home of a 55-year-old, 230-lb man who is complaining of chest pain. According to his wife, the patient was exercising when he began having substernal chest pain. Your assessment reveals that he is alert and oriented; has a respiratory rate of 18; a blood pressure of 182/98; warm, moist skin; and a pulse oximetry reading of 93%. Auscultation of the chest reveals clear bilateral lung sounds. You note that there is no peripheral edema or external jugular vein distention. The patient denies any shortness of breath or nausea and is reported to have a history of hypertension, for which he takes methyldopa, and angina, for which he takes nitroglycerin. According to the patient's wife, he has taken three nitroglycerin tablets, which seems to have eased the chest pain. You attach the ECG monitor to reveal sinus tachycardia.

98. This patient is suffering from:
    a. indigestion
    b. AMI
    c. angina
    d. muscle strain

99. Which of the following treatments would be correct for this patient?
    a. delivering 15 L/min via nasal cannula
    b. administering atropine, 0.5 to 1.0 mg, IV push
    c. administering nitroglycerin, 0.3 to 0.5 mg, SL
    d. establishing an IV line of 5% dextrose in water or normal saline, KVO

It is 3:30 on Friday afternoon when you are called to a local shopping mall for a 61-year-old, 180-lb sales clerk who is complaining of dizziness and "chest palpitations." She states that she has been feeling ill for the past week or so but has not seen her physician. Her fellow workers called today because she seems to be getting worse. The patient denies chest pain and shortness of breath. Assessment reveals that she is well oriented; has a respiratory rate of 20; a blood pressure of 176/102; warm, dry skin; and a pulse oximetry reading of 90%. She has a medical history of diabetes that is diet controlled and hypertension, for which she takes Apresoline. Also, you note that she has an allergy to narcotic agents. You attach the ECG monitor and see sinus rhythm with PVCs.

100. This patient is suffering from:
    a. indigestion
    b. a cardiac dysrhythmia
    c. angina
    d. muscle strain

101. Treatment for this patient includes:
    a. administering atropine, 0.5 to 1.0 mg, IV push
    b. establishing an IV line with 5% dextrose in water and a macrodrip administration set
    c. administering high-concentration oxygen via nonrebreather mask
    d. administering nitroglycerin, 0.3 to 0.5 mg, SL

It is Wednesday afternoon when you are called to a downtown hotel where a 62-year-old man is complaining of substernal chest pain. The patient denies shortness of breath or nausea. Assessment reveals that the patient is confused; has a respiratory rate of 18; a blood pressure of 80/60; cool, diaphoretic skin; and a pulse oximetry reading of 80%. Auscultation of the chest reveals clear bilateral lung sounds. There is no external jugular vein distention or peripheral edema. You determine that the patient has a history of diabetes for which he takes daily insulin. You attach the ECG monitor to see a slow, regular rhythm with round upright P waves preceding each QRS complex. The PR intervals appear longer than normal.

102. This patient is suffering from:
    a. cardiogenic shock
    b. CHF
    c. third-degree AV heart block
    d. sinus bradycardia with first-degree AV heart block

103. You have begun administering 15 L/min of oxygen via nonrebreather mask and placed an IV line of normal saline at a KVO rate. It is 3:46; you should now do which of the following?
    a. administer atropine, 0.5 mg, IV push
    b. administer nitroglycerin, 0.3 to 0.5 mg, SL
    c. defibrillate the patient at 200 J
    d. administer lidocaine, 1.0 to 1.5 mg/kg, IV push, followed by an appropriate maintenance dose

104. The patient's condition remains the same despite the above treatment. It is now 3:50; you should administer:
    a. atropine, 0.5 mg, IV push
    b. nitroglycerin, 0.3 to 0.5 mg, SL
    c. epinephrine, 1 mg, slow IV push
    d. naloxone, 2 mg, IV push

The patient's *(see above)* blood pressure is now 130/82, and he is becoming more oriented.

You have been called to a local community college for a 52-year-old, 160-lb professor who was complaining of chest pain before he passed out. According to several students, the patient "grasped his chest and slumped to the floor" while lecturing. Your assessment reveals that the patient is semiconscious; has shallow breathing at a rate of 34 breaths/min; a blood pressure of 60/40; cold, diaphoretic skin; and a pulse oximetry reading of 60%. Auscultation of the chest reveals bilateral rales, and you note slight external jugular vein distention. You are able to determine that the patient has a history of asthma for which he uses an Isuprel medihaler. You attach an ECG monitor to reveal sinus tachycardia.

105. This patient is most likely experiencing:
    a. aortic aneurysm
    b. cardiogenic shock
    c. electromechanical dissociation
    d. CHF

106. Which of the following treatments would be correct for this patient?
    a. assisting his breathing with a ventilatory device capable of delivering 100% oxygen
    b. administering 1 mg of atropine, IV push
    c. administering 0.3 mg of nitroglycerin, SL
    d. inserting an oropharyngeal airway

It is a snowy December day when you receive a call for a 61-year-old man who is complaining of chest pain. On your arrival you find the patient sitting in the living room of his home smoking a cigarette. The patient states that he was shoveling snow when he began having substernal chest pain. He describes the pain as a crushing-type pain that radiates to his left arm. He states it started approximately half an hour ago and is unaffected by position or by breathing. He acknowledges some shortness of breath and nausea. The patient has a medical history of a pacemaker, open-heart surgery (double bypass) 10 years ago, and diabetes for which he takes Inderal, Thorazine, and Diabinese. Assessment of the patient reveals that he is well oriented; has a respiratory rate of 14; an irregular pulse rate of 74; a blood pressure of 160/94; cool, diaphoretic skin; and a pulse oximetry reading of 88%. Auscultation of the chest reveals clear bilateral lung sounds.

107. This patient is most likely suffering from:
    a. cardiogenic shock
    b. an AMI
    c. right-sided heart failure
    d. pneumonia

You have begun administering 15 L/min of oxygen to the patient and are preparing to establish an IV line. As you explain the procedure and apply a venous tourniquet to his right arm, he states that "they have difficulty getting IVs in me." You can see why as you note swelling of both hands and lateral aspects of his lower arms. Despite this difficulty, you are able to cannulate a vein on the inner aspect of his left wrist.

108. Treatment of this patient should include:
    a. monitoring the ECG rhythm
    b. having him drink hot coffee
    c. administering lidocaine, 1 mg/kg, IV push
    d. transporting him to the hospital with emergency lights and siren

CROSSWORD PUZZLE EXERCISE

109. Complete the following crossword puzzle.

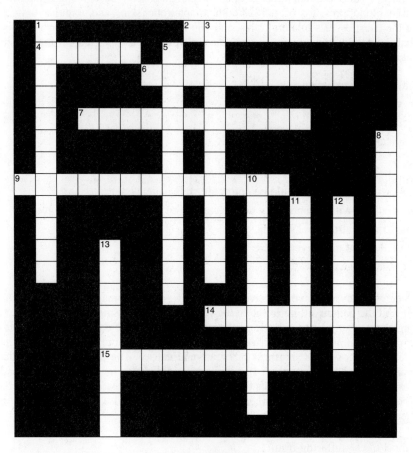

ACROSS

2. Two lower chambers of the heart.
4. Muscular, cone-shaped organ, and its function is to pump blood throughout the body.
6. The heart muscle.
7. Hypercholesterolemia means elevated serum _____ levels.
9. Hypertriglyceridemia means elevated _____.
14. When this is reached, depolarization of the entire cell occurs.
15. Node where the impulse originates that stimulates the heart to beat.

DOWN

1. Involves rate of contraction.
3. Ability to respond to an appropriate electrical stimulus.
5. Major risk factor of IHD.
8. Is determined by the total resistance within the arteriolar bed.
10. Inner lining cells of the heart.
11. Lubricating fluid that allows the heart to contract and expand smoothly within the chest cavity.
12. The relaxation phase.
13. Valve that is situated between the right atrium and right ventricle.

25 Diabetic Emergencies

CHAPTER TERMINAL OBJECTIVES

On completion of this chapter, the EMT-Intermediate will be able to use assessment findings to formulate a field impression and implement a treatment plan for the patient with a diabetic emergency.

For the multiple-choice questions, select the single best answer to each question. For the matching questions, select the best corresponding answer for each item. Because there are sometimes more items than corresponding answers in the matching questions, some items may not be used.

1. Diabetes mellitus is a chronic disease of the _____ system caused by a _____ in the secretion or activity of the hormone _____ .
   a. endocrine; decrease; insulin
   b. circulatory; increase; calcium
   c. nervous; decrease; glucagons
   d. lymphatic; decrease; ADH

2. Insulin:
   a. is released from the beta cells of the pancreas
   b. aids in the breakdown of fat tissue in the body
   c. increases the blood sugar
   d. is a counterregulatory hormone

3. Describe the role of glucagon and epinephrine in the regulation of glucose in the body and from where each is secreted.

   _____
   _____
   _____
   _____
   _____

4. T F Persons with diabetes metabolize glucose too quickly.

5. T F Hyperglycemia is an abnormally low blood sugar level.

6. T F Although the cells use glucose as their primary "food source," they will turn to fat, then to muscle, if a lack of insulin prevents the inward movement of glucose.

7. When the body metabolizes fats:
   a. the glucagon levels increase
   b. ketones and ketoacids result
   c. protein levels increase
   d. alkalosis develops

8. Describe the effect a lack of glucose has on the central nervous system.

   _____
   _____
   _____
   _____
   _____

9. Match the types of diabetes with the correct characteristic. Items may be used more than once.

   Condition
   a. Type 1
   b. Type 2

   Sign/Symptom
   _____ Patients typically have disease onset at a younger age
   _____ Non–insulin-dependent
   _____ Insulin-dependent
   _____ Prone to diabetic ketoacidosis (DKA)
   _____ Usually onset is after the teenage years
   _____ Less prone to DKA

10. List four complications of diabetes.

    _____
    _____
    _____
    _____

11. List seven causes of hypoglycemia.

    _____
    _____
    _____
    _____
    _____
    _____
    _____

12. The most common causes of hypoglycemia in a diabetic patient are when he or she takes his or her insulin and does not eat enough _____ .

13. Hypoglycemia generally develops _____ .

14. T F If a known diabetic patient has an altered level of consciousness or neurological symptoms, you should assume that he or she has low blood glucose.

15. T F The signs and symptoms of mild to moderate hypoglycemia include shakiness, weakness, diaphoresis, rapid pulse, and increased respiratory rate.

16. T F In the field setting the EMT-I can easily differentiate hypoglycemia from a stroke.

17. Match the following signs and symptoms with either hypoglycemia or hyperglycemia. Items may be used more than once.

    Condition
    a. Hypoglycemia
    b. Hyperglycemia

    Sign/Symptom
    _____ Diaphoresis
    _____ Frequent urination
    _____ Thirst
    _____ Slurred speech
    _____ Seizures
    _____ Fruity, acetone-like odor to the breath
    _____ Nausea and vomiting
    _____ Kussmaul respirations
    _____ Shakiness, weakness

18. Two questions the EMT-I should always ask the diabetic patient are:

    _____

    _____

It is 12:30 PM when you are called to a local library for a 24-year-old, 140-lb man who is reported to be experiencing a "diabetic emergency." You find the patient pacing back and forth in the restroom. He is disoriented and agitated, has a respiratory rate of 20 breaths/min, an irregular pulse, a blood pressure of 152/96, and cool, diaphoretic skin. Auscultation of the chest reveals clear bilateral lung sounds. Your physical assessment fails to detect anything else abnormal, although the blood glucose reading is 50 mg/dL. According to his friends, the patient takes insulin for diabetes.

19. This patient is experiencing:
    a. hyperventilation syndrome
    b. DKA
    c. cocaine overdose
    d. hypoglycemia

20. Treatment for this patient includes all of the following *except:*
    a. administering high-concentration oxygen via nonrebreather mask
    b. helping him take his insulin
    c. administering 50% dextrose, 50 mL, IV push
    d. establishing an IV line of normal saline

21. Fifty percent dextrose:
    a. can be safely administered in the presence of cerebral ischemia or stroke
    b. administration should be followed by thiamine in the patient who has a history of alcoholism
    c. should be administered rapidly
    d. can cause tissue necrosis if it is allowed to leak from the vein

22. Describe how DKA occurs.

    _____

    _____

    _____

    _____

    _____

23. The most common reason a diabetic person develops DKA is _____ .

24. DKA includes all of the following *except:*
    a. hypoglycemia
    b. dehydration
    c. accumulation of ketones and ketoacids
    d. increased urination

25. A 39-year-old patient is experiencing "DKA," apparently brought on by a failure to take his insulin. He is displaying Kussmaul respiration (respiratory rate is 34 and deep), his pulse rate is 140, and blood pressure is 100/80. This patient will typically have:
    a. metabolic acidosis
    b. respiratory alkalosis
    c. respiratory acidosis
    d. a and b

26. T F DKA has a relatively slow onset.

27. T F The patient with DKA usually has slow, sighing respirations.

28. List the treatment for the patient experiencing DKA.

_____

_____

_____

_____

_____

_____

_____

29. Persons with hyperglycemic hyperosmolar nonketotic coma (HHNC):
    a. have poor underlying health
    b. are typically younger than 50 years of age
    c. have rapid deterioration in mental status over 1 to 2 hours
    d. have an acetone odor to their breath

CROSSWORD PUZZLE EXERCISE

30. Complete the following crossword puzzle.

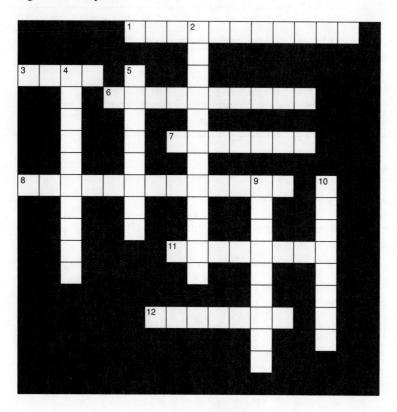

ACROSS

1. Disease of the kidney.
3. State where blood sugar is markedly elevated but no acidosis or accumulation of ketones is present.
6. Battery-operated glucose monitoring system.
7. Sole source of oxidative metabolism (nutrition) for the central nervous system.
8. Abnormally high blood glucose level.
11. Disease of endocrine system resulting from a lack of insulin.
12. Hormone that moves glucose molecules from the blood into the cells.

DOWN

2. Abnormally low blood glucose level.
4. Nerve disease.
5. A counterregulatory hormone.
9. Most common reason a diabetic person develops DKA.
10. Rapid, deep, sighing respirations.

26 Allergic Reactions

CHAPTER TERMINAL OBJECTIVES

On completion of this chapter, the EMT-Intermediate will be able to use assessment findings to formulate a field impression and implement a treatment plan for the patient with an allergic or anaphylactic reaction.

For the multiple-choice questions, select the single best answer to each question. For the matching questions, select the best corresponding answer for each item. Because there are sometimes more items than corresponding answers in the matching questions, some items may not be used.

1. Describe what causes an allergic reaction.

   _____

   _____

   _____

   _____

   _____

2. Define the term *anaphylaxis*.

   _____

   _____

   _____

   _____

   _____

3. When a/an _____ to which one is sensitive enters the body, it is attacked by a substance known as a/an

   _____ .

4. Five types of antibodies are formed by the immune system and reside on the surface of _____ cells, a type

   of _____ blood cell.

5. Antibodies are also called _____ and are abbreviated as _____ followed by a letter.

6. The _____ antibody is the only one involved in an anaphylactic reaction.

7. List three responses the release of histamine may cause.

_____

_____

_____

8. The table below lists the four primary ways in which allergens enter the body. Fill in examples of each.

Skin contact	
Injections	
Inhalation	
Ingestion	

9. T F The largest concentrations of mast cells are in the skin and the respiratory and the gastrointestinal tracts.

10. T F Stridor indicates lower airway constriction.

11. Which of the following is *not* a life-threatening condition of an allergic reaction/anaphylactic shock?
    a. urticaria
    b. airway edema
    c. vascular collapse
    d. severe bronchospasm

12. Diphenhydramine (Benadryl):
    a. is used as the primary medication to treat anaphylaxis
    b. is contraindicated in patients who have facial swelling
    c. blocks the effects of histamine
    d. is a beta-2 selective agent

You are called to the scene where a 31-year-old woman was stung by a wasp while working in the garden. Assessment reveals that she is awake and oriented, has a respiratory rate of 16 breaths/min, a bounding pulse of 96 beats per minute (BPM), a blood pressure of 138/64, and flushed skin. You note the presence of facial swelling (particularly around the eyes) and hives on her back and posterior arms. Auscultation of the chest reveals clear bilateral lung sounds. You determine that the patient has a previous medical history of allergies and asthma.

13. This patient is experiencing:
    a. an acute asthma attack
    b. sepsis
    c. a mild allergic reaction
    d. anaphylactic shock

14. Treatment for this patient includes:
    a. administering diphenhydramine (Benadryl), slow intravenous (IV) push or intramuscularly (IM)
    b. administering high-concentration oxygen, 10 to 15 L/min via nasal cannula
    c. placing an IV line and running it wide open
    d. administering epinephrine, 1:1000 solution, subcutaneously (SQ)

15. With anaphylaxis:
    a. the patient in respiratory distress will usually prefer a supine position
    b. the progression to death can be extremely rapid, sometimes within minutes
    c. rapid transport to a trauma center is required
    d. the patient should receive 6 L of oxygen via nasal cannula

16. IV lines used in the management of anaphylaxis should:
    a. be established using a small-bore catheter
    b. consist of either 5% dextrose in water or lactated Ringer's solution
    c. be run wide open if the patient's blood pressure is less than 90 systolic
    d. include a microdrip administration set

17. Epinephrine (1:1000):
    a. is administered at a dose of 1 to 5 mL, SQ
    b. is a first-line treatment of allergic reaction
    c. administration may be repeated, five or more times, at 10-minute intervals
    d. is used in the treatment of anaphylaxis

18. Describe how a bee stinger should be removed from a patient's skin.

19. Describe treatment that should be provided if wheezing or stridor is present in the patient experiencing anaphylaxis and hemodynamic compromise.

27 Poisoning and Overdose Emergencies

CHAPTER TERMINAL OBJECTIVES

On completion of this chapter, the EMT-Intermediate will be able to use assessment findings to formulate a field impression and implement a treatment plan for the patient with a toxic exposure.

For the multiple-choice questions, select the single best answer to each question. For the matching questions, select the best corresponding answer for each item. Because there are sometimes more items than corresponding answers in the matching questions, some items may not be used.

1. T F About 10% of poisonings involve prescription drugs.

2. T F Poisoning is most common among children younger than 5 years.

3. T F In adults, most poisonings are suicide attempts or drug abuse.

4. Define the term *overdose*.

   _____

   _____

   _____

5. List the three generic types of toxicological emergencies.

   _____

   _____

   _____

6. Match the type of poisoning with the correct characteristic.

   Type of Poisoning
   a. Dosage errors
   b. Idiosyncratic reactions
   c. Childhood poisoning
   d. Environmental exposures
   e. Occupational exposures

   Characteristic
   _____ Usually the result of an unforeseen leak or explosion, resulting in the widespread release of toxic materials absorbed by unprotected workers

   _____ Examples include carbon monoxide in a school with inadequate ventilation, chemical exposure when driving near a freshly sprayed crop field, or smoke inhalation in persons living downwind from a large fire in progress

   _____ May occur by the prescribing physician, treating emergency medical services (EMS) provider, nurse, physician assistant, or pharmacist. Patients or their families may also be responsible for mistakes.

   _____ Untoward side effects that are unpredictable and different from that common to any particular drug

   _____ Most are the result of caregiver inattention and innate childhood curiosity

7. Describe the precautions the EMT-I should take when responding to a call where poisons may be present.

   _____
   _____
   _____
   _____
   _____

8. Regional Poison Control Centers (PCCs):
   a. are mostly found in large urban centers
   b. are usually contacted via 800-MHz radio
   c. are a reliable and up-to-date source of information on the assessment and treatment of toxicological emergencies
   d. can be contacted only with permission of medical direction

9. List four routes of exposure to a poison.

   _____
   _____
   _____
   _____

10. Of the four routes, which is the most common route of poisoning?

11. List five examples of exposure potentials that are geographically specific.

12. List four items of information that should be acquired when caring for a poisoning patient.

13. List four physical findings that may help identify the poison involved.

14. Activated charcoal administered orally is contraindicated in all of the following situations *except:*
    a. 30-year-old man who has taken an overdose of sleeping pills and is semiconscious
    b. 45-year-old woman who has experienced a convulsion after ingesting brownies that were laced with marijuana; she is now postictal
    c. 22-year-old man who has accidentally ingested drain cleaner and is alert and well oriented
    d. 16-year-old girl who has ingested a handful of barbiturates and is unconscious

15. Cholinergic agents:
    a. lead to suppression of the parasympathetic nervous system
    b. prevent the breakdown of acetylcholine by acetylcholinesterase
    c. include pesticides (organophosphates, carbamates) and nerve gas agents (sarin, soman)
    d. are easily absorbed through the respiratory system but not the skin

16. Signs of exposure to cholinergic agents include all of the following *except:*
    a. tachycardia
    b. myosis
    c. coma
    d. convulsions

17. Fill in the meaning of each letter in the mnemonic SLUDGE.

    S: _____

    L: _____

    U: _____

    D: _____

    G: _____

    E: _____

18. Atropine used to treat exposure to cholinergic agents:
    a. directly blocks the parasympathetic nervous system from further stimulation by acetylcholine that cannot be degraded
    b. is given at slightly higher total doses (4 to 5 mg IV) than those used in cardiac patients
    c. is delivered via prefilled syringes containing 1 mg/10 mL of the medication
    d. is given to suppress seizures, severe muscle cramps, and tremors

19. T F The EMT-I does not need to wear protective equipment when treating persons exposed to cholinergic agents.

20. T F Many antihistamines, antispasmodics, and tricyclic antidepressant drugs have anticholinergic actions, especially when taken in excess.

21. Describe what causes the "red, hot, hyper, and mad" appearance of patients with anticholinergic poisoning.

    _____

    _____

    _____

    _____

22. A patient is found deeply unconscious, breathing slowly and shallowly, and has pinpoint pupils. You should first suspect:
    a. stroke
    b. the postictal phase of a seizure
    c. intracranial hemorrhage
    d. narcotic overdose

23. Naloxone reverses the effects of all of the drugs below *except:*
    a. opiates
    b. heroin
    c. meperidine
    d. valium

24. The initial dose for naloxone administration in drug overdose is:
    a. 0.1 mg/kg
    b. 0.2 to 0.3 mg
    c. 0.4 to 2 mg
    d. 5 to 10 mg

25. The patient who has inhaled a toxic substance may be expected to display all of the following *except:*
    a. hoarseness
    b. wheezing
    c. chest tightness
    d. bradypnea

You are called to the scene where a 30-year-old man is attempting suicide by sitting in a closed garage with the car engine running. It is estimated that the patient had been in the garage for approximately 15 minutes before being found by his girlfriend. On your arrival the patient is still sitting in the car.

26. The first thing you should do is:
    a. remove the patient to fresh air
    b. do an initial assessment of the patient
    c. begin administering oxygen
    d. open the patient's airway

Your assessment reveals that the patient is drowsy, has a respiratory rate of 20, a weak pulse rate of 110, a blood pressure of 120/84, and cool, diaphoretic skin. Auscultation of the chest reveals bilateral rales and rhonchi. The patient tells you that he has a severe headache.

27. This patient is experiencing:
    a. carbon dioxide intoxication
    b. cyanide poisoning
    c. carbon monoxide poisoning
    d. nitrogen overdose

28. This condition develops because carbon monoxide:
    a. has a much greater affinity for the hemoglobin of the red blood cells, interferes with the normal oxygen-carrying capability of the blood, and subsequently causes tissue hypoxia
    b. alters the normal breathing pattern and decreases the brain's responsiveness to increases in carbon dioxide; subsequently, carbon dioxide accumulates and causes respiratory depression and arrest
    c. interferes with the cells' ability to utilize oxygen, subsequently causing cellular hypoxia and death
    d. impairs the substance that inactivates the neurotransmitter of the parasympathetic nervous system; subsequently, the parasympathetic nervous system causes a decrease in the heart rate, cardiac output, blood pressure, and so on

29. The patient's pulse oximetry reading shows 100% saturation. You should:
    a. withhold oxygen administration unless the patient's oxygen saturation decreases
    b. administer 2 to 4 L of oxygen via nasal cannula
    c. intubate the patient
    d. administer 15 L/min of oxygen via nonrebreather mask

30. List the four physiological properties of snake venom.

_____

_____

_____

_____

31. Treatment of a victim who has been bitten by a poisonous snake includes:
    a. elevating the extremity
    b. applying an arterial tourniquet
    c. applying ice to the site
    d. keeping the victim quiet

CROSSWORD PUZZLE EXERCISE

32. Complete the following crossword puzzle.

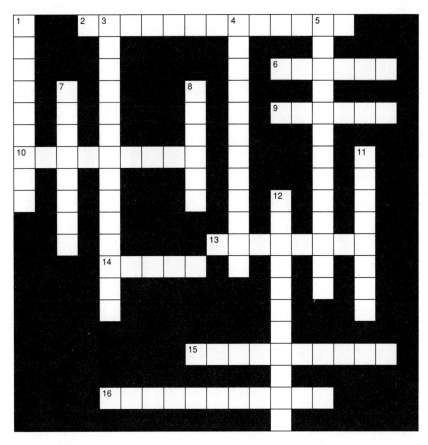

ACROSS

2. The major cholinergic neurotransmitter.
6. Acronym for signs seen with organophosphate poisoning.
9. Droopy eyelid.
10. These gases cause direct irritation to tissues.
13. Directly blocks parasympathetic nervous system from further stimulation by acetylcholine.
14. These gases generally cause no direct tissue toxicity.
15. Substances passing through the skin into bloodstream.
16. Specifically reactivates acetylcholinesterase, acting as an antidote to cholinergic agents.

DOWN

1. Exposure to substance that is generally only harmful and has no usual beneficial effects.
3. Produces decreased cardiac output and blood pressure.
4. Coagulant, anticoagulant, hemolytic, platelet problems.
5. Produces paresthesias, paralysis, and neuromuscular transmission disturbances.
7. Excessive exposure to a substance that has normal treatment uses.
8. Small pupils.
11. May be helpful for seizures and severe muscle cramps and tremors.
12. Agents that lead to stimulation of the parasympathetic nervous system.

28 Neurological Emergencies

CHAPTER TERMINAL OBJECTIVES

On completion of this chapter, the EMT-Intermediate will be able to utilize assessment findings to formulate a field impression and implement a treatment plan for the patient with a neurological emergency.

For the multiple-choice questions, select the single best answer to each question. For the matching questions, select the best corresponding answer for each item. Because there are sometimes more items than corresponding answers in the matching questions, some items may not be used.

1. Alertness, awareness, and a normal wakeful state ("consciousness") are maintained by:
   a. cognitive systems
   b. cerebral homeostasis
   c. motor control
   d. sensation control

2. A major goal of cerebral _____ is to maintain brain perfusion and oxygenation despite fluctuations in the mean arterial blood pressure.

3. Describe the process of cerebral autoregulation.

   _____

   _____

   _____

   _____

   _____

4. Alterations in the motor control systems result in a variety of conditions, including:
   a. loss of feeling in an area
   b. localized random movements
   c. inability to remember the date, time, or place
   d. inappropriate fluctuations in the blood pressure

5. List the meaning of each letter of the mnemonic VINDICATE.

   V: _____

   I: _____

   N: _____

   D: _____

   I: _____

   C: _____

   A: _____

   T: _____

   E: _____

6. A/An _____ is a condition that results from a disruption of circulation to the brain, causing ischemia and damage to brain tissue.

7. There are two types of strokes, _____ and _____.

8. Signs and symptoms of stroke include:
   a. sudden onset of unilateral weakness, numbness, and inability to walk
   b. chest pain that is unrelieved with rest
   c. weak, thready pulse
   d. cold, clammy, and diaphoretic skin

9. An unconscious stroke patient is making snoring sounds. After repositioning the head and neck, the snoring sounds are still present. You should now:
   a. ventilate every 5 seconds
   b. suction vigorously
   c. perform the Sellick maneuver
   d. insert an oropharyngeal or nasopharyngeal airway

10. A seizure is a:
    a. sudden episode of abnormal brain cell electrical activity resulting in a period of atypical muscular activity or abnormal behavior
    b. strokelike neurological deficit that completely resolves within minutes to hours
    c. progressive degenerative brain condition resulting in a tremor, progressive loss of motor control, and speech difficulty
    d. partial or complete loss of consciousness, from which the patient recovers

11. Seizures spontaneously recurring over a span of years are termed:
    a. tonic-clonic seizure movements
    b. generalized major motor seizures
    c. epilepsy
    d. status epilepticus

12. List the four types of seizures.

   _____

   _____

   _____

   _____

13. Seizures are not a _____, but a symptom of an underlying _____.

14. Seizures may be _____ (no demonstrable cause) or _____ (caused by a brain lesion or metabolic abnormality).

15. List five causes of central nervous system (CNS) origin seizures.

   _____

   _____

   _____

   _____

   _____

16. A continuous seizure lasting more than 30 minutes or a series of seizures during which the patient does not regain consciousness is referred to as:
    a. status epilepticus
    b. epilepsy
    c. clonic seizures
    d. grand mal seizures

You are called to a downtown hotel for a 33-year-old bartender who experienced an apparent seizure. On your arrival at the scene, you find the patient sitting behind the bar. The patient is awake but has difficulty responding to your questions; he remembers his name but cannot remember the time or date. He has a respiratory rate of 16 breaths/min, a pulse rate of 112, a blood pressure of 182/100, and warm, moist skin. During your assessment, you find a medical alert bracelet that indicates that the patient has epilepsy. You also note that he is carrying an empty prescription bottle for phenytoin (Dilantin). A glucose meter reading reveals a blood glucose level of 120 mg/dL. Just as you start administering oxygen using a nonrebreather mask, the patient suddenly loses consciousness and begins convulsing.

17. This phase of a convulsive episode is referred to as the:
    a. aura
    b. tonic-clonic phase
    c. petit mal phase
    d. postictal phase

18. Treatment for this patient includes:
    a. administering an initial dose of 50% dextrose, IV push
    b. inserting an oropharyngeal airway
    c. restraining the patient to prevent injury
    d. placing him on an electrocardiograph (ECG) monitor

19. Before a seizure, some patients will notice a warning sign consisting of seeing, hearing, or smelling something unusual before losing consciousness. This is called a/an:
    a. postictal state
    b. coma
    c. aura
    d. preseizure sensation

20. Diazepam:
    a. is administered to the seizure patient between active seizures
    b. is also referred to as Ativan
    c. has a CNS depressant action of 1.5 to 2.0 hours
    d. is a benzodiazepine agent

21. The most common serious side effect of diazepam and lorazepam is:
    a. allergic reaction
    b. respiratory depression
    c. severe vasodilation
    d. shortness of breath

22. Coma is a:
    a. period of confusion and forgetfulness
    b. state of unconsciousness during which the patient is responsive to pain and verbal stimulus
    c. state of unconsciousness characterized by the absence of spontaneous eye movements, response to painful stimuli, and vocalization
    d. period of apnea, followed by rapid breathing, and then apnea

23. List five causes of coma that originate from within the brain.

    _____

    _____

    _____

    _____

    _____

24. List seven causes of coma arising outside the nervous system.

    _____

    _____

    _____

    _____

    _____

    _____

    _____

25. Unequal pupils associated with a comatose patient are indicative of:
    a. stroke
    b. hyperglycemia
    c. drug abuse
    d. liver disease

26. The *most* important priority in caring for a comatose patient is to:
    a. establish an IV line—normal saline or lactated Ringer's TKO or heparin lock
    b. give high-concentration oxygen via nonrebreather mask
    c. administer 1 ampule (25 g) of D_{50}, IV push
    d. establish and maintain a patent airway

27. Unconscious patients should be placed in a _____ position.
    a. supine (with legs elevated 10 to 12 inches)
    b. prone
    c. coma
    d. right lateral recumbent

28. The recommended initial dosage for naloxone administration in the coma patient is _____ mg.
    a. 0.2 to 1.0
    b. 0.4 to 2.0
    c. 2 to 10
    d. 5 to 10

29. Describe *syncope*.

    _____

    _____

    _____

30. The most important management consideration in a syncopal episode is to monitor the patient for:
    a. cardiac dysrhythmias
    b. dehydration
    c. hypoglycemia
    d. hypertension

31. When persons faint, they often have jerking movements called:
    a. psychomotor seizures
    b. tonic-clonic movements
    c. myoclonal jerks
    d. palpitations

32. List five causes of headache caused by potentially serious conditions.

___

33. Which of the following causes of headache is vascular in nature?
    a. muscle spasm
    b. meningitis
    c. tumor
    d. stroke

34. Eye pain with bright light is called:
    a. photophobia
    b. diplopia
    c. ataxia
    d. vasculitis

35. List the treatments that may be provided to the patient complaining of headache.

___

It is 3:30 PM when you are called to the home of a 40-year-old man who is disoriented. According to family members, the patient was fine yesterday, but when he awoke this morning he seemed confused and agitated. During the day, he became more and more disoriented. You are able to determine that the patient has a medical history of hypertension. Assessment reveals that he is unable to recall the time, date, or place; has a grip deficit on the right side; becomes dizzy and complains of a severe headache every time he attempts to sit up; has a respiratory rate of 24; a pulse rate of 106; a blood pressure of 170/98; and ashen, diaphoretic skin. Pupils are unequal, the left pupil being fixed and dilated, whereas the right pupil is constricted.

36. This patient is experiencing:
    a. hypertensive crisis
    b. a stroke
    c. insulin shock
    d. an overdose of antihypertensive medication

37. Treatment includes:
    a. administering high-concentration oxygen
    b. placing him in a supine position
    c. delaying transport until a paramedic unit is at the scene to assist with care
    d. administering 50% dextrose, IV push

CROSSWORD PUZZLE EXERCISE

38. Complete the following crossword puzzle.

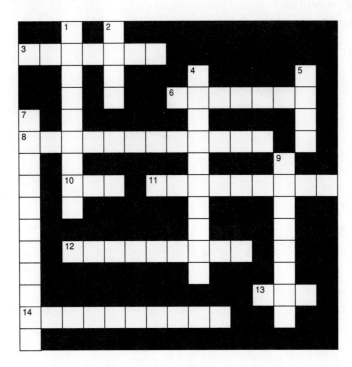

ACROSS

3. Sudden episode of abnormal brain cell electrical activity.
6. Spinning of the room.
8. Infection of the brain tissue itself.
10. Temporary disruption in the circulation to the brain.
11. Systems that maintain alertness, awareness, and a normal wakeful state.
12. Stroke caused by a blockage in a blood vessel resulting from either an atherosclerotic plaque or an embolus.
13. Abbreviation for central nervous system.
14. No demonstrable cause.

DOWN

1. Mnemonic that helps you remember the many conditions that can lead to CNS disorders.
2. Seeing, hearing, or smelling something unusual before losing consciousness.
4. Inflammation of the membranes surrounding the brain.
5. Unconsciousness with no spontaneous eye movements, response to painful stimuli, vocalization.
7. Stroke caused by bleeding into brain tissue resulting from rupture of a weakened blood vessel.
9. Pupils seen in altered level of consciousness that suggest drug overdose or intracranial bleeding.

29 Nontraumatic Abdominal Emergencies

CHAPTER TERMINAL OBJECTIVES

On completion of this chapter, the EMT-Intermediate will be able to utilize assessment findings to formulate a field impression and implement a treatment plan for the patient with nontraumatic abdominal pain.

For the multiple-choice questions, select the single best answer to each question. For the matching questions, select the best corresponding answer for each item. Because there are sometimes more items than corresponding answers in the matching questions, some items may not be used.

1. The abdominal cavity:
    a. contains the organs of digestion, the organs of the urinary and reproductive tracts, the vertebral column, and major blood vessels
    b. extends from the umbilicus to the pelvic bones and is surrounded by a large muscle mass
    c. is divided into six quadrants
    d. is lined by the pericardium

2. For the list of abdominal organs below, identify in which quadrant each is located by placing RUQ (right upper quadrant), LUQ (left upper quadrant), RLQ (right lower quadrant), or LLQ (left lower quadrant) in front of it (some may have more than one).
    _____ Liver
    _____ Spleen
    _____ Stomach
    _____ Appendix
    _____ Gallbladder
    _____ Pancreas
    _____ Small intestine
    _____ Large intestine
    _____ Kidney
    _____ Ovary
    _____ Uterus
    _____ Urinary bladder
    _____ Ureter

3. List five common causes of acute abdominal pain.

    _____

    _____

    _____

    _____

    _____

4. _____ is usually caused by infection in the bowel, the surrounding peritoneal cavity, or both.
   a. Obstruction
   b. Peritoneal inflammation
   c. Chemical contamination
   d. Bacterial contamination

5. Match the following diseases that cause acute abdominal pain and are immediately life threatening with the appropriate characteristics.

   Condition
   a. Acute myocardial infarction
   b. Ruptured abdominal aortic aneurysm
   c. Ruptured ectopic pregnancy
   d. Ruptured viscus

   Characteristic
   _____ Occurs when the fertilized egg implants outside the uterus. Internal structures may rupture, causing severe internal bleeding.
   _____ Rupture of any hollow organ; produces sudden onset of sharp epigastric pain and shock—the abdomen is rigid.
   _____ An outpouching of the abdominal portion of the aorta caused by atherosclerosis. Severe abdominal and back pain, as well as shock, results. The patient may easily bleed to death.

6. Gnawing upper abdominal pain and nausea that is often relieved with food or antacids is characteristic of:
   a. gastritis
   b. appendicitis
   c. peptic ulcer disease
   d. cholecystitis

7. Which of the following signs or symptoms is associated with pancreatitis?
   a. severe abdominal pain with radiation from the umbilicus to the back and shoulders
   b. vomiting of large amounts of bright red blood
   c. yellow skin
   d. pulsating abdominal mass

8. Gastritis is characterized by:
   a. intermittent pain located in the right upper quadrant and accompanied by nausea
   b. lower abdominal pain with fever and chills
   c. cramplike abdominal pain in the left lower quadrant that may be accompanied by fever, diarrhea, or constipation
   d. loss of appetite, nausea, vomiting, and epigastric discomfort after eating

9. Match the following conditions with the appropriate characteristics.

   Condition
   a. Appendicitis
   b. Cholecystitis
   c. Pyelonephritis
   d. Diverticulitis
   e. Bowel obstruction

   Characteristic
   _____ Blockage of the intestinal tract that produces cramping pain, vomiting, abdominal tenderness, and distention of the abdomen
   _____ Kidney infection that leads to flank pain, which may radiate to the abdomen, discomfort with urination, nausea, and vomiting

_____ Infection of small, saclike outpouchings in the intestine that causes cramplike abdominal pain in the left lower quadrant. May be accompanied by fever, diarrhea, or constipation.

_____ Occlusion of the gallbladder duct, leading to inflammation and pain. The pain is usually intermittent, located in the right upper quadrant, and accompanied by nausea. Pain may radiate to the posterior scapula or right shoulder.

_____ Results from obstruction of the lumen of the appendix. The patient initially has pain around the umbilicus that then localizes to the right lower quadrant. Loss of appetite (anorexia) is common.

10. T F The abdominal organs have nerve receptors for pain.
11. T F Conditions that originate in the abdomen can cause pain in distant locations such as the neck, shoulder, chest, or flank.
12. T F You should ask the patient when his or her last meal was only when there is an indication a meal may have been recently ingested.

13. Describe the general appearance of the patient with an acute abdominal condition.

_____
_____
_____
_____
_____

14. The abdomen may be soft, _____, or _____. There may be localized or diffuse _____ to palpation. _____ means that the abdomen feels rigid to palpation. _____ is voluntary or involuntary resistance to your touch.

15. T F The position of comfort for patients experiencing abdominal pain is typically on their side with their legs straight.
16. T F Patients experiencing abdominal pain who are dehydrated or hypotensive should receive an IV line and a fluid bolus of normal saline or lactated Ringer's solution.
17. T F The EMT-I should always check distal pulses bilaterally in all patients with abdominal pain.

18. A pulsating mass in the abdomen suggests:
    a. abdominal aortic aneurysm
    b. kidney stones
    c. bowel obstruction
    d. diverticulitis

19. List three common causes of upper GI bleeding.

   _____

   _____

   _____

20. List four common causes of lower GI bleeding.

   _____

   _____

   _____

   _____

21. The common cause of upper GI bleeding in alcoholic patients is esophageal _____.

   It is 12:30 PM when you are called to the scene where a 69-year-old woman is "throwing up" blood. On your arrival, you find the woman sitting at the dining room table, slumped over with her head and arms resting on the table. She is moaning in discomfort. Your initial assessment reveals that she is alert; has cold, clammy, pale, diaphoretic skin; a blood pressure of 80/60; a pulse rate of 120; and a respiratory rate of 26. According to the patient, she had diarrhea this morning that appeared dark and coffee-ground–like. She then had acute lower abdominal pain and vomited bright red blood with clots. Assessment reveals that the abdomen is soft without mass, but palpation reveals lower abdominal pain. The patient has a history of heart and respiratory problems. She takes theophylline, quinidine, verapamil (Calan), and just recently began taking indomethacin (Indocin). She is allergic to meperidine (Demerol).

22. This patient is suffering from:
    a. gastrointestinal bleeding
    b. appendicitis
    c. a bowel obstruction
    d. pancreatitis

23. Treatment includes:
    a. administering high-concentration oxygen
    b. placing the patient into a semisitting position on the cot
    c. starting an IV line of 5% dextrose in water
    d. applying the pneumatic antishock garment (PASG) and inflating the abdominal section

24. You are moving the patient to the cot when she suddenly begins vomiting. You should:
    a. remove the PASG if it is in place
    b. hyperventilate the patient with a bag-mask device and 100% oxygen
    c. decrease the flow rate of the IV
    d. switch over to a nasal cannula, and administer 4 to 6 L/min of oxygen

25. The patient experiencing _____ should be placed in a supine position with legs elevated if he or she is _____.
    a. chest pain; disoriented
    b. a diabetic emergency; hypoglycemic
    c. hypertensive crisis; experiencing a diastolic pressure of more than 120 mm Hg
    d. gastrointestinal bleeding; hypotensive

26. _____ is the presence of bright red blood in the stool. _____ is black, tarry stool caused by digested blood passing slowly through the GI tract. _____ is the vomiting of blood.

CROSSWORD PUZZLE EXERCISE

27. Complete the following crossword puzzle.

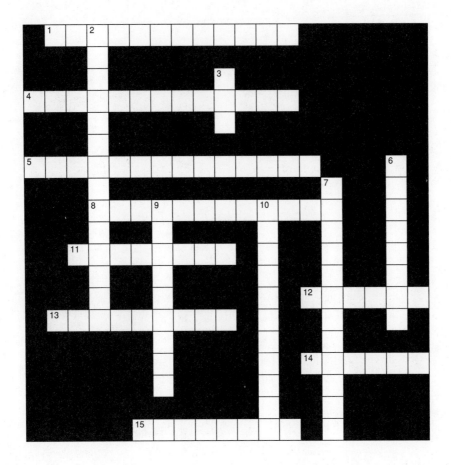

ACROSS

1. Inflammation of the appendix.
4. Occlusion of the gallbladder duct, leading to inflammation and pain.
5. Infection of saclike outpouchings in the intestine.
8. Presence of bright red blood in the stool.
11. Abdomen feels hard and firm to palpation.
12. Black, tarry stool caused by digested blood passing slowly through the GI tract.
13. Inflammation of the lining of the stomach resulting from drugs, alcohol, or infection.
14. General term for any hollow organ.
15. An outpouching of the abdominal portion of the aorta caused by atherosclerosis.

DOWN

2. Kidney infection.
3. Inflammation of the female internal genitalia, usually caused by sexually transmitted disease.
6. Voluntary or involuntary resistance to your touch.
7. Inflammation of the pancreas caused by either alcohol or stones that block the ducts.
9. Cavity that extends from the diaphragm to the pelvic bones.
10. Irritation of the esophagus.

30 Environmental Emergencies

CHAPTER TERMINAL OBJECTIVES

On completion of this chapter, the EMT-Intermediate will be able to utilize assessment findings to formulate a field impression and implement a treatment plan for the patient with an environmentally induced or exacerbated emergency.

For the multiple-choice questions, select the single best answer to each question. For the matching questions, select the best corresponding answer for each item. Because there are sometimes more items than corresponding answers in the matching questions, some items may not be used.

1. Define the term environmental emergency.

   _____
   _____
   _____
   _____
   _____

2. List five preexisting risk factors that make environmental emergencies dangerous.

   _____
   _____
   _____
   _____
   _____
   _____

3. List four environmental factors that may cause illness or exacerbate a preexisting illness.

   _____
   _____
   _____
   _____
   _____

4. Environmental illnesses can be divided into two categories, _____ and _____. Regarding emergency care, _____ problems are more potentially harmful than are _____ ones.

5. Which of the following is a systemic environmental illness?
   a. frostbite
   b. sunburn
   c. snakebite
   d. heatstroke

6. T F The normal body temperature is at or near 37° C.

7. T F A tympanic temperature most accurately measures core temperature.

8. _____ refers to normal body means of heat loss and gain. Heat is generated by muscular _____ and through _____ reactions in the body.

9. Match the following heat-dissipating mechanisms with the correct description. Some items may be used more than once.

   Mechanism
   a. Radiation
   b. Conduction
   c. Convection
   d. Evaporation

   Characteristic
   _____ Transmission of heat from warmer to cooler objects in direct contact
   _____ Loss of heat at the surface from vaporization of liquid
   _____ Examples are touching a cold surface or lying on a cold floor
   _____ Transmission of heat through space
   _____ Examples are sweating, spraying water mist on the body to keep cool while sunbathing
   _____ Examples are wind chill, cold water exposure

10. Describe another way heat is lost from the body.

    _____
    _____
    _____
    _____
    _____

11. At room temperature:
    a. in humans, conduction is a major mechanism of heat loss
    b. 75% of heat dissipation is by radiation and convection
    c. the loss of moisture from the lungs and skin accounts for about 50% of heat loss
    d. convection is enhanced by clothing

12. T F As the ambient temperature approaches body temperature, radiation becomes the most effective means of dissipating heat.

13. T F At high temperatures and high humidity, evaporation quickly dissipates heat.

14. Heat illness is defined as _____ core body temperature (CBT) as a result of inadequate _____ .

15. Describe how extremes of age, underlying disease, and medications affect temperature regulation.

___

16. Heat cramps are:
    a. cramps or pains in the muscles, especially of the chest and lower extremities
    b. caused by dehydration and overexertion that occur during normal temperatures
    c. the least common of the heat injury syndromes
    d. caused by excessive loss of salt and water in the sweat

17. List the signs and symptoms associated with heat cramps.

___

18. Signs and symptoms associated with heat exhaustion include:
    a. flushed skin
    b. temperature greater than 105° F
    c. diaphoresis
    d. coma, convulsions

19. Treatment of heat exhaustion includes all of the following *except:*
    a. giving the patient salt pills
    b. giving a high concentration of oxygen by nonrebreather mask
    c. removing the patient from the hot environment to a cool environment
    d. placing an IV line and administering a fluid bolus of normal saline

It is a hot summer day when you are called to an apartment complex for a 58-year-old woman who is complaining of abdominal cramps, weakness, and nausea. Apparently she was locked in her apartment for several days during unusually hot weather. Your assessment reveals the patient is disoriented, has a respiratory rate of 26, a pulse rate of 130, a blood pressure of 106/92, and flushed, dry skin that is hot to the touch. According to the landlord, the patient has a history of hypertension for which she takes several medicines.

20. This patient is experiencing:
    a. cardiogenic shock
    b. heat stroke
    c. heat exhaustion
    d. heat cramps

21. Treatment includes all of the following *except:*
    a. having her rest
    b. moving her to a cool environment
    c. administering 6 L/min of oxygen via nonrebreather mask
    d. cooling her immediately by applying ice packs to the neck, axillae (armpits), wrists, and groin

22. Generalized hypothermia is a condition in which the core or internal body temperature is less than _____ ° F because of either decreased production of _____ or increased heat _____ from the body.

23. List the three primary causes of hypothermia.
    _____
    _____
    _____

24. T F   Drowning is the principal cause of death following boating accidents.

25. T F   With the exception of wool, wet clothing loses 90% of its insulating value. Thus soaked individuals are effectively nude.

26. T F   Cold stress among the aged, intoxicated, or debilitated can cause fatal hypothermia.

27. A patient with hypothermia usually has a CBT of:
    a. 97° F
    b. 98° F or less
    c. 95° F or less
    d. 100° F or greater

28. List seven predisposing factors of hypothermia.
    _____
    _____
    _____
    _____
    _____
    _____
    _____

29. T F   Medications that predispose the patient to hypothermia include narcotics, phenothiazines, barbiturates, anti-seizure medications, antihistamines, and other allergy medications.

30. T F   Victims of hypothermia stop shivering when the body temperature is below 92° F.

31. Mild hypothermia is defined as the presence of signs and symptoms with a:
    a. CBT greater than 90° F
    b. CBT less than 90° F
    c. normal CBT
    d. higher than normal CBT

32. It is midmorning when you are called to a residence where a 76-year-old man fell down the basement stairs to the floor below. He was unable to get up off the floor all night. You determine he is hypothermic. This is classified as:
    a. chronic onset
    b. subacute onset
    c. acute onset
    d. delayed onset

You have been called to the scene where a 50-year-old man has fallen through the ice of a local pond during his attempt to rescue a dog. Several bystanders have formed a human chain to try to reach the man. You arrive just in time to assist pulling the patient from the water. Your assessment of the patient reveals that he is awake but seems confused, has a respiratory rate of 30, a pulse rate of 124, a blood pressure of 112/90, and cold, pale skin. You also note that he has intense, uncontrollable shivering and difficulty speaking. Your physical examination reveals no fractures. You determine that the patient has a history of asthma that he uses an inhaler to treat.

33. While in the water the patient lost heat through:
    a. convection
    b. conduction
    c. evaporation
    d. radiation

34. This patient is experiencing what stage of hypothermia?
    a. mild
    b. severe
    c. compensated
    d. subacute

35. Treatment for this patient includes:
    a. withholding oxygen unless the cylinder can be warmed
    b. having the patient walk around to generate heat
    c. providing aggressive rewarming
    d. removing all wet clothing

It is a cold winter night when you are called to a local freeway where a 31-year-old man was found unconscious in his car. Police state they found the man as they were checking on a report of an abandoned auto. The patient is unconscious, has a respiratory rate of 6 breaths/min, a pulse rate of 30 beats per minute (BPM), an "inaudible" blood pressure, and his skin is ice cold. The patient also seems "stiff," and his eyes seem to have a glassy stare. Your examination of the patient reveals no obvious injuries and no medical alert tags.

36. The patient is most likely suffering from which of the following?
    a. cardiac arrest
    b. hypoglycemia
    c. severe hypothermia
    d. diabetic coma

37. Treatment includes:
    a. delivering cardiopulmonary resuscitation (CPR)
    b. rewarming the patient with hot packs and warm blankets
    c. performing endotracheal intubation
    d. assisting the patient's breathing

38. Cold may affect the _____ of first-line _____ drugs. There is no increased risk of inducing ventricular fibrillation (VF) from _____ or _____ intubation as long as the patient is _____ adequately _____ handling, however, *can* induce VF.

39. T F The most common dysrhythmias in hypothermia-associated cardiac arrest are pulseless electrical activity (PEA) and asystole.

40. T F The hypothermic heart is often resistant to defibrillation.

41. T F Lidocaine and procainamide should be used in hypothermia because they increase the VF threshold, making successful defibrillation more likely.

42. T F VF often occurs as a patient is being rewarmed when the heart temperature rises above 86° F.

43. Describe when defibrillation should be done in the hypothermic cardiac arrest patient.
    _____
    _____
    _____
    _____
    _____

44. Describe the difference between drowning and near-drowning.
    _____
    _____
    _____
    _____
    _____

45. The most common factor in adult drowning is:
    a. the presence of medical conditions such as diabetes, seizures, and heart disease
    b. hyperventilation in preparation for a long underwater submersion
    c. swimmer exhaustion
    d. use of alcohol and mind-altering drugs

46. Match the following types of drowning with the correct description. Some items may be used more than once.

Drowning Type
a. Dry
b. Wet
c. Secondary

Characteristic
_____ These victims have the best chance of survival.
_____ Involves 80% to 90% of cases
_____ Asphyxiation is caused by anoxia as a result of laryngeal spasm that prevents the entrance of water, as well as air, into the lungs. This leads to cerebral anoxia, edema, and unconsciousness.
_____ Victim makes a violent respiratory effort and fluid fills the lungs.
_____ Recurrence of respiratory distress (usually in the form of pulmonary edema or aspiration pneumonia) after successful recovery from the initial incident

47. With saltwater drowning:
    a. there is a washout of surfactant in the alveoli
    b. the presence of a concentrated fluid in the lung causes an influx of hypotonic serum into the alveoli, leading to pulmonary edema
    c. alveolar dehydration occurs as the inhaled saltwater and lung fluids are drawn into the bloodstream
    d. hypoxia occurs as a result of collapse of the alveoli

48. List seven signs of near-drowning.

_____
_____
_____
_____
_____
_____
_____

It is a cool spring afternoon when you are called to a local lake for a drowning. You arrive to find park rangers delivering oxygen to a 17-year-old male teenager who was pulled from the water after being submerged for approximately 5 minutes. He was unconscious, apneic, cyanotic, and pulseless but regained a pulse and spontaneous breathing after several minutes of CPR. He is now starting to wake up and wants to go home.

49. This patient experienced:
    a. saltwater near-drowning
    b. severe hypothermia
    c. freshwater near-drowning
    d. status epilepticus

50. Treatment for this patient includes:
    a. administering high-concentration oxygen via nonrebreather mask
    b. placing him in a head-dependent position
    c. applying subdiaphragmatic thrusts
    d. placing an IV of 5% dextrose in water

51. Describe why the patient should not be allowed to go home without first being assessed at the hospital.

_____
_____
_____
_____

Your patient is a 27-year-old woman who became severely dyspneic after a breath-holding ascent while scuba diving. She is disoriented; the skin is cold, clammy, and diaphoretic with cyanosis around the lips; blood pressure is 60 by palpation; pulse is weak and thready; respirations are 30; lung sounds are diminished on the left side; and you notice tracheal deviation to the right.

52. This patient is experiencing:
    a. tension pneumothorax
    b. microembolism
    c. acute pulmonary edema
    d. nitrogen narcosis

53. Treatment for this patient includes:
    a. placing an IV of normal saline and running it at a wide open rate
    b. immediately performing emergency needle thoracostomy
    c. limiting oxygen administration to 2 to 3 L/min via nasal cannula
    d. placing her in a semisitting position

54. Describe what is meant by the term acute mountain sickness (AMS).

_____
_____
_____
_____

55. List five signs and symptoms of acute mountain sickness.

_____
_____
_____
_____

56. High-altitude pulmonary edema (HAPE):
    a. often results in symptoms 4 to 6 hours after exposure
    b. is caused by increased pulmonary artery pressure that develops in response to hypoxia
    c. progresses to high-altitude cerebral edema (HACE) if not treated quickly
    d. leads to bronchospasm, acute hypoxia, and hypercarbia

57. HACE:
    a. is the most severe form of acute high-altitude illness
    b. is caused by decreased intracranial pressure
    c. occurs almost immediately after exposure to high altitude
    d. is easy to differentiate from acute mountain sickness

58. Initially with frostbite the affected area:
    a. appears yellowish white and waxy or bluish white
    b. becomes flushed with a red to purple-burgundy color
    c. feels frozen to the touch
    d. swells two to three times the normal size

59. Treatment of frostbite includes:
    a. rewarming in 110° F to 115° F water
    b. rubbing the affected area
    c. having the patient smoke a cigarette
    d. transporting the patient to the hospital as soon as possible

CROSSWORD PUZZLE EXERCISE

60. Complete the following crossword puzzle.

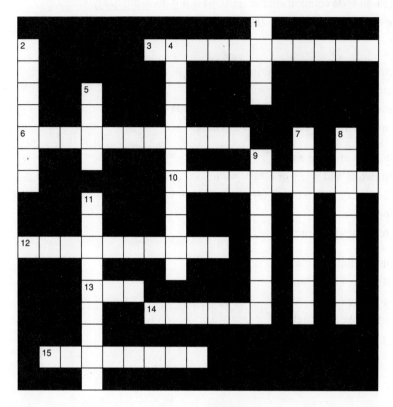

ACROSS

3. Refers to normal bodily means of heat loss and gain.
6. Loss of heat at the surface from vaporization of liquid.
10. Heat _____ is a more severe loss of fluid and salt than occurs in heat cramps.
12. Transmission of heat from warmer to cooler objects in direct contact.
13. Abbreviation of acute mountain sickness.
14. Hypothermia where there are signs and symptoms and a CBT of less than 90° F.
15. Death caused by asphyxiation during an immersion episode.

DOWN

1. Inner body temperature.
2. Law that states that the volume of a gas varies inversely with the absolute pressure.
4. Condition in which CBT is less than 95° F.
5. Abbreviation for high-altitude pulmonary edema.
7. Reflex vasodilation seen with rewarming.
8. Formation of ice crystals within the tissues.
9. Onset of hypothermia that comes on over minutes to hours.
11. Transmission of heat through space.

31 Behavioral Emergencies and Substance Abuse

CHAPTER TERMINAL OBJECTIVES

On completion of this chapter, the EMT-Intermediate will be able to utilize assessment findings to form a field impression and implement a management plan for patients with behavioral or drug abuse emergencies.

For the multiple-choice questions, select the single best answer to each question. For the matching questions, select the best corresponding answer for each item. Because there are sometimes more items than corresponding answers in the matching questions, some items may not be used.

1. Define the term *behavior*.

   _____
   _____
   _____
   _____
   _____

2. Abnormal behavior:
   a. consists of actions that conform to society's norms and expectations
   b. interferes with a person's well-being and ability to function, although an individual may not be aware of it
   c. is typically harmful to the patient or other people
   d. is also referred to as adaptive behavior, indicating that a person is unable to properly adapt to various challenging circumstances

3. Define the term *behavioral emergency*.

   _____
   _____
   _____
   _____
   _____

4. List three causes of behavioral emergencies.

   _____
   _____
   _____

5. A significant proportion of acute behavioral emergencies are caused by:
   a. the increased use of electricity
   b. breakdown of the ozone layer
   c. drug and substance abuse
   d. death of a loved one

6. T F The EMT-I should avoid establishing a rapport with the patient experiencing a behavioral emergency until after the patient has been restrained.

7. T F The EMT-I should prevent the patient from expressing anger and frustration verbally.

8. T F The EMT-I should avoid making eye contact with a patient who is experiencing a behavioral emergency.

9. List five clues that a patient may develop violent behavior.

_____

_____

_____

_____

_____

10. As part of interviewing the patient experiencing a behavioral emergency, the EMT-I should:
    a. remove the patient from the crisis or disturbing situation
    b. argue with the patient if he or she becomes loud or abusive
    c. loudly discount any delusions the patient experiences
    d. attempt to interpret the patient's statements

11. List seven things the EMT-I should pay attention to during assessment of the behavioral emergency patient.

_____

_____

_____

_____

_____

_____

_____

12. _____ is an abnormal anxiety reaction to a perceived fear. There is no basis, in reality, for that fear.

    _____ is when the patient has no concept whatsoever of reality. The person truly believes his or her situation or condition is real—often the person hears voices.

13. In drug-induced _____, hallucinogens or stimulant agents cause the patient to lose touch with reality.

14. List three signs and symptoms that indicate a person is depressed.

_____

_____

_____

You are called to the home of a 29-year-old man who was found unconscious in the bedroom. According to family members who found him, he has been despondent over breaking up with his girlfriend. Your initial assessment reveals that he is unconscious and does not respond to verbal or painful stimuli, has a respiratory rate of 8 breaths/min, a pulse rate of 50 beats per minute (BPM), and a blood pressure of 72/40. His skin is cool and sweaty, and his pupils are pinpoint. You find an empty sleeping pill bottle lying beside the bed.

15. This case is considered a _____.
    a. suicide
    b. suicide gesture
    c. suicide attempt
    d. psychotic episode

16. Treatment includes:
    a. administering high-concentration oxygen via nonrebreather mask
    b. administering syrup of ipecac to induce vomiting
    c. administering activated charcoal to dilute the drug
    d. inserting an oropharyngeal airway

17. Suicide is more common in which of the following?
    a. young men between the ages of 15 and 35
    b. married men
    c. single women
    d. elderly men who are recently widowed

18. T F The term alcohol abuse means the same as alcoholism.

19. T F Ingestion of alcohol in combination with other drugs such as sleeping pills can be fatal.

20. Signs and symptoms of alcohol intoxication include:
    a. unequal pupils
    b. steady gait
    c. slurred, loud, and inappropriate speech
    d. cold, clammy skin

21. Serious conditions that mimic alcohol intoxication include all of the following *except:*
    a. hypoglycemia
    b. head injury
    c. hypoxia
    d. cardiogenic shock

22. Describe the reason that severely intoxicated patients should be transported to the hospital.

_____

_____

_____

_____

_____

23. Delirium tremens:
    a. refers to a condition of glucose deficiency in the body
    b. includes signs and symptoms such as gross tremors, increasing agitation, hallucinations, confusion, seizures, tachycardia, fever, and hypertension
    c. may be treated adequately "at home" rather than requiring transport to the hospital
    d. is treated with an IV of 5% dextrose in water run at a wide open rate

24. _____ _____ is a condition characterized by an overwhelming desire to continue taking a drug to which one has become "hooked" through repeated consumption because it produces a particular effect.

25. _____ _____ is a psychological craving for, or a psychological reliance on, a chemical agent, resulting from abuse or addiction.

26. _____ _____ is a set of signs and symptoms that develop in a person following abrupt cessation of taking a drug.

27. Match the following classes with the appropriate drugs and symptoms.

    Class
    a. Stimulants (uppers)
    b. Narcotics
    c. Hallucinogens
    d. Depressants (downers)

    Symptom

    _____ Includes heroin, morphine, methadone, meperidine (Demerol), hydromorphone (Dilaudid), pentazocine (Talwin), codeine, hydrocodone (Vicodin), and propoxyphene (Darvon). Symptoms include drowsiness, coma, impaired coordination, sweating, respiratory depression, constricted pupils, shock, convulsions, and coma. Respiratory and cardiac arrest is possible.

    _____ Includes marijuana, barbiturates, sleeping pills, tranquilizers, and antidepressant pills. Symptoms include sluggishness, poor coordination, slurred speech, decreased respiration or respiratory arrest, and impaired memory and judgment.

    _____ Includes cocaine, amphetamines, and "ice." Symptoms include hyperactivity, euphoria, tachycardia, hypertension, dilated pupils, diaphoresis, sleeplessness, seizures, and disorientation. Cocaine causes hypertensive crises, seizures, myocardial infarction, and stroke.

    _____ Lysergic acid diethylamide (LSD), mescaline, psilocybin, and phencyclidine (PCP or angel dust). Symptoms include hallucinations, unpredictable behavior, tachypnea, nausea, dilated pupils, and increased pulse and blood pressure.

You have been called to the scene where a 19-year-old man was found unconscious in the restroom of a local shopping mall. Your assessment reveals that he is unresponsive to verbal or painful stimuli, has shallow respirations at a rate of 6 breaths/min, a weak thready pulse, a blood pressure of 108/90, and pinpoint pupils. According to his friends, the patient has no history of medical problems.

28. This patient is suffering from:
    a. insulin shock
    b. crack overdose
    c. opiate overdose
    d. head injury

29. Treatment includes:
    a. performing tracheal suctioning
    b. administering 0.4 to 2.0 mg of naloxone, IV push
    c. assisting the patient's breathing using a bag-mask device with 6 L/min of supplemental oxygen
    d. administering syrup of ipecac

CROSSWORD PUZZLE EXERCISE

30. Complete the following crossword puzzle.

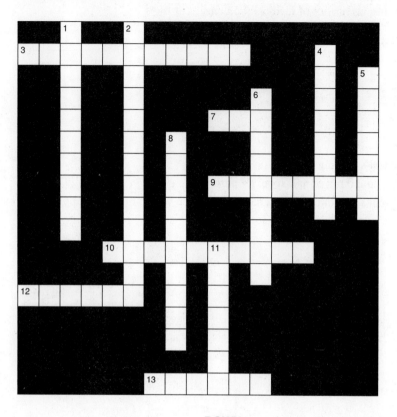

ACROSS

3. Abnormal behavior.
7. Severe state of delirium, hallucinations, and autonomic nervous system hyperactivity.
9. Defined as how a person acts.
10. Common reaction to major life stresses.
12. These occur within 24 hours of drinking cessation.
13. These drugs stimulate the central nervous system.

DOWN

1. Chronic condition characterized by dependence on alcohol.
2. These drugs induce a sense of euphoria and hallucinations.
4. Abnormal anxiety reaction to a perceived fear.
5. These drugs depress the central nervous system.
6. When the patient has no concept whatsoever of reality.
8. Seizures that occur within 24 to 48 hours of stopping drinking alcohol.
11. The intentional taking of one's life.

32 Gynecological Emergencies

CHAPTER TERMINAL OBJECTIVES

On completion of this chapter, the EMT-Intermediate will be able to utilize assessment findings to formulate a field impression and implement the management plan for the patient experiencing a gynecological emergency.

For the multiple-choice questions, select the single best answer to each question. For the matching questions, select the best corresponding answer for each item. Because there are sometimes more items than corresponding answers in the matching questions, some items may not be used.

1. For the illustration of the female reproductive system anatomical structures below, label the name of each shown. Then use colored pens or pencils to color the illustration according to the following: A-blue, B-red, C-orange, D-pink, and E-tan.

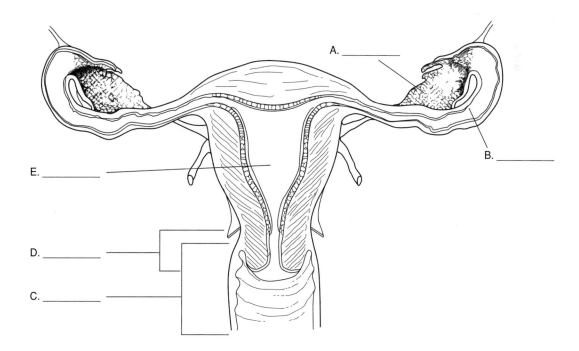

2. The menstrual cycle:
    a. occurs when an egg implants in the uterus
    b. is vaginal bleeding that typically occurs every 28 days
    c. generally lasts 7 to 10 days
    d. occurs when the normal hormonal regulation causes the inner lining of the vagina to shed

3. Menarche:
    a. occurs anywhere from the age of 35 up until 60 years
    b. typically occurs at age 16
    c. is the first menstrual cycle that the woman experiences
    d. is a time at which there is no further menstrual bleeding

429

4. Describe what normally happens if sperm fertilizes an egg.

_____

_____

_____

_____

_____

5. T F Women experiencing acute gynecological emergencies are at little risk of developing shock.

6. T F The organs of fertility located in the pelvis are close to other abdominal organs.

7. T F Assessment of any woman with a possible disorder of the bladder, urinary tract, gastrointestinal tract, and other abdominal organs should also consider the possibility of a gynecological origin.

8. List nine questions that should be asked of patients experiencing gynecological emergencies.

_____

_____

_____

_____

_____

_____

_____

_____

_____

9. Hypotension in the patient experiencing an acute gynecological emergency is most commonly caused by:
   a. internal hemorrhage in the pelvis
   b. external bleeding noted from the vagina
   c. severe peripheral vasodilation
   d. a and b

10. Warm and flushed skin seen in patients experiencing an acute gynecological emergency indicates:
    a. respiratory insufficiency
    b. severe anemia
    c. dehydration
    d. overwhelming infection

11. List five causes of tachycardia in patients experiencing an acute gynecological emergency.

___

12. T F The initial evaluation of the abdomen in patients experiencing an acute gynecological emergency should be simple observation to see whether the abdomen appears distended or whether it is flat and normal in shape.

13. T F Abdominal guarding is indicative of masses within the abdominal cavity.

14. T F Pain while the EMT-I is pressing down on the abdomen is considered a positive rebound tenderness test.

15. Describe how to elicit rebound tenderness during abdominal assessment.

___

You are called to the apartment of a 20-year-old woman who is complaining of lower abdominal pain. She says the pain started several days ago and has gotten worse. She reports pain with intercourse and vaginal discharge. Assessment reveals that she is alert, has a respiratory rate of 14, a pulse rate of 90, a blood pressure of 130/80, and warm, flushed skin. The pulse oximetry reading is 96% on room air. You note there is intense pain with minimal palpation, abdominal guarding, and the patient cannot lie completely supine. The patient has no significant medical history other than a miscarriage the previous year.

16. The patient is experiencing:
    a. ectopic pregnancy
    b. a miscarriage
    c. acute appendicitis
    d. pelvic inflammatory disease (PID)

17. Treatment for this patient includes:
    a. administering oxygen via nasal cannula
    b. placing her in a lateral recumbent position
    c. placing a large-bore IV line and running it wide open
    d. administering morphine sulfate, 1 to 3 mg, slow IV push

18. Describe how a ruptured ovarian cyst occurs.

_____

_____

_____

_____

_____

19. Embryo implantation occurring outside the body of the uterus, such as in the fallopian tube, is referred to as:
    a. spontaneous abortion
    b. ruptured uterus
    c. ectopic pregnancy
    d. ovarian cyst

A 16-year-old female patient is complaining of severe abdominal pain. Assessment reveals that she is alert and oriented, has a respiratory rate of 20, a pulse rate of 100, a blood pressure of 90/70, and cool, pale skin. The patient reports that she missed her period and has had intermittent spotting over the past 6 to 8 weeks. She also states that she has had breast tenderness, nausea, vomiting, fatigue, and shoulder pain. The patient reports a previous medical history of PID. The abdominal examination reveals a normal-sized abdomen with significant tenderness, particularly in the lower left quadrant. Questioning of the patient reveals that she may be pregnant.

20. Your patient is experiencing:
    a. ectopic pregnancy
    b. an elective abortion
    c. acute appendicitis
    d. abruptio placentae

21. Treatment for this patient includes:
    a. administering 100% oxygen via nonrebreather mask
    b. placing her in a semisitting position
    c. performing a vaginal examination
    d. administering diazepam, 5 to 10 mg, slow IV push

22. Which of the following is true regarding initiating IV therapy in this case?
    a. Eighteen- to 20-gauge needles should be used.
    b. The IVs should be infused at a TKO rate.
    c. Normal saline or lactated Ringer's solution should be used.
    d. Microdrip administration sets are preferred.

23. An abortion that starts of its own accord is referred to as:
    a. spontaneous
    b. therapeutic
    c. elective
    d. criminal

24. Management of the female patient with vaginal bleeding in the prehospital setting includes:
    a. packing the vagina with dressings to tamponade or slow the bleeding
    b. placing her in a sitting position
    c. establishing a second IV line if shock is present
    d. administering 4 to 6 L of oxygen per minute via nasal cannula

25. Which of the following is part of managing sexual assault victims?
    a. having them change clothes before being taken to the receiving facility
    b. having them take a shower as soon as possible
    c. cleansing any areas of traumatic injury
    d. ensuring the environment is safe, quiet, and provides as much psychological support as possible

CROSSWORD PUZZLE EXERCISE

26. Complete the following crossword puzzle.

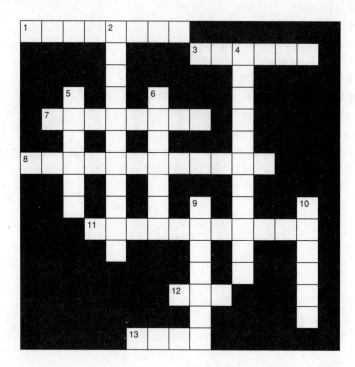

ACROSS

1. Injuries occurring when a female falls or strikes an object with both legs abducted.
3. Muscular pelvic structure that protects and nourishes the fetus during development.
7. First menstrual cycle that a woman experiences.
8. Pain with menses.
11. Spontaneous demise of the pregnancy.
12. Infection involving pelvic structures including the uterus and fallopian tubes.
13. Total number of live births.

DOWN

2. Pain with intercourse.
4. Inner lining of the uterus.
5. Occurs approximately every 28 days in most women.
6. Pregnancy located outside the uterus, usually in the fallopian tubes.
9. Total number of pregnancies.
10. Any assault crime that involves the genitalia of either party.

33 Obstetrical Emergencies

CHAPTER TERMINAL OBJECTIVES

On completion of this chapter, the EMT-Intermediate will be able to apply and utilize the assessment findings to formulate and implement a treatment plan for normal and abnormal labor.

For the multiple-choice questions, select the single best answer to each question. For the matching questions, select the best corresponding answer for each item. Because there are sometimes more items than corresponding answers in the matching questions, some items may not be used.

1. Match the following reproductive organs with the correct description.

   Organ
   a. Ovaries
   b. Fallopian tubes
   c. Uterus
   d. Cervix
   e. Vagina
   f. Perineum

   Description
   _____ Hollow, muscular organ shaped like an inverted pear located in the pelvic cavity

   _____ Inferior narrow portion of the uterus where it opens into the vagina; dilates to allow the baby and placenta to pass into the birth canal during labor

   _____ The birth canal or passageway between the uterus and the external opening in a female.

   _____ Walnut-sized pair of glands located on each side of the uterus in the upper pelvic cavity; produce mature eggs and secrete primarily female sexual hormones

   _____ External female genital region between the urinary opening (urethra) and the anus or rectal opening

   _____ Pair of muscular tubes that extend from the uterus to the pelvic cavity; provide a passageway for the transport of sperm to the egg (ova) and transport of the ova back to the uterus by wavelike, muscular contractions

2. The placenta:
   a. develops late in pregnancy
   b. provides for the exchange of respiratory gases and transport of nutrients from the mother to the fetus
   c. is attached to the developing fetus by the renal artery
   d. produces several important energy sources for the fetus

3. During pregnancy, the fetus grows in the mother's:
   a. bladder
   b. cervix
   c. uterus
   d. vagina

4. The amniotic sac:
   a. consists of membranes that surround and protect the developing fetus
   b. contains approximately 300 mL of amniotic fluid
   c. will normally rupture before the beginning of labor
   d. contains fluid that is brown

5. With fetal circulation:
   a. there is intermittent exchange of nutrients between the mother and fetus
   b. blood passes through the heart of the fetus the same way as it does in the adult
   c. unoxygenated blood is returned from the fetus to the placenta via the umbilical arteries
   d. oxygenated blood is carried from the placenta to the fetus via the umbilical arteries

6. For the illustration of the pregnant patient below, label the name of each anatomical structure shown.

   Then use colored pens or pencils to color the illustration according to the following: A-red, B-blue, C-tan, D-pink, E-orange, and F-yellow.

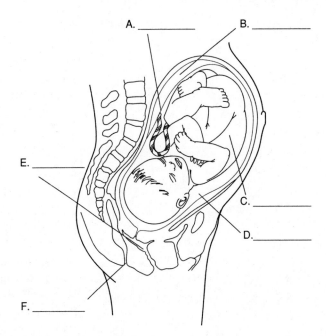

7. Match the following terms with the correct definition.

   Term
   a. Postpartum
   b. Primipara
   c. Gravidity
   d. Natal
   e. Multipara

   Definition
   _____ A woman who has delivered her first child
   _____ The number of times a woman has been pregnant
   _____ The time after delivery of the infant
   _____ A woman who has had two or more deliveries
   _____ Means birth

8. A woman who is currently pregnant with her third child, has delivered two previous live births, and had one miscarriage would be described as a
   a. G3P2A1
   b. G4P2A1
   c. G2P3A1
   d. G1P3A2

9. Common signs and symptoms of early pregnancy include:
    a. missed or late menstrual period
    b. nausea and vomiting that occurs in the evening
    c. breast shrinkage
    d. infrequent urination

10. Cardiovascular changes seen in pregnancy include:
    a. pulmonary functional residual capacity increases
    b. uterine blood flow increases from 2% to 20% of cardiac output
    c. maternal heart rate, minute volume, and oxygen consumption are decreased
    d. maternal blood volume and cardiac output are increased up to 10%

11. Describe why the mother is more likely to vomit and aspirate in the later stage of pregnancy.

    _____
    _____
    _____
    _____
    _____

12. Define what is meant by supine hypotensive syndrome.

    _____
    _____
    _____
    _____
    _____

13. The pregnant patient who is 20 weeks' gestation or more should be placed:
    a. in a supine position
    b. in a prone position
    c. on her left side
    d. on her right side

14. Appendicitis:
    a. occurs in about 1 of every 5000 pregnancies
    b. is caused by the appendix being displaced posteriorly
    c. is more difficult to assess during pregnancy
    d. is treated by placing the pregnant patient in a prone position

15. Eclampsia is present when a pregnant patient experiences:
    a. visual disturbances
    b. excessive weight loss
    c. hypotension
    d. coma and convulsions

16. Treatment of a patient experiencing eclampsia includes:
    a. administering low-flow oxygen
    b. administering diazepam, 10 to 15 mg, intravenous (IV) push
    c. placing an IV line and running it wide open
    d. avoiding the use of emergency lights or sirens during transport

17. Placenta previa is a condition in which the:
    a. placenta separates from the uterine wall
    b. fertilized egg becomes implanted outside the uterus
    c. placenta is formed in an abnormal location
    d. fetus and placenta deliver before the twenty-eighth week of pregnancy

18. List four factors that predispose patients to placenta previa.

    _____

    _____

    _____

    _____

19. Describe the typical presentation of patients experiencing placenta previa.

    _____

    _____

    _____

    _____

    _____

It is a warm, spring evening when you are called to a scene where a 23-year-old woman who is 8 months' pregnant is complaining of severe, constant abdominal pain. She tells you that the pain feels like a tearing sensation. Your assessment reveals that she is alert, has a respiratory rate of 18 breaths/min, a pulse rate of 120 beats per minute (BPM), a blood pressure of 124/98, and cool, clammy skin. There is heavy, dark red vaginal bleeding.

20. Your patient is most likely experiencing:
    a. placenta previa
    b. eclampsia
    c. abruptio placentae
    d. Braxton-Hicks contractions

21. Treatment for this patient includes:
    a. administering high-concentration oxygen via nonrebreather mask
    b. performing a vaginal examination
    c. administering diazepam, 5 mg, slow IV push
    d. applying and inflating all three compartments of the pneumatic antishock garment

22. List seven signs or symptoms that may be seen with a patient in labor.

___

23. The first stage of labor begins with _____ and ends with _____.
    a. the baby entering the birth canal; delivery of the placenta
    b. regular contractions and the thinning and gradual dilation of the cervix; the cervix completely dilated
    c. the baby being born; the afterbirth being delivered
    d. thinning and gradual dilation of the cervix; the baby being born

24. Match the following terms with the correct description.

    Term
    a. Crowning
    b. Breech birth
    c. Cephalic delivery
    d. Third stage of labor
    e. Contraction time

    Description
    _____ Situation in which the buttocks or both feet of the baby deliver first
    _____ The time from the beginning of contraction to when the uterus relaxes
    _____ Occurs when the presenting part of the baby first bulges from the vaginal opening
    _____ Head-first delivery of the newly born
    _____ The time from the delivery of the baby to the delivery of the placenta

25. Describe when delivery is imminent in the woman with her first pregnancy.

___

You have been called to the scene where a 31-year-old woman is in labor. On your arrival at the patient's home, you find her sitting at the dining table. Assessment reveals that the patient is alert and oriented, has a respiratory rate of 18, a pulse rate of 102, and a blood pressure of 140/88. According to the patient's husband, this is her first pregnancy, she has been having contractions for the past 4 hours, and her water just broke. You time the contractions and find they are 60 seconds in duration and approximately 2 minutes apart. An examination reveals crowning.

26. This patient is in what stage of labor?
    a. first stage
    b. second stage
    c. first trimester
    d. third stage

27. Treatment for this patient includes:
    a. rapidly transporting her to the hospital
    b. administering 15 L/min of oxygen via nasal cannula
    c. placing her in a birthing position and waiting at the scene until the baby is born
    d. performing a vaginal exam

28. Which of the following lists the correct steps, in the correct order, for delivering a baby?
    a. Control the head with gentle pressure as it crowns; ensure that the umbilical cord is not wrapped around the baby's neck; suction the baby's mouth and nose; deliver the baby's anterior shoulder and then the posterior shoulder; dry, warm, and stimulate the baby; administer oxygen; perform an Apgar score.
    b. Stimulate the baby; ensure that the umbilical cord is not wrapped around the baby's neck; deliver the baby's anterior shoulder and then the posterior shoulder; suction the baby's mouth and nose; dry and warm the baby; perform an Apgar score.
    c. Control the head with gentle pressure as it crowns; suction the baby's mouth and nose; deliver the baby's anterior shoulder and then the posterior shoulder; administer oxygen; perform an Apgar score; dry, warm, and stimulate the baby as necessary.
    d. Deliver the baby's anterior shoulder, then the posterior shoulder; dry and warm the baby; suction the baby's nose and mouth; administer oxygen.

29. When the umbilical cord is wrapped around the baby's neck during delivery, you should do all of following *except:*
    a. avoid applying excessive tension on the cord
    b. slip the cord over the baby's head
    c. clamp the cord in two places and cut it between the clamps
    d. apply steady pressure on the infant's head to delay delivery until after arrival at the hospital

30. You have delivered a baby girl. Assessment reveals that she has a pulse rate of 110, slow breathing, and a pink body with blue hands and feet. She is active with some motion in the extremities. Nasal stimulation prompts grimace. The Apgar score for this baby is:
    a. 2
    b. 4
    c. 5
    d. 7

31. An Apgar score should be performed:
    a. immediately after birth only
    b. 1 minute after delivery and then repeated in 5 minutes
    c. 5 minutes after delivery and then repeated in 10 minutes
    d. 10 minutes after delivery only

32. Which of the following is true regarding the presence of meconium during delivery?
    a. Meconium aspiration is seldom a cause of neonatal death.
    b. The first step in managing an infant in which meconium staining is present is to stimulate the infant.
    c. Endotracheal intubation is contraindicated in the presence of meconium staining.
    d. The presence of meconium indicates fetal respiratory distress.

33. To reduce postpartum bleeding, the EMT-I should:
    a. place the patient in a semisitting position
    b. withhold the baby from the mother
    c. massage the mother's upper abdomen
    d. encourage the mother to breast-feed

34. If spontaneous breathing is absent after delivery, you can stimulate the infant by all of the following *except:*
    a. rubbing the infant's back gently
    b. slapping or flicking the soles of the infant's feet
    c. delivering six quick breaths with a bag-mask device
    d. drying and suctioning the infant

35. T F If the infant fails to respond to normal techniques to stimulate breathing, the EMT-I should assist ventilations at a rate of 40 to 60 breaths/min.

36. T F To insert an oropharyngeal airway in the infant, it should be rotated at a 180-degree angle as is done for adults.

37. To cut the umbilical cord, the *first* clamp should be placed:
    a. approximately 2 inches from the baby's abdomen
    b. right next to the baby's abdomen
    c. proximal to the placenta
    d. approximately 4 inches from the baby's abdomen

38. To maintain the newly born infant's temperature, the EMT-I should:
    a. keep the head uncovered
    b. dry the baby with a clean towel
    c. vigorously rub the extremities
    d. apply hot packs directly to the torso

39. Following delivery, cardiopulmonary resuscitation (CPR) should be delivered to the newly born when:
    a. the heart rate is less than 100 BPM
    b. the heart rate is between 80 and 100 BPM and does not improve despite 30 seconds of positive-pressure ventilation and supplemental oxygenation
    c. the heart rate is less than 60 BPM
    d. the Apgar score is less than 10

40. In the newly born, cardiac compressions should be delivered at a rate of _____ per minute.
    a. 60
    b. 80
    c. 100
    d. 120

41. A breech birth:
    a. is identified by a single limb protruding from the vagina
    b. is impossible to perform in the field setting
    c. is treated by placing the mother in a head-down position and administering a high concentration of oxygen
    d. is when the umbilical cord presents through the birth canal before delivery of the head

42. Match the following conditions with the correct descriptions and treatments. Terms may be used more than once.

    Term
    a. Breech delivery
    b. Prolapsed cord
    c. Abruptio placentae
    d. Placenta previa
    e. Preeclampsia

    Description/Treatment

    _____ Two fingers of a gloved hand are inserted into the vagina to raise the presenting part of the fetus off the cord; the cord is checked for pulsations; and the mother is placed in a Trendelenburg or knee-chest position

    _____ Gloved hand is placed into the vagina with the palm toward the infant's face; a "V" is formed with the index and middle fingers on either side of the infant's nose; and the vaginal wall is pushed away from the infant's face to allow unrestricted respiration

    _____ Disorder of pregnancy marked by hypertension, abnormal weight gain, edema, headache, protein in urine, epigastric pain, and occasionally visual disturbances

    _____ The attachment of the placenta very low in the uterus so that it partially or completely covers the internal cervical opening

    _____ Most common sign associated with this condition is painless, bright red vaginal bleeding

    _____ Premature detachment of a normally situated placenta

43. Describe *cephalopelvic disproportion*.

    _____

    _____

    _____

    _____

    _____

44. List three things that may cause postpartum hemorrhage.

    _____

    _____

    _____

CROSSWORD PUZZLE EXERCISE

45. Complete the following crossword puzzle.

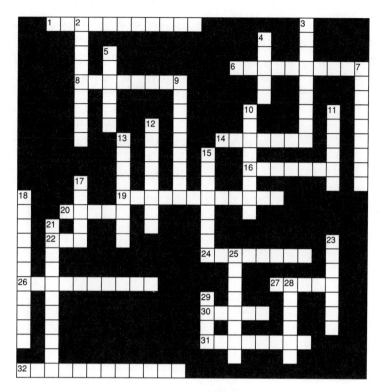

ACROSS

1. Occurs when the weight of the pregnant uterus compresses the inferior vena cava while the mother is in a supine position.
6. Maternal period before delivery.
8. Premature detachment of a normally situated placenta.
14. Refers to the number of pregnancies including the current pregnancy.
16. Type of pregnancy that occurs when a fertilized egg implants itself anywhere outside the uterus, usually in the fallopian tube.
19. Condition that is more difficult to assess during pregnancy, especially in the last two trimesters.
20. Stage of labor that includes beginning of regular contractions to complete dilation of the cervix (10 cm).
22. Abbreviation for intrauterine device.
24. Fetal waste substance produced by a baby in distress—if aspirated during delivery, the baby may suffer severe respiratory damage.
26. Occurs close to delivery, patient may panic and be "out of control" with overwhelming contractions.

DOWN

2. When the umbilical cord is the presenting part during delivery.
3. Defined as the occurrence of seizures in addition to the syndrome of preeclampsia.
4. Unborn child.
5. Inferior narrow portion of the uterus where it opens into the vagina.
7. The menstrual cycle between approximately the ages 35 and 60 years, when a woman's reproductive years come to an end.
9. Egg is released by an ovary on approximately the fourteenth day of the cycle.
10. Disk-shaped spongy organ that develops in the uterus during pregnancy.
11. Includes any delivery in which the buttocks or feet present first rather than the head of the baby.
12. Double vision.
13. Existing or occurring before birth.
15. External female genital region between the urinary opening (urethra) and the anus or rectal opening.

ACROSS—cont'd

27. Score that is used to evaluate infant's physical condition after birth.
30. Without breath.
31. Protective membranous sac that insulates and protects the fetus during pregnancy.
32. Defined as an abnormal state during pregnancy characterized by hypertension and fluid retention.

DOWN—cont'd

17. Stage of labor that includes delivery of the baby to delivery of the placenta.
18. Serves as the site of implantation of the fertilized egg, as well as the organ of menstruation.
21. Sudden unexpected loss of pregnancy.
23. Type of rupture that occurs most commonly after the onset of labor.
25. Appearance of the baby's head bulging at the perineum close to delivery.
28. Abnormal positioning of the placenta within the uterus.
29. Refers to the number of previous live births.

34 Neonatal Resuscitation

CHAPTER TERMINAL OBJECTIVES

On completion of this chapter, the EMT-Intermediate will be able to utilize assessment findings to formulate a field impression and implement the treatment plan for the resuscitation of a neonatal patient.

For the multiple-choice questions, select the single best answer to each question. For the matching questions, select the best corresponding answer for each item. Because there are sometimes more items than corresponding answers in the matching questions, some items may not be used.

1. A neonate is a:
   a. recently born baby during the first few hours of life
   b. baby during the first 28 days of life
   c. baby during the first 6 months of life
   d. baby in the mother's womb

2. The leading cause of death in the neonatal period is associated with infants who:
   a. are born to unwed mothers
   b. experience long birth times
   c. are born at low birth weight
   d. have a gestational age of between 32 and 34 weeks at birth

3. The younger the newly born's gestational age at birth, the _____ the mortality risk, especially if the infant is less than _____ weeks of gestation.

4. List five intrauterine events that result in low birth weight.

   _____

   _____

   _____

   _____

   _____

5. Describe why there is a higher incidence of prematurity and low birth weight in infants born to teenagers.

   _____

   _____

   _____

   _____

   _____

6. Narcotic use by the mother may cause a neonate to have _____ after delivery.
   a. respiratory depression
   b. heightened excitability
   c. cardiac failure
   d. airway edema

7. The onset of _____ is the most critical and immediate physiological change required of the newly born.
   a. digestion
   b. circulation
   c. breathing
   d. endocrine function

8. The primary stimulus(i) that help initiate respiration in the neonate after delivery is(are)
   a. low oxygen and high carbon dioxide levels, and a low pH
   b. the fetus leaving a cooler environment and entering a warm atmosphere
   c. the presence of surfactant in the alveoli
   d. closure of the foramen ovale

9. Describe how the fluid that fills the fetal lungs and alveoli is removed during the delivery process.

   _____
   _____
   _____
   _____

10. A substance produced by the alveolar epithelium that coats the alveolar surface and reduces surface tension is called:
    a. mucus
    b. protein
    c. plasma
    d. surfactant

11. The transition from fetal circulation to postnatal circulation involves the functional closure of the _____ _____ and ductus _____.

12. The most important factor controlling ductal closure is the increased _____ concentration of the blood.

13. Next to establishing respiration, _____ regulation is most critical to the newly born's survival.

14. T F A full-term newly born has a blood volume of about 80 to 85 mL/kg of body weight. Immediately after birth, the total blood volume averages 150 mL.

15. T F Depending on how long the newly born is attached to the placenta, as much as 100 mL can be added to the blood volume.

16. T F The majority of newly borns who are full term will not require any advanced life support intervention.

You are called to a local shopping mall where a 21-year-old woman is in active labor. You find her sitting on a bench in the food court. Your assessment reveals that she is alert and oriented, has a respiratory rate of 20, a pulse rate of 114, and a blood pressure of 150/82. According to her mother, who accompanied her on the shopping trip, this is her third pregnancy. She has a 3-year-old son and 1-year-old daughter at home. Apparently she has been having contractions during the past couple of hours, and her water just broke. You note the contractions are 60 seconds in duration and approximately 2 minutes apart. You move her to the patient module of the ambulance, where your examination reveals crowning. You prepare to deliver the baby.

17. As the head is delivered, you should suction the baby's:
    a. mouth, then the nose, with a bulb syringe for up to 15 seconds at a time
    b. nose with a bulb syringe for up to 10 seconds at a time
    c. nose and mouth simultaneously with a soft-tip catheter attached to a portable suction unit
    d. mouth using the on-board suction for up to 15 seconds at a time

18. As the body is delivered, you determine the newly born is a boy. You should position him on his:
    a. back with the head slightly lower than the rest of the body
    b. stomach with the head slightly lower than the rest of the body
    c. side with the head slightly higher than the rest of the body
    d. back with the head level with the rest of the body

19. The next action that should be taken is:
    a. administering oxygen to the mother at 15 L/min using a nonrebreather mask
    b. drying the baby's head, face, and body thoroughly
    c. covering the baby's head with a blanket, towel, or hat to prevent heat loss
    d. establishing an intravenous (IV) line of normal saline for the mother

20. Describe how the newly born can be kept warm.

    _____
    _____
    _____
    _____
    _____

21. The baby is not breathing; he should be stimulated by:
    a. administering 100% oxygen
    b. spanking his buttocks
    c. providing several breaths with an infant bag-mask device
    d. gently rubbing the soles of his feet or the back

22. Describe the differences in treating primary apnea and secondary apnea.

    _____
    _____
    _____
    _____

23. Describe the procedure for opening the airway of this newly born.

    _____
    _____
    _____
    _____

24. The newly born remains apneic despite your efforts to warm and stimulate him and open his airway. You should now:
    a. ventilate the newly born with a bag-mask device with 100% oxygen at a rate of 40 to 60 breaths/min
    b. administer 100% oxygen via a nonrebreather mask
    c. ventilate the newly born with a bag-mask device with 100% oxygen at a rate of 20 to 40 breaths/min
    d. deliver two slow breaths using a bag-mask device with 100% oxygen

25. T F To insert an oropharyngeal airway in the newly born, it should be rotated at a 180-degree angle as is done for an adult.

26. T F The infant who is crying and active has an adequate heart rate.

27. T F If the heart rate is below 100 beats per minute (BPM) and the patient is breathing, the first course of action is to provide 100% oxygen via nonrebreather mask.

28. Following delivery, cardiopulmonary resuscitation (CPR) should be initiated if the baby's pulse is absent or below _____ BPM.
    a. 40
    b. 60
    c. 80
    d. 100

29. Acrocyanosis:
    a. is a bluish color to the trunk and face
    b. is a bluish color to the hands and feet
    c. requires treatment with 100% oxygen
    d. seldom lasts more than 10 to 15 minutes following birth

30. Describe when oxygen administration is necessary in the newly born.

_____
_____
_____
_____

31. Babies most often experience cardiopulmonary arrest because of:
    a. cardiogenic shock
    b. sudden death syndrome
    c. hypoxia
    d. congenital heart defects

32. Fill in the following pyramid representing actions taken during newly born resuscitation.

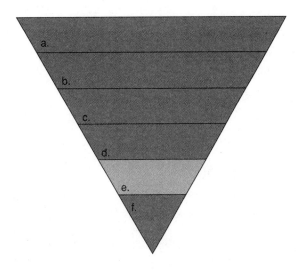

33. Which of the following medications should *not* be used to treat the newly born who is in cardiac arrest?
    a. atropine
    b. epinephrine
    c. verapamil
    d. naloxone

34. Describe the delivery of IV fluid therapy in the newly born.

_____
_____
_____
_____

35. Describe how meconium aspiration syndrome (MAS) occurs and the effect it has on the newly born.

_____

_____

_____

_____

_____

36. T F Infants who have released meconium in utero for some time before birth are stained from green meconium stools.

37. T F Newly borns experiencing severe meconium aspiration will be in respiratory arrest at birth.

You arrive at the home of a 30-year-old woman who is in active labor. Assessment reveals that the infant is crowning and the amniotic fluid is stained with thick meconium. The infant is delivered blue, limp, and apneic.

38. The first treatment you should provide to the newly born is:
    a. deep hypopharynx and tracheal suctioning
    b. ventilatory support using a bag-mask device
    c. drying and stimulating the infant
    d. administering epinephrine, 1 mg (1 mL of a 1:1000 solution), endotracheally

39. A premature baby is one that:
    a. weighs less than 6 lb at birth
    b. is born before the thirty-seventh week of gestation
    c. requires little additional care
    d. has a smaller head in proportion to its body

CROSSWORD PUZZLE EXERCISE

40. Complete the following crossword puzzle.

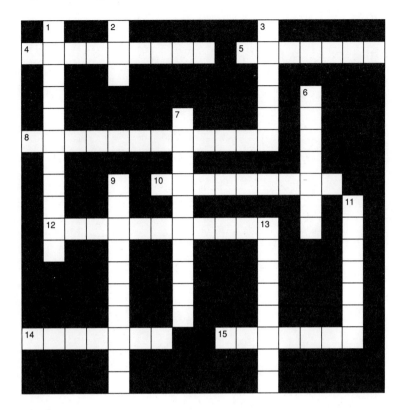

ACROSS

4. Infant born before completion of 37 weeks' gestation.
5. A recently born baby.
8. Bluish color to the hands and feet.
10. Apnea that will not reverse with simple stimulation techniques and requires assisted ventilation.
12. As the baby is being born.
14. Apnea that can be reversed by touching and stimulating the baby as when drying the newly born.
15. Cardiac arrest in most newly borns is usually secondary to respiratory _____.

DOWN

1. Heart rate seen with hypoxic infant.
2. Occurs when fetus or newly born inhales thick, sticky meconium.
3. Generalized bacterial infection in the bloodstream.
6. Cyanosis of the trunk and face.
7. Before the baby is born.
9. Substance produced by alveolar epithelium that coats alveolar surface.
11. A baby during the first 28 days of life.
13. Thick, greenish-black material.

35 Pediatric Emergencies

CHAPTER TERMINAL OBJECTIVES

On completion of this chapter, the EMT-Intermediate will be able to utilize assessment findings to formulate a field impression and implement the treatment plan for a pediatric patient.

For the multiple-choice questions, select the single best answer to each question. For the matching questions, select the best corresponding answer for each item. Because there are sometimes more items than corresponding answers in the matching questions, some items may not be used.

1. In children between the ages of 5 and 14 years, the most common reason for being seen by emergency medical services (EMS) is:
    a. asthma
    b. trauma
    c. cardiac arrest
    d. medical illness

2. The term "child" is used to refer to those individuals:
    a. under the age of 1 year
    b. between the ages of 3 and 7 years
    c. from age 1 to age 8
    d. from age 8 to age 16

3. T F The key to determining medication dosages and providing treatments in pediatric cases is the patient's age.

4. Important anatomical feature(s) of the airway to consider in infants and children is(are):
    a. the overall size of the airway is bigger than in the adult
    b. the airway of a child younger than 8 years includes a smaller tongue in comparison with the size of the mouth
    c. the airway of a child younger than 8 years includes a large and floppy epiglottis
    d. the narrowest part of the infant's airway is the glottic opening

5. The vocal cords of a child sit more _____ and _____ on the cervical spine than an adult. In infants, the cords are located at approximately the _____ (or second) cervical vertebra. As the child grows, the cords begin to move _____ closer to the level of the third vertebra.

6. Label and color the following illustration of the upper airway in the child. Use colored pencils or pens to color the illustration according to the following: A-orange, B-red, C-green, D-tan, E-gray, and F-yellow.

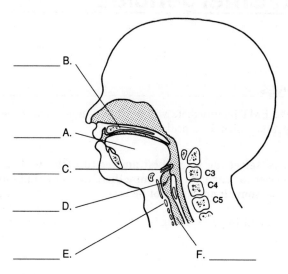

7. Describe the reason that many childhood injuries involve head injury.

_____
_____
_____
_____
_____

8. Which of the following is true regarding the fontanelles?
   a. Infants have fontanelles, or soft spots, on the backs of their heads.
   b. Fontanelles are spaces between the bones of the infant's cranium that are covered by a thin bone.
   c. The anterior fontanelle can be palpated until approximately 18 to 24 months of age.
   d. The fontanelles will be depressed with any increase in intracranial pressure and be bulged when dehydration is present.

9. T F An injury to a child's bone is more likely to produce a "bending" of the bone than a break.

10. T F In a child, an underlying lung injury is unlikely without an overlying rib fracture.

11. T F An infant or child is better able to move out of the way when an object suddenly comes at him or her than an adult.

12. The parents of the injured child:
    a. are seldom considered as part of the child's psychological environment
    b. must be isolated so they are not exposed to the severity of the child's condition
    c. often require psychological assistance in dealing with their injured or ill child
    d. seldom feel responsible for the child receiving the injuries

13. Describe how the EMT-I should handle the parents of an injured or ill child.

___

14. List the three components of the pediatric assessment triangle.

___

15. The first sign of respiratory distress in an infant is usually:
    a. nasal flaring
    b. head bobbing
    c. tachypnea
    d. diminished breath sounds

16. Describe the significance of a slow or irregular respiratory rate in an acutely ill infant or child.

___

17. In infants and children:
    a. the heart rate is normally 60 to 80 beats per minute (BPM)
    b. tachycardia can occur as a result of stress caused by hypovolemia, hypoxia, anxiety, fever, pain, increased carbon dioxide, or cardiac impairment
    c. bradycardia usually occurs when the child is receiving adequate oxygenation
    d. proper oxygenation will cause the heart rate to decrease, thus decreasing the child's cardiac output

18. The proper location for palpating a pulse in the infant is the _____ artery.
    a. carotid
    b. femoral
    c. radial
    d. brachial

19. T F The appropriate method of opening the child's airway is the head-tilt/chin-lift or jaw-thrust maneuver.

20. T F The primary cause of airway obstruction in the infant or child is swelling of the epiglottis.

You are working the "A" shift at a local fire department and are assigned to the rescue squad. Your first call of the day is for a 4-year-old who is acutely dyspneic. You find the child sitting upright, leaning forward, and clutching her throat. She appears frightened, is coughing and gasping for air, and has inspiratory stridor, suprasternal retractions, a pulse rate of 180 BPM, and warm, moist skin. According to her mother, she was playing with her older brother's marbles when the problem occurred. The mother reports that the child is allergic to bee stings.

21. This child is experiencing:
    a. an acute asthma attack
    b. epiglottitis
    c. an upper airway obstruction caused by a foreign body
    d. an allergic reaction

22. Place a checkmark beside the treatment(s) listed below that is(are) considered appropriate in the *initial* management of this child.

    _____ Administering subdiaphragmatic abdominal thrusts (Heimlich maneuver)

    _____ Administering epinephrine, 0.01 mg/kg (1:10,000)

    _____ Performing blind finger probes

    _____ Delivering back blows

    _____ Reassuring and encouraging the child to cough

    _____ Administering albuterol (Ventolin) via nebulizer

    _____ Performing endotracheal (ET) intubation

23. List four indications for intubating a child.

    _____

    _____

    _____

    _____

24. The correct size ET tube for a 6-year-old child is _____ ID (mm).
    a. 3.0
    b. 4.0
    c. 4.5
    d. 5.5

25. Uncuffed ET tubes should be used in children:
    a. between the ages of 6 and 10
    b. younger than 8 years of age
    c. older than 8 years of age
    d. between the ages of 5 and 14

26. When ventilating a child with a bag-mask device:
    a. oxygen should be attached to the device and set to at least 10 L/min
    b. use one that has a capacity of at least 250 cc
    c. it must be done with two hands
    d. breaths should be delivered at rate of 40 per minute

27. T F When opening the airway of an infant, the head should be placed in a hyperextended position.

28. T F When using a nasal cannula in a child, the appropriate flow rate per minute is 6 to 8 L/min.

29. With intraosseous infusion:
    a. intravenous (IV) fluids are infused into the marrow cavity of the bone
    b. the amount of fluid resuscitation is less than IV therapy
    c. only fluids may be administered; drugs should be given IV
    d. a seesaw motion is used to advance the needle through the bone

30. When administering fluid resuscitation therapy in a pediatric patient:
    a. large volumes of dextrose-containing solutions should be used
    b. one or two 40-mL/kg boluses should be administered to promptly address the volume deficit
    c. frequent reassessments are necessary to determine the need for additional fluid boluses
    d. all of the above

31. The leading cause of cardiopulmonary arrest in children is:
    a. cardiac dysrhythmias
    b. meningitis
    c. respiratory compromise
    d. trauma

You are working as an EMT-I for a local hospital-based EMS system. It is a warm Saturday morning when you are called to the home of an 8-month-old baby who is unresponsive. You determine the infant is apneic and pulseless. The mother states she just laid the baby down for a nap when she stopped breathing. Apparently, the infant has been suffering from an upper respiratory infection for the past 2 days. You attach the electrocardiogram (ECG) monitor to reveal:

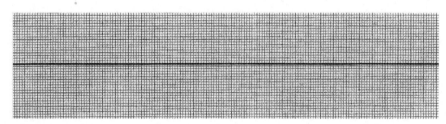

32. This baby is suffering from:
    a. pulseless electrical activity (PEA)
    b. cardiogenic shock
    c. ventricular fibrillation
    d. asystole

33. Place a checkmark beside the treatments indicated for this baby:

    _____ Perform ET intubation using a number 3.5 to 4.0 ID uncuffed ET tube.

    _____ Ventilate her with a bag-mask device supplied with high-concentration oxygen.

    _____ Establish an IV line using normal saline (or lactated Ringer's) solution.

    _____ Defibrillating one time 2 J/kg (maximum of 200 J), immediately resume cardiopulmonary resuscitation (CPR).

    _____ Administer epinephrine at an initial dose of 0.01 mg/kg (1:10,000) for the IV/intraosseous routes and 0.1 mg/kg (1:1000) for the ET route.

    _____ Administer lidocaine, 1 mg/kg IV or intraosseous route.

    _____ Administer atropine, 0.02 mg/kg IV or intraosseous route.

You are called to treat a 9-year-old boy who collapsed while playing outside with his friends. You arrive on scene to find the mother providing CPR to the child. You determine the patient is pulseless and apneic and has a healing sternotomy scar. His mother states he has some kind of "heart problem" and had surgery 2 months ago. The ECG shows:

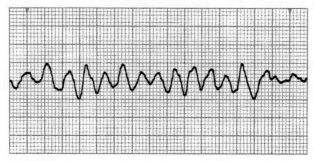

coarse VF

34. Treatment of this child includes:
    a. defibrillating one time 2 J/kg (maximum of 200 J), immediately resume CPR
    b. administering epinephrine, IV infusion
    c. placing an IV line using normal saline
    d. performing ET intubation using a number 3.5 ID ET tube

Following your placement of an ET tube, administration of epinephrine, and repeated defibrillations, you reestablish effective circulation in the child. While still unconscious and apneic, the patient now has a palpable pulse with a heart rate of 174 BPM and his color is returning to normal. As you load him into the back of the ambulance, you note that he is becoming blue and mottled despite your continuing ventilatory support. Auscultation of the chest reveals lung sounds only on the right side. The ECG now shows a heart rate of 38 BPM.

35. Which of the following has likely occurred?
    a. The ET tube has advanced into the right mainstem bronchi.
    b. The ET tube has become obstructed by a mucous plug.
    c. The ET tube has been displaced into the esophagus.
    d. The bag-mask device has malfunctioned.

36. This 9-year-old boy is suffering from:
    a. hypoxia
    b. paroxysmal supraventricular tachycardia
    c. ventricular fibrillation
    d. PEA

37. To relieve this problem, you should:
    a. remove the ET tube and reattempt intubation
    b. suction the ET tube
    c. withdraw the ET tube until lung sounds are heard on both sides of the chest
    d. replace the bag-mask device

You are assigned to a hospital-based EMS ambulance when you are called to an apartment to evaluate a 4-month-old boy who has a fever, cough, increased respiratory rate, retraction, and nasal flaring. According to the mother, the baby has no history of foreign body airway obstruction or trauma. While obtaining a brief history from the mother, the child becomes mottled and blue, the breathing appears more labored, and his heart slows to 40 BPM.

38. This patient is experiencing:
    a. congestive heart failure
    b. septic shock
    c. tension pneumothorax
    d. respiratory failure

39. Treatment for this child includes:
    a. administering 6 to 8 L/min of oxygen via nasal cannula
    b. assisting his breathing with a bag-mask device
    c. rapidly administering 0.01 mg/kg of atropine, IV push
    d. placing an IV line using normal saline and a 14- to 16-gauge intraosseous needle

40. Complete the following table regarding epiglottitis and croup.

	Epiglottitis	Croup
Cause		
When it occurs		
Age groups seen in		
Type of onset		
How the patient presents		
Type of cough		
Presence of drooling?		
Temperature		

It is a cold afternoon when you respond to a call where a 4-year-old girl is having trouble breathing. You find the child sitting on her bed in a "tripod position." The family states she has been sick since morning, starting with a sore throat and progressing to severe dyspnea. Examination reveals she has labored respirations at a rate of 38 breaths/min; a high-pitched, stridorous sound that is heard on inspiration; a blood pressure of 100/60; and hot, dry skin. You note that the patient is drooling and refuses to swallow anything.

41. The patient is most likely suffering from:
    a. croup
    b. an acute asthma attack
    c. bronchitis
    d. epiglottitis

42. Treatment of this patient includes:
    a. examining her oropharynx with a tongue blade and penlight
    b. administering humidified oxygen
    c. administering epinephrine, 0.1 mg (1:10,000 solution), subcutaneously
    d. inserting an oropharyngeal airway

You are called to a cookout in a neighborhood park where a 9-year-old girl is experiencing shortness of breath. Her father states that the problem began several hours ago and has gotten progressively worse. You determine that the child is agitated and unable to speak in full sentences, has labored respirations at a rate of 26 breaths/min, a blood pressure of 134/94, a pulse rate of 110 BPM, and cold, clammy, diaphoretic skin. You note that the patient has intercostal retraction and accessory muscle usage. Auscultation of the chest reveals bilateral wheezing on expiration. The father is unsure about the girl's previous medical history, but you are able to determine that the child uses some sort of handheld inhaler.

43. This child is most likely experiencing:
    a. epiglottitis
    b. an acute asthma attack
    c. croup
    d. congestive heart failure

44. Treatment for this child includes:
    a. establishing an IV of lactated Ringer's or normal saline solution
    b. administering epinephrine, 1.0 mg (1.0 mL of a 1:1000 solution) subcutaneously
    c. administering atropine, 1.0 mg, IV push
    d. withholding oxygen unless the patient becomes cyanotic

45. Prehospital treatment for pediatric patients experiencing respiratory distress caused by bronchiolitis includes:
    a. ET intubation
    b. administering a bronchodilator agent by nebulization
    c. administering aminophylline by IV infusion
    d. delivering 2 to 3 L/min of oxygen by nasal cannula

46. Complete the following table regarding the differences between asthma and bronchiolitis.

	Asthma	Bronchiolitis
Age affected		
Time occurs		
Caused by		
Family history		
Effect of medications		

You are working the afternoon shift on an ambulance that is based out of a hospital emergency department. As you are returning from a call where the patient refused transport, a car comes to a screeching halt in front of you. A mother frantically waves for you to help her 18-month-old daughter. Your initial examination reveals that the infant is listless; has a respiratory rate of 40 breaths/min; equal bilateral breath sounds; absent distal pulses and faint femoral pulses at a rate of 170; cool, cyanotic extremities; decreased skin turgor; eyes that appear dull and sunken; dry mucous membranes; a depressed anterior fontanelle; and a capillary refill time of 4 seconds. The mother states that during the past 2 days the child has experienced diarrhea, vomiting, and poor feeding, and is going through fewer diapers than normal. She remarks that her "baby has lost weight."

47. This child is experiencing:
    a. ketoacidosis
    b. shock
    c. drug overdose
    d. meningitis

48. Initial treatment of this child includes:
    a. establishing an IV line of 5% dextrose and water
    b. delivering a fluid bolus of 20 mL/kg, and repeating it as necessary
    c. administering epinephrine (1:1000), 0.5 to 1.0 mg, IV push
    d. administering a low concentration of oxygen

You are called to a hotel where a mother reports that her 2-year-old daughter experienced a convulsion. You perform an assessment that reveals the child is irritable, has a rapid pulse, rapid respirations, profuse perspiration, and a rectal temperature of 105° F. The mother states that she has been sick since morning.

49. This child is likely experiencing:
    a. febrile seizures
    b. septicemia
    c. hypoglycemia
    d. epilepsy

50. Which of the following would be used to treat this child?
    a. sponging her with 4 × 4-inch gauze pads moistened with tepid water
    b. forcing a bite block between the child's clenched teeth
    c. starting an IV of normal saline
    d. administering 2 to 3 L/min of oxygen via simple face mask

51. A continuous seizure lasting more than 30 minutes or a series of seizures during which the patient does not regain consciousness is referred to as:
    a. status epilepticus
    b. grand mal seizures
    c. partial seizures
    d. postictal state

52. T F Meningitis is defined as an inflammation of the peripheral nervous system.

53. T F Meningitis cases can develop seizures.

54. Place a checkmark beside those signs and symptoms of meningitis.

    _____ Vomiting

    _____ Headache (in infants younger than 1 year old)

    _____ Bradycardia and hypoventilation

    _____ Stiff neck (in children older than 2 years old)

    _____ Increased appetite

    _____ Bulging fontanelle (in infants younger than 1 year old)

    _____ Lethargy and irritability

55. List the most common types of poisons ingested by children.

    _____

    _____

    _____

    _____

    _____

56. List the causes of pediatric injuries, categorized from most to least common.

    _____

    _____

    _____

    _____

    _____

You are called to a playground where a 4-year-old girl was hit in the head with a stone. You arrive to find the child lying supine on the ground. Your assessment reveals she is unconscious, has a respiratory rate of 10 breaths/min, a strong radial pulse at a rate of 52, a blood pressure of 136/74, pale skin, and a capillary refill time of 3 seconds. Auscultation of the chest reveals clear breath sounds. The pupils are unequal. You attach the ECG to reveal a regular rhythm with narrow complexes. There is a large hematoma in the right occipital area. You note that there is no blood or cerebrospinal fluid leaking from her nose or ears.

57. This child is suffering from:
    a. a concussion
    b. a basilar skull fracture
    c. neurogenic shock
    d. increased intracranial pressure

58. Treatment for this child includes:
    a. administering oxygen with a nonrebreather mask
    b. assisting her breathing with a bag-mask device
    c. administering D_{50}, IV push
    d. placing an IV line of 5% dextrose in water

Your patient is an 8-year-old boy who was shot by one of his friends. Apparently, the two were looking at a gun when it accidentally discharged. Your examination reveals an entrance wound just below his right nipple; there is no exit wound. The patient is awake but apprehensive, has labored breathing at a rate of 28 breaths/min, a weak and thready pulse at a rate of 142, hypotension, and cold, clammy skin. You note cyanosis about his lips. Auscultation of the chest reveals diminished lung sounds on the left side and none on the right. The trachea seems to be moving to the left of the midline.

59. This patient is most likely experiencing:
    a. cardiac tamponade
    b. a ruptured diaphragm
    c. a tension pneumothorax
    d. a lacerated trachea

60. Treatment for this patient includes:
    a. administering 6 to 8 L/min of oxygen via nasal cannula
    b. performing emergency pericardiocentesis
    c. rapidly transporting him to the hospital
    d. establishing two IV lines with 5% dextrose in water using 14- to 16-gauge needles

61. List two signs of blunt trauma to the abdomen in the pediatric patient.

_____

_____

You are called to the scene where a 10-year-old girl was hit by a car as she crossed the street on her way to school. According to her mother, the car was going about 25 mph when it struck the girl, throwing her to the ground. Your assessment reveals the child is awake and crying (reportedly there was no loss of consciousness), has a respiratory rate of 26 breaths/min, a weak pulse rate of 150 BPM, a blood pressure of 106/72, and pale skin. Auscultation of the chest reveals clear breath sounds. Capillary refill in upper extremities is 4 seconds. Your physical exam reveals deformity, swelling, and angulation of the right upper leg and bruising on the right flank. The right dorsalis pedis pulse is present but weak, and capillary refill is 5 seconds in the injured extremity. You note that the abdomen is diffusely tender, especially in the right upper quadrant. The child is crying for her mother.

62. This patient is suffering from:
    a. a fractured femur
    b. neurogenic shock
    c. a lacerated spleen
    d. respiratory failure

63. Treatment for this child includes:
    a. administering 4 to 6 L/min of oxygen via nasal cannula
    b. immobilizing the injured leg with a pediatric traction splint
    c. administering epinephrine, IV infusion
    d. placing an IV line using normal saline and a 16- or 18-gauge intraosseous needle in the injured extremity

It is a cold winter day when you are called to winter sports camp where an 11-year-old boy is reportedly lost. It is several hours before searchers find the boy lying at the bottom of a steep ravine. The child is unconscious, has a respiratory rate of 6 breaths/min, a pulse rate of 30 BPM, an "inaudible" blood pressure, and his skin is ice cold. The patient seems "stiff," and his eyes have a glassy stare. Your examination of the patient reveals no obvious injuries and no medical alert tags. You note that his clothing is wet from lying in the snow.

64. The patient is most likely suffering from which of the following?
    a. cardiac arrest
    b. congestive heart failure
    c. diabetic coma
    d. severe hypothermia

65. Treatment for this patient would include:
    a. removing his wet clothes
    b. having him drink a shot of alcohol
    c. placing an endotracheal tube
    d. delivering CPR

66. Your partner suggests that the patient be placed on a full backboard. His rationale for doing this might be that the:
    a. backboard will be more comfortable for the patient
    b. patient may have a neck and/or back injury
    c. backboard is a better "insulator" than the cot
    d. backboard can be more easily cleaned than the cot

67. If a child dies within 24 hours of a submersion incident, it is called a _____ - _____ _____ .

68. T F Behaviors inflicted on the child that are degrading, terrorizing, isolating, or rejecting are referred to as physical abuse.

69. T F Neglect is a failure to meet a child's emotional needs.

70. List five indicators of child abuse or maltreatment.

71. Describe the treatment of an occluded tracheostomy tube in the child.

36 Geriatrics

CHAPTER TERMINAL OBJECTIVES

On completion of this chapter, the EMT-Intermediate will be able apply the necessary knowledge and skills to properly assess and manage geriatric patients.

For the multiple-choice questions, select the single best answer to each question. For the matching questions, select the best corresponding answer for each item. Because there are sometimes more items than corresponding answers in the matching questions, some items may not be used.

1. T F Most geriatric patients reside in nursing homes.

2. T F Assisted living facilities provide constant nursing support.

3. List seven resources for elderly persons in need.

   _____
   _____
   _____
   _____
   _____
   _____
   _____
   _____

4. Some of the most significant problems that people face as they age involve difficulties with _____,

   _____. Because of difficulties with ambulation, coordination, and strength, the incidence of

   _____ is greatly increased.

5. List five consequences decreased mobility has on elderly patients.

   _____
   _____
   _____
   _____
   _____

6. Describe important psychological implications associated with the patient who experiences decreased mobility.

_____
_____
_____
_____

It is Sunday morning when you are called to the home of an 84-year-old woman who "fell and needs help getting up." You find her sitting on the floor next to the dining room table. She tells you that she was on her way to get a glass of water when she slipped on a kitchen rug. Your initial assessment reveals that she is alert; has warm, dry skin; a blood pressure of 152/94; regular pulse at a rate of 78 beats per minute (BPM); and a respiratory rate of 16 breaths/min. According to the patient, she slid to the floor and did not fall. She says she has no pain anywhere and just wants help getting back up. Your detailed examination reveals no injuries, and the patient has good range of motion in all extremities. The patient has a history of heart failure for which she takes quinidine, furosemide, and nitroglycerin.

7. To deal with this situation you should next:
    a. transport her to the hospital against her will
    b. call for police to assist in convincing her to go to the hospital for evaluation
    c. identify if she has particular high risks for falls and subsequent additional injuries
    d. have her sign a refusal form and return to service

8. Two significant changes in vision in persons more than 40 years of age are _____ and _____.

9. Describe some problems that can occur in the older population when they do not have their eyeglasses.

_____
_____
_____
_____

10. T F There is only minimal decay in hearing as the aging process progresses.

11. T F Central nervous system (CNS) insults from strokes and anatomical derangements in the larynx or pharynx can impair the patient's ability to properly conduct speech.

12. T F The pain mechanism in elderly patients is often depressed.

13. List three problems created by the decreased ability of the elderly population to hear.

_____
_____
_____

14. Incontinence:
    a. is the inability to prevent urination or bowel movements
    b. is caused by prostate gland enlargement
    c. can be controlled through proper nutrition
    d. can be caused by inadequate fluid intake, improper diet, or medications

15. Describe what problems can occur when incontinence is not cared for appropriately.

    _____

    _____

    _____

    _____

    _____

16. Constipation in the elderly population can result from:
    a. inadequate fluid intake, improper diet, or medications
    b. chronic use of pain control medications
    c. inflammatory disorders such as diverticulitis or malignancy such as colorectal cancer
    d. all of the above

17. List four communication strategies that can be used to provide psychological support in elderly patients.

    _____

    _____

    _____

    _____

    _____

18. Airway management problems in the elderly population include:
    a. dentures or partial dentures, which may impair intubation attempts
    b. adequate bag-mask ventilation, which may be difficult if dentures are left in place
    c. patients experiencing acute syncopal events; they often lose their ability to adequately protect their own airway
    d. all of the above

19. Many patients in the elderly population have _____ or _____ veins. This may make venipuncture and intravenous (IV) access _____.

20. Caution should be used in the _____ of IV fluid administered to patients who have any history of cardiac disease, especially _____ _____ failure.

21. Describe what the Emergency Medical Technician–Intermediate (EMT-I) should look for to determine whether IV fluids are being infused too quickly or at too high an amount.

_____

_____

_____

_____

_____

22. Medications administered to the elderly patient:
    a. are metabolized more effectively than in the middle-aged adult
    b. may compete with the normal metabolic process
    c. are typically broken down rapidly
    d. may exhibit shortened length of action and effect

23. For each of the following drugs that have greater or prolonged effects in the elderly population, list the class of medications to which it belongs.

Drug	Class
Ibuprofen	
Morphine	
Meperidine	
Diltiazem	
Lidocaine	
Propranolol	
Verapamil	
Furosemide	
Diazepam	

24. T F Elderly patients typically experience fewer adverse reactions to prescription medications than younger patients.

25. T F Lidocaine metabolism by the liver is significantly reduced in the elderly population, and a standard adult dose may have a greater and potentially toxic effect.

26. T F Every effort should be made to transport the elderly patient in the position of most comfort.

27. List four significant changes in the patient's respiratory status that occur with the aging process.

_____

_____

_____

_____

28. List three common causes of respiratory disease in the elderly population.

_____

_____

_____

You have been called to a local diner for an 83-year-old woman who is having trouble breathing. Your assessment reveals that she is alert and oriented, has labored respirations at a rate of 20 breaths/min, an irregular pulse at a rate of 136, a blood pressure of 162/108, and cool, diaphoretic skin. You auscultate her chest to find bilateral wheezes and rales. You note that she has a barrel-shaped chest, has intercostal retraction and accessory muscle usage, and is breathing through pursed lips. Examination of her lower extremities reveals slight bilateral edema. The pulse oximetry shows a Sao_2 of 90%. According to her friends she has a history of respiratory and heart problems for which she is taking medications. The patient reports no recent infections or fever.

29. The pulse oximetry reading:
    a. is normal
    b. indicates she is hypoxic
    c. is probably inaccurate
    d. indicates high CO_2 levels

30. The patient is suffering from:
    a. a pulmonary embolus
    b. spontaneous pneumothorax
    c. pneumonia
    d. chronic obstructive pulmonary disease (COPD) exacerbation

31. Treatment includes:
    a. assisting the patient's breathing with a bag-mask device and 100% oxygen
    b. administering bronchodilator therapy
    c. placing an IV line and running it at a wide-open rate
    d. transporting her in a supine position

32. A high percentage of EMS calls relate to patients being evaluated for _____ pain or _____.

   As individuals age, arteries tend to become more _____. Patients with _____ can further

   have cardiac and vascular damage because of the effects of the _____ blood pressure.

33. List four things the EMT-I should do when gathering the history of present illness in the patient experiencing a possible neurological emergency.

___

34. Describe prehospital management of most acute neurological events.

___

It is Wednesday morning when you are called to the home of a 77-year-old man who reports passing bloody stool. You find him sitting on the edge of the bathtub; he appears to be in significant discomfort, leaning forward, holding his abdomen. Your initial assessment reveals he is alert; has cool, pale, moist skin; a blood pressure of 94/70; a pulse rate of 134 BPM; and a respiratory rate of 20 breaths/min. According to the patient, his bowel movement this morning was dark red and coffee ground–like. Assessment reveals the abdomen is soft without mass, but there is lower abdominal pain on palpation. The patient has a history of heart problems for which he takes nitroglycerin, antihypertensive agents, and diuretics.

35. Dark, tarry bowel movements are called:
    a. hematemesis
    b. melena
    c. anemia
    d. thrombosis

36. This patient is suffering from:
    a. gastrointestinal bleeding
    b. appendicitis
    c. bowel obstruction
    d. pancreatitis

37. Treatment includes:
    a. administering 100% oxygen
    b. placing the patient into a semisitting position on the cot
    c. starting an IV line of 5% dextrose in water
    d. applying the pneumatic antishock garment and inflating the abdominal section

38. Match the following characteristics with the corresponding condition.

   Condition
   a. Alzheimer's disease

   b. Parkinson's disease

   Characteristic

   _____ Slowly progressing degenerative disorder of the nervous system

   _____ Progressive loss of cognitive function and has been associated with anatomical changes within the cerebral cortex

   _____ Represents approximately 65% of all the dementias in the elderly population

   _____ Typically distinguished by a tremor at rest, sluggish initiation of movements, and muscle rigidity

   _____ Primary site of insult is an area of the brain known as the basal ganglia, which helps to initiate actions such as lifting an arm and other movements

   _____ Typically has a subtle onset, with patients noticing diminished performance in normal tasks—memory loss, episodes of depression, fear, and anxiety may occur

   _____ Some cases may be caused by infection or insults from drugs or toxins

39. T   F   On average, elderly patients take two or three prescription medications routinely.

40. T   F   Prescription medications may not be absorbed as well in the gastrointestinal tract of elderly patients because of hypomotility within the bowel.

41. T   F   For any given drug, geriatric patients are less likely to have as many significant side effects from the medication compared with the younger population.

42. T   F   Many older patients suffer from depression or anxiety and may turn to intoxicants for some form of comfort.

43. T   F   Large amounts of intoxicants are needed to achieve significant levels of impairment in the geriatric patient.

44. List six signs of substance abuse in the elderly population.

_____

_____

_____

_____

_____

_____

45. Describe why patients with dementia or delirium are at risk of hypothermia.

_____
_____
_____
_____
_____

46. Hyperthermia can result from inadequate _____ intake and _____ ambient temperatures.

    The _____ population represents the vast majority of fatalities that occur during heat waves.

47. T F Osteoporosis contributes to a significant number of orthopedic fractures in the elderly population.

48. T F More energy is needed to fracture a long bone, spinal bone, or pelvis in an elderly patient than in a normal healthy adult.

49. In elderly patients:
    a. cardiac function and cardiac output are reduced
    b. compensatory mechanisms normally activated when shock or other blood loss occurs are more pronounced
    c. cardiac medications may limit the heart's ability to maintain adequate organ perfusion following a traumatic insult
    d. all of the above

50. T F Generalized cerebral atrophy causes the brain to be more mobile within the skull.

51. T F Serious burns can cause significant mortality in the elderly population.

52. Describe some of the complications that elderly patients may experience as a result of serious burns.

_____
_____
_____
_____
_____

53. Describe how to immobilize elderly patients who require cervical and long board immobilization when previous neurological injuries or orthopedic conditions prohibit the patient from lying completely flat.

_____
_____
_____
_____
_____

CROSSWORD PUZZLE EXERCISE

54. Complete the following crossword puzzle.

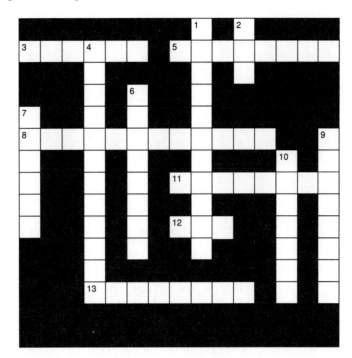

ACROSS

3. Also referred to as a cerebral vascular accident.
5. Organic brain dysfunction resulting in confusion, abnormal behavior, or hallucinations.
8. The inability to prevent urination or bowel movements.
11. Progressive loss of intellectual function.
12. Most common orthopedic condition encountered in the elderly population.
13. Type of hematomas that are more common after blunt head injury in elderly patients.

DOWN

1. Blood noted within the vomitus.
2. Acute neurological deficit that resolves over time.
4. Loss of calcium in the bone.
6. Opacities within the lens of the eyes, distorting and preventing light sensation.
7. Type of hernia where there is protrusion of stomach through the diaphragm.
9. Presence of an elevated intraocular pressure within the eye that can lead to vision loss.
10. Loss of brain tissue.

37 Patients with Special Challenges

CHAPTER TERMINAL OBJECTIVES

On completion of this chapter, the EMT-Intermediate will be able to integrate pathophysiological and psychosocial principles to adapt the assessment and treatment plan for diverse patients and those who face physical, mental, social, and financial challenges.

For the multiple-choice questions, select the single best answer to each question. For the matching questions, select the best corresponding answer for each item. Because there are sometimes more items than corresponding answers, some items may not be used.

1. Describe why it is important for the EMT-Intermediate to develop the necessary knowledge and skills to interact with and treat patients with special challenges.

    _____

    _____

    _____

    _____

2. _____ is a complete or partial inability to hear.

3. Match the type of hearing loss with the correct characteristics.

    Type of hearing loss
    a. Conductive
    b. Sensorineural
    c. Mixed

    Characteristics
    _____ Most common
    _____ Also called perceptive or nerve deafness
    _____ Combination of conductive and sensorineural
    _____ Distortion of sound and problems with discrimination of sound
    _____ Result of problems with inner ear or auditory nerve
    _____ Interference with loudness of sound
    _____ Related to problems of the outer or middle ear
    _____ Interference with transmission of sound in the middle ear and along the neural pathways

4. A ringing, roaring sound, or hissing in the ears that is usually caused by certain medicines or exposure to loud noise is called:
    a. otosclerosis
    b. spina bifida
    c. tinnitus
    d. vertigo

5. List six things you can do to communicate with persons who are hearing impaired.

   _____
   _____
   _____
   _____
   _____
   _____

6. Match the type of vision loss with the correct description.

   Type of vision loss
   a. Partially sighted
   b. Low vision
   c. Legally blind
   d. Totally blind

   Description
   _____ Refers to individuals who are unable to read a newspaper at the usual viewing distance even if they use glasses or contact lenses
   _____ Refers to a person who has less than 20/200 vision in at least one eye or has a very limited field of vision
   _____ Refers to a patient who has some type of visual problem who may need assistance
   _____ Refers to anyone who has no vision and uses nonvisual media or reads via Braille

7. List five things you can do to assist persons who are visually impaired.

   _____
   _____
   _____
   _____
   _____

8. T F Language disorders usually result from stroke, head injury, or brain tumor, which cause damage to the language centers of the brain.

9. T F Aphasia affects only adults.

10. A speech disorder in which the person has difficulty saying what he or she wants to say in a correct and consistent manner is called:
    a. aphasia
    b. apraxia
    c. dysarthria
    d. tinnitus

11. List four things you can do to assist persons who have speech impairment.

    _____

    _____

    _____

    _____

12. Which of the following should be done when assessing, treating, or transporting a patient who is obese?
    a. Use a regular size blood pressure cuff
    b. Request extra personnel as necessary to move the patient to the ambulance and from the ambulance into the hospital
    c. Minimize the length of time used to gather the patient's history of present illness and past medical history
    d. To ease any tension that may exist, joke with the patient about his or her weight

13. _____ is weakness or paralysis of both legs and possibly the trunk. _____ is weakness or paralysis affecting the level below the neck and chest area, involving all four extremities.

14. Paralysis is considered to be _____ when there is no voluntary movement or sensation below the level of the injury.

15. T F The cause of paralysis is trauma.

16. When performing airway skills on a patient with spina bifida, the head should be in _____ position.
    a. neutral, in-line
    b. hyperextended
    c. flexed forward
    d. rotated laterally

17. Which one is the most common cause of school absences among children?
    a. epilepsy
    b. transplant recipients
    c. heart disease
    d. asthma

18. A person with spina bifida is prone to _____ allergy.

38 Assessment-Based Management

CHAPTER TERMINAL OBJECTIVES

At the end of this chapter, the EMT-Intermediate will be able to integrate the principles of assessment-based management to perform an appropriate assessment and implement the management plan for patients with common complaints.

For the multiple-choice questions, select the single best answer to each question. For the matching questions, select the best corresponding answer for each item. Because there are sometimes more items than corresponding answers in the matching questions, some items may not be used.

1. The most important skill that any medical practitioner can possess is the ability to:
   a. place an intravenous (IV) line
   b. perform endotracheal intubation
   c. effectively assess the patient
   d. interpret electrocardiogram (ECG) dysrhythmias

2. Describe the consequence of the failure to perform an adequate assessment.

   _____
   _____
   _____
   _____
   _____

3. Effective assessment skills involve the continuous _____, _____, and ongoing _____ of the information that the Emergency Medical Technician–Intermediate (EMT-I) learns from the _____ and the patient.

4. List three things an effective assessment will allow the EMT-I to do.

   _____
   _____
   _____

5. One of the most important and critical steps in gathering information regarding the patient is learned from the:
   a. patient history
   b. physical examination
   c. initial assessment
   d. general impression

481

6. The history is *most often* gained from the:
   a. family members
   b. patients themselves
   c. friends
   d. medical records at the patient's home

7. An effective history-taking process involves asking _____ and _____ questions regarding certain components of the patient's _____ and _____ throughout the history taking.

8. These _____ questions should be focused toward the _____ _____ and _____ problems that are learned during the history-taking process.

9. T F Knowledge of the disease or injury process does little to direct the EMT-I as to what questions should be asked of the patient.

10. T F Once the EMT-I reaches a working diagnosis, he or she should stick to it even in the face of conflicting information.

11. The second key component of information gathering is the:
    a. focused history
    b. general impression
    c. physical examination
    d. working diagnosis

12. Describe what the physical examination should do.

    _____
    _____
    _____
    _____
    _____

13. Even in situations that limit the EMT-I's ability to perform a complete physical examination, a focused physical examination should be done and include the:
    a. vital signs and attention to the body systems associated with the chief complaint
    b. field impression and a treatment plan
    c. detailed physical examination and assessment of the chief complaint
    d. neurological and cardiovascular assessments

14. Describe how a working diagnosis is formed.

15. Describe the relationship of a proper working diagnosis to the selection of the appropriate treatment protocol.

16. List three factors the EMT-I uses to form a proper attitude.

17. T F The EMT-I has a responsibility to be the advocate for the patient, caretaker for the patient, and uphold the desires of society in treating people in need.

18. T F If the EMT-I has a judgmental attitude during assessment it will not interfere with the necessary information gathering as long as he or she remains focused on the task at hand.

19. Describe the problems that can arise if the EMT-I has a judgmental attitude.

20. Describe the effect that an uncooperative patient, friends, or family members can have on the assessment.

___

21. Another component of the EMT-I's attitude in patient assessment is the _____ put into each component of the _____ _____ process.

22. Describe the problem that can occur when the EMT-I "locks on" to a specific working diagnosis early in the assessment process.

___

23. Describe why an organized team approach to treatment and assessment is important.

___

24. T F Developing and practicing a preplan is one way of ensuring that each emergency medical service (EMS) response to a call for help results in a coordinated, seamless patient care assessment and intervention.

25. T F Team members should be assigned roles once they arrive on the scene.

26. T F Each EMS crew member should perform the same duties for each patient encounter.

27. List eight responsibilities of the team leader.

   _____

   _____

   _____

   _____

   _____

   _____

   _____

   _____

28. Describe why critical equipment must be brought in with each patient encounter.

   _____

   _____

   _____

   _____

   _____

29. Place a checkmark beside those items the EMS team must bring in with them to manage the high-acuity patient.

   _____ Oxygen tank and regulator

   _____ Cot

   _____ Laryngoscope and a selection of laryngoscope blades

   _____ Long backboard

   _____ Suction devices, including rigid and flexible suction catheters

   _____ Bag-mask device

   _____ Cardiac monitor/defibrillator

30. The EMT-I should approach the patient appearing _____ and _____ _____.

31. The EMT-I must portray a high degree of _____ and _____ to the patient to establish and maintain a level of trust.

32. Describe problems that can result with patients who have concern over the abilities of a caregiver.

   _____
   _____
   _____
   _____

33. Describe three ways the EMS team can come across as strong, confident, and highly skilled.

   _____
   _____
   _____

34. Describe how the team member who is obtaining history and interacting with the patient should carry out that responsibility.

   _____
   _____
   _____
   _____
   _____

35. Match the following type of approach with the correct characteristics. Letters may be used more than once.

   Approach
   a. Evacuation
   b. Resuscitative
   c. Uncomplicated

   Characteristic
   _____ Initial assessment identifies that immediate interventions are needed and can be initiated by the EMT-I
   _____ A more "relaxed" patient history, physical assessment, and intervention can be undertaken
   _____ Typically involve patients who may have cardiac or respiratory arrest, respiratory failure or distress, unstable cardiac dysrhythmias, and so on
   _____ Most commonly used in trauma patients with penetrating injuries to the thorax or abdomen
   _____ Patients typically do not need immediate intervention
   _____ With the initial assessment, the EMT-I determines that critical life-saving interventions are needed that cannot be provided by on-scene caregivers

36. The systematic approach to patient assessment:
    a. calls for the EMT-I to proceed directly to assessing the patient's vital signs
    b. helps the EMT-I identify key, life-threatening conditions that may require immediate intervention
    c. is used mostly in the clinical setting by physicians and nurses
    d. begins with the initial assessment

37. List the five components of the systematic patient assessment.

    _____

    _____

    _____

    _____

    _____

    _____

    _____

38. Multitasking is:
    a. the ability to process multiple pieces of information, determine actions that need to be taken, and perform these actions while continuing to assess the patient
    b. a technique that should be used by all prehospital providers
    c. done only in patients experiencing critical illnesses or injuries
    d. used only in adult patients who are experiencing multiple complaints and when there are sufficient crew members to properly manage all aspects of the assessment and patient care

39. Failure to effectively _____ is often identified as one of the weakest links in the prehospital-to-hospital transition of patient care.

40. Utilizing effective communication skills will help the EMT-I gain more _____ and _____ within the health care system.

41. List five highlights of effective prehospital-to-hospital communications.

    _____

    _____

    _____

    _____

    _____

    _____

CROSSWORD PUZZLE EXERCISE

42. Complete the following crossword puzzle.

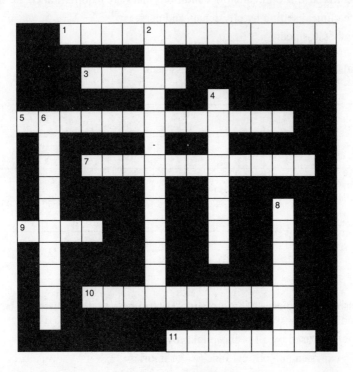

ACROSS

1. With this approach, patients typically do not need immediate intervention.
3. Following formulation of this impression a plan of action must ensue.
5. This approach is used when patients need immediate interventions and they can be initiated.
7. An important characteristic of equipment used in the field setting.
9. An oxygen _____ and regulator are critical need items.
10. This type of attitude will flaw any patient assessment.
11. Type of diagnosis based on available information and subject to modification.

DOWN

2. Ability to process information to formulate multiple decisions and actions simultaneously.
4. Practiced approach to patient assessment includes proper _____ at the beginning of the encounter.
6. This approach is most commonly used in patients with penetrating thorax or abdomen injuries.
8. Organized, predetermined approach to commonly encountered situations.

39 First Responder Procedures with Weapons of Mass Destruction

CHAPTER TERMINAL OBJECTIVES

On completion of this chapter, the EMT-Intermediate will be able to discuss the role of emergency medical services (EMS) in responding to threats by terrorism and weapons of mass destruction.

For the multiple-choice questions, select the single best answer to each question. For the matching questions, select the best corresponding answer for each item. Because there are sometimes more items than corresponding answers, some items may not be used.

1. Describe what is meant by the term *terrorism*.

   _____

   _____

2. List the three classes of terrorists:

   _____

   _____

   _____

3. Describe how you, as a first responder, may be the first to detect an act of bioterrorism.

   _____

   _____

   _____

4. Match the type of chemical agent with the correct description.

   Type of Chemical Agent
   a. Organophosphate nerve agents
   b. Vesicants
   c. Chemical asphyxiants

   Description
   _____ Inhibit deoxyribonucleic acid (DNA) replication
   _____ Interfere with the use and metabolism of oxygen in the body
   _____ Produce an overload of acetylcholine by blocking acetylcholinesterase, the enzyme that breaks down acetylcholine in the body

5. Which of the following is an organophosphate agent?
   a. Lewisite
   b. Mustard
   c. Cyanide
   d. Sarin

6. List what signs the mnemonic SLUDGE represents.

7. Which of the following provides adequate protection for first responders who are part of the response to a terrorist use of chemical agents?
   a. latex gloves
   b. surgical mask
   c. chemical-resistant garments
   d. infection control aprons

8. Describe the term *barrier protection*.

9. List the three medications that are used in the treatment of exposure to organophosphate nerve agents.

10. List the contents of a Mark I kit.

11. To treat exposure to organophosphate nerve agents, up to _____ Mark I kits can be delivered in the field.
    a. 2
    b. 3
    c. 5
    d. 10

12. The medications used to treat exposure to organophosphate nerve agents are supplied in _____ and delivered by _____ injection.

13. The term vesicant refers to the chemical's ability to cause:
    a. blisters in the skin and airways
    b. birth defects
    c. SLUDGE
    d. severe hypoxia

14. Which of the following is a blister agent?
    a. Lewisite
    b. VX
    c. Cyanide
    d. Sarin

15. Describe why mustard is more *sinister* than Lewisite.

16. Describe the treatment for cyanide poisoning.

17. Describe the most efficient way to spread biological weapons.

18. T F When aerosolized disease-causing microbes or toxins are released, the condition a first responder is likely to see is pneumonia.

19. List the five conditions or types of diseases that may be caused by biological agents.

20. List eight biological agents that can be aerosolized.

_____
_____
_____
_____
_____
_____
_____
_____

21. List four protective measures the first responder should take to ensure that no further spread of a disease caused by a biological agent occurs.

_____
_____
_____
_____

22. Pinpoint, round red spots that indicate bleeding under the skin are called:
    a. blotching
    b. petechiae
    c. botulism
    d. red eye

23. A simple radiological source:
    a. combines a radioactive source with a conventional bomb to create a low-level contamination event
    b. causes blast casualties, and the radioactive contamination complicates the rescue process
    c. continues to do damage until detected
    d. spreads contamination over a large area

24. T F Identification of radiological exposure is primarily done through identification of presenting signs and symptoms of those persons exposed.

25. T F Radiation in high doses or in lower doses over time causes damaging effects on DNA replication in dividing cells.

26. T F Victims, first responders, and their vehicles must be decontaminated if they are exposed to harmful chemicals, infectious disease, or radiation contamination.

27. T F Decontamination can be achieved by using copious amounts of water and soap or a decontamination solution.

28. T F Ambulatory patients should never attempt to decontaminate themselves.

40 Incident Command

CHAPTER TERMINAL OBJECTIVES

On completion of this chapter, the EMT-Intermediate will be able to discuss the role of emergency medical services (EMS) in situations when an incident command management system is in effect.

For the multiple-choice questions, select the single best answer to each question. For the matching questions, select the best corresponding answer for each item. Because there are sometimes more items than corresponding answers, some items may not be used.

1. Describe what is meant by the term incident command system (ICS).

   _____

   _____

2. Describe the benefits of using the ICS.

   _____

   _____

   _____

3. T F The incident management system is used mainly by EMS.

4. T F Once a major incident has been declared, an incident commander is identified.

5. T F Usually the initial incident commander is the oldest EMT-I on scene.

6. Which of the following is true regarding the incident commander?
   a. the incident commander need not be aware of the incident management system, the available resources, and operations procedures if he or she is a strong leader
   b. there may be two persons assigned to the role of incident commander if the communication system supports their use
   c. the incident commander should be clearly identified on the scene
   d. once assumed, the command position is not transferred until the incident is resolved

7. During major incidents, several _____ are established, each with unique _____.

8. List the seven recognized EMS sectors:

   _____
   _____
   _____
   _____
   _____
   _____
   _____

9. Which of the following is true regarding sectors?
   a. each sector has a leader or sector officer
   b. only supervisory level personnel are assigned to sector officer positions
   c. all seven recognized sectors are established for all incidents
   d. the sector officer performs specific tasks

10. A method of categorizing patients according to treatment and transport priorities is called:
    a. prioritizing
    b. sorting
    c. organizing by severity
    d. triage

11. Match the priority levels with the correct conditions.

    Priority Level   **Conditions**
    a. Highest priority   _____ Burns without airway compromise
    b. Second priority   _____ Airway or breathing difficulties
    c. Lowest priority   _____ Uncontrolled or severe bleeding
                                    _____ Minor soft tissue injuries
                                    _____ Prolonged respiratory arrest
                                    _____ Back injuries with or without spinal cord damage
                                    _____ Signs and symptoms of shock (hypoperfusion)
                                    _____ Cardiopulmonary arrest
                                    _____ Decreased or altered mental status

12. T F Transport decisions from large-scale emergencies and/or disasters are based on patient priority, the receiving hospital's capabilities and capacity, and transportation resources.

41 Tactical Emergency Medical Support

CHAPTER TERMINAL OBJECTIVES

On completion of this chapter, the EMT-Intermediate will be able to discuss the role of emergency medical services (EMS) in tactical operations and describe how it operates.

For the multiple-choice questions, select the single best answer to each question. For the matching questions, select the best corresponding answer for each item. Because there are sometimes more items than corresponding answers, some items may not be used.

1. Describe what is meant by the term *Tactical Emergency Medical Support (TEMS)*.

   _____

   _____

   _____

2. Describe the rationale for using TEMS.

   _____

   _____

   _____

3. T F Unlike normal EMS operations, in which patient care is the primary objective, the TEMS objective is the successful completion of the tactical mission.

4. With a tactical team:
   a. the senior paramedic is in charge of all patient care delivery
   b. EMS serves in a support and advisory role
   c. the tactical commander is in charge of only the law enforcement agencies involved in the tactical operation
   d. EMS has a key role in decision making

5. Match each of the following tactical environment zones with the appropriate description(s).

   Zone
   a. Cold zone
   b. Warm zone
   c. Hot zone

   Description
   _____ Area of potential threat
   _____ Sometimes referred to as the Kill Zone
   _____ Area of no threat
   _____ Sometimes referred to as the Safe Zone
   _____ Area of direct or immediate threat

6. List six responsibilities of TEMS.

_____

_____

_____

_____

_____

_____

7. *Medical intelligence* refers to:
    a. the amount of training the TEMS is required to provide to first responders
    b. the mental awareness of the TEMS members
    c. information about medical and psychological conditions of perpetrators or hostages
    d. the aptitude of the TEMS members

8. TEMS members with necessary training accompany the team during entries and into hot zones. Which of the following is true?
    a. quick initiation of treatment of injuries cannot be done
    b. it is safer in this zone
    c. more equipment can be brought into this zone
    d. evacuation of injured or ill patients may be difficult if the environment is hostile

9. The _____ phase is the most dangerous.

10. Typical TEMS equipment is carried in _____ or _____ bags to limit visibility during operations.

11. The TEMS member:
    a. must be able to think quickly and clearly in very loud and chaotic situations
    b. is required to contact medical direction before performing most skills
    c. is only required to provide care to law enforcement officers who are injured or who become ill
    d. is required to carry a weapon

12. T F The TEMS operational preplan should include already identified closest trauma centers, burn units, and acute care hospitals.

Answer Keys and Rationales

CHAPTER 1

1. **b**

2. **d:** The EMT-I **uses additional skills, including advanced airway adjuncts, intravenous therapy, and defibrillation.** EMT-Is are also trained to monitor and interpret basic cardiac dysrhythmias, as well as to administer some medications including epinephrine, 5% dextrose, naloxone, aerosol bronchodilators, first-round cardiac drugs such as atropine and lidocaine, and others. Because of the advanced level of care provided, many states *require* EMT-Is to work under medical direction. The typical EMT-I training program ranges between *300 and 400 hours.*

3. **a**

4. What you learned from your research will determine the answer to this question.

5. **b**

6. **True**

7. **False:** To become recertified, EMT-Is *may* be required to participate in a refresher course, obtain a specific amount of continuing education each year, and/or successfully complete written or skill testing.

8. **Continuing education can help the EMT-I reach full competency. The EMT-I curriculum does not provide extensive knowledge in hazardous materials, bloodborne pathogens, emergency vehicle operations, or rescue practices in unusual environments. Continuing education helps reduce the erosion of knowledge and skills. Also, continuing education keeps the EMT-I current on new procedures and treatments, allows a sharing of real-life experiences with other prehospital care providers, and encourages further professional development.**

9. **d**

10. **c:** EMS journals keep the EMT-I aware of the latest changes in a constantly evolving industry, highlight tips that can be used on the job, and provide excellent sources of continuing education to sharpen knowledge and skills. They also list employment opportunities and calendars identifying available EMS seminars and conferences, provide details about new products and equipment, and review various EMS-related books, videos, and films. **EMS journals do not meet all the requirements for recertification.**

11. Teaching done by an EMT-I can **serve as a source of continuing education credit and establish the EMT-I as a leader and resource person in the community and can fill a much needed void in having CPR and first responder qualified persons trained in the community.**

12. **c:** The EMT-I *does not need to be paid* to be a professional. Professionalism is necessary to promote high-quality patient care, to instill pride in the prehospital environment, to promote high standards, and to earn the respect of other members of the health care team.

13. Professional behaviors include **being well-groomed; wearing a clean, pressed, and well-fitting uniform; addressing patients by their proper names; attending continuing education; practicing skills, reading EMS-related literature, and participating in quality improvement activities; working well as a member of the prehospital team; sharing equally in the workload.**

    Unprofessional behaviors include **smoking while treating patients; having outbursts when persons call for EMS unnecessarily; referring to your place of employment as being a terrible place to work; not keeping the ambulance and equipment clean; falsifying run reports; and arguing with nurses at a hospital where a patient has been transported.**

    One of the most professional things one can do as an EMT-I is show compassion toward every patient. Patients should always be treated the way the EMT-I would want to be treated if he or she were in need of help.

14. **d:** Responsibilities of the EMT-I include **interacting with first responders who are already on the scene providing care, rapidly assessing and managing life-threatening illnesses and injuries, recognizing when the limits of field care have been reached and when prompt transportation is needed,** performing a careful patient assessment, recognizing the nature and seriousness of illnesses or injuries, determining the requirements for emergency medical care, and providing prompt and efficient care for life-threatening illnesses or injuries, among others.

15. **d:** Ethics **deal with the EMT-I's relationship with his or her peers, patients, the patient's family, and society in general,** are set standards for the *rightness and wrongness* of human behavior, and are *principles* governing one's conduct as an EMT-I.

16. The following are considered examples of unethical behavior: **giving an attorney's business card to a victim who has fallen on icy steps in front of a public building, discouraging a patient from going to the hospital because he or she cannot pay, and failing to maintain patient confidentiality.**

17. **c:** Ethical decisions should *not* be based on what other people think is right or wrong, and emotion should *not* be a factor when making an ethical decision. Also, an EMT-I should *avoid* doing anything that is considered morally wrong.

18. **a**

19. **d**

20. **True**

21. **c**

22. An emergency medical service (EMS) system is an **organized** approach to providing **emergency care** to the **sick** and **injured.**

23. **The primary responsibilities of an EMS system are to respond to requests for medical assistance, provide life-saving or stabilizing treatment, and transport patients to definitive medical care.**

24. **b: Definitive trauma care** is not a component of today's EMS systems. This care is provided by specialized hospital facilities such as trauma centers. Regulation and policy, resource management, human resources and training (including continuing education), transportation, facilities, communications, trauma systems, public information and education, medical direction, and evaluation are all considered components of today's EMS systems.

25. **c:** The *system medical director* is ultimately responsible for all the medical care provided by his or her service.

26. **False:** When the EMT sees a patient and contacts his or her medical direction base for instructions *before* rendering certain care, it is referred to as on-line medical direction.

27. **True**

28. **False:** Patient care protocols are typically developed by the *EMS physician* in cooperation with *expert EMS personnel.*

29. **c**

30. **Duties of an EMS physician include educating and training EMS personnel; participating in personnel selection process; participating in equipment selection; developing clinical protocols in cooperation with expert EMS personnel; participating in quality improvement and problem resolution; providing direct input into patient care; serving as an interface between EMS systems and other health care agencies; being an advocate for EMS within the medical community; serving as the "medical conscience" of the EMS system; and being an advocate for high-quality patient care.**

31. **c:** Continuous quality improvement **compares the care delivered with the accepted standard of care** and is the evaluation of *EMS performance.* Processes should be in place to monitor and evaluate the delivery of care. *Research* is defined as scientific study, investigation, and experimentation to establish facts and determine their significance. It can also prove that prehospital care makes a difference and is valuable.

32. **b**

33. **Continuous quality improvement reveals problems that may not otherwise be recognized when the EMS system is viewed from the surface. It can propel changes in treatment protocols. It can help support the EMS system to acquire additional resources at budget time. It allows the EMS system management and medical direction to evaluate and fix system problems.**

34. **Four things that should be checked for on the patient care reports include completeness; accuracy of charting and assessment; adherence to system treatment protocols; and patterns of error or system-related problems.**

35. **a**

36. EMS research **can eliminate much of the uncertainty associated with prehospital care. It can prove which patient care protocols and techniques are useful and beneficial. Also, changes in professional standards can be based on empirical data, rather than "great ideas" or "new gadget" models.**

37. **Research has the immediate potential of saving lives or limiting morbidity by improving current and future patient care delivered in the field. It can prove that prehospital care makes a difference and is valuable. It enhances recognition and respect for EMS professionals.**

38. This exercise gave you a chance to apply what you learned. Therefore there are no absolutely right or wrong answers. Here are some examples of possible reporting mechanisms and preventive measures:

Reporting Mechanisms	Preventive Measures
• Monitor EMS run reports and police reports to identify incidents. • Have the local coroner's office report any identified cases. • Perform queries of the computer-aided dispatch database. • Have the dispatch center report all such incidents to identified administrative personnel.	• Develop a public information campaign that includes public service announcements on the radio and television, informational flyers, etc. • Conduct educational programs in the community to make parents aware of the risk of leaving children unattended in cars. • Enlist local hospitals to conduct programs to educate parents of newly borns and children on these hazards. • Educate all EMS, fire, and police personnel on the problem and encourage them to identify and report incidents.

39. Four reasons why EMS providers can play an important role in education and prevention activities are **there are more than 600,000 widely distributed EMS providers in the United States; the EMS provider may be the most medically educated individual in some communities; EMS providers are high-profile role models who are considered champions of the customer; and EMS providers are welcome in schools and other environments and are considered authorities on injury and prevention.**

40. Epidemiology is the **study of the elements that influence the frequency, distribution, and causes of injury, disease, and other health-related events in a population.**

41. An injury is the **intentional or unintentional damage to a person that is produced by acute exposure to thermal, mechanical, electrical, radiological, or chemical energy or from the lack of such essentials as heat or oxygen.**

42. **False:** Trauma is the leading cause of death in persons ages *1 to 44.*

43. **True**

44. **False:** *Fifty percent* **of deaths occur immediately after the trauma event.**

45. **The EMT-I can help reduce the incidence of injury by educating the public on illness and injury prevention, such as safe driving and accident avoidance practices.**

46. a: Accidental injuries **are referred to as unintentional.** Injuries that occur because of purposeful actions are called *intentional injuries*. Approximately one third of all injury deaths are the result of *intentional* injuries.

47.

Case	Lost Productive Years
33-year-old female...	32
41-year-old male...	24
19-year-old male...	46
61-year-old female...	4

48. Injury terms: **a. injury risk:** real or potential hazardous situations that put individuals in danger of sustaining injury; an example is using power tools without wearing eye protection. **b. injury surveillance:** ongoing systematic collection, analysis, and interpretation of injury data. **c. primary injury prevention:** keeping an injury from occurring. **d. secondary and tertiary prevention:** care and rehabilitation activities (respectively) that prevent further problems from an event that has already occurred. **e. teachable moment:** time after an injury has occurred when the patient remains acutely aware of what has happened and may be receptive to instruction about how event or illness could be prevented.

49. EMT-Is identify injury causes

↓

Information reported through EMS run reports or other data-collection documents

↓

These data are disseminated to those who need to know in a timely manner

↓

These data are applied to prevention and control

50. Answers to crossword puzzle

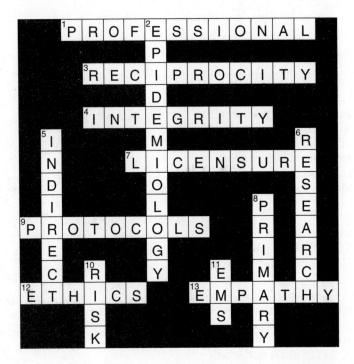

CHAPTER 2

1. **b**

2. A contagious disease is **any disease that can be spread from person to person.**

3. **False:** Persons who are carrying pathogens for a disease often exhibit *no noticeable signs* of the illness.

4. **False:** In the normal course of their duties EMT-Is are at risk of being exposed to infection through various means.

5. **True**

6. Ways an EMT-I can be exposed to an infectious disease during the normal course of performing their duties include **being splashed by blood; stuck by a needle; allowing blood or body fluids to come in contact with broken or scraped skin or the mucous membranes of the eyes, nose, or mouth; and through surface contamination or orally (as a result of improper hand washing).**

7. To decrease the chance of being exposed or infected, **follow recommended engineering and work practices; maintain good personal health and hygiene habits; keep your immunizations up to date; receive periodic tuberculosis screening; and use body substance isolation/standard (universal) precautions.**

8. **a**

9. **d**

10. **False:** Hand washing should be done even when you do not come in contact with body fluids or when protective gloves are worn (after removing the gloves).

11. **False:** Latex or vinyl gloves should never be reused.

12. **True**

13. **Use waterless soaps,** which are often carried on the emergency vehicle, to clean your hands when you do not have access to running water.

14. "PPE" stands for **personal protective equipment.**

15. There are three basic types of gloves, **nitrile, latex,** and **vinyl.** Nitrile or vinyl gloves should be used if you are allergic to latex. An indication that you may be allergic is if you experience a **rash** after wearing latex gloves.

16. If your gloves become contaminated during a call, you should **replace them as soon as it is safe to do so.**

17. **a**

18. **d**

19. Four indicators of TB include **fever; weight loss; night sweats; and a continual cough.**

20. Groups at high risk for TB include **nursing home patients; those who are institutionalized; alcoholics; homeless persons (living in a shelter); indigent elderly persons; AIDS patients; and immigrants from countries having a high TB rate.**

21. **Placing a surgical mask on the patient can cut down on the release of droplets into the air that occurs with coughing.** This should be done only if the patient's airway is patent and no breathing difficulty is noted.

22. **False:** Disposable medical devices that become contaminated with blood or other body fluids can be placed in a red *bag or container marked with a biohazard seal.* Once the contaminated material is placed in an appropriate bag or container, it should be handled according to your system's procedures for disposing of biohazardous waste.

23. **True**

24. **c**

25. Five actions that should be taken if you are exposed to blood or body fluids or stuck by a needle include **immediately and thoroughly wash the area of contact; get a medical evaluation; if appropriate, take the proper immunization boosters; document the situation in which the exposure occurred;** and **complete any required medical follow-up.**

26. Immunization is the **process of rendering a person immune or of becoming immune.**

27. **True**

28. Four factors that play a major role in maintaining physical health are **good nutrition, physical fitness and weight control, adequate sleep, and prevention of disease and injury.**

29. **Eating mostly fast foods that contain high percentages of fat** is a poor nutritional habit.

30. The six categories of nutrients are **carbohydrates, fats, proteins, vitamins, minerals,** and **water.**

31. **False:** Food groups include sugar, fats, proteins, dairy products, vegetables, fruits, and *grains.*

32. **False**

33. **False**

34. **True**

35. **False:** Alcoholic beverages should be avoided or consumed *only in moderation.*

36. **EMT-Is are required to perform physically demanding tasks as part of their day-to-day duties.** For these reasons, physical fitness and weight control are important to them.

37. **c**

38. Overweight EMT-Is face the following problems. **Performing related work tasks requires more energy, thus making the EMT-I susceptible to tiring and fatigue, and can contribute to a host of injuries. Also, people who are overweight tend to be at greater risk for developing high blood pressure, diabetes mellitus, heart disease, some cancers, and other illnesses.**

39. **c**

40. **d**

41. **a**

42. **d**

43. Signs of stress include **irritability with co-workers, family, friends, or patients; inability to concentrate; physical exhaustion; difficulty sleeping or nightmares; anxiety; indecisiveness; guilt; loss of appetite; loss of interest in sexual activities; isolation; loss of interest in work; increased substance use or abuse (alcohol, medications, illegal drugs);** and **depression.**

44. **d**

45. Answers to crossword puzzle

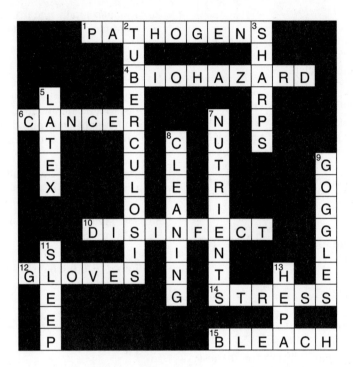

CHAPTER 3

1. **a: Adhere to state and local guidelines concerning prehospital care** (including appropriate use of on- and off-line medical control), *not* perform procedures that you are not certified in or allowed to do within protocols or guidelines, and provide thorough and accurate patient care documentation as required by your EMS system.

2. **b:** This is unethical.

3. **c**

4. **a. Criminal law:** prohibits the performance of any act that is considered damaging to the public. Violation of these laws results in *crimes,* and violators may be prosecuted in a *criminal proceeding*—a trial before a judge, and sometimes a jury, where evidence is heard and a verdict of guilty or not guilty is reached. If a person is found guilty, a fine, imprisonment, or both may result. Typical criminal acts cover offenses such as robbery, assault, and murder. **b. Tort law:** also called *civil law,* covers a private or public wrong or injury that occurs as a result of a breach, or break, of a legal duty or obligation. Under tort law, the *plaintiff,* or injured person, files a *lawsuit* or legal action against the *defendant,* or person accused of committing the breach of duty. If the plaintiff successfully proves that the defendant caused him or her harm by violating a legal duty, the plaintiff may collect *damages.* Injuries include medical bills, loss of employment, pain, suffering, and loss of ability to be with others.

5. **Civil law:** A paramedic is sued for failing to intubate a patient who was in cardiac arrest; an ambulance company fails to live up to its contract; an EMT-I makes untrue and malicious remarks about a patient. ***Criminal law:*** An EMT-I is called as a witness in

a drive-by shooting; an EMT-I is charged with taking an unconscious patient's money; two EMT-Is assault an intoxicated patient; an EMT-I practices medicine without a license.

6. **c:** Medical Practice Acts are laws that govern the provision of medicine within a state. They define the limits for the scope of practice of the EMT-I (what assessment and treatment skills an EMT-I may legally perform).

7. **d**

8. **b:** Examples of things the EMT-I may have an obligation to report include suspected abuse or neglect of elderly persons or children, alleged rape, gunshot and/or stab wounds, and animal bites. The EMT-I is not required to report **a 16-year-old who is pregnant and unmarried.** Generally, these laws provide immunity from lawsuits for providers who reported these problems in good faith.

9. **a:** The standard of care **is the degree of medical care and skill that is expected of a reasonably competent EMT-I acting in the same or similar circumstances,** is measured by matching the EMT-I's performance to others with *similar* training and experience, and is based on *community practice; federal, state, and local laws;* scientific literature; and EMS system standards.

10. Answers to crossword puzzle.

11. **c**

12. **b:** EMS system medical directors **are not protected** from liability through each state's Medical Practice Act. Some states provide some degree of immunity, but it is not universal to all states.

13. **a. Negligence:** This is conduct that falls below the standard of care. This may entail either doing something that should not have been done, or failing to do something that should have been done. **b. Duty to act:** Obligation to provide care. **c. Proximate cause:** Something that is directly responsible for damage.

14. **Ordinary negligence is an act of omission that occurs in an attempt to deliver proper care, whereas gross negligence is the willful and reckless giving of care that causes injury to the patient.**

15. The EMT-I must have had a duty to act; the act or omission must have been below the standard of care; an injury must have occurred to the patient; the act or omission of the EMT-I must have been the proximate (direct) cause of injury.

16. **a**

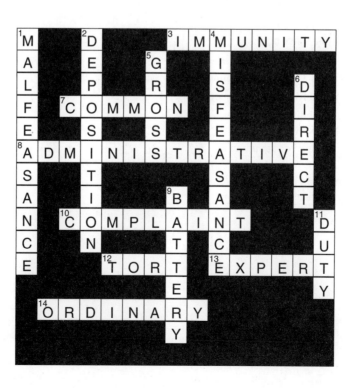

17. Possible conclusions to Case 1

Conclusion	Agree or Disagree	Justify Your Answer
EMT-Is Landford and Jones had a duty to act.	Agree	Both EMT-Is had a duty to act because the fire department is the agency responsible for providing emergency medical service to this community.
The care the EMT-Is provided fell below the standard of care.	Agree	The EMT-Is failed to deliver the care required for this condition.
Mr. Alfonzo suffered a myocardial infarction that led to cardiac arrest and his subsequent death because of the actions of EMT-Is Landford and Jones.	It can be argued both ways	Based on the present history it appears Mr. Alfonzo suffered a myocardial infarction, and that prompted him to call for help. As such the EMT-Is had nothing to do with the initial "injury." However, the actions of the EMT-Is in not providing the necessary care and walking him to the ambulance may have worsened his condition, which led to cardiac arrest and his subsequent death.

18. Things EMT-Is Jones and Landford did wrong and whether they are considered misfeasance, malfeasance, or nonfeasance.

Action	Type of Breach of Duty
Walking the patient to the ambulance. This is in direct violation of the section of the protocol that says, *"Do not walk the patient to the vehicle."*	Malfeasance
Failing to provide the patient care identified in the treatment protocol, including: • Administering high flow oxygen, 10 to 15 L (85% to 100%) by nonrebreather mask • Providing continuous ECG monitoring • Administering nitroglycerin, 0.3 to 0.4 mg, sublingually • Contacting medical command for further instruction • Under the direction of medical direction administering morphine sulfate, 2 to 4 mg, slow IV push • Moving patient to the ambulance or squad on a stair chair or cot • Placing the patient in a position of comfort based on his or her physiological needs	Nonfeasance

19. Possible arguments regarding whether the EMT-Is in this case are grossly negligent

Why he is not correct	It can be argued that although the EMT-Is walked the patient to the ambulance and did not provide the care that was required by protocol, their actions did not cause the patient to experience cardiac arrest. The basis for this argument is that studies show there are a substantial percentage of patients who experience cardiac arrest solely as a result of acute myocardial infarction. In other words, there is no evidence that what the EMT-Is did or did not do caused injury to the patient. Further, although the EMT-Is appear to be negligent, the plaintiff would have to show that they were "willful and wanton" (grossly negligent) in their actions.
Why he is correct	It can be argued that the lack of treatment allowed the infarction to worsen and cardiac dysrhythmias to develop. Further, having the patient walk to the ambulance caused more injury to his already damaged heart and led directly to the cardiac arrest. This is evidenced by the fact he had adequate cardiac output before his being walked to the ambulance. Because the protocol and the standard of care (for patients experiencing acute myocardial infarction) so clearly spell out what the EMT-Is are required to do and the fact the patient informed the EMT-Is he did not feel he had the strength to walk to the ambulance, it is clear they were purposeful in their actions.

In this case, the EMT-Is had a duty to act. Because they failed to do what was required by protocol they did not meet the standard of care. Although they did not cause the patient to have a heart attack, their actions could be considered causal to a patient experiencing cardiac arrest.

There is no absolute answer as to which side would prevail in this case. A lot depends on the skill of the attorneys on both sides, the quality of the expert witnesses, and how the jurors perceive each party. However, the outcome of this case does not appear favorable to the defendants.

20. **b:** He or she can talk about patient care issues, protocols, and the required standard of care. Further, someone who can speak to the effects of myocardial ischemia/infarction such as a cardiologist will likely be solicited to serve as an expert witness.

21. Possible conclusions to Case 2

Conclusion	Agree or Disagree	Justify Your Answer
EMT-Is Lukas and Smith fulfilled their duty to act.	Agree	The EMT-Is responded to the scene, assessed the patient appropriately, and then offered to provide treatment and transport to the hospital.
The care the EMT-Is provided met the standard of care.	Agree	Because the patient is alert and oriented, he can decline treatment and transport. By having the patient sign a refusal form the EMT-Is can demonstrate they made an effort to convince the patient that he should allow treatments to be given and to be transported to the hospital. The EMT-Is also involved medical direction in attempting to get the patient to go to the hospital for treatment. This further substantiates they put forth the necessary effort to properly care for the patient.
Mr. Taylor experienced cardiac arrest, but his death was not because of the actions of EMT-Is Lukas and Smith.	Agree	The patient's death is unfortunate, but the action of the EMT-Is did not cause it. However, some might argue the patient should have been taken against his will to the hospital because he could have been under duress (because of his condition) and not able to make a rational decision. To avoid problems and offer a greater degree of protection, your protocol should spell out how to handle these complicated problems.

22. **b:** Whereas Good Samaritan laws vary greatly from state to state in scope of their coverage or requirements, under certain circumstances the EMT-I may be immune from being successfully sued for negligence.

23. **False:** Good Samaritan laws *do not prevent* the EMT-I from being sued. Many questions remain to be answered regarding Good Samaritan legislation. These include concerns as to vagueness in the laws and the true definition of "fee for service."

24. **False:** Good Samaritan laws are not equal from state to state in scope of their coverage or requirements.

25. **True**

26. **b:** Laypersons and medical personnel are likely to be protected by Good Samaritan laws when **they are charged with ordinary negligence** but not gross negligence; they give care *without* charging a fee for service; and they give care that is appropriate *only* for their certification level.

27. **c:** Separate (individual) malpractice insurance is also recommended for those EMT-Is whose EMS systems *lack* adequate insurance.

28. While providing medical direction, physicians may face liability in the areas of **on-line** (providing orders over the phone or radio) and **off-line** (protocols including standing orders) medical direction and through **indirect supervision** ("borrowed servant" doctrine).

29. **d**

30. **b**

31. **c**

32. **c**

33. **Limit oral reporting to appropriate personnel; avoid slang terms—describe the person's behavior, not your opinion of his or her condition; regard all information about patient encounters and care, whether written or verbal, as confidential.**

34. **False:** Emergency department physicians and hospitals are subject to the provisions of the Consolidated Omnibus Budget Reconciliation Act of 1985 (EMTALA; formerly called COBRA; *42 U.S.C. § 1392dd*). EMTALA specifies several responsibilities of the emergency department that must be met before transferring a patient, including providing a medical screening examination to determine whether the patient is suffering from an emergency medical condition or is in active labor.

35. **False**

36. **True:** Patients in active labor may be transferred to another hospital if the appropriate treatment facilities are not available at the initial institution. Unstable patients (or those in active labor) are not to be transferred unless the patient or representative so requests. Before transfer, all patients must first be stabilized unless the risk of waiting to attempt stabilization outweighs the potential benefit of transferring the patient to a more specialized facility. The treatment given at the transferring facility must be documented.

37. **True**

38. **False:** Conscious and mentally competent adult patients have the right to accept or refuse *any* examination, care, or transportation offered, *regardless of their condition*.

39. **False:** The EMT-I who performs assessment, care, or transport without appropriate patient consent *risks legal action*.

40. **c:** Expressed consent exists when the patient gives verbal or written consent for the EMT-I to examine, care for, and transport him or her to an appropriate facility.

41. **d**

42. **b:** This applies to unconscious patients or those who cannot make informed decisions. In these instances, it is **implied** that a patient who is severely ill or injured would wish for care to be provided.

43. Informed consent means that **the patient makes a decision to give expressed consent only after he or she has all the information necessary to understand his or her condition, the risks and benefits of care, and the risks and benefits of refusal of care.**

44. **The EMT-I's assessment of the situation based on his or her field impression; what care is being considered and why; an explanation of the benefits and possible risks (including potential side effects) of accepting or refusing examination, care, or transportation.**

45. **b**

46. **b:** Emancipated minors have been legally freed from the need for parental consent—most often this occurs if a minor becomes married or joins the armed forces.

47. **False:** A patient who has been legally determined mentally incompetent *cannot* consent to care. In these cases, consent is usually given by a legal guardian.

48. **False:** If the legally responsible party is not available, the patient can be cared for under the *implied* consent standard.

49. **True:** Patients experiencing alcohol or substance intoxication, emotional (psychiatric) problems, or certain medical conditions can be cared for under the implied consent standard. It is always better to err on the side of caring for patients who appear to be mentally incompetent, regardless of the reason, because they may be suffering from a serious medical problem that, without care, can result in serious harm to the patient.

50. **c:** Conscious, adult patients have the right to refuse examination, care, and transport by the EMT-I. In many cases, a well-worded explanation of the possible consequences of refusing care may change the patient's mind. A family member, friend, or medical command physician may be able to assist you in convincing the patient to cooperate. It is extremely important to accurately document when a patient refuses care. Obtain a written refusal from the patient on a standardized form; when possible, have the refusal witnessed by a family member, police officer, or firefighter. If a patient refuses to sign the form, record the details in narrative fashion on the run report.

51. **d**

52. **a. Assault:** creation of the fear of immediate bodily harm in a person, without his or her consent (does not require that the person be touched by the perpetrator); **b. Battery:** criminal offense of attempting to inflict bodily injury on another; **c. False imprisonment:** intentional and unjustifiable detention of a person against his or her will; **d. Abandonment:** when the EMT-I–patient relationship is terminated by the EMT-I without ensuring continuity of care; **e. Libel:** when you injure a person's character, name, or reputation by false and malicious writings.

53. **c:** Once you begin care, remain with the patient until care is continued by equal or more highly trained personnel; the patient is delivered to an appropriate care facility and you are certain that transfer has been accepted; or the patient makes an informed decision to sign a refusal statement.

54. **a**

55. **c:** The legality of accepting living wills or DNR orders varies from state to state. Some states require the EMT-I to comply with the provisions in a living will or DNR order, whereas other states do not. If the patient's or physician's intentions are not *clearly and legally documented,* the safest course of action is to proceed with care.

56. **a**

57. **When a critically ill patient is identified as a potential organ donor, establish communication with medical direction as soon as possible. Based on medical direction, provide emergency care that will help maintain viable organs.**

58. **b**

59. **a:** Do not touch, kick, or move anything (including vehicles or debris) unless it is absolutely necessary to facilitate patient care. Both patient care and preservation of evidence can be accomplished, but patient care is the first priority.

60. **b:** EMT-Is have a legal mandate to report suspected child abuse, and failure to do so may be subject to fines, imprisonment, and loss of state certification to practice. Handle these matters after transporting the child to the hospital. All states have laws that protect health care professionals from liability for reporting, in good faith, suspected child abuse.

61. **a:** Legally, the initial responsibility for patient care rests with the on-line medical direction physician. If the on-scene physician documents his or her licensure and ability to deal with the situation, some medical direction facilities will allow an on-scene physician to take over care, provided he or she is willing to accompany the patient to the hospital. EMS systems that do not have the ability to contact on-line medical control should have written protocols in place to deal with on-scene physicians. These protocols should require that if a licensed physician wishes to take control, he or she must ride in the ambulance with the patient to the hospital and sign all necessary care forms, including the run report. The EMT-I must then record the physician's name, state where he or she practices, and his or her medical license number on the run sheet.

62. **c**

63. **d**

64. Answers to crossword puzzle

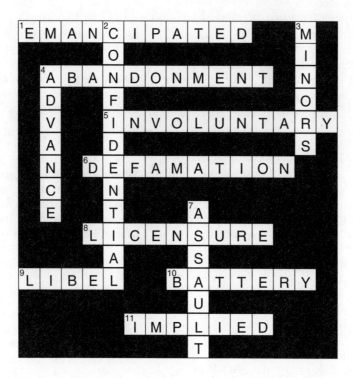

CHAPTER 4

1. anatomy: **study of the structure of an organism and its parts;** physiology: **study of an organism's normal bodily functions;** pathophysiology: **study of disease mechanisms.**

2. **False:** The human body consists of *many increasingly complex* levels of organization.

3. Organizational levels of the body are as follows: organelles, cells, tissue, organs, and organ systems. As a point of information, some references describe the *molecular level* as the most basic level in the body. *a. System:* group of organs that have a common function and purpose; **b. Cells:** the basic building blocks of all life; **c. Tissue:** groups of similar cells working together for a common function; **d. Organelles:** carry out the processes necessary for life within each cell; **e. Organs:** composed of different types of tissues.

4. Homeostasis is **the normal state of balance among all of the body's systems.**

5. **a. Prone:** lying on your stomach with your face down. **b. Frontal:** the plane that vertically divides the body into a front and back portion. **c. Caudal:** pertaining to the lower part of the spinal column. **d. Lateral:** farther away from the midline or toward the side. **e: Dorsal:** toward the back. **f. distal:** farthest from point of attachment. **g. superior:** above or in a higher position.

6. **a:** Remember, the front portion of the body is referred to as ventral, or anterior, and the back is dorsal, or posterior.

7. **a**

8. **A. sagittal plane; B. frontal plane; C. midsagittal plane; D. transverse plane.**

9. **d**

10. The knee is the **proximal** portion of the lower leg, whereas the ankle is the **distal** portion. The terms *superior* (instead of *proximal*) and *inferior* (instead of *distal*) can also be used here.

11. **a:** A person lying on his or her back is in a **supine** position. In the lateral recumbent position, the patient is lying on either the *right or left side*.

12. Body cavities are **hollow** areas within the body that contain **organs** and **systems.**

13. **a. Thoracic:** between the base of the neck and the diaphragm, is formed by the roughly circular

508

Answer Keys and Rationales

boundary of the rib cage; major structures belong to the cardiovascular and respiratory systems—the heart, major blood vessels, and lungs. **b. Spinal:** travels through the vertebral column and contains the spinal cord. **c. Cranial:** has a domed top and a base composed of several bones; it houses the brain. **d. Abdominal:** is a single large cavity that extends from the diaphragm to the pelvic bones; contains the organs of digestion and excretion, which comprise the gastrointestinal and urinary systems. **e. Pelvic:** comprises the lower portion of the abdominal cavity and is bounded by the ilium, ischium, pubis, sacrum, and coccyx; includes organs of the gastrointestinal, reproductive, and urinary systems.

14. **d**

15. **A. cranial cavity; B. spinal cavity; C. thoracic cavity; D. abdominal cavity; E. pelvic cavity**

16. **c:** Between the lungs is a space known as the mediastinum, which contains **the heart, trachea, part of the esophagus,** mainstem bronchi, and large blood vessels.

17. **a:** the **peritoneum,** a double-layered smooth membrane of connective tissue.

18. **b**

19. The abdomen is divided into imaginary quadrants. The umbilicus (navel) serves as the central reference point. The diaphragm is the top of the abdominal cavity and the pelvic bones, the bottom. The quadrants are divided by a set of imaginary perpendicular lines intersecting at the umbilicus. The major organs in each quadrant are **right upper quadrant (RUQ)**—liver, gallbladder, part of the large intestine, right kidney; **left upper quadrant (LUQ)**—stomach, spleen, pancreas, part of the large intestine, left kidney; **right lower quadrant (RLQ)**—appendix, part of the large intestine, right ovary, right ureter, uterus, urinary bladder; **left lower quadrant (LLQ)**—part of the large intestine, left ovary, left ureter, uterus, urinary bladder.

20. Answers to crossword puzzle

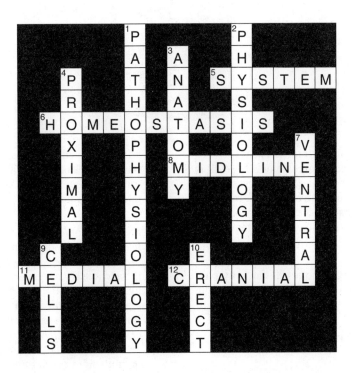

21. **a**

22. **b:** Smaller molecules such as water diffuse *more easily* than do larger molecules such as protein. *Water* is the one molecule allowed to pass freely back and forth across the cell membrane. Electrolytes, on the other hand, *may have difficulty* passing through the membrane because of their electrical charge.

23. **a. Diffusion:** movement of particles from an area of higher concentration to one of lower concentration until the substances scatter themselves evenly throughout an available space; **b. Facilitated diffusion:** requires the assistance of a helper protein; **c. Osmosis:** occurs when water moves from an area of lesser solute concentration to an area of higher solute concentration.

24. The direction particles move during diffusion

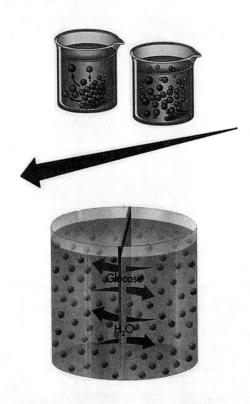

25. **d:** This energy is obtained from a chemical substance called adenosine triphosphate or ATP. ATP is produced in the mitochondria (located inside each cell) from nutrients and is capable of releasing energy that in turn enables the cell to work. The other processes are *passive*—they *do not* require the expenditure of energy.

26. **a:** Glucose, being a larger molecule, can only pass through the cell membrane with the assistance of the hormone insulin.

27. **A. hypotonic; B. isotonic; C. hypertonic**

28. **d:** Solutions are described by their tonicity (the number of particles present per unit volume). An isotonic solution has an osmotic pressure **equal to that within the cell.** This means that solutions are equal on both sides of the cell membrane. Examples of isotonic IV solutions are 0.9% (normal) saline and lactated Ringer's solution.

29. **a:** A hypotonic solution **has an osmotic pressure less than that of normal bodily fluids,** will be *drawn out of the vascular space* when administered intravenously, and has *more solvent than solutes*. A hypertonic solution has an osmotic pressure greater than that of normal body fluids. When the concentration of a given solute is greater on one side of the cell membrane than the other it draws water into the solution until the solute-to-solution ratio is equal on both sides (even though the volumes differ).

30. **b**

31. The arrows below show the direction water moves across a semipermeable membrane. In osmosis, water (the solvent) moves across a semipermeable membrane from an area of lesser solute concentration to an area of greater solute concentration.

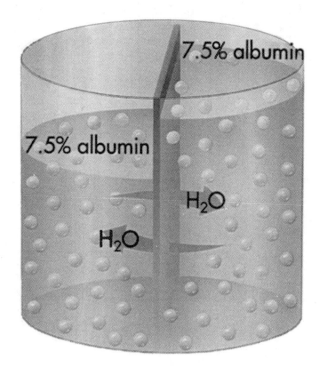

32. **b**

33. **d**

34. *Metabolism* is the **combination of all chemical processes that take place in the body resulting in growth, generation of energy, elimination of wastes, and other bodily functions.**

35. **False:** The *Krebs cycle* yields more ATP stores than does glycolysis.

36. **c**

37. **b**

38. Cellular respiration takes place in the **mitochondria** of the cells.

39. Answers to crossword puzzle

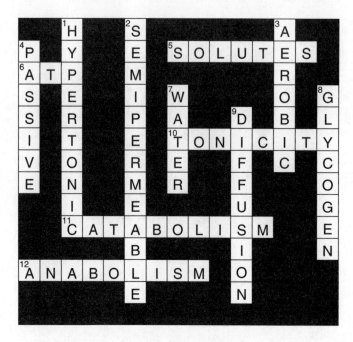

40. The four types of tissue are **epithelial, connective, muscle,** and **nerve.**

41. **a:** Epithelial tissue **covers all external surfaces of the body** and **lines the hollow organs,** provides a protective barrier and aids in the absorption of food (in the intestines), and secretes various body substances (in the sweat glands). *Connective tissue* binds other types of tissues together. Types of *connective tissue* include bone, cartilage, and adipose (fat) tissue. Muscle tissue contracts, leading to movement of body structures. Nerve tissue includes the brain, spinal cord, and all the nerves that pass from these to various parts of the body. *Nerves* generate and transmit impulses throughout the body that control all bodily processes.

42. Three major layers of skin

Layer	Location	Contains
Epidermis	Outermost layer of skin	Rich in hair (in many locations), openings from sweat and oil glands; also contains some blood vessels and nerves
Dermis	A thick layer that lies below the epidermis	Connective tissue, hair follicles, glands, nerve endings (for temperature, touch, pain, and pressure), most nerves, and blood vessels
Subcutaneous	Lies below the skin (epidermis and dermis)	Attaches the skin to the underlying bone or muscle; contains much of the body's fat stores

43. **d**

44. **c**

45. The skeletal system **provides the body's framework; protects internal organs and, with muscles, enables movement; serves as a storage site for minerals, particularly calcium; and has a role in the formation of certain blood cells.**

46. **a**

47. **c**

48. The skeletal system is divided into two major components, the **axial skeleton** and the **appendicular skeleton.** The axial skeleton runs the length of the torso. Attached to the axial skeleton is the appendicular skeleton, which consists of the **extremities**—the arms and legs—as well as the **girdles,** or bony belts that attach the limbs to the body.

    A. parietal bone
    B. occipital bone
    C. cervical vertebrae
    D. thoracic vertebrae
    E. ribs
    F. lumbar vertebrae
    G. coccyx
    H. clavicle
    I. scapula
    J. humerus
    K. coxal (hip) bone
    L. ulna
    M. radius
    N. sacrum
    O. carpals
    P. metacarpals
    Q. phalanges
    R. femur
    S. tibia
    T. fibula
    U. tarsals
    V. metatarsals
    W. phalanges
    X. frontal bone
    Y. skull
    Z. orbit
    AA. nasal bone
    BB. maxilla
    CC. mandible
    DD. sternum

49. **a**

50. **c:** There are **7** cervical vertebrae in the neck; 12 thoracic vertebrae in the posterior chest; 5 lumbar vertebrae in the lower back; 5 sacral vertebrae, fused into a platelike bone, the sacrum, that forms the posterior portion of the pelvic bone; and 4 vertebrae fused into the coccyx, or tailbone, which is attached to the lower portion of the sacrum.

51. **False:** The first vertebra directly beneath the skull is called the *atlas* (C1) and supports the head. The *next* vertebra, C2, is known as the axis and is the point at which the head turns. The remaining cervical vertebrae are simply numbered C3 through C7 and have no special names.

52. **False:** Twelve pairs of ribs form the rib cage. Each is attached to a thoracic vertebra posteriorly. The upper 10 pairs attach directly to the sternum, or breastbone. The remaining 2 pairs of ribs, called floating ribs, are held in place by cartilage.

53. **b**

54. **d**

55. **d:** The acetabulum is the **socket of the hip bone.** Other terms include *patella:* knee cap; *ischium:* inferior, posterior portion of the pelvis; *ilium:* superior bone of the pelvis that contains the iliac crest.

56. **a: Cartilages:** plates of shiny connective tissue that aid movement (of the joints). b. **Tendons:** connect muscles to bones. **c: Joints:** where two or more bones articulate (meet). **d. Ligaments:** tough white bands of tissue that bind joints together, connecting bone and cartilage.

57. **immovable:** joints that normally allow no motion between bones; **slightly movable:** allow only a small amount of movement between bones; **freely movable:** allow a wide variety of movement between bones.

58. **a**

59. Three types of muscle are **skeletal, cardiac,** and **smooth muscle.**

60. Answers to crossword puzzle

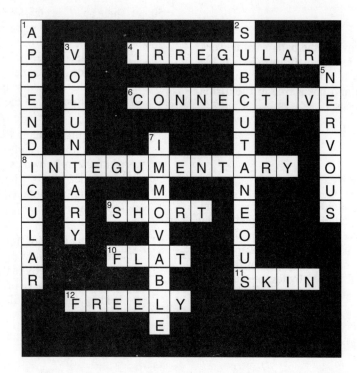

61. The nervous system is an **extensive network of cells that conducts information that controls and coordinates all the functions of the body.**

62. The nervous system is divided into two parts: the **central** nervous system, and the **peripheral** nervous system.

63. **a. Cell body:** main part of the neuron containing the nucleus and surrounding tissues; **b. Synapse:** the region surrounding the point of contact between two neurons or between a neuron and its effector organ; **c. Axon:** cylinder-like extension of a neuron that carries impulses away from the cell body; **d. Dendrite:** branching process that extends from the cell body of a neuron.

64. **Sensory** nerves transmit nerve impulses toward the spinal cord and the brain. **Motor** nerves transmit impulses from the brain and the spinal cord to the muscles and glands.

65. d

66. Depolarization occurs **when sodium and calcium move inward while potassium moves into the fluid surrounding the cell.** It occurs quickly and results in the interior of the cell becoming less negatively charged (i.e., more positive) than during the resting state.

67. **a. Cerebrum:** top portion of the brain that consists of the left and right hemispheres; controls thinking, sensation, and voluntary movement; **b. Cerebellum:** its primary function is to control the body's coordination; **c. Medulla:** most inferior portion of the brain; is part of the brainstem; contains important centers that control involuntary respiration, heart, and blood vessel function.

68. **True**

69. **False:** The spinal cord *receives* motor nerve impulses *from the brain* and transmits them to the body, causing muscles to contract and movement to occur.

70. **False:** The brain and spinal cord are covered by three layers of *membranes known as meninges.*

71. **a:** The outer meningeal layer is called the **dura mater.** The *middle* layer is called the arachnoid membrane, and the *inner* layer, which is closely adherent to the brain tissue, the pia mater.

72. **a:** Cerebrospinal fluid **circulates between the pia mater and the arachnoid in the subarachnoid space.** It fills and protects the cranial and spinal cavities, cushioning the brain and spinal cord. Cerebrospinal fluid is normally *clear* and is produced *in* the brain. In the adult there is normally about 140 mL of CSF.

73. The **autonomic nervous system** is a specialized subdivision of the peripheral nervous system that regulates involuntary functions of the body. Examples include activity of the heart and smooth muscle.

74. There are **two** divisions of the autonomic nervous system—the **sympathetic** and the **parasympathetic** nervous systems.

75. **d:** Stimulation of the parasympathetic nervous system causes **slowing of the heart rate.** In contrast, stimulation of the *sympathetic* nervous system causes constriction of blood vessels, elevation of the blood pressure and heart rate, and a feeling of nervousness.

76. Answers to crossword puzzle

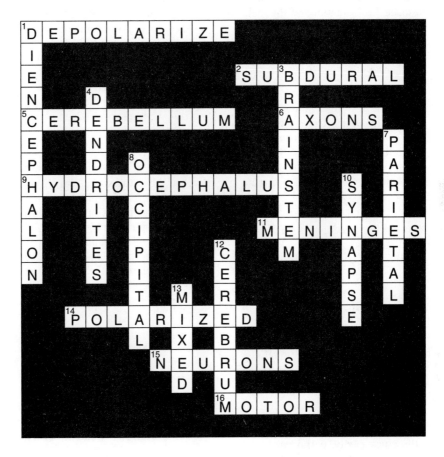

77. **a. Pituitary:** located in base of the skull, regulates all other endocrine glands; **b. Adrenal:** hormones produced include adrenaline; **c. Pancreas:** regulates glucose metabolism and other functions; hormones produced include insulin; **d. Ovary:** regulates sexual function, characteristics, and reproduction; located in the female pelvis.

78. These endocrine glands secrete **proteins,** called **hormones,** directly into the blood.

79. An example of a negative feedback mechanism is as follows: **In response to a lack of or too much of something, hormones are produced and released into the bloodstream. On achieving the desired result, "feedback" is sent to the hypothalamus, causing it to cease production of further stimulating factors. The hypothalamus may also secrete inhibitory factors that terminate pituitary gland production of "stimulating factors."**

80. Hormones **regulate many body functions, such as growth, reproduction, temperature, metabolism, and blood pressure.**

81. **c:** Although insulin and glucagon have opposite effects, both function to maintain a normal blood sugar (glucose) level. Insulin causes the blood glucose to decrease because it causes absorption of glucose into the cells. **Glucagon, on the other hand, causes adrenergic stimulation, leading to an increase in the blood sugar level.**

82. Norepinephrine is the most common **sympathetic neurotransmitter.** It is closely related to epinephrine (adrenaline), **which also functions as a sympathetic branch neurotransmitter.**

83. **b:** The adult male has about **5 to 6** L of blood. This amounts to approximately 10 to 12 pints.

84. **a. Plasma:** pale, straw-colored fluid; **b. Platelets:** small cells that, when ruptured, release chemical factors needed to form blood clots; **c. White blood cells:** also called leukocytes; involved in destroying germs and producing substances called antibodies that help the body resist infection; **d. Red blood cells:** also called erythrocytes; carry oxygen to the tissues.

85. **d**

86. White blood cells (leukocytes) fight infection and help eliminate foreign materials from the body. There are five types of leukocytes: **a. Eosinophils and basophils:** important in allergic reactions; **b. Neutrophils:** fight bacterial infections; **c. Lymphocytes and monocytes:** help eliminate viruses and fungal infections.

87. If the body's blood-clotting mechanisms fail, the patient will not be able to form blood clots. Because of this, bleeding will likely continue, and serious blood loss can result.

88. The primary components of the circulatory system are the **heart, blood vessels, and blood.**

89. **c:** The heart is **located behind the sternum;** it is a muscular, *cone*-shaped organ about the size of a *closed fist.* Further, *roughly two thirds of the heart* lies in the left side of the chest cavity.

90. **d:** The pericardizal sac **allows the heart to contract smoothly within the chest cavity.** If fluid or blood accumulates in the sac as a result of injury or illness, it can impede contraction of the heart muscle, and cardiac output is compromised. This condition is called cardiac tamponade and can be life threatening.

91. A. superior vena cava
    B. aortic semilunar valve
    C. pulmonary semilunar valve
    D. right atrium
    E. tricuspid valve
    F. papillary muscles
    G. inferior vena cava
    H. right ventricle
    I. left ventricle
    J. bicuspid valve
    K. left atrium
    L. pulmonary veins
    M. pulmonary arteries
    N. aorta

92. **a:** The left ventricle of the heart **pumps oxygen-rich blood to the cells** and is the *strongest and largest* of the four cardiac chambers (because it must pump blood through thousands of miles of arterial blood vessels).

93. **a**

94. Blood moving from the right atrium to the right ventricle passes through the **tricuspid** valve. As the blood moves from the right ventricle to the pulmonary artery it passes through the **pulmonic** valve. Blood moving from the left atrium to the left ventricle passes through the **mitral** valve. As the blood moves from the left ventricle into the aorta it passes through the **aortic** valve.

95. **a**

96. The right main coronary artery—the nodal artery—supplies **the sinoatrial [SA] node**; the descending right artery supplies the **anterior right ventricle**; and the posterior descending artery supplies the **posterior heart wall.**
    The left main coronary artery—left anterior descending artery—supplies the anterior wall of the left ventricle; the diagonal artery usually supplies the lateral left ventricular wall; and the circumflex artery usually supplies the superior left ventricle.

97. Deoxygenated venous blood from the heart drains into **five** different coronary veins that empty into the right atrium via the **coronary sinus.**

98. The cardiac cycle is the **repetitive pumping process of blood that begins with the onset of cardiac muscle contraction and ends with the beginning of the next contraction.**

99. **a**

100. **b:** The first heart sound **is referred to as the "lub."** It is caused by vibrations resulting from the sudden closure of the mitral and tricuspid valves at the start of ventricular systole.

101. **a**

102. A. SA node
     B. intraatrial conductive pathways
     C. AV node
     D. bundle of His
     E. right bundle branch
     F. left bundle branch
     G. Purkinje fibers

103. **1:** The electrical impulse originates in the **sinus node** (high in the right atrium).

   2: It then travels throughout the atria via the **intra-atrial pathways**.

   3: It reaches the **atrioventricular node** (AV node), where there is a slight delay in conduction of the impulse.

   4: It then passes into the **bundle of His**.

   5: Next, the impulse passes through the **right and left bundle branches**.

   6: Finally, the impulse travels through the very small **Purkinje fibers** to the individual ventricular myocardial cells.

104. Illustration of the factors affecting cardiac output

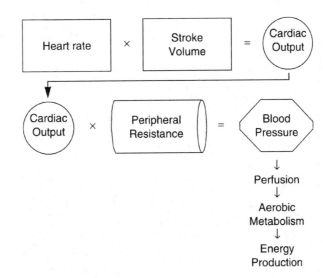

105. **c:** Control of the heart's rate and strength of contraction comes partially from the brain, via the *autonomic* nervous system, from **hormones of the endocrine system,** and from the heart tissue.

106. **Baroreceptors** respond to changes in pressure, usually within the heart or the main arteries. **Chemoreceptors** sense changes in the chemical composition of the blood.

107. If the heart is stretched, the muscle contracts **harder.**

108. **d**

109. **a. Arteries:** blood vessels that carry blood away from the heart to the body; **b. Veins:** transport blood from the body back to the heart; **c. Arterioles:** small branches of an artery; **d. Capillaries:** microscopic thin-walled vessels.

110. **Oxygen, carbon dioxide, and other nutrients and waste products are exchanged** in the capillaries.

111. **c**

112. **d**

113. The main pulmonary artery branches to each lung. In the lungs **the blood is oxygenated and waste products are removed.**

114. **c**

115. **a**

116. **a:** They may be used as a cannulation site, particularly when the peripheral veins of the arm are not available.

117. Blood pressure is **the pressure exerted by the circulating blood on the walls of the arteries, the veins, and the chambers of the heart.**

118. **c**

119. **False:** The body tissues are bathed in a plasmalike fluid called *lymph.*

120. **False:** Lymph comes from excess cellular fluid and circulates through the body in thin-walled lymph vessels that travel close to the major *veins.*

121. **True**

122. The immune system **defends the body against bacteria, viruses, and other foreign matter.**

123. **d:** Chemicals such as histamine work by **promoting inflammation in response to foreign invaders in the body.** *Mechanical barriers, such as the skin, prevent the entry of many bacteria. White blood cells (leukocytes)* ingest and destroy bacterial invaders and foreign matter.

124. **d**

125. Answers to crossword puzzle

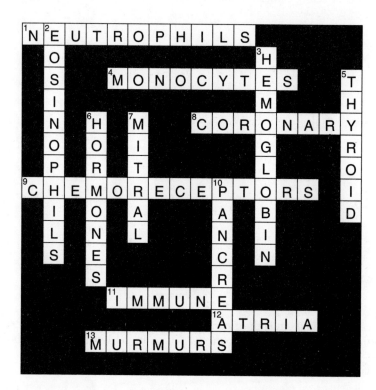

126. The function of the respiratory system is to **bring oxygen into the body and excrete carbon dioxide.**

127. **a. Oropharynx:** inside of the mouth posterior to the tongue leading to the throat; **b. Nasopharynx:** area between the nasal passages and the oropharynx; *c. Epiglottis:* flap of tissue that covers the glottic opening of the trachea when swallowing or gagging takes place; **d. Larynx:** voice box that holds the vocal cords and the glottic opening to the trachea; **e. Trachea:** tube in the front of the throat that carries air into the lungs.

128. A. nasal cavity
  B. nasopharynx
  C. oropharynx
  D. epiglottis
  E. larynx
  F. trachea
  G. bronchus
  H. lungs
  I. alveolus
  J. pulmonary capillaries

129. **c:** The alveoli are **tiny sacs of lung tissue where gas exchange takes place.** Each is about *0.3* mm in diameter, surrounded by *capillaries,* and the most *distal* portion of the respiratory tree.

130. **b:** The lungs are covered with two connective tissue membranes known as the pleura. These membranes envelop each lung and line the inner borders of the rib cage, or pleural cavity. The membrane closer to the lung is referred to as the visceral pleura. The membrane that lines the thoracic cavity is called the **parietal pleura.** There is a potential space between the visceral and parietal pleura, known as the pleural space. Normally the two membranes are close together and a space does not exist, other than a small amount of lubricating fluid.

131. The right lung consists of **three** lobes, whereas the left lung has **two** lobes.

132. The process of inhalation occurs when **the diaphragm and intercostal muscles contract, creating a negative pressure in the chest cavity. This negative pressure "sucks" in air, expanding the lungs.**

133. **c**

134. **d**

135. Inspired air contains about **21%** oxygen, whereas expired air contains about **16%** oxygen.

136. Oxygen goes from the alveolus to the hemoglobin molecule of the red blood cell. Carbon dioxide flows from the blood into the alveolus. When an individual exhales, carbon dioxide is breathed into the atmosphere and eliminated from the body.

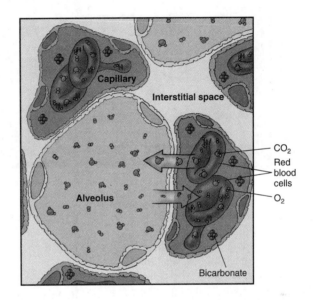

137. **b**

138. **d**

139. **a: Excess levels of carbon dioxide** stimulate breathing, whereas decreased levels slow it. The brain also responds to levels of oxygen in the blood, but in a far less predictable fashion than its response to carbon dioxide.

140. Answers to crossword puzzle

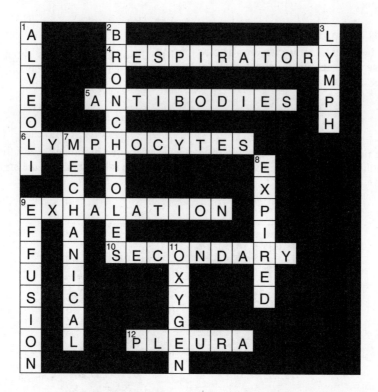

141. **a. Small intestine:** where chemical digestion is completed and absorption of foods takes place; **b. Appendix:** hollow fingerlike projection situated at the beginning of the large intestine (it has no proven function); **c. Large intestine:** where the collection and removal of wastes from the digestive system occur (includes the colon, rectum, and anus); **d. Gallbladder:** pear-shaped reservoir for bile, located on the posterior undersurface of the liver; **e. Stomach:** where the initial chemical breakdown of food begins, producing a semisolid substance called *chyme*.

142. **d:** Hollow abdominal organs include the *esophagus,* stomach, small intestine, large intestine, appendix, and gallbladder. *Solid organs* include the liver, *spleen, pancreas, and kidneys.*

143. **a. Kidneys:** filter blood, excrete body wastes in the form of urine, and are important in the regulation of the body's fluid balance and blood pressure; **b. Ureters:** thick-walled, hollow tubes that carry urine from the kidneys to the urinary bladder; **c. Urethra:** hollow, tubular structure that drains urine from the bladder, passing it to the outside; **d. Urinary bladder:** hollow, muscular sac in the midline of the lower abdominal area that stores urine until it is excreted.

145. A. ovary
     B. fallopian tube
     C. vagina
     D. cervix
     E. uterus

145. **False:** Water is the *most abundant* substance in the human body. The average adult has a total body water content of approximately 50% to 60% of body weight. In a newly born, total body water may be as high as 75% to 80% total body weight.

146. **True**

147. **True:** These solutes can be classified as either electrolytes or nonelectrolytes.

148. a. intravascular fluid (4.5%) red
     b. interstitial fluid (10.5%) blue
     c. intracellular fluid (40% to 45%) green

149. **c**

150. **d:** Extracellular fluid (outside the cells) makes up *15% of the body weight and approximately 25% of the body fluids.*

151. **b:** The body's water **distribution in the three body compartments remains relatively constant.** Water coming into the body is referred to as intake, whereas water that is excreted from the body is referred to as output. To maintain relative homeostasis, *intake must equal output.* Input and output averages 2500 mL each day. Antidiuretic hormone (ADH), secreted by the pituitary gland, causes the kidney tubules to *reabsorb* more water into the blood and excrete less urine.

152. When the fluid volume decreases, the pituitary gland secretes antidiuretic hormone (ADH). **ADH causes the kidney tubules to reabsorb more water into the blood and excrete less urine. This action allows fluid volume in the body to build up.**

153. **b:** Thirst **helps regulate fluid intake.** The sensation of thirst occurs when body fluids become *decreased,* stimulating the person to take in more fluids. Conversely, when too many fluids enter the body, the kidneys are activated and more urine is excreted, thus eliminating the excess fluid. The body also maintains fluid balance by shifting water from one compartment to another.

154. **a. Acid:** substance that increases the concentration of hydrogen ions in a water solution; when in greater concentration it lowers the pH; **b. Base:** substance that decreases the concentration of hydrogen ions; when in greater concentration it increases the pH; **c. pH:** mathematical expression of hydrogen ion concentration.

155. **b:** The acid-base balance of the body is highly dynamic. It varies because of wide fluctuations in the intake of and production of acids. The body depends on three principal lines of defense that work to maintain this narrow range of pH, including (from fast to slowest) **buffer systems, lungs,** and **kidneys.** These key body systems must continually readjust to maintain acid-base balance.

156. **a. Buffer system:** provides almost immediate protection against changes in the hydrogen ion concentration of the extracellular fluid; acts as a chemical sponge, absorbing H^+ ions when they are in excess and donating H^+ ions when they are depleted; **b. Respiratory system:** regulates the concentration of carbon dioxide and subsequently the amount of carbonic acid (H_2CO_3) in the body; **c. Renal system:** excretes hydrogen ions and forms bicarbonate ions in specific amounts as indicated by the pH of the blood.

157. **b:** One side of the buffering system uses a weak base to convert a strong acid to a weak acid. The buffer used to convert metabolic acids into "weak acids" is **bicarbonate.**

158. **c: H_2CO_3 (carbonic acid)** is produced by the metabolic acid–buffering process. The carbonic acid can then further dissociate to release water (H_2O) and carbon dioxide (CO_2).

159.

$$H^+ + HCO_3^- \leftrightarrow H_2CO_3 \leftrightarrow H_2O + CO_2$$

(strong acid) **(bicarbonate)** (weak acid) (water) **(carbon dioxide)**

160. Equation showing the changes that occur with increased breathing.

$$\uparrow \text{breathing} \to \downarrow CO_2 \to \downarrow H_2CO_3 \to \downarrow H^+ \to \uparrow pH$$

Increased ventilation decreases carbon dioxide. This leads to a decrease in carbonic acid and hydrogen ions in the blood. The blood pH is therefore increased.

161. Equation showing the changes that occur with decreased breathing.

$$\downarrow \text{breathing} \to \uparrow CO_2 \to \uparrow H_2CO_3 \to \uparrow H^+ \to \downarrow pH$$

Decreased ventilation increases carbon dioxide. This leads to an increase in carbonic acid and hydrogen ions in the blood. The blood pH is therefore decreased.

Patients who are not breathing or breathing inadequately are most likely to be acidotic because of an inadequate removal of CO_2. In these cases, treatment must be directed to improving ventilation.

162. **a:** When the plasma pH decreases (becomes more acidic), hydrogen ions (acid) are excreted, and bicarbonate ions (base) are formed and retained. Conversely, when the plasma pH increases (becomes more alkaline), hydrogen ions are retained in the body, and bicarbonate ions are excreted.

163. **a:** The pH of the human body is normally slightly alkaline, about **7.35 to 7.45.**

164. **d:** A pH of the body fluid greater than **7.45** is considered alkalosis, whereas a pH less than 7.35 is referred to as acidosis.

165. **b:** In addition to *increasing* the blood CO_2 level and *decreasing* the blood pH, this creates a carbonic acid excess in the body. Hypoventilation (decreased respiration) is its general cause. Two major conditions that cause hypoventilation are central nervous system depression and obstructive lung disease. Morphine poisoning and anesthesia are examples of central nervous system depression, whereas asthma and emphysema are obstructive lung diseases. Treatment is aimed at improving ventilation.

166. **b:** Respiratory acidosis occurs when the exhalation of CO_2 is inhibited. This leads to a *decrease* in the pH. The $PaCO_2$ may be normal or decreased (because of hyperventilation). Starvation, renal impairment, and diabetes mellitus are among the conditions that flood the plasma with acid metabolites. Treatment is aimed at eliminating CO_2 by ventilation. In severe cases, the administration of a bicarbonate, such as sodium bicarbonate, may be required.

167. **a. Respiratory acidosis:** a 19-year-old who has taken an overdose of sleeping pills and is breathing 6 breaths/min; **b. Respiratory alkalosis:** a 30-year-old who is experiencing "hyperventilation syndrome" brought on by an argument; **c. Metabolic acidosis:** a 39-year-old diabetic patient who is suffering from diabetic ketoacidosis; **d. Metabolic alkalosis:** a 53-year-old who has been ingesting excessive baking soda to relieve indigestion.

168. Answers to crossword

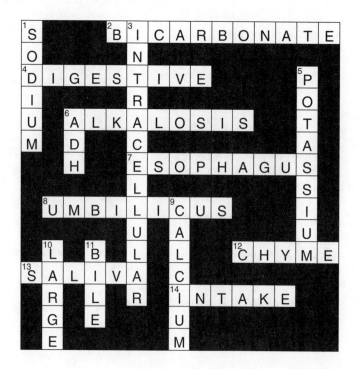

CHAPTER 5

1. A drug is **any substance that, when taken into the body, changes one or more of the body's functions.** Pharmacology is **the study of drugs, their actions, dosages, and side effects.** Pharmaceutical companies are required to list the chemical compound, actions, dosages, side effects, indications, and contraindications of the drugs they manufacture.

2. Drug terms with descriptions: **a. Trade:** name is registered by the U.S. Patent Office and has the office mark of the patent office after its name (symbol ®); **b. Chemical:** compound makeup; **c. Official:** name listed in the *United States Pharmacopeia (USP)*; **d. Generic:** name assigned to a drug before it becomes officially listed.

3.

Generic Name	Trade Name
Lidocaine	**Lidocaine HCl**
Nitroglycerin	**Nitro-Bid**
Diazepam	**Valium**

4. **c:** Furosemide is a **generic** name. A trade name for furosemide is Lasix.

5. Acts with descriptions: **a. Pure Food and Drug Act of 1906:** enacted to prevent the manufacture and trafficking of mislabeled, poisonous, or harmful food and drugs; **b. Harrison Narcotic Act of 1914:** the first federal legislation designed to stop drug addiction or dependence; *c. Controlled Substances Act of 1970:* regulates the manufacture and distribution of drugs whose use may result in dependency; **d. Federal Food, Drug, and Cosmetic Act of 1938:** requires that labels be used to list the possible habit-forming properties and side effects of drugs.

6. **a**

7. Drug schedules with descriptions and examples

Schedule	Description	Example
I	Have the highest potential for abuse and have no currently accepted medical use in the United States	Heroin, marijuana, LSD, peyote, and mescaline
II	Have a high potential for abuse; these drugs have a current accepted medicinal use in the United States but with severe restrictions	Morphine, codeine, Seconal, cocaine, amphetamines, Dilaudid, and Ritalin
III	Have a limited potential for psychological or physiological dependence	Paregoric, Tylenol with codeine, and Fiorinal
IV	Have a lower potential for abuse than those in schedules II and III	Librium, Valium, Darvon, and Phenobarbital
V	Have a lower potential for abuse than those in schedules I, II, III, and IV	Lomotil, Dimetane expectorant-DC, and Robitussin-DAC

8. **b**

9. **c**

10. **c:** The majority of drugs on the market today are synthetically derived. Three other sources of drugs include animals, plants, and minerals. *Insulin,* commonly used in the management of diabetes, is prepared from the pancreas of cows and pigs, whereas *mineral* drugs, such as sodium bicarbonate and calcium chloride, are derived from inorganic sources. Until the early 1900s most drugs came from medicinal plants. Today, drugs are still derived from different plant parts, including dried bark, roots, leaves, flowers, and seeds.

11. **a**

12. Sources with various drugs: **a. Plant:** atropine, digitalis, morphine; **b. Animal:** insulin, oxytocin; **c. Mineral:** iodine, calcium; **d. Synthetic:** lidocaine.

13. Two drugs derived from microorganisms are **penicillin** and **streptomycin**.

14. The three categories of drugs are **body system, class of agent,** and **mechanism of action.**

15. - The *Physicians' Desk Reference (PDR)* is widely used as a reference for drugs in current use. It contains such information as a drug's indications, therapeutic effects, dosages, administration, warnings, contraindications, precautions, side effects and drug interactions, and photographs of various drugs.
    - *American Hospital Formulary Service (AHFS)* is distributed to practicing physicians and contains concise information that is arranged according to drug classifications.
    - *Compendium of Drug Therapy* is published annually and is distributed to practicing physicians. It includes photographs of the drugs and telephone numbers of major pharmaceutical companies and poison control centers. It also includes copies of some package inserts.
    - *American Medical Association Drug Evaluation.* Drugs are evaluated according to the American Medical Association's standards.
    - *Drug inserts.* These are found in all drug packages. They supply detailed information about the drug. Many drug inserts contain the same information that is contained in the *PDR.*
    - The *United States Pharmacopeia (USP)* is two paperback volumes providing drug information for the health care provider. It defines drugs with respect to sources, chemistry, physical properties, tests to identity, storage, and dosage. It also provides directions for compounding and general use.

16. **b**

17. **True**

18. **False:** During pregnancy the metabolism in the liver is *delayed,* and the rate of drug excretion may be increased because of the *increased* cardiac output that occurs.

19. **True**

20. Drugs that are **ingested, inhaled,** or absorbed by the mother have the potential to harm the fetus by crossing the **placenta** or through **lactation.**

21. The Food and Drug Administration has established a scale, with categories **A, B, C, D,** and **X,** to indicate drugs that may have documented problems in animals or humans during pregnancy.

22. **a**

23. **Infants have immature livers and kidneys, so it is difficult for them to metabolize and eliminate the same dosages of drugs as adults.**

24. **As people age they experience an increase in percentage body fat, a decrease in lean body mass, and a decrease in total body water. Drugs that are adjusted according to body weight appear in significantly higher concentration in a 70-year-old patient than in a 30-year-old patient.**

25. **Renal function and renal blood flow both decrease with age. Blood flow through the liver also declines with age, particularly in the presence of congestive heart failure. The liver also decreases in size. Because most drugs are eliminated through the kidneys or metabolized by the liver, drug clearance in elderly persons is adversely affected. Drugs like digoxin, lidocaine, and lithium, which have a narrow therapeutic index, must be administered in decreased dosages as a patient ages.**

26. Proper procedures for using drug therapy: **Use correct precautions and techniques. Observe and document the effects of drugs. Keep your knowledge base current with changes and trends in pharmacology. Establish and maintain professional relationships. Understand pharmacology. Perform evaluations to identify drug indications and contraindications. Seek drug reference literature. Take a drug history from the patient, including prescribed medications (name, strength, and daily dosage), over-the-counter medications, vitamins, herbal preparations, and drug reactions. Consult with medical control.**

27. Features of the parasympathetic and sympathetic systems

Feature	Parasympathetic	Sympathetic
Other name	**Cholinergic**	**Adrenergic**
Neurotransmitter	**Acetylcholine**	**Norepinephrine, epinephrine**
Primary nerve(s)	**Vagus**	**Nerves from the thoracic and lumbar ganglia**
Stimulating drug(s)	**Reserpine**	**Isoproterenol, norepinephrine, epinephrine, dopamine**
Blocking drug(s)	**Atropine**	**Propranolol**

28. **b:** Stimulation of the beta-1 receptors will cause **increased heart rate,** *increased contractility,* and *increased automaticity.*

29. **b:** Effects of beta-2 receptor stimulation include **bronchodilation.**

30. **d**

31. **a:** Stimulation of the parasympathetic nervous system results in **decreased heart rate** and *decreased AV conduction velocity.*

32. **d**

33. Their effects on bodily **functions** commonly categorize drugs.

34. All drugs cause cellular change, which is their **drug action**, and a degree of physiological change, which is their **drug effect.**

35. **True**

36. **False:** Drugs generally *exert multiple actions* rather than a single effect.

37. **False:** Drugs do not confer any new functions on a tissue or organ; they *only modify existing functions.*

38. **b**

39. **b:** Tablets will usually dissolve high in the gastrointestinal tract.

40. Answers to crossword puzzle

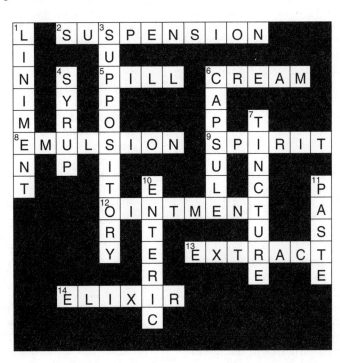

41. **c:** The digestive system is referred to as the enteral system. Therefore the **p.o.** drug administration route is not a parenteral route. Intramuscular, subcutaneous, intravascular, and endotracheal routes are referred to as parenteral because they are outside the digestive tract. Parenteral preparations must be sterile because they are introduced directly into the body.

42. Characteristics of medication administration: **a. Intradermal:** medication is injected into the dermal layer of the skin; **b. Transdermal:** medication is placed on the skin, where it is absorbed; **c. Intravenous:** medication is administered directly into a vein; **d. Endotracheal:** medication is absorbed through the pulmonary capillaries of the lungs; **e. Intramuscular:** medication is injected into the muscle tissue; **f. Subcutaneous:** medication is injected into the fatty tissue underneath the skin that overlies the muscle; **g. Sublingual:** medication is absorbed into the vast capillary network directly under the tongue.

43. **b**

44. Five reasons for administering drugs by a certain route: **may be administered by only one route; may be toxic if given by a particular route; may not be effective if given by a certain route; may be given for either their local or systemic effects; and can be absorbed only by a certain route.**

45. **b**

46. **c**

47. Terms with descriptions: **a. Distribution:** refers to the manner in which a drug is transported by the bloodstream to various areas of the body; **b. Biotransformation:** the physical and chemical alterations that a drug undergoes within the blood; **c. Excretion:** the process in which drugs are removed from the body in either their original form or as metabolites; **d. Absorption:** the process involved in transferring drug molecules from the place where they are deposited in the body to their movement through the capillary walls and into the bloodstream.

48. Factors affecting drug absorption: **nature of the absorbing surface; blood flow to the site of administration; solubility of the drug; pH; drug concentration; dosage form; routes of administration; and bioavailability.**

49. Diffusion: **the constant movement of molecules from an area of higher to an area of lower concentration;** osmosis: **the physical property that allows water to proceed from one side of a membrane to another;** and filtration: **the movement through a pressure gradient of a liquid that prevents some or all of the substances in the liquid from passing through.**

50. **d**

51. **False:** *Almost* all drugs are capable of crossing the placenta from the mother to the fetus except a few drugs with large molecules.

52. **False:** The most vulnerable time for drug-induced birth defects is the *first* trimester, when fetal organs are developing. During the third trimester any drugs taken may have a residual effect on the fetus.

53. **True**

54. **c:** Drug tolerance has to do with an improved ability of the liver to metabolize a given drug. The problem that develops is that there is less drug available to contact the receptors, and higher doses are needed to achieve the same physiological effect as previously experienced.

55. **a**

56. **d:** Elderly people have *slower* metabolic processes that extend the breakdown and excretion times in these patients.

57. **Women and men have different reactions to some drugs because of different body compositions and hormone levels. A woman's hematocrit (concentration of red blood cells per unit of volume) measurements are lower than a man's. Men have a lower proportion of subcutaneous fat than women. Men and women also have differences in the proportion of water volume per body weight. A woman's ability to receive medication is affected by pregnancy and considerations of the medication's effect on an unborn fetus. The use of some medications by pregnant women may cause birth defects in their children.**

58. **a. Side effect:** an effect that is unintended; **b. Drug allergy:** occurs in a person who has been previously exposed to the drug and has developed antibodies; **c. Idiosyncratic reactions:** an abnormal or unexpected reaction to a drug peculiar to a certain patient; **d. Synergism:** one drug helps the action of another drug to produce an effect that neither produces alone; *e. Cross tolerance:* tolerance that increases to other drugs in the same class; **f. Iatrogenic responses:** administration of many drugs can lead to symptoms that mimic naturally occurring disease states; **g. Drug dependence:** physical state in which withdrawal symptoms occur when a person discontinues use of the drug; **h. Drug toxicity:** results from overdosage, ingestion of a drug intended for external use, or buildup of the drug in the blood because of impaired metabolism or excretion; **i. Cumulative effect:** occurs when a repeat dose of drug is administered before the initial dose(s) is excreted. It is caused by a buildup of the drug in the blood.

59. Answers to crossword puzzle

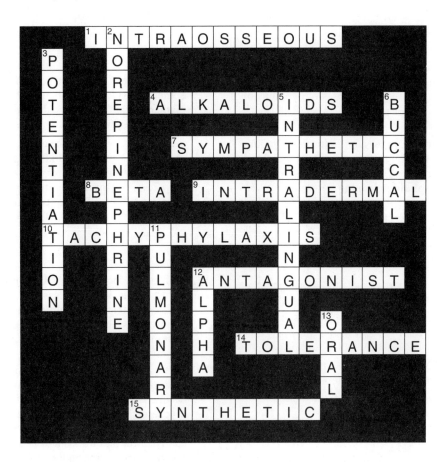

60. Drug interactions may occur **when two or more drugs are taken simultaneously and when one drug increases, decreases, or cancels the effects of the other.** There are many variables that influence drug interaction, such as intestinal absorption, competition for plasma protein binding, drug metabolism or biotransformation, action at the receptor site, renal excretion, and alteration of electrolyte balance.

61. When storing any drug the EMT-I should keep in mind that **drug potency can be affected by temperature, light, moisture, air exposure, and shelf life.** Further, state regulations commonly require that drugs be secured in a locked compartment in the ambulance.

62. **Controlled substances must be locked in a secure box in a locked cabinet in the ambulance. The number of crew members with access to the keys or to the cabinet should be limited. Inventory forms should be kept in the cabinet with the drugs. If controlled substances are administered, records must be maintained separate from the patients' charts and must be readily available for inspection by the authorities of the DEA.**

63. Components of a drug profile: **drug names; body system; class of agent; mechanism of action; drug actions, pharmacokinetics, and indications; contraindications and side effects; dosage; routes of administration; how supplied; and special considerations.**

64. **c**

65. **b:** Amiodarone is an **antidysrhythmic** drug.

66. To treat cardiac arrest, amiodarone is given **IV/IO push** at a dose of **300 mg.**

67. **d**

68. **c: Nervousness** is a side effect of bronchodilators such as albuterol sulfate. Increased myocardial oxygen consumption is another.

69. *Albuterol* works by relaxing bronchial smooth muscle, resulting in bronchodilation.

70. **d**

71. **b**

72. **a**

73. **d:** Atropine is used to **increase the heart rate in life-threatening bradycardia.** This in turn increases the blood pressure in cases of hypotension caused by a slow heart rate.

74. Indications for atropine administration include **symptomatic bradycardia, asystole,** pulseless electrical activity (PEA) where there is a slow rate, and **organophosphate poisoning.**

75. **c**

76. **b**

77. The indications for the administration of 50% dextrose are **hypoglycemia, coma of unknown origin, altered level of consciousness, and seizure of unknown origin.**

78. **False:** Given the amount of glucose present in $D_{50}W$, it can be administered to patients experiencing ketoacidosis without any adverse effects.

79. **True**

80. **True:** Because localized venous irritation may occur with the administration of D_{50}, it should be delivered via a large vein. Because D_{50} is so viscous (thick) it should be administered through a large IV cannula (16 to 18 gauge). Keep this in mind when you are establishing an IV line in patients who are likely to receive $D_{50}W$.

81. To deliver 50 g of $D_{50}W$, you will need to administer **2 prefilled syringes.**

82. **d:** Epinephrine increases myocardial oxygen demand, is a potent alpha and beta *stimulant*, contains *1* mg of medication in 10 mL of normal saline, and is used to convert *fine* ventricular fibrillation to *coarse* ventricular fibrillation.

83. Four indications for epinephrine use include **cardiac arrest (VF, pulseless VT, asystole, PEA); symptomatic bradycardia (after atropine and transcutaneous pacing); acute bronchospasm (bronchiolitis, asthma, chronic obstructive pulmonary disease);** and **anaphylaxis.**

84. **b:** Epinephrine used to treat cardiac arrest is given at a dose of 1.0 mg (1:10,000 dilution), repeated every 3 to 5 minutes. When used in the treatment of asthma and acute anaphylaxis, it is typically administered subcutaneously at a dosage of 0.1 to 0.5 mg (1:1000 dilution).

85. **c**

86. The number of milliliters needed to deliver 0.3 mg of epinephrine (1:1000) subcutaneously is **0.3 mL.** The mathematical formula used to determine this answer is shown below.

    Step 1: Multiply the desired dosage by the volume on hand: 0.3 mg × 1.0 mL = 0.3 mg/mL

    Step 2: Divide the answer obtained in Step 1 by the concentration on hand: 0.3 mg/mL ÷ 1.0 mg = 0.3 mL

87. **c**

88. Indications for the use of lidocaine include **cardiac arrest from VF/pulseless VT, hemodynamically stable ventricular tachycardia,** and **ventricular ectopy.** It is also used following successful conversion of ventricular fibrillation with defibrillation.

89. **False:** Lidocaine *increases* the fibrillation threshold, making it less likely the patient will experience ventricular fibrillation. This is particularly useful in acute myocardial infarction and following defibrillation in which the fibrillation threshold tends to be significantly lower and the patient is prone to deterioration into ventricular fibrillation.

90. **True**

91. **False:** A 75- to 100-mg bolus of lidocaine will typically maintain adequate therapeutic blood levels for *only up to 20 minutes.* Therefore in the patient who has adequate cardiac output, a bolus of lidocaine should be followed by a 1 to 4 mg/min infusion to ensure therapeutic blood levels.

92. **False:** Premature ventricular complexes occurring in conjunction with bradycardia are usually compensatory in nature and should not be suppressed with lidocaine. Instead, the heart rate should be increased with atropine or transcutaneous pacing, followed by dopamine (or epinephrine or isoproterenol) if the atropine fails to resolve the bradycardia. If the PVCs are still present after increasing the heart rate, lidocaine can then be used.

93. **b:** Adverse reactions seen with lidocaine include drowsiness, tremor, and respiratory depression. Other reactions include numbness, confusion, headache, dizziness, restlessness, irritability, seizures, blurred vision, hearing loss, nausea, vomiting, hypotension, bradycardia, cardiovascular collapse, cardiac arrest, dyspnea, rash, urticaria, edema, and swelling.

94. The correct dosage and number of milliliters needed is **84** mg, **4.2** mL. The mathematical formula used to arrive at this answer is shown below.
    Step 1: Divide the weight in pounds by 2.2: 185 pounds ÷ 2.2 = 84 kg
    Step 2: Multiply the weight in kilograms × the prescribed dosage: 84 kg × 1 mg = 84 mg
    Step 3: Multiply the desired dosage × the volume on hand: 84 mg × 5 mL = 420 mg/mL
    Step 4: Divide the answer obtained in Step 3 by the dose on hand: 420 mg/mL ÷ 100 mg = 4.2 mL

95. The drop rate per minute needed to administer 2 mg/min of lidocaine is **30.** The mathematical steps used to determine this drop rate per minute are shown below.
    Step 1: Multiply volume of IV bag × dose desired: 500 mL × 2 mg/min = 1000 mL/mg/min
    Step 2: Convert the drug concentration to a lower unit: 2 g = 2000 mg.
    Step 3: Divide the answer identified in Step 2 by the drug dose on hand: 1000 mL/mg/min ÷ 2000 mg = 0.50 mL/min
    Step 4: Multiply the answer determined in Step 3 by the drop rate of the administration set: 0.50 mL/min × 60 gtt/mL = 30 gtt/min

96. **c:** The trade name for naloxone is **Narcan.** Other trade names are Inotropin (dopamine), Osmitrol (mannitol), and Dobutrex (dobutamine).

97. **Overdoses caused by narcotics or synthetic narcotic agents and acutely depressed levels of responsiveness.**

98. Naloxone may be used to treat overdoses of **Talwin, heroin, paregoric, morphine, and Demerol,** as well as Percodan, Dilaudid, fentanyl, codeine, methadone, Nubain, Stadol, and Darvon.

99. To deliver 2 mg of naloxone, **2 mL** must be administered.

100. **c:** Naloxone can be administered **subcutaneously, intravenously, intramuscularly,** and endotracheally.

101. c

102. **True**

103. **True**

104. **a:** Side effects of nitroglycerin include **throbbing headache**, postural hypotension, tachycardia, collapse, nausea, vomiting, pallor, sweating, flushing, and dizziness.

105. To deliver 0.6 mg of nitroglycerin you would need to administer **2 tablets.**

106. **a:** Furosemide is a loop diuretic, is used to treat *pulmonary edema and congestive heart failure,* and is given *slow* IV push.

107. **a**

108. **Furosemide may exacerbate hypovolemia, precipitate hyperglycemia (because of hemoconcentration), precipitate hypokalemia, and decrease the response to pressors.**

109. A trade name for furosemide is **Lasix.**

110. **b:** Morphine sulfate, a *narcotic,* **elevates the pain threshold,** is used to treat *myocardial infarction and pulmonary edema; it is used for analgesia, especially in patients with burns, or renal colic,* and it *increases* venous capacitance.

111. **True**

112. **False:** Morphine sulfate is usually given *IV* in the field.

113. **Naloxone** should be used to reverse respiratory depression that follows morphine sulfate administration.

114. **Adenocard** is a brand name for adenosine.

115. Adenosine is used to treat **supraventricular tachycardia.**

116. Adenosine is not effective in conversion of **atrial fibrillation, flutter,** or **ventricular tachycardia.**

117. Adenosine may cause **bronchoconstriction** in asthmatic patients.

118. Adenosine **slows conduction time through the AV node, can interrupt reentrant pathways through the AV node, slows the sinus rate, and has a direct effect on supraventricular tissue.**

119. The dosage for adenosine in the adult patient is **6-mg IV bolus as rapidly as possible, followed by flushing the IV line; if rhythm does not convert within 2 minutes, repeat using a 12-mg bolus. May give a third dose at 12 mg 1 to 2 minutes later.**

120. Answers to crossword puzzle

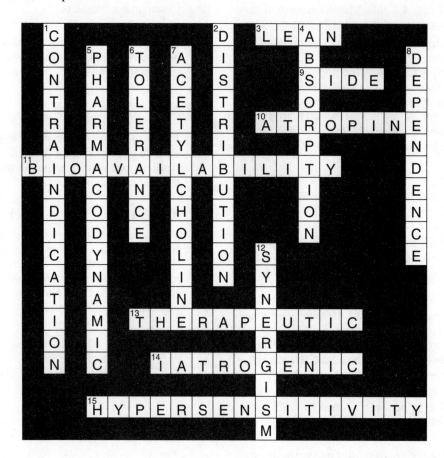

CHAPTER 6

1. **b**

2. **d:** Primary reasons for intravenous cannulation in the prehospital setting include **administering medications,** blood, and/or fluids directly into the circulatory system and to obtain venous blood specimens for laboratory determinations.

3. **False:** Because IV fluids are drugs, permission by on-line medical direction or standing orders is typically *required* for the EMT-I to administer them.

4. **True**

5. Four common indications for IV therapy are **cardiac disease, hypoglycemia, seizures,** and **shock.** As a precautionary measure, an IV can be placed in patients who are in stable condition but whose deterioration is anticipated. This may be for the purpose of medication access, volume replacement, or both.

6. **c**

7. **Giving a drug intravenously places it directly into the bloodstream.** This results in a more rapid onset of action than is achieved through any other administration route.

8. **b:** Contraindications for IV cannulation at a particular site include **burned extremities,** sclerotic veins, areas where an arterial pulse is palpable close to the vein, veins near joints where immobilization will be difficult, or veins near injured areas and edematous extremities. Circulatory problems in an extremity such as dialysis fistula or a history of mastectomy should also prompt the EMT-I to select another IV site. If possible, the patient's nondominant hand should be used.

9. **False:** Attempts at IV therapy *should not* significantly delay transporting critically ill or injured patients to the hospital. Rather, the IV should be started *while en route* to the hospital.

10. **True**

11. **a:** Whenever IV cannulation is performed: **used needles must be placed in a puncture-resistant (sharps) container as quickly as possible,** *gloves* must be worn, and the EMT-I must wash his or her hands *before* and *after* the procedure. If there is any possibility of blood or body fluids splashing, additional barrier protection such as a gown, mask, and eyewear should be worn. Also, needles should *not* be recapped.

12. Needlestick injuries can be avoided by **not bending, breaking, or recapping needles; separating them from the syringe; or manipulating them by hand.**

13. HBV is **hepatitis B virus.**

14. The equipment and supplies needed to establish and maintain an IV line include **the IV solution, administration set, extension set, needles/catheters (assorted sizes), protective gloves, gown and goggles, tourniquet (venous constricting band), tape, antibiotic swabs/ointment, gauze dressings (2 × 2s, 4 × 4s), 10- to 35-mL syringes, a Vacutainer holder with a multisample IV Luer-Lok adapter fitted to it, assorted blood collection tubes, and padded armboards.**

15. IV administration set components:
    A. **piercing spike**
    B. **drip chamber**
    C. **drug administration port**
    D. **connector end**
    E. **flow clamp**

16. **c:** Containers for IV solutions used in the prehospital setting are typically clear plastic bags that collapse as they empty, come in 100- to 250-mL sizes, which are used for medical emergencies and drug administration, and a 1000-mL size, which is used for fluid replacement and trauma emergencies. The IV bag has two ports at the bottom, **one with a rubber stopper for the infusion of medications,** and the other with a plastic tab that is removed to insert the spiked piercing end of the IV administration set tubing.

17. **b:** The usual solutions for fluid replacement in the field setting are normal saline (0.9%) and lactated Ringer's solution. Both are isotonic **crystalloid solutions.**

18. **b:** Two thirds of a crystalloid solution is lost to the interstitial space within 1 hour when administered intravenously. The reason is that they contain no proteins or other high molecular-weight solutes. When introduced into the circulatory system, the dissolved ions cross the cell membrane quickly, followed by the IV solution water. Normal saline and lactated Ringer's solution are examples of crystalloids. The amount of IV fluid administered in the field setting should be limited to 2 to 3 L.

19. **d:** It is necessary to administer **3 L** of IV crystalloid solution for every liter of blood lost when treating patients who have experienced hypovolemic shock (3:1 ratio).

20. **Colloids contain large molecules, such as protein, that do not readily pass through the capillary membrane, causing these solutions to remain in the intravascular space for extended periods.** In addition, the presence of the large molecules in colloids results in an osmotic pressure that is greater than the osmotic pressure of interstitial and intracellular fluid. This causes fluid to move from the interstitial and intracellular spaces into the intravascular space. For this reason, colloids are often referred to as volume expanders. **Colloids are not commonly used in the prehospital setting because they are expensive, have short half-lives, and often require refrigeration.**

21. **c**

22. **True:** Dextran provides immediate volume expansion, but its use may cause clotting problems and interfere with type and crossmatching of blood. Also, allergic reaction is a possible side effect.

23. **True**

24. **False:** D_5W is a glucose solution that is isotonic in the container but hypotonic after it enters the circulatory system. The reason is that glucose quickly moves from the circulation, leaving free water. This free water then moves from the circulatory space into the interstitial and intracellular spaces.

25. **b: 5% dextrose in water is one of the IV solutions often used in the management of medical emergencies.** However, the American Heart Association ACLS Guidelines for cardiac arrest no longer lists it as the preferred solution given poor neurological outcomes associated with increased glucose levels in patients who survive. Also, because it does not remain in the circulatory system for long, it is not used in the management of trauma or volume-depleted patients.

26. IV solutions with make-up

IV Solution	1 L Contains
0.9% sodium chloride solution (normal saline)	154 mEq of sodium ions (Na$^+$) and 154 mEq of chloride ions (Cl$^-$)
Lactated Ringer's solution (LR)	130 mEq of sodium (Na$^+$), 4 mEq of potassium (K$^+$), 3 mEq of calcium (Ca^{2+}), 109 mEq of chloride ions (Cl$^-$), and 28 mEq of lactate

27. Components of IV administration sets: **a. Piercing spiked end:** portion of the administration set that is inserted into the tubing insertion port of the IV bag; **b. Drip chamber:** clear, cylindrical portion of the tubing where the drops passing through the administration set can be viewed and counted; **c. Flow clamp:** plastic housing with a roller-type clamp that is used to control the amount of fluid the patient receives; **d. Drug administration port:** consists of a rubber stopper and a Y-shaped inlet; **e. Connector end:** part of the IV administration set that is inserted into the hub of the IV catheter; **f. IV administration set:** clear plastic tubing that connects the IV bag to the catheter. It provides easy viewing in case of air bubbles or precipitation of certain medications administered through the tubing.

28. Administration sets with characteristics

	Also Referred to as	Drops Equal to 1 mL	Used for What Situation
Microdrip	Mini or pediatric administration set	Usually 60 drops are equivalent to 1 mL	Children, adults who require minimal fluid, and when medications are administered via an IV infusion
Macrodrip	Regular or standard administration set	Usually 10, 15, or 20 drops are equivalent to 1 mL	Preferred device for administering fluids to treat patients experiencing hypovolemia

29. **c:** The **flow clamp** controls the rate of fluid delivery to the patient. It is located below the drip chamber.

30. The term TKO means **a "to keep open" rate of infusing an IV solution.** It is also referred to as KVO (keep vein open). It is equal to approximately 8 to 15 gtt/min.

31. **d:** In trauma or other situations in which IV fluids are used to replace circulatory volume, the flow rate is based on the patient's response to the IV infusion, including in the **pulse, blood pressure, cerebral function,** and capillary refill (in children less than 6 years old).

32. Using large amounts of IV fluids when there is uncontrolled bleeding can **cause an increase in blood pressure that can lead to more bleeding.** Further, infusing large amounts of IV fluid dilutes the clotting effect of the blood, allowing more bleeding to occur.

33. d

34. The spiked piercing and connector ends of the IV administration set are packaged with protective caps to prevent them from being contaminated before use.

35. **a:** Volutrol chamber IV tubing is used when **specific amounts are to be administered.** It is more commonly used for infant and pediatric infusions.

36. **Extra IV tubing may slow the IV flow rate.** Therefore it should be used carefully in trauma patients. **In addition, the extra length of tubing may get caught under the stretcher when removing the patient from the ambulance.**

37. Three types of IV catheters are **hollow needles (butterfly type); plastic catheters inserted over a hollow needle (e.g., Angiocath, Quickcath, and Jelco); and plastic catheters inserted through a hollow needle or over a guidewire (Intracath).** Plastic catheters are generally preferred over hollow needles in advanced life support.

38. **b:** The catheter-over-needle **can be better anchored than most other cannulation devices,** permits *freer* movement of the extremity in which it is placed, and is the *same size* as the puncture site. It is the preferred device for cannulating veins. Because the device has both a catheter and needle, it is more difficult to insert than winged steel needles. It also has a flashback chamber at the proximal end of the needle that allows the EMT-I to see blood return when the vein is penetrated.

39. **d:** The larger the gauge number, the smaller the diameter of the shaft (e.g., a 22-gauge catheter is small, whereas a 14-gauge catheter is large).

40. **b:** A large-diameter catheter (14 gauge) provides much greater fluid flow than does a small-diameter catheter (22 gauge).

41. **True:** Large-bore devices (14 to 16 gauge) should be used for patients in shock, cardiac arrest, or with other life-threatening emergencies in which rapid fluid replacement may be required. When using a large catheter, be sure to choose a large enough vein to accommodate it.

42. **a**

43. Catheter gauge with characteristics: **a. 14 to 16:** used in adolescents and adults for volume replacement such as in trauma, when viscous medications such as 50% dextrose are to be administered; painful insertion, requires large vein; **b. 20:** used in older children, adolescents, average-size adult patients, suitable for most IV infusions; **c. 22:** used for fragile and/or small veins and where lower rates must be maintained but is more difficult to insert through tough skin.

44. **c:** Smaller catheters reduce the risk of clotting, cause *less* trauma to the vein, invite *fewer* complications, and are *better* tolerated in elderly patients' veins.

45. **b:** A larger-gauge IV catheter can increase the IV flow rate. In contrast, the longer the catheter, the slower the flow rate. For cannulation of a peripheral vein, a needle and catheter length of 1.5 to 2 inches (5 cm) is adequate.

46. **b**

47. Blood vessels with characteristics: **a. Arteries:** run deep and are usually surrounded by muscle that provides them the protection they need; pulsation is present; **b. Veins:** color of blood is dark red because of decreased oxygen concentration; lie just under the skin and drain the skin and superficial fascia; have valves that keep blood flowing toward the heart; otherwise, muscular pressure would cause backing up of blood supply; direction of blood flow is toward the heart.

48. **b**

49. **c:** In cardiac arrest, the preferred sites for IV cannulation are the **peripheral veins of the antecubital fossa** because they are among the largest, most visible, and easily accessible in the arm.

50. **c**

51. **b**

52. Veins of the arm:
    A. cephalic vein
    B. radial vein
    C. digital veins
    D. metacarpal vein
    E. median antebrachial vein
    F. basilic vein
    G. subclavian vein

53. Veins with characteristics: **a. Digital veins:** cannot be used if dorsal hand veins are already being used; **b. Metacarpal veins:** insertion is more painful because of increased nerve endings in hands; wrist movement is limited unless a short catheter is used; **c. Accessory cephalic vein:** readily accepts large-bore needles, and its position on the forearm creates a natural splint for the needle and adapter; is sometimes difficult to position catheter flush with skin; **d. Antecubital veins:** may be uncomfortable for patient because the arm must be kept straight; otherwise, the catheter could kink or slide in and out of the vein, damaging it; often visible or palpable in children when other veins will not dilate.

54. Four things that should be explained to the patient before IV cannulation: **the need for the IV; how venipuncture is performed; how much discomfort will be felt; and how therapy will limit his or her activities.**

55. **False:** Any IV bag that is leaking or appears cloudy *should be discarded*. The EMT-I must make sure the proper solution has been selected and is not outdated.

56. **c:** To prepare an IV administration set, the EMT-I should remove the administration set from its

protective wrapping or box and slide the flow control valve close to the drip chamber, close off the flow control valve, **using sterile technique insert the spiked piercing end of the administration set into the tubing insertion port of the IV bag,** turn the IV bag right side up, and squeeze the drip chamber of the administration set two or three times to fill it halfway. Last, open the control valve to flush IV solution through the entire tubing. This should force out all the air.

57. **b:** Before IV cannulation, place the patient's selected extremity **lower than the heart.** This helps distend the distal veins.

58. **b:** To reduce pain and discomfort, release the tourniquet as soon as the venipuncture device has been placed and blood samples have been drawn. Also, avoid keeping it in place for more than 2 minutes; keep it as flat as possible; and make it snug but not uncomfortably tight. Loosen and retighten the tourniquet if the patient complains of severe tightness.

59. Three ways veins can be distended are **having the patient open and close the fist tightly five or six times; flicking the skin over the vein with one or two sharp snaps of the fingers;** and **rubbing or stroking the skin upward toward the tourniquet.**

60. **Using a firm circular motion, cleanse the site thoroughly with povidone-iodine or alcohol wipe. It should be allowed to dry before penetrating the skin.**

61. **Stabilize the vein by anchoring it with your thumb and stretching the skin downward. This makes the venipuncture site taut.** Stabilizing the vein helps ensure successful cannulation of the vein the first time.

62. **c**

63. **True**

64. **False:** The tourniquet should not be released before penetrating the skin with the needle.

65. **False:** Meeting a great deal of resistance as the needle is advanced through the skin is indicative of a problem and should prompt the EMT-I to stop and attempt venipuncture at a new site using a new venipuncture device.

66. **True**

67. **True:** Be careful not to enter too fast or too deeply because the needle can go through the back wall of the vein.

68. **d**

69. The venipuncture device is advanced another 1 to 2 cm **so that the tip of the catheter is well within the vein** because the catheter is slightly shorter than the needle and blood backflow sometimes occurs with just the needle in the vein. Advancing the venipuncture device a bit helps ensure the catheter is correctly situated in the vein.

70. **a**

71. Once the needle tip is within the catheter, **apply pressure to the vein beyond the catheter tip with the little finger to prevent blood from leaking out of the catheter hub once the needle is completely withdrawn.**

72. **b:** Once the IV tubing is connected to the IV catheter hub, open the flow clamp and adjust it accordingly. Also, the cannula and tubing are taped in place; the IV site is covered with a sterile dressing; and the size of the cannula and time and date of insertion can be written on the tape.

73. **d**

74. **c:** When infiltration occurs, the tissue around the site is typically cool and swollen. The catheter should be removed and discarded and a sterile dressing placed on the site; venipuncture should be attempted at another site using sterile equipment.

75. **c:** Armboards must be long enough to prevent flexion or extension at the tip of the venipuncture device, are *not* used in every case, do *not* prevent rotation or movement of the patient's arm, and should be covered with a *soft material and applied with tape* that is padded with folded gauze or tissue.

76. The correct drip rate to deliver 1000 mL of normal saline in 4 hours using an administration set that delivers 10 gtt/mL is **40 gtt/min.**

    The mathematical formula used to arrive at this answer:
    1000 mL × 10 gtt/mL ÷ 240 minutes = 40 gtt/min

77. The correct drip rate to deliver 750 mL of normal saline in 2 hours using an administration set that delivers 10 gtt/mL is **60 gtt/min.**

    The mathematical formula used to arrive at this answer:
    750 mL × 10 gtt/mL ÷ 120 minutes = 60 gtt/min

78. The correct drip rate to deliver 50 mL of 5% dextrose in water in 30 minutes using an administration set that delivers 60 gtt/mL is **100 gtt/min.**

    The mathematical formula used to arrive at this answer:
    50 mL × 60 gtt/mL ÷ 30 minutes = 100 gtt/min

79. The correct drip rate to administer an infusion of 1250 mL of lactated Ringer's solution over 2 hours using an administration set that delivers 10 gtt/mL is **100 gtt/min.**

    The mathematical formula used to arrive at this answer:
    1250 mL × 10 gtt/mL ÷ 120 minutes = 100 gtt/min

80. The correct drip rate to administer an infusion of 20 mL of 5% dextrose in water over 20 minutes using an administration set that delivers 60 gtt/mL is **60 gtt/min.**

    The mathematical formula used to arrive at this answer:
    20 mL × 60 gtt/mL ÷ 20 minutes = 60 gtt/min

81. **c**

82. **d:** When an IV is started, the following must be documented on the run report: **date and time of the venipuncture, type and amount of solution, number of insertion attempts (if more than one), venipuncture site,** type of venipuncture device used (including the length and gauge), venipuncture site IV flow rate, any adverse reactions and the actions taken to correct them, and the name or identification number of the EMT-I initiating the infusion. In addition to documenting correct IV placement, unsuccessful attempts should also be documented.

83. **False:** Some local protocols call for the EMT-I to document the date and time of insertion, type and gauge of needle or catheter, and initials of the EMT-I who placed the device on the tape that is used to secure the venipuncture device and administration set tubing in place. To do this properly, cut a piece of tape and place it on a flat surface. Write the information on it, and then apply it over the dressing. Never label the tape after it has been applied over the dressing because doing so will irritate the venipuncture site.

84. **d:** The IV will not flow if the venous constricting band has been left in place, if the IV bag is too low, or if there is infiltration into the tissues. The flow regulator being in a closed position and the tip of the catheter positioned against a valve or wall of the vein will also result in an absence of IV fluid.

85. **a**

86. Complications of IV therapy include **pain, catheter shear, circulatory overload, cannulation of an artery, infiltration/hematoma, local infection, pyrogenic reaction, air embolism, as well as thrombosis, phlebitis, sepsis,** and **pulmonary thromboembolism.**

87. **To avoid the possibility of catheter shear,** *never* **withdraw the catheter back over or through the needle.** Always withdraw the needle first and then the catheter.

88. **d:** The following are indicative of circulatory overload: **shortness of breath, rales,** tachypnea, coughing, engorgement of neck veins, headache, flushed skin, rapid pulse, and increased blood pressure. Constantly watch all patients receiving IV fluids for signs of developing congestive heart failure in which case the IV flow rate should be significantly reduced or terminated.

89. **d:** Bright red blood spurting from the IV cannula is indicative of accidental arterial placement. If this occurs, the device should be completely removed and direct pressure applied to the puncture site for at least 10 minutes, until the bleeding has stopped.

90. **c:** Air embolism can occur if **the IV tubing becomes dislodged from the catheter hub.** It can also occur during central vein cannulation or when air is not cleared from the IV administration set appropriately.

91. **a:** Pyrogenic reaction **occurs when foreign proteins, capable of producing fever, are present in the administration set or IV solution,** is characterized by the abrupt onset of fever (100° F to 106° F), chills, backache, headache, nausea, vomiting, face flushing, and sudden pulse change. Cardiovascular collapse may also result. The reaction usually occurs within 30 minutes of the IV therapy being initiated. If a pyrogenic reaction is suspected, the IV should be immediately terminated and established in the other arm using a new administration set and solution.

92. **b**

93. **1. Apply a venous tourniquet, and select a suitable vein by palpation and sight.**

2. Cleanse the site thoroughly with an alcohol wipe (or povidone-iodine) using a firm circular motion.
3. Stabilize the vein by anchoring it with your thumb and stretching the skin downward.
4. Tell the patient there will be a small poke or pinch as the needle enters the skin.
5. Hold the end of venipuncture device between the thumb and index/middle fingers.
6. Depending on the type of venipuncture device and manufacturer's recommendations, hold the needle at a 15-, 30-, or 45-degree angle to the skin.
7. Penetrate the skin with the bevel of the needle pointed up, and enter the vein with the needle from either the top or side.
8. Note when blood fills the flashback chamber of the needle, and lower the venipuncture device and advance it another 1 to 2 cm until the tip of the catheter is well within the vein.
9. While holding the needle stable between the first/middle fingers and thumb, use the first finger and thumb of the other hand to slide the catheter into the vein until the hub is against the skin.
10. Once the needle tip is within the catheter, apply pressure to the vein beyond the catheter tip with the little finger to prevent blood from leaking out of the catheter hub once the needle is completely withdrawn.
11. Draw a blood sample and release the tourniquet from the patient's arm.
12. Reapply pressure to the vein beyond the catheter tip with the little finger to prevent blood from leaking out of the catheter hub once the blood-drawing device is disconnected.
13. Disconnect the syringe or Vacutainer device from the hub of the catheter by holding the hub between the first finger and thumb and pulling the device free with the other hand.
14. Connect the IV tubing to the catheter hub, being careful not to contaminate either the hub or connector before insertion and open the IV flow control valve. Run the IV for a brief period to ensure the line is patent.
15. Cover the IV site with povidone-iodine ointment (if called for by local protocol) and a sterile dressing or an adhesive bandage, and secure the catheter, administration set tubing, and sterile dressing in place with tape or a commercial device.
16. Adjust the flow rate as is appropriate for the patient's condition, and dispose of the needle(s) in a proper biomedical waste container.

94. **d:** When making subsequent attempts to cannulate a vein, select a site that is proximal to the first venipuncture site. If there are no adequate sites on the same extremity, the other extremity should be assessed for possible cannulation.

95. **b:** To discontinue an IV line, stop the IV fluid flow completely by closing the flow clamp. Taking care not to disturb the catheter, carefully untape and remove the dressing. Hold a 2 × 2 sterile gauze dressing just above the site, and withdraw the catheter by pulling straight back. Immediately cover the IV site with the 2 × 2 sterile dressing, and hold it against the vein until the bleeding has stopped. Tape the dressing in place.

96. **a:** The external jugular vein **is usually easy to cannulate,** is considered a peripheral vein, provides direct access to the central circulation, and lies superficially along the lateral portion of the neck.

97. **d:** When cannulating the external jugular vein, **turn the patient's head away from you.** Also, align the cannula in the direction of the vein with the point aimed at the midclavicular line. The vein should be penetrated at a 45-degree angle; the puncture should be made midway between the angle of the jaw and midclavicular line; and the vein should be "tourniqueted" by applying slight pressure to it with the index finger just above the clavicle.

98. **a**

99. **b:** In trauma patients, **the IVs should be started while en route to the hospital;** 14- to 16-gauge needles should be used; normal saline or lactated Ringer's solution should be used; macrodrip administration sets are preferred; and the IVs should be infused at a wide-open rate.

100. **d:** IV lines used in the management of cardiac arrest should **be elevated above the level of the heart.** This facilitates the passage of medications into the central circulation. In addition, IV lines should be placed in an *antecubital fossa vein,* consist of a *normal saline solution,* and be run at a *keep open rate* unless volume depletion is suspected.

101. Answers to crossword puzzle

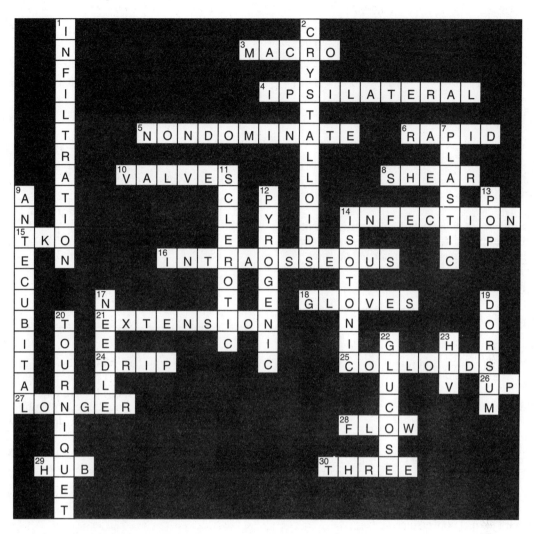

CHAPTER 7

1. A fraction is a number that expresses **part** of a group.

2. **c:** To administer ½ of a prefilled syringe containing 10 mL you would deliver 5 mL.

3. **a:** To administer ⅕ of a prefilled syringe containing 5 mL you would deliver 1 mL.

4. Answers to decimal exercise:

0.75 + 0.25 = **1.0**	0.66 − 0.2 = **0.46**	12.5 × 10 = **125**	14.8 ÷ 2 = **7.4**
1.24 + 0.33 = **1.57**	1.65 − 0.94 = **0.71**	1.23 × 0.75 = **0.9225**	0.48 ÷ 0.6 = **0.8**
8.76 + 1.28 = **10.04**	44.32 − 1.16 = **43.16**	7.52 × 1.23 = **9.2496**	12.6 ÷ 4.2 = **3.0**
7.2 + 3.82 = **11.02**	9.13 − 0.71 = **8.42**	0.55 × 16.53 = **9.0915**	198.4 ÷ 12.8 = **15.5**

5. There are two systems of measuring drug dosage: the **metric** system and the **apothecary** system.

6. The metric system is based on multiples of **10**.

7. Terms with correct abbreviation: **a. gram:** g; **b. liter:** L; **c. kilogram:** kg; **d. milliliter:** mL; **e. milligram:** mg; **f. cubic centimeter:** cc; **g. microgram:** mcg

8. Units with conversions:

Unit	Conversion
5 mL	**0.005** L
3 L	**3000** mL
1 g	**1000** mg
4 mg	**4000** mcg
1 cc	**1** mL
8 mcg	**0.008** mg
100 mg	**0.1** g

9. **c:** One kilogram is equal to **2.2** pounds.

10. Pounds converted to kilograms:

Pounds	Kilograms
100	**45** (45)
85	**38** (39)
220	**99** (100)
170	**77** (77)
150	**68** (68)

The first number is the result of dividing the pounds in half and then subtracting 10%. The number in parentheses is the result of dividing the pounds by 2.2. For the purpose of calculating drug dosages, the numbers shown above would be further rounded up or down: 45 kg rounded down to 40 kg or up to 50 kg; 38 kg rounded up to 40 kg; 99 kg rounded up to 100 kg; 77 kg rounded up to 80 kg; and 68 kg rounded up to 70 kg.

11. Table with correct conversions

Grams (g)	Milligrams (mg)	Micrograms (mcg)
1	1000	1,000,000
0.4	400	400,000
0.001	1	1000
2	2000	2,000,000
0.05	50	50,000
0.000004	0.004	4
25	25,000	25,000,000
0.8	800	800,000

12. **d:** With a microdrip administration set, **60** drops is equal to 1 mL.

13. To administer 0.5 mg of epinephrine **0.5 mL** is needed. The formula shown below demonstrates how this answer was reached.
    Step 1: Multiply the desired dosage by the volume on hand: 0.5 mg × 1.0 mL = 0.5 mg/mL
    Step 2: Divide the answer obtained in Step 1 by the dose on hand: 0.5 mg/mL ÷ 1 mg = 0.5 mL

14. To administer 5 mg of diazepam **1 mL** is needed. The formula shown below demonstrates how this answer was reached.
    Step 1: Multiply the desired dosage by the volume on hand: 5 mg × 2 mL = 10 mg/mL
    Step 2: Divide the answer obtained in Step 1 by the dose on hand: 10 mg/mL ÷ 10 mg = 1 mL

15. To administer 3 mg of morphine sulfate **0.3 mL** is needed. The formula shown below demonstrates how this answer was determined.
    Step 1: Multiply the desired dosage by the volume on hand: 3 mg × 1 mL = 3 mg/mL
    Step 2: Divide the answer obtained in Step 1 by the dose on hand: 3 mg/mL ÷ 10 mg = 0.3 mL

16. Answers to weight/dose math exercise

Weight (lb)	Step 1	Step 2	Step 3	Step 4
230	230 ÷ 2.2 = 104 kg	104 kg × 1 mg = 104 mg	104 mg × 5 mL = 520 mg/mL	520 mg/mL ÷ 100 mg = **5.2 mL** (to be given)
128	128 ÷ 2.2 = 58 kg	58 kg × 1 mg = 58 mg	58 mg × 5 mL = 290 mg/mL	290 mg/mL ÷ 100 mg = **2.9 mL** (to be given)
94	94 ÷ 2.2 = 43 kg	43 kg × 1 mg = 43 mg	43 mg × 5 mL = 215 mg/mL	215 mg/mL ÷ 100 mg = **2.15 mL** (to be given)
198	198 ÷ 2.2 = 90 kg	90 kg × 1 mg = 90 mg	90 mg × 5 mL = 450 mg/mL	450 mg/mL ÷ 100 mg = **4.5 mL** (to be given)

17. Answers to weight/dose math exercise

Weight (lb)	Step 1	Step 2	Step 3	Step 4
254	254 ÷ 2.2 = 115 kg	115 kg × 0.5 mg = 57 mg	57 mg × 4 mL = 228 mg/mL	228 mg/mL ÷ 40 mg = **5.7 mL** (to be given)
112	112 ÷ 2.2 = 51 kg	51 kg × 0.5 mg = 25 mg	25 mg × 4 mL = 100 mg/mL	100 mg/mL ÷ 40 mg = **2.5 mL** (to be given)
76	76 ÷ 2.2 = 34 kg	34 kg × 0.5 mg = 17 mg	17 mg × 4 mL = 68 mg/mL	68 mg/mL ÷ 40 mg = **1.7 mL** (to be given)
172	172 ÷ 2.2 = 78 kg	78 kg × 0.5 mg = 39 mg	39 mg × 4 mL = 156 mg/mL	156 mg/mL ÷ 40 mg = **3.9 mL** (to be given)

18. Answers to math exercise

Step 1	Step 2	Step 3	Step 4
500 mL × 3 mg/min = 1500 mL/mg/min	2 g = 2000 mg	1500 mL/min ÷ 2000 = 0.75 mL/min	0.75 mL/min × 60 drops per mL = **45 gtt/min** (to be given)

19. Number of drops per minute required to deliver the number of milligrams listed in the column to the left.

Dose	Infusion Rate
1 mg/min	15 gtt/min
2 mg/min	30 gtt/min
3 mg/min	45 gtt/min
4 mg/min	60 gtt/min

20. When converting Fahrenheit to centigrade, first **subtract** 32, and then **multiply** by 5/9. When converting centigrade to Fahrenheit, first multiply by **9/5,** then add **32.**

CHAPTER 8

1. **b**

2. **False:** Gowns are indicated when splashes of blood or body fluids may occur but not when administering a medication.

3. **False:** After you administer a medication and remove your gloves, you should also wash your hands because gloves are *not* an absolute barrier to bacteria and viruses.

4. **True**

5. **Medical asepsis practices interrupt a chain of events necessary for the continuation of an infectious process by preventing the transfer of pathogenic organisms from person to person, place to place, or person to place.**

6. **c**

7. **False:** Compared with that which is obtainable in an operating room, it is virtually impossible to achieve sterile technique in the prehospital setting.

8. Ten medically clean procedures and techniques are used to reduce the patient's risk of infection in the prehospital setting:
   - Hand washing
   - Changing gloves whenever they become contaminated
   - Gowning and wearing facial masks when appropriate
   - Cleaning all sites used for medication injection such as the skin or the injection port of an IV administration set
   - Careful handling of medications (which have been packaged sterile) to keep them clean and uncontaminated until they are used
   - Discarding any supplies or equipment that becomes accidentally contaminated (i.e., such as when the uncovered connector end of an IV administration tubing or an unsheathed IV needle comes into contact with an unclean surface in the ambulance)
   - Discarding equipment or supplies found to be in opened packages
   - Separating clean from contaminated or potentially contaminated materials
   - Keeping the ambulance and patient care equipment as clean as possible
   - Using antiseptics and disinfectants when indicated

9. **Disinfectants are toxic to living tissue, whereas antiseptics are not.** For this reason antiseptics can be applied to skin and mucous membranes to prevent infections or to cleanse a local area before penetrating it with a needle. Disinfectants are applied to the surface of nonliving objects and can be used to clean such things as the inside of the ambulance, laryngoscope blades, backboards, and reusable splints.

10. Extreme **care** should be taken when handling needles, scalpels, lancets, and other sharp instruments or devices; when handling sharp instruments after procedures; when cleaning used instruments; and when disposing of **used** needles.

11. **d:** Disposable syringes and needles should be **placed in a puncture-resistant container** immediately after use. The Centers for Disease Control and Prevention recommends that needles *not* be recapped after use because recapping often results in needle-stick injuries. Needles should *not* be cut or bent for disposal.

12. **False:** Dispensing drugs by standing orders or by a direct order from a physician places *tremendous responsibility on an EMT-I.* If the EMT-I's knowledge of a drug is incomplete or the wrong dosage or drug is given, he or she may be exposed to liability.

13. **True:** The EMS run report should include the type, dosage, and time each medication was administered. It should also report the effect that the drug had on the patient.

14. The six rights of drug administration are:
    1. "right" patient
    2. "right" drug
    3. "right" dose
    4. "right" route
    5. "right" time
    6. "right" documentation

15. **b:** The EMT-I **should not talk when drawing up or administering a drug.** It is important to remain attentive during this task.

16. It is important to check the strength of the medication and the route of administration before delivering a drug **because some medications are too concentrated to be administered any other way than what is specified.** An example is epinephrine 1:1000, which is normally delivered subcutaneously. If it were administered directly into the circulatory system (e.g., IV push) it could cause the patient to experience an adverse reaction.

17. Four causes of common medication errors: **giving the wrong drug; an error in drug calculations; drugs administered through the wrong route;** and **giving the drug to the wrong patient.**

18. Six things the EMT-I should do when a medication error occurs include **accept professional responsibility; immediately advise medical direction or the supervisor; assess and carefully monitor the patient for effects of the drug; document the medication error as required by local and state drug administration policies and those of the medical direction institution; modify personal practice to avoid a similar error in the future;** and **follow EMS agency procedures for documentation and quality improvement activities.**

19. Labeled syringe used for medication administration is shown below.

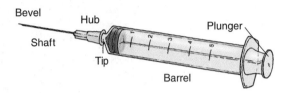

20. The other types of syringes used for parenteral administration besides the hypodermic syringe are the **tuberculin** and **insulin.**

21. Needle gauge varies from **18** to 27; the **higher** the number, the **smaller** the gauge.

22. **True**

23. **False:** Subcutaneous injections generally are given using a *short, small-gauge needle—25 gauge, ⅝ inch or 23 gauge, ½ inch.*

24. **c**

25. **c**

26. Answers to crossword puzzle

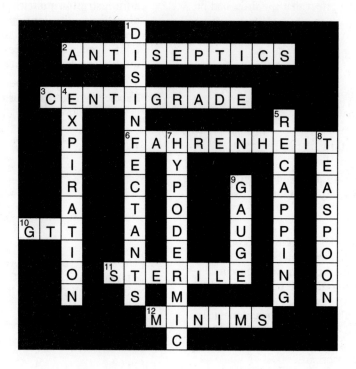

27. The tuberculin syringe is narrow and has a total capacity of **1** mL. There are **100** calibration lines marking the capacity. Each line represents **0.01** mL. Every tenth line is longer than the others to indicate **0.1** mL.

28. Prefilled syringes contain a **premeasured** amount of a medication in a **disposable** cartridge with a needle attached.

29. **a:** An **ampule** is a small sterile glass container that contains a single-dose injectable medication and is drawn up by use of a syringe and needle. Vials are *multiple-dose* glass containers that are sealed with a rubber stopper and used to store a sterile liquid or powdered drug preparation. In the emergency setting, prefilled syringes are used to administer the majority of parenteral medications. A Tubex brand syringe is a *reusable* device that is used to administer medications that are contained in *disposable cartridges*.

30. **a**

31. **False:** To open an ampule, the base should be held between the forefinger and thumb of one hand while the top is held *between the forefinger and thumb of the other hand*. Force, directed away from the body, is then used to snap off the top of the ampule. To prevent injury, hold the ampule with a 4 × 4 gauze dressing while snapping off the top.

32. Medication container tag terms:
    A. **name**
    B. **dosage**
    C. **concentration**
    D. **administration route**

33. **d:** To prepare a preloaded medication the following steps should be performed: remove the protective caps from the medication container and from the needle housing; engage the medication container into the needle housing and rotate it clockwise until it is securely fastened; point the needle upward and tap the medication container portion of the syringe until the air bubbles rise to the top; and uncap the needle and with the syringe needle pointed *upward*, expel the excess air until only the medication remains in the syringe. **Pointing the syringe needle downward is incorrect.**

34. **d:** To withdraw medication from a vial you should clean the rubber stopper with *alcohol*, determine the amount to be withdrawn, *draw that volume* of air into the syringe, invert the vial, **insert the needle through the rubber stopper,** *inject the air into the vial,* **withdraw the desired amount of solution,** and remove the needle from the vial.

35. a

36. Medication administration routes with descriptions: **a. Oral:** generally the most popular method of drug administration for nonemergency situations; **b. Rectal:** have a local or systemic action and are usually in the form of suppositories or solutions instilled through the enema procedure; *c. Endotracheal:* because of the large surface area of the alveoli and vast blood supply of the pulmonary capillary beds that return blood to the left heart, drugs administered through the trachea are rapidly absorbed and delivered to the heart for distribution; **d. Intramuscular:** involves the injection of small quantities of a drug into the muscle; *e. Intravenous push:* drug is injected directly into the bloodstream; **f. Sublingual:** medications are placed in the mouth, under the tongue; **g. Aerosol:** allow drugs to act directly on the structures of the lung or be absorbed into the systemic circulation; **h. Subcutaneous:** involves the injection of a drug into the fatty tissue beneath the skin.

37. **It is convenient; it is inexpensive; and there is a large surface area, mixing of contents, and differences in pH that act to enhance absorption.**

38. Problems that can occur with administering medications orally: **The acids and enzymes of the gastrointestinal tract can inactivate some medications before they can be absorbed and others are so irritating to the gastrointestinal tract that they should be taken only after eating a meal.**

39. You can assist a patient swallow a tablet or pill **by giving him or her water to drink.**

40. **b**

41. **c:** To administer a drug rectally open the suppository package and drop it onto an *unsterile gauze*, use one hand to separate the buttocks exposing the *anus*, **insert the suppository about 1 to 1.5 inches until it passes through the internal anal sphincter**, hold the buttocks closed following insertion, and instruct the patient *not to* bear down.

42. **True**

43. **False:** When administering a medication sublingually, the patient should be directed to place the tablet *beneath his or her tongue so that it may dissolve* and not be swallowed or chewed.

44. **b**

45. **c:** For patients **older than 5 years of age** a mouthpiece is more effective than a mask when administering an aerosolized drug.

46. **b:** To administer an aerosolized drug you should pour the prescribed drug into the *nebulizer* using aseptic technique; **adjust the oxygen flow meter to 4 to 6 L/min to produce a steady, visible mist;** instruct the patient to *inhale slowly and deeply;* continue administering the treatment until *the aerosol canister is depleted of the medication.*

47. If changes in heart rate or dysrhythmias are noted during delivery of an aerosolized medication, **nebulization should be stopped and medical direction contacted for further orders.**

48. **True**

49. **False:** When preparing to insert the needle during subcutaneous medication administration, the skin should be pulled *away from the underlying muscle.*

50. **True**

51. **True:** If blood is seen (indicating that the needle is in a blood vessel), the needle should be withdrawn and the medication administered in another location. Administering the concentrations (of medication) used for subcutaneous injection directly into the circulatory system will likely produce a severe adverse reaction.

52. Common sites for SQ injection

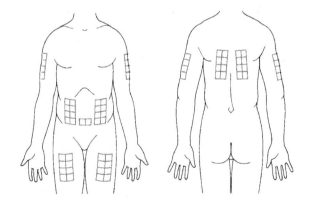

53. **d**

54. **d**

55. **False:** A venous constricting band is *unnecessary* when administering medications intramuscularly.

56. **False:** Typically, *no more than 1 mL* of medication is injected into the deltoid muscle. However, up to 10 mL of medication can be administered into the *gluteal* muscle.

57. **True**

58. Common sites for IM injection

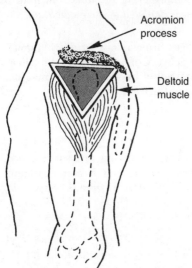

59. **True**

60. **False:** Before injecting the IV medication, stop the IV flow by pinching the IV tubing *above* the injection site. Closing the tubing leading to the IV bag prevents the medication from flowing up into the IV bag instead of into the patient.

61. **False:** Following injection of the IV medication, the needle and syringe should be disposed of in *an appropriate sharps container.*

62. Flush the IV tubing **by briefly running it wide open or following the drug bolus with a 20-mL bolus of IV fluid.**

63. The administration of medication through the intraosseous route is the same as for the intravenous route **except that after a drug has been administered by intraosseous infusion, it must be followed by a 5-mL saline flush to make sure the drug is delivered into the systemic circulation.**

64. Answers to crossword puzzle

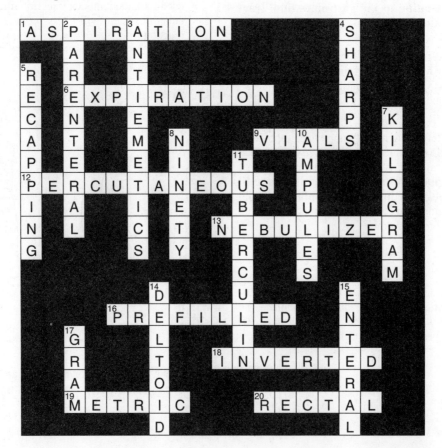

CHAPTER 9

1. The primary objective in emergency care is to **ensure each patient has a patent airway and optimal ventilation. This provides for the intake of oxygen and removal of carbon dioxide.**

2. **a:** Commonly neglected airway skills in the prehospital setting include failing to create an effective seal with a bag-mask device, improper positioning of the patient's head and neck, and not reassessing the patient's condition. All of these can lead to inadequate oxygenation and ventilation. **Inserting an oropharyngeal airway too deeply** is not one of the commonly neglected airway skills.

3. **d**

4. **b**

5. **d:** The nose **has two openings to the outside of the body that are referred to as nostrils,** is the *uppermost* aspect of the airway, has a part that protrudes from the face that is made up of a *bony and cartilaginous framework covered by skin,* and is surrounded by the *maxilla* along the sides and below at its base.

6. **b:** The turbinates create turbulent airflow through the nose. This causes the inspired air to rebound in several directions during its passage, trapping finer particles that the cilia of the mucous membrane propel back to the pharynx to be swallowed.

7. **False:** Air enters the nose through the *anterior nares* (nostrils). The majority of breathing occurs through the nose.

8. **True:** As such, serious bleeding can occur with injury.

9. **False:** The cartilaginous structure that separates the right and left cavities of the nose is referred to as the *nasal septum.*

10. **b:** The **nares**, cartilage, nasal bones, maxilla, and vascular supply are considered part of the nasopharynx. The two posterior nares serve as a passageway into the nasopharynx.

11. Anatomical structures with description: **a. Laryngopharynx:** extends from the hyoid bone at the base of the tongue to the esophagus, posteriorly, and to the trachea, anteriorly; **b. Vallecula:** depression or "pocket" formed by the base of the tongue and the epiglottis; **c. Soft palate:** extends posteriorly from the hard palate to separate the nasopharynx from the rest of the pharynx; **d. Nasopharynx:** located immediately behind the nasal cavity; **e. Mouth:** consists of the lips, cheeks, gums, teeth, and the hard and soft palates; **f. Oropharynx:** extends from the soft palate in the back of the mouth to the hyoid bone below the mandible; **g. Nose:** separated into right and left cavities by a cartilaginous structure (the septum).

12. The tongue is attached to the **mandible** and to the **hyoid** bone through a series of muscles and ligaments. Movement of the mandible anteriorly moves the tongue forward, away from the posterior oropharynx. This is the basis for using the head-tilt/chin-lift procedure in semiconscious or unconscious patients.

13. The three regions of the pharynx are the **oropharynx, nasopharynx,** and **laryngopharynx** (also called the hypopharynx).

14. Functions of upper airway structures: **trachea:** conducts air between the larynx and the lungs; **pharynx:** serves as the passageway for air into the respiratory tract (anteriorly) and food and liquid into the digestive system (posteriorly); **vocal cords:** vibrate to produce sound as expired air passes over them; **nose:** serves as the primary passageway for air entering and leaving the respiratory tree; cleans, humidifies, and warms the inspired air; **larynx:** protects the lower airway and produces voice; and **tongue:** assists with speech and the swallowing of food.

15. **c:** The hyoid bone is **suspended from the temporal bone by ligaments,** shaped like a U, and located *just under* the chin. It is unique in that it is the *only bone of the axial skeleton that does not articulate with any other bone.*

16. **a:** The epiglottis serves as an important landmark for the EMT-I who is using a laryngoscope to perform endotracheal intubation or performing the task digitally. Another important consideration is that this structure can be pushed into an obstructing position by an oropharyngeal airway that is too long.

17. The epiglottis lies **superior** to (above) the larynx.

18. The space between the base of the tongue and the epiglottis is referred to as the **vallecula.** This is where the tip of a curved laryngoscope blade is placed during orotracheal intubation.

19. On either side of the epiglottis is a recess called the **piriform sinus.** This is where endotracheal tubes sometimes get hung up during insertion, so great caution must be exercised.

20. **False:** The epiglottis is connected to the *hyoid bone and mandible* by a series of muscles and ligaments. Remember, the tongue and mandible are also connected to the hyoid bone. As such, lifting the mandible anteriorly pulls the tongue *and* epiglottis away from the posterior oropharynx.

21. **True**

22. **c:** The **thyroid cartilage** consists of two large shield-shaped pieces that form the anterior wall of the larynx and give it its V-shaped appearance. The posterior wall is open and consists of muscle.

23. **b:** The cricoid cartilage is **attached to the first ring of tracheal cartilage,** located *below (inferior to)* the thyroid cartilage, a *complete ring* (shaped like a signet ring with the bulky portion located posteriorly), and is the narrowest part of the upper airway in *children.*

24. **d:** The two pyramidal cartilages lie on the rear surface of the cricoid cartilage, attach to the vocal folds and pharyngeal wall, and by their action open and close the vocal cords.

25. **b:** The esophagus is the passageway leading to the stomach and **is distensible.** In the prehospital setting, the EMT-I may use certain airway adjuncts to occlude the esophagus. This is done to prevent regurgitation of stomach contents and gastric distention that may otherwise occur with efforts to ventilate the patient. In addition, the EMT-I must be careful not to misplace the endotracheal tube in this anatomical structure because no air exchange will take place and the patient will likely die.

26. A. nasal cavity
    B. palate
    C. oral cavity
    D. tongue
    E. mandible
    F. hyoid bone
    G. vallecula
    H. vocal cords
    I. thyroid cartilage
    J. cricoid cartilage
    K. trachea
    L. nasopharynx
    M. soft palate
    N. oropharynx
    O. laryngopharynx
    P. esophagus

27. The **vocal cords** are fibrous bands that control the passage of air through the **larynx** and the production of sound.

28. Anatomical structures with locations: **a. Esophagus:** swallowing tube; carries food and liquid from the pharynx to the stomach; **b. Pharynx:** superior to the larynx; **c. Tongue:** superior and anterior to the larynx; **d. Cricoid cartilage:** a complete ring of cartilage shaped like a signet ring with the bulky portion located posteriorly; below the thyroid cartilage; **e. False vocal cords:** slightly superior of the true vocal cords.

29. **d:** The true vocal cords **can vibrate to produce sound as expired air passes over them,** lie *inferior* to (below) the false vocal cords, and are cordlike structures. The *false* vocal cords consist of elastic connective tissue covered by folds of mucous membrane. When these cords come together, they stop air from leaving the lungs (as when a person holds his or her breath) and prevent foreign materials such as food or liquids from entering the airway.

30. **c:** The **glottic opening** is the space between the vocal cords. It is the narrowest part of the airway in the adult and where the tip of a tube is passed through during endotracheal intubation.

31. **True:** Because of the degree of vagal innervation, stimulation of the pharyngeal and laryngeal mucous membranes (by a laryngoscope or endotracheal tube) can cause bradycardia, hypotension, and a decreased respiratory rate.

32. **b:** The lower airway consists of the **trachea, right and left mainstem bronchi,** secondary bronchi, bronchioles, and **alveoli.**

33. **b:** The trachea **attaches to the larynx at the cricoid cartilage,** connects the larynx to the *mainstem bronchi,* is maintained in an open position by C-shaped cartilaginous rings that extend throughout its length, lies *anterior* to the esophagus, is lined by a respiratory epithelium that contains cilia and mucus-producing cells, and bifurcates *at the carina* into the right and left mainstem bronchi. It is approximately 10 to 15 cm long.

34. **True:** Because the right mainstem bronchus is shorter, wider, and more in line with the trachea, aspirated foreign bodies—or mispositioned endotracheal tubes—are more likely to enter the right mainstem bronchus than the left.

35. **True:** Irritation of these structures can lead to bronchospasm and decreased airflow.

36. **a:** The alveoli are hollow and surrounded by the thin alveolar membrane, which is often only one or two cell layers thick, serve as the primary site for

exchange of oxygen and carbon dioxide, and are in contact with a rich capillary network arising from the pulmonary artery.

37. **False:** The left lung is composed of the *upper and lower lobes.* The *right* lung is composed of the upper, middle, and lower lobes.

38. **False:** The *parietal* pleura lines the inside of the thoracic cavity. The membrane enclosing the lungs is referred to as the visceral pleura.

39. **False:** The space between the visceral pleura and parietal pleura is called the *pleural* space.

40. c

41. c

42. **The overall size of the pediatric airway is smaller. Because of this the airway of an infant or child is more likely to become occluded by foreign bodies, blood, vomit, loose teeth, or swollen tissue. A child less than 8 years of age has a larger tongue compared with the size of the mouth. A proportionately smaller jaw can cause the tongue to encroach on the airway. Also, the child has a large, floppy, omega-shaped epiglottis, and the teeth may be absent or delicate. Because of their inability to hold the various anatomical structures clear of the airway, the weak muscles of the neck may allow obstruction to occur.**

43. **a**

44. **b:** Retching or striving to vomit is called **the gag reflex.** It is a normal reflex triggered by touching the soft palate or the throat.

45. **a:** The exchange of gases between a living organism and its environment is referred to as **respiration.** Pulmonary ventilation is the process that moves air in and out of the lungs.

46. c

47. **a:** When stimulated by the brain to contract, the **diaphragm** flattens downward against the abdominal structures, thus increasing the intrathoracic space. Normal quiet breathing is accomplished almost entirely by this muscle.

48. c

49. Phases of breathing: **a. Inspiration:** the respiratory center in the medulla of the brain signals the muscles of respiration to increase the size of the chest cavity; the diaphragm and intercostal muscles are stimulated to contract; the intercostal muscles lift the rib cage upward and outward, thus increasing the horizontal and transverse dimensions of the thoracic cavity; a potential vacuum draws air into the enlarged lungs, filling them. **b. Expiration:** is a passive act (unless forced); the diaphragm and respiratory muscles relax, and the chest cavity decreases in size; the decreasing thoracic volume increases the intrathoracic pressure, and air is forced out of the lungs.

50. The respiratory minute volume (air exchanged over the course of 1 minute) equals the respiratory **rate** times the **tidal volume.** On average, adults breathe in and exhale between 500 and 800 mL of air, 12 to 20 times every minute. The average minute volume ranges between 6000 and 16,000 mL. These volumes of air are necessary to remove carbon dioxide that is produced as a part of metabolism and to bring in sufficient supplies of oxygen.

51. Air reaching the alveoli for gas exchange equals **350 mL.**

52. **c:** The amount of air **in the inspired and expired air with each breath** is the tidal volume. Normally, it is between 500 and 800 mL of air.

53. a

54. **d:** Field use of the PEFR allows the EMT-I to evaluate the **effectiveness of treatments such as bronchodilators** used in the treatment of patients experiencing respiratory distress.

55. **d:** When inspired air reaches the alveoli **it interfaces with capillary venous blood oxygen that has a P_{O_2} of 40 mm Hg,** the partial pressure of oxygen is *104 mm Hg,* and it contains *more oxygen* and *less carbon dioxide.* In a physiological process called diffusion, oxygen moves across the alveolar/capillary membrane into the bloodstream until gas pressures are equal on both sides.

56. **d:** Each gram of saturated hemoglobin is considered saturated to its fullest extent when carrying 1.34 mL of oxygen. Blood that is fully saturated with oxygen is bright red or scarlet; during the time blood is in the alveolar capillary it absorbs enough oxygen to increase its partial pressure to *104 mm Hg;* a small portion (3%) of oxygen is carried by *plasma,* whereas the majority (97%) is carried by *hemoglobin;* and oxygen carried by hemoglobin is reflected in the blood saturation (Sa_{O_2}).

57. **d**

58. **b:** Once blood that is pumped through the systemic circulation reaches the capillaries it comes into contact with tissues having a Po_2 of close to *40 mm Hg*, and **oxygen diffuses from the bloodstream into the tissues.** *Oxygen* then moves to the cells, where it plays an essential role in the production of energy. The amount of oxygen released from the blood is influenced by several factors. More oxygen is released if the partial pressure of oxygen in the tissues is low, the partial pressure of carbon dioxide is high, the pH is low, and the temperature is high. Consequently, as an example, during periods of physical exercise, more oxygen is released to the skeletal muscles.

59. **a**

60. **a:** Carbon dioxide is carried in the blood dissolved in plasma (produces the Pco_2 of the blood), coupled with hemoglobin, and combined with water as carbonic acid and its component ions.

61. The amount of carbon dioxide in the body is dependent on **ventilatory effectiveness.** Under normal conditions, if ventilations are increased, the carbon dioxide will **decrease.** If ventilations are decreased, the carbon dioxide will **increase.**

62. **a:** The main nervous centers for controlling the rate and depth of breathing **are located in the medulla oblongata and the pons of the brainstem,** are sensitive to slight changes in the concentration of *carbon dioxide* in the blood plasma, and increase respirations when the carbon dioxide concentration in the blood is *elevated.* The *cerebral cortex* can influence respiration by allowing a person to voluntarily speed up or slow down the breathing rate.

63. **d:** The peripheral chemoreceptors **sense changes in CO_2 and O_2 concentrations of the arterial blood.** They are located peripherally in the *aortic arch and carotid bodies.* When stimulated, these receptors send nerve impulses to the respiratory control centers in the medulla that in turn modify the respiratory rate.

64. Seven factors that increase or decrease respiration include **body temperature—respirations increase with fever; drug and medications—may increase or decrease respirations depending on their physiological action; pain—increases respirations; emotion—increases respirations; hypoxia—increases respirations; acidosis—respirations increase as a compensatory response to increased CO_2 production; and sleep—respirations decrease.**

65. Modified forms of respiration: **a. Cough:** forceful, spastic exhalation of a large volume of air from the lungs; **b. Sneeze:** sudden forceful exhalation from the nose that clears the nasopharynx; **c. Sigh:** involuntary slow, deep breath followed by prolonged expiration; **d. Hiccough:** sudden inspiration caused by spasmodic contraction of the diaphragm and intermittent spastic closure of the glottis; **e. Gag reflex:** spastic pharyngeal and esophageal reflex that results from stimulus of the posterior pharynx; may bring about nausea and vomiting.

66. **a**

67. **a**

68. In addition to **protective latex or vinyl gloves and eyewear, you should wear a mask and protective gown.**

69. **c:** The first thing to do with an unconscious patient is to determine whether an open airway is present. If airway compromise is identified, it must be resolved. Once a patent airway is ensured, breathing must be assessed. If the patient is not breathing adequately, the EMT-I must provide assisted breathing. Following that, circulatory effectiveness must be evaluated and measures taken to resolve any life-threatening deficiencies.

70. Five indications of respiratory function include **airway patency, appearance of the neck, breathing efforts, color of the skin, breath sounds, outward signs (flaring of the nares, retraction, noisy breathing), air movement at the nose and mouth, compliance (felt with ventilatory assistance provided with a bag-mask device), and the pulse rate.** Devices such as the pulse oximetry unit can be used to determine the oxygen saturation. Silence is another sign of respiratory function; it indicates a complete absence of air movement.

71. **a**

72. Three signs found in the neck that indicate a likely respiratory problem are **distended jugular veins, tracheal shift,** and **tugging.**

73. **d:** Pulsus paradoxus is **indicative of an increase in the intrathoracic pressure.** The increase in pressure within the thoracic cavity interferes with the ability of the ventricles to fill properly, leading to a decrease in blood pressure. Pulsus paradoxus is an indicator of *respiratory distress,* is present when the systolic blood pressure *decreases* greater than 10 mm Hg during inspiration (a change in pulse quality may also be detected), and is seen in *chronic obstructive pulmonary disease (COPD).*

74. **b:** Pulse oximetry **detects trends in a patient's oxygenation status within 6 seconds;** is a simple, *noninvasive* procedure used to determine effectiveness of patient oxygenation; allows for continuous monitoring; works by measuring transmission of red and near-infrared light through *arterial* capillary beds; and is *unreliable* in carbon monoxide poisoning and states of hypoperfusion.

75. **b:** Disposable colorimetric end-tidal CO_2 detectors **detect the presence of carbon dioxide in the intubated patient's expired air,** indicate proper placement of the endotracheal tube in the trachea by turning *yellow* with patient expiration, and are not always *reliable* in cardiac arrest because adequate circulation and pulmonary perfusion are required to obtain diffusion of CO_2 from the pulmonary capillary bed.

76. **b**

77. After the endotracheal tube is placed and before any ventilation attempts, the device is attached (with the compression plunger fully inserted into the syringe barrel) to the endotracheal tube. The compression plunger is then withdrawn. **If the tube is in the esophagus, its soft, unsupported walls will collapse around the end of the endotracheal tube, preventing air from being drawn out of the device.** The bulb-type esophageal detector device works in a similar way. It is compressed before it is attached to the endotracheal tube. As compression on the bulb is released, a vacuum is created. **If the tube is in the esophagus, the bulb will not reinflate.**

78. Four factors that can produce false readings when using the esophageal intubation detector are **morbid obesity, late pregnancy, status asthmaticus,** and **copious tracheal secretions.**

79. Four things that indicate a likely respiratory problem are **the presence of nasal flaring (nostrils wide open during inspiration), tracheal tugging, retraction of the intercostal muscles,** and **use of the diaphragm and neck muscles to assist with inspiration.**

80. **b**

81. The sites of the chest that are usually auscultated include (1) just beneath the right and left clavicles (apexes of the lungs) and (2) the right and left lateral sides of the chest in the midaxillary line (at the level of the eighth or ninth intercostal space).
    At each site, the EMT-I should listen to one side of the chest and then the other. This helps compare airflow in and out of each lung.

82. **False:** At *each* site, you should listen to first one side of the chest and then the other.

83. **True**

84. **False:** The presence of airflow with auscultation over the sternal notch reveals the *correct* placement of an endotracheal tube in the *trachea*.

85. **True**

86. Gastric distention indicates **inadequate hyperextension of the head, too much pressure being generated by the ventilatory device,** and **improperly placed airway adjuncts.**

87. **c**

88. Tachycardia usually accompanies hypoxemia, whereas **bradycardia** suggests anoxia with imminent cardiac arrest.

89. **b:** Hypoxia **is defined as a decreased or inadequate supply of oxygen.** It leads to *anaerobic* metabolism, metabolic acidosis, cellular depression, and eventually cellular death. It also leads to swelling of the brain, cardiac dysrhythmias, decreased cardiac output, and *increased myocardial and respiratory workloads.*

90. Causes of hypoxia: **insufficient oxygen in the inspired air; failure of the ventilatory mechanism; upper airway compromise; lower airway compromise; circulatory deficiency;** and **cellular deficiency.**

91. To clear an oxygen supply cylinder of dust or dirt, **stand to the side of the main valve opening, and open (crack) the cylinder valve slightly for just a second. This should clear any dirt or dust out of the delivery port or threaded outlet.**

92. The **pressure** in a full oxygen cylinder is approximately **2000** psi. This pressure is too **high** to be **safely** delivered to a patient. Therefore a pressure **regulator** is attached to the **cylinder** to deliver a safe working pressure of **30** to **70** psi.

93. **c**

94. Petroleum-based substances or adhesive tape **that comes into contact with the valve stem of the oxygen cylinder or the oxygen regulator can contaminate the oxygen and contribute to spontaneous combustion when mixed with the pressurized oxygen.**

95. Common signs for oxygen cylinders used in the prehospital setting are:

    D: **400 L**

    E: **660 L**

    M: **3450 L**

96. **a:** The constant flow selector valve **is the type of regulator commonly used on portable units,** has *no* gauge, and controls the liter flow per minute through a *dial that has stepped increments (2, 4, 6, or 15 L or more per minute)*. It can be accurately used with any type of oxygen delivery device and with any size oxygen cylinder. It is *rugged* and functions *at any angle*. The *pressure-compensated flow meter* is more fragile than the Bourdon gauge and must be operated in an upright position.

97. The correct order for attaching a regulator to an oxygen cylinder and connecting an oxygen delivery device.
    1. **Select an oxygen cylinder.**
    2. **Place the cylinder in an upright position, and stand to one side.**
    3. **If present, remove the plastic wrapper or cap protecting the cylinder outlet.**
    4. **Crack the valve for 1 second to clear any dust or dirt.**
    5. **Line up the pins in the regulator yoke to the corresponding holes in the cylinder valve (smaller tanks) or the threads of the regulator to the oxygen cylinder outlet (larger tanks).**
    6. **Tighten the regulator to the cylinder valve.**
    7. **Attach oxygen tubing and delivery device.**

98. First subtract 200 psi (safe residual pressure) from 1500—this leaves 1300 psi. Next, multiply 1300 psi by 0.16 (the tank factor)—this equals 208 psi. Now divide 208 psi by 15 L/min to yield a time of **13.86 (rounded off to 14) minutes.**

99. **True**

100. **False:** Oxygen humidifiers *do not* produce an adverse effect. However, there is a risk of infection if the water is not changed and the reservoir is not kept clean.

101. **True**

102. **Patients are usually more comfortable when given humidified oxygen. This is particularly true in patients who have COPD and in children.**

103. Oxygen delivery devices with concentration each delivers: **b. 80% to 100%:** nonrebreather mask, 10 to 15 L/min; **d. 24% to 44%:** nasal cannula, 2 to 6 L/min; **e. 35% to 60%:** simple face mask, 6 to 10 L/min.

104. **d:** The recommended oxygen concentration is 24% to 28% delivered by Venturi mask. Alternatively, a nasal cannula supplied with a liter flow rate of 1 to 3 L can be used. If a patient develops respiratory depression, the breathing must be supported with a bag-mask device supplied with 15 L of oxygen (85% to 100%) or another ventilatory device.

105. **d**

106. **b**

107. Oxygen delivery devices with characteristics: **a. Nasal cannula:** flow rate should be limited to 6 L/min; should be used when the patient is frightened or feels suffocated with other delivery devices; offers the benefit of not interfering with assessment because the patient's response to questions can be more easily heard; **b. Simple face mask:** no less than 6 L should be administered through the device because expired carbon dioxide can accumulate, resulting in hypercarbia; has holes in the side of the mask that allow air to be drawn into the mask during inspiration and expired air to be passed to the outside; **c. Nonrebreather mask:** at least 10 L of oxygen is needed to move sufficient oxygen into the reservoir bag and remove exhaled carbon dioxide; recommended for the treatment of severely hypoxic patients (e.g., respiratory compromise, shock, acute myocardial infarction, trauma, and carbon monoxide poisoning); the reservoir bag should not be allowed to totally deflate because the patient can suffocate; **d. Venturi mask:** with this device the same amount of ambient air is always entrained regardless of the rate or depth of respirations; the device delivers oxygen concentrations of 24%, 28%, 35%, or 40%.

108. 1. **Attach tubing of the nonrebreather mask to oxygen flow meter nipple, and prefill the reservoir by using your finger to cover the exhaust portal (the connection between the mask and reservoir).**

2. Adjust the flow meter to deliver 10 to 15 L/min.
3. Apply the mask by placing it over the patient's nose, mouth, and chin.
4. Press the flexible metal nosepiece so that it fits the bridge of the nose.
5. Tighten the mask by adjusting the elastic strap on both sides simultaneously until the mask is secure.
6. Make sure the one-way flaps are secure and functioning, and observe the reservoir bag as the patient breathes (if it collapses more than slightly during inspiration, increase the flow rate). Keep the reservoir from kinking or twisting.
7. Continuously monitor the oxygen level in the tank.

109. **a:** A decrease in either the respiratory rate or volume will lead to a reduction in the respiratory minute volume. This is referred to as hypoventilation. Hypoventilation leads to **the accumulation of carbon dioxide** (also referred to as hypercarbia), development of hypoxia, and a *lowered* pH. Too little air exchange takes place because of an overall reduction in respiratory minute volumes. Ultimately, if left uncorrected, respiratory and/or cardiac arrest can occur.

110. Patients with decreased levels of consciousness and respiratory rates of less than **10** or greater than **30** breaths/min should receive ventilatory assistance.

111. **b**

112. **a**

113. **c:** When providing mouth-to-mouth ventilation, **you may be exposed to communicable disease.** For this reason, you should use a protective barrier.

114. **b**

115. **b:** The pocket mask is a clear plastic device that covers the patient's mouth and nose, thereby preventing contact between the EMT-I and patient. **This eliminates exposure to the patient's exhaled air** and reduces the risk of contamination during resuscitation. Mouth-to-mask breathing has been shown to be more effective at delivering adequate tidal volumes than when a bag-mask device is used. Mouth-to-mask breathing, combined with an oxygen flow rate of 10 L/min, can deliver an inspired oxygen concentration of approximately 50%.

116. Components of the bag-mask device include: **A.** nonrebreathing valve; **B.** bag; **C.** oxygen supply tubing; **D.** oxygen reservoir; **E.** intake valve; and **F.** face mask.

117. **a:** Bag-mask devices **convey a sense of compliance of a patient's lungs to the rescuer.** In addition, only *trained* individuals should use these devices. Because of the potential for skill degradation after only a short while, ventilating with a bag-mask device should be practiced on a CPR mannequin with appropriate frequency. The bag-mask device has a *standard 15 mm/22 mm* fitting that allows for attachment of the device to a standard mask, endotracheal tube, or dual lumen airway. When equipped with a *reservoir* and *supplied with 10 to 15 L of oxygen, the bag-mask device will deliver approximately 85% to 100% oxygen.*

118. **d:** When ventilating a patient with a bag-mask device, the **mask must be held firmly to the patient's face to prevent air from leaking,** the bag should be squeezed until the patient's *chest* rises, the patient's neck must be *hyperextended,* and *attachment of the device to an endotracheal tube is preferred.*

119. 1. Select the appropriate size mask, and place it on the patient's face with the narrow end (apex) over the bridge of the nose and the wide end (base) in the groove between the lower lip and chin.
2. Obtain a tight seal by applying firm downward pressure over the mask with your thumb on the dome and index and middle fingers on the base.
3. Hook the last two or three fingers under the jaw, and then pull the chin backward to maintain the head tilt.
4. Squeeze the bag between one hand and your arm, chest, or thigh (if kneeling), using a smooth, steady action. Between each compression the bag should be allowed to refill completely.
5. Watch for the patient's chest to rise during ventilation and collapse during passive exhalation.
6. Auscultate the chest to make sure that appropriate ventilation is occurring.

7. Connect the reservoir and oxygen tubing to the oxygen inlet of the bag-mask device, and deliver oxygen at 12 to 15 L/min.
8. **Ventilate the patient with a tidal volume of approximately 6 to 7 mL/kg or 500 to 600 mL over 1 second (until the chest rises).** Breaths should be delivered at a rate of at least 8 to 10 times per minute if the patient is pulseless and 10 to 12 times per minute if the patient has a perfusion rhythm.

120. Volumes for three sizes of bag-mask devices:
Adult: **capable of storing between 1000 and 1600 mL of air**
Child: **capable of storing 500 to 700 mL of air**
Infant: **capable of storing 150 to 240 mL of air**

121. **c:** When gastric distention occurs in the field setting and is interfering with ventilations, measures must be taken to relieve it. **After turning the patient onto his or her side, one hand should be placed over the epigastrium, between the umbilicus and the rib cage, and moderate pressure exerted.** A suction unit should be available to clear the airway in case of regurgitation.

122. **c:** Two- or three-person bag-mask ventilation **offers the advantage of maintaining a superior mask seal and volume delivery.** It is especially useful for cervical spine–immobilized patients or when you are having difficulty obtaining or maintaining an adequate mask seal. Disadvantages of the procedures include that they require additional personnel and may be difficult to perform in tight quarters such as in the back of an ambulance.

123. When ventilating with a bag-mask device using two EMT-Is **one holds the mask in place and maintains an open airway while the other squeezes the bag with two hands.**

124. **d:** The flow-restricted, oxygen-powered ventilation device **depends on an oxygen source.** In addition it is a *manually triggered, oxygen-powered (delivering 100% oxygen at 40 to 60 L/min)* ventilatory device and creates *high* airway pressures. Because of the sudden high pressure it provides, it should not be used in pediatric patients (under the age of 16) or in patients who are endotracheally intubated. On the delivery end, it can be attached to a face mask.

125. **b**

126. **True**

127. **False:** Automatic transport ventilators are equipped with a *standard 15 mm inside diameter/22 mm outside diameter adapter* that allows them to be attached to various airway devices and masks.

128. **False:** Automatic transport ventilators are often equipped with *two controls: one that regulates the ventilatory rate and one that regulates tidal volume.*

129. **True**

130. Four conditions in which pop-off valves on automatic transport ventilators may be detrimental are **cardiogenic pulmonary edema, adult respiratory distress syndrome (ARDS), pulmonary contusion, bronchospasm,** and **other disorders in which high airway pressures must be exerted.**

131. Four advantages of an automatic transport ventilator are that **it frees personnel to perform other tasks; it is lightweight, portable, durable, and mechanically simple; it has an adjustable tidal volume and rate; and it adapts to a portable oxygen tank.**

132. The automatic transport ventilator **cannot detect tube displacement, does not detect increasing airway resistance, is difficult to secure, and is dependent on oxygen tank pressure.**

133. **d**

134. Cricoid pressure **compresses the esophagus between the cricoid ring and the cervical spine.**

135. Cricoid pressure moves **the larynx posteriorly, making visualization of the glottic opening and passage of the endotracheal tube easier.**

136. **d**

137. **c**

138. **d:** When ventilating infants and toddlers with a bag-mask device, maintaining the head in a neutral, *sniffing position without hyperextension* is usually adequate for infants and toddlers. **A folded towel can be placed under the patient's shoulders to help maintain the sniffing position.** The ventilation rate for infants and children is at least *20* breaths/min. It is best to use a bag-mask device that provides at least *450* cc of volume and is *not* equipped with a pop-off valve on pediatric patients. Infant bag-mask devices that provide only approxi-

mately 250 cc should **NOT** be used in infants and neonates because they cannot give enough tidal volume and provide a longer time for inspiration.

139. **Steps for using a bag-mask device or mouth-to-stoma technique to provide ventilatory assistance to a patient with a stoma are as follows: Locate the stoma site and expose it. Obtain a tight seal around the stoma site, and deliver ventilation as you normally would. Check for adequate ventilation with each breath. Be sure to seal the mouth and nose if you note air leaking from these sites. When using the mouth-to-stoma technique it is preferable to use a pocket mask to cover the stoma.**

140. Answers to crossword puzzle

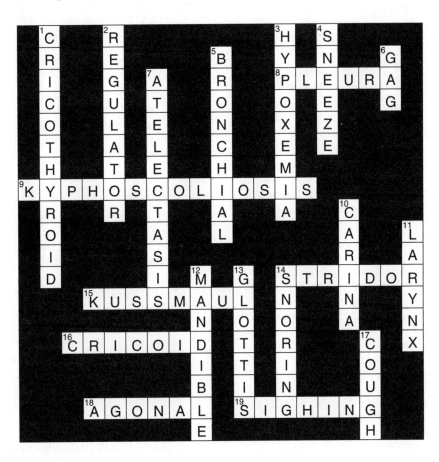

141. **a. Tongue:** most common cause of upper airway obstruction; occurs when muscle tone is depressed or absent in the supine patient (the tongue relaxes and falls back against the pharynx and occludes airflow); **b. Laryngeal edema:** in adults, can result from anaphylaxis, epiglottitis, and inhalation of superheated air, smoke, or toxic substances. In children, upper airway obstruction is typically caused by epiglottitis or croup; **c. Trauma:** clotted blood, facial bones, teeth, fractured larynx; **d. Foreign body:** "café coronary" (occurs when a person swallows a large piece of food, typically meat), loose teeth, dentures, and toys.

142. **b:** Lifting the mandible forward displaces the hyoid *anteriorly,* **pulls the tongue forward,** and keeps the epiglottis elevated *away* from the back of the throat and glottic opening.

143. **d**

144. **a:** Caution must be used whenever trauma is suspected. Those cases require use of the chin-lift without head-tilt maneuver or modified jaw thrust to open the airway.

145. **c:** To perform the head-tilt/chin-lift maneuver the EMT-I should **place one hand on the patient's forehead and apply firm, backward pressure with the palm to tip the head back.** Next, the patient's chin should be grasped with the rescuer's

hand by placing the thumb on the front of the jaw and positioning the index finger under the jaw. The jaw should then be lifted anteriorly to open the airway.

146. **d:** The jaw thrust without head tilt is the preferred technique. The reason is that the patient may have sustained a cervical spine injury, and this procedure will not hyperextend or flex the neck. If the modified jaw thrust or chin lift without head tilt is unsuccessful, the head should be slightly tilted back until the airway is opened.

147. **d**

148. **False:** The oropharyngeal airway should only be used in *unconscious patients.* Placement of an oropharyngeal airway in those who are conscious, semiconscious, or who have an active gag reflex may precipitate vomiting and as such should not be used.

149. **False:** The oropharyngeal airway fits over the tongue, extending back into the pharynx. It is used to hold the tongue in place so that it does not fall back against the posterior oropharynx and obstruct the airway. It *does nothing* to prevent regurgitation of stomach contents.

150. **False:** Oropharyngeal airways are available in a *variety of sizes including* 0, 1, 2, 3, 4, 5, and 6 (size 0 is the smallest, 6 is the largest). Sizes 4 and 5 fit the average-size adult. The EMT-I should be careful to select a proper sized airway because one that is too large or too small for a particular patient can obstruct the airway. As a means of checking for proper sizing, the oropharyngeal airway should be measured against the patient's face before insertion. The proximal (top) end should be even with the center of the mouth, and the distal (bottom) end should be even with the angle of the jaw (mandible).

151. **True**

152. **One that is too short fails to hold the tongue forward and may push it back against the posterior oropharynx. An oropharyngeal airway that is too long can press the epiglottis against the laryngeal entrance, thereby obstructing the airway.**

153. **b:** An oropharyngeal airway is indicated for a **16-year-old patient who is unconscious from a drug overdose.** It is contraindicated in the presence of lower facial trauma and is of no value in patients who have a stoma (because they breathe through a permanent hole in their neck). When the possibility of epiglottitis exists, no airway adjunct should be inserted into the oropharynx because it may precipitate fatal tracheal obstruction.

154. **c:** The nasopharyngeal airway **is an uncuffed soft plastic tube, extends from the nostril to the posterior pharynx just below the base of the tongue,** and **should not be used when basilar skull fracture is likely present** because the tube can be inadvertently passed into the brain. Use of the nasopharyngeal airway should be avoided in patients who have nasal obstructions, are prone to nosebleeds, or when there are indications of nasal injury. Advantages of the nasopharyngeal airway are that it may be used when a gag reflex is present, in the presence of injuries to the oral cavity (trauma to the mandible, maxilla, or significant soft tissue damage to the tongue or pharynx), and when the patient's teeth are clenched.

155. **b:** The proper size nasopharyngeal airway extends from the **tip of the nose to the tip of the ear lobe.** It is slightly smaller in diameter than the opening of the patient's nostril (about the diameter of the patient's little finger).

156. Selecting the appropriate size nasopharyngeal airway is important because **a tube that is too short will not extend past the tongue.** Conversely, **a tube that is too long may pass into the esophagus, resulting in hypoventilation and gastric distention when artificial ventilation is delivered.**

157. **Endo**tracheal means *within the trachea.*

158. **c:** Endotracheal intubation is the preferred technique for airway control in patients who are unable to maintain a patent airway in all types of medical and trauma emergencies. It is typically accomplished using specialized equipment through one of two routes—orotracheal or nasotracheal.

159. Seven indications for endotracheal intubation are **when the EMT-I is unable to ventilate an unconscious patient with conventional methods, when patients cannot protect their airway (coma, respiratory and cardiac arrest), when prolonged artificial ventilation is needed, in patients experiencing or likely to experience upper airway compromise, unconscious patients who lack a gag reflex, when there is decreased tidal volume because of slow respirations,** and **airway obstruction resulting from foreign bodies, trauma, or anaphylaxis.**

160. **a:** Endotracheal intubation prevents gastric insufflation as air is delivered directly into the trachea during positive-pressure ventilation, facilitates ventilation and oxygenation because a tight face seal is *not* required, provides a direct route into the trachea that allows for easy suctioning of the trachea and bronchi, provides an effective route for administration of some

medications, is a complicated skill requiring extensive initial and ongoing training to ensure proficiency, and usually requires *specialized equipment and visualization of vocal cords to place the tube.*

161. **b**

162. **d:** Endotracheal intubation is contraindicated in patients **with epiglottitis.** The reason is that insertion and manipulation of the laryngoscope into the upper airway may precipitate life-threatening laryngospasm. Instead, in this condition, the patient's breathing should be assisted with a bag-mask device until more definitive airway procedures can be performed.

163. **The laryngoscope is used to move the tongue and epiglottis out of the way. This allows visualization of the vocal cords and placement of an endotracheal tube.**

164. Components of the laryngoscope with the function of each

Name of Component	Function
A. Handle	Holds several batteries that serve as the energy source for the light
B. Light	Illuminates the airway so the upper airway structures can be seen
C. Hooked indentation	Where blade is attached to handle
D. Tip	Area of blade that is inserted deep into airway

165. **b:** The straight laryngoscope blade is inserted **posterior to the epiglottis.** When the handle is lifted anteriorly the epiglottis is lifted out of the way, exposing the glottic opening.

166. Types of laryngoscope blades with characteristics:
a. Curved: Its tip is inserted into the vallecula (in this position, the tongue and epiglottis are raised out of the way when the laryngoscope handle is lifted anteriorly); also referred to as a MacIntosh blade; permits more room for visualization of the glottic opening and tube insertion; is associated with less trauma and reflex stimulation (because many of the sensitive gag receptors are located on the posterior surface of the epiglottis); **b. Straight:** also referred to as a Miller, Wisconsin, or Flagg blade; is preferred in infants (because it provides greater displacement of the tongue and better visualization of the glottis, which lies higher and more anterior).

167. **d:** Laryngoscope blades come in a variety of sizes ranging from #1 for the infant to #4 for the large adult patient.

168. Components of endotracheal tube with the functions of each

Name of Component	Function
a. Standard 15-mm adapter	Can be connected to various devices for delivery of positive-pressure ventilation
b. One-way inflating valve	Accepts a syringe for inflation of distal cuff
c. Pilot balloon	Reveals whether the distal cuff is inflated
d. Inflating tube	Used to inflate distal cuff
e. Tube	Flexible, translucent tube that is open at both ends
f. Balloon cuff	When inflated, occludes the remainder of the tracheal lumen, preventing aspiration around the tube and minimizing air leaks
g. Beveled end	Facilitates placement between the vocal cords

169. The abbreviation ID means **internal diameter.** This is the standard for measuring endotracheal tubes that come in graduated sizes from 3 to 9 mm.

170. **c:** An **8.0 to 8.5** i.d. endotracheal tube is recommended for the average size adult male. When immediate placement of an endotracheal tube is required, a 7.5 i.d. tube may be used for both adult female and male patients.

171. **A tube that is too small provides too little airflow and may lead to inadequate ventilatory volumes being delivered. It may also produce a negative pressure in the lungs that can lead to pneumothorax and pulmonary edema. An endotracheal tube that is too large can cause tracheal edema and/or damage to the vocal cords.**

172. **Uncuffed endotracheal tubes are used for infants and children younger than 8 years of age because the round narrowing of the cricoid cartilage serves as a functional cuff.**

173. **b:** The distal cuff of an endotracheal tube should be inflated with **5 to 10** mL of air. Use only the minimum amount of air necessary to create an effective seal. Determine how much air is needed by listening for the sound of air leaking around the tube before distal cuff inflation. The cuff should be inflated only to the point where air leakage stops.

174. **Because the stylet can cause tissue damage, it should be recessed at least 0.5 inch from the distal tip of the endotracheal tube.**

175. **c:** Magill forceps resemble a bent pair of scissors with circular tips at their distal end (can be used to grasp objects). They are used to **guide endotracheal tubes into place during nasotracheal intubation** and extract foreign objects from the posterior pharynx.

176. **False:** The distal cuff should *always* be examined for leaks before placement in the trachea. Withdraw the plunger of a 10-cc syringe to pull in 5 to 10 cc of air. Insert the tip of the syringe into the port of the one-way inflation valve that is connected to the distal cuff. Push the entire contents of the syringe into the distal cuff. It should be firm and have no leaks.

177. **True:** The bulb should appear bright white. A yellow, flickering light provides insufficient illumination of the upper airway and suggests the laryngoscope batteries are in need of replacement. If the light fails to go on, suspect that the batteries are dead or the bulb is loose. Infrequently, the problem may lie in the contact point(s) or the wire traveling through the blade to the bulb.

178. **c:** Each attempt at endotracheal intubation should not take longer than **30** seconds.

179.

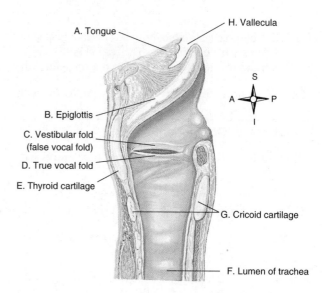

180. Cricoid pressure used during intubation is performed **by applying firm downward pressure on the patient's neck in the region of the cricoid cartilage. This action pushes the larynx backward, allowing better visualization.**

181. The term **oro**tracheal means *through the mouth.*

182. The advantage of the orotracheal route over nasotracheal intubation is that **it allows the EMT-I to directly observe the endotracheal tube being passed between the vocal cords.** This is an essential step for ensuring correct placement.

183. **a:** The patient's head should be placed in a **sniffing** position when performing endotracheal intubation. This aligns the three axes of the mouth, pharynx, and trachea.

184. 1. **Place the patient's head and neck into an appropriate position.**
   2. **Using the left hand, grasp the laryngoscope by its handle, and insert the blade into the right side of the patient's mouth. Using a sweeping motion, displace the tongue to the left.**
   3. **Move the blade slightly toward the midline, and advance it until the distal end is positioned at the base of the tongue. Visualize the tip of the epiglottis, and then place the laryngoscope blade into the proper position.**

4. Lift the laryngoscope slightly upward and forward to displace the jaw and airway structures without allowing the blade to touch the teeth. Suction any vomitus or secretions lying in the posterior pharynx.
5. Keeping the left wrist straight, use the shoulder and arm to continue lifting the mandible and tongue at a 45-degree angle to the ground until the glottis is exposed.
6. Grasp the endotracheal tube in the right hand, holding it the same way a pencil is grasped. Advance it through the right corner of the patient's mouth, directing the distal end of the tube up or down to pass it into the larynx.
7. Insert the endotracheal tube into the glottic opening, and advance it until the distal cuff disappears slightly (0.5 to 1 inch) past the vocal cords. Observe the tube enter the glottic opening. Hold it in place with the left hand. Do not release the endotracheal tube before it is secured in place.
8. Inflate the distal cuff with between 5 and 10 cc of air. Use only the minimum amount of air necessary to create an effective seal.
9. Attach a ventilatory device to the 15/22-mm adapter of the tube, and deliver several breaths.
10. Listen over the epigastrium to ensure there are no sounds when ventilations are delivered.
11. Auscultate the chest for the presence of equal bilateral lung sounds.
12. Ventilate the patient with 100% oxygen, and insert an oropharyngeal airway to serve as a bite block.
13. Secure the endotracheal tube in place with umbilical tape or a commercial device while continuing ventilatory support.

185. **a:** You can facilitate intubation of a patient with an anterior trachea by **having a partner apply firm downward pressure on the patient's neck in the region of the cricoid cartilage.** This pushes the larynx backward, allowing better visualization. A stylet may be useful in this situation because the tube can be more easily directed anteriorly.

186. **False:** If a tube is inserted between the vocal cords, *no* sound can be generated.

187. **True**

188. **d**

189. **c:** Accidental esophageal intubation is identified by **gurgling sounds heard over the epigastric area,** an *absence* of breath sounds, and a patient who becomes *increasingly more cyanotic.*

190. **a**

191. Complications of endotracheal intubation: **a. Hypoxia:** occurs when intubation attempts are longer than appropriate or the EMT-I fails to provide ventilatory support between procedures; **b. Injury to teeth and tissue:** when manipulating the jaw anteriorly, use upward traction rather than following the natural inclination to rotate and flex the wrist; **c. Vallecula misplacement:** occurs when the tube is allowed to slip too far anteriorly and becomes lodged in the space between the epiglottis and base of the tongue; slightly withdraw and redirect the tube posteriorly; **d. Endobronchial misplacement:** occurs when the endotracheal tube is inserted too far; withdraw the tube until lung sounds are heard equally on both sides of the chest; **e. Esophageal intubation:** occurs when the endotracheal tube is misplaced posteriorly.

192. **True**

193. **False:** The biggest concern with extubation is that patients who are awake are at high risk of laryngospasm immediately following extubation, and it is difficult to reintubate a laryngospastic patient.

194. **True**

195. Four indications for intubation of a child are **inadequate central nervous system control of ventilation; functional or anatomical airway obstruction; excessive work of breathing leading to fatigue; the need for high peak inspiratory pressure or positive end-expiratory pressure to maintain effective alveolar gas exchange.**

196. **c**

197. Four ways of confirming proper endotracheal tube placement in a pediatric patient are to **observe for symmetrical chest expansion, auscultate the epigastrium for sounds during ventilation (there should be an absence of sounds), auscultate for equal breath sounds over each lateral chest wall high in the axillae, note the presence of improved heart rate and color,** and **apply an end-tidal carbon dioxide detector.** Also, pulse oximetry can be used to assess proper tube placement.

198. Because children have more soft tissue in the oropharynx, extra care must be used when inserting the laryngoscope so as not to cause injury. The child's larger tongue must be swept out of the way as completely as possible to keep it from blocking your line of sight. Also, the larynx is higher in the pediatric patient than in the adult, and the epiglottis is floppy, making visualization of the cords more difficult.

199. When properly inserted, the **cream-colored cuff will rest in the pharynx and effectively seal off the oropharynx and nasopharynx when inflated.** The tube will come to rest in either the trachea or esophagus. When the distal cuff is inflated and air is delivered through the appropriate tube, the lungs will be inflated.

200. **d:** The ETC airway is different from the PtL airway in that the ETC **has a self-adjusting, self-positioning posterior pharyngeal balloon,** is a *double* lumen tube having two balloon cuffs, *allows immediate suctioning* of gastric contents (because there is no stylet in the distal lumen), and *allows a spontaneously breathing patient to breathe through multiple small ports* in the unused lumen in undiagnosed tracheal placement.

201. 1. **Connect the blue-tipped syringe (drawn up with at least 100 mL of air) to the blue one-way valve marked tube "No. 1." Then connect the white-tipped syringe (drawn up with at least 15 mL of air) to the white one-way valve marked tube "No. 2."**
    2. If a spinal injury is not likely, open the airway by hyperextending the patient's head and neck.
    3. Direct the ventilator to move to the side of the patient's head while you assume a position above the patient. Insert the thumb of the right hand deep into the patient's mouth, grasping the tongue and lower jaw between the thumb and index finger. Lift the tongue and lower jaw anteriorly, away from the posterior pharynx.
    4. Hold the ETC so that it curves in the same direction as the natural curvature of the pharynx. Insert the tip into the mouth along the midline, and advance it carefully along the tongue. Gently guide the ETC along the base of the tongue and into the airway. When the ETC is at the proper depth, the teeth or alveolar ridge will be between the heavy black lines.
    5. Inflate the blue pilot balloon (and flesh-colored cuff) with the predrawn 100 mL blue-tipped syringe.
    6. Once that cuff is inflated and the pilot balloon is tense, immediately inflate the white pilot balloon (and the distal cuff) with the smaller predrawn 15-mL syringe. The ETC may move forward a little bit, but this is normal.
    7. Ventilate the patient through the blue tube.
    8. Observe the patient's chest, and listen for lung sounds. If the chest rises and falls and breath sounds are heard, the ETC is in the esophagus. Thus the patient is being ventilated as with an EOA/EGTA. When this is the case, continue to ventilate through the blue tube.
    9. If the chest does not rise and breath sounds are not heard, the ETC is in the trachea. In this case, attach the bag-mask device or other ventilatory device to the shorter clear tube, and ventilate the patient through it. Again, listen for breath sounds in all lung fields and in both axillae. Also, listen over the stomach.
    10. Continue ventilating the patient with a bag-mask device or other ventilatory device.

202. **b:** Pharyngotracheal airways are designed to deliver lung ventilation *when placed either in the trachea or the esophagus,* are *inserted blindly* into the oropharynx and esophagus or trachea, and may be inserted by an EMT-I.

203. The first is a short, wide tube that has a large cuff along its lower portion. When inflated, this cuff seals off the oropharynx, and air introduced through the tube at its proximal end enters the pharynx. A second, longer tube travels through the first, extending past its distal end. Because of its longer length, it can be passed into either the trachea or the esophagus. At the distal end of the longer tube is a cuff that, when inflated, seals off whichever anatomical structure it is in. When the longer tube is in the esophagus, the device acts like an EOA and the patient is ventilated through the first tube. When the longer tube is in the trachea, the device acts like an endotracheal tube and the patient is ventilated through it.

204. **a: PtL has a longer tube that acts like an EOA when it is inserted into the esophagus,** has 15/22-mm connectors at its *proximal* end for attachment of a standard ventilatory device, *eliminates* the need for a face mask to maintain a face seal because the oropharyngeal cuff seals off the oropharynx, and *does not* keep the patient from aspirating foreign materials (such as blood or vomitus) present in the upper airway when the longer tube is in the esophagus.

205. Close the relief port with the small white cap, and open the slide clamp and blow air into the inflation valve to check the proximal and distal cuffs for proper inflation. Once this is done, remove the small white cap and deflate both cuffs fully. Then replace the white cap on the relief port.

206. 1. Tell the rescuer who is providing ventilatory support to move to the side of the patient's head while you assume a position above the patient.
    2. Place the patient's head into a hyperextended position if there are no suspected spinal injuries. When spinal injury is suspected, the patient's head and neck should be kept in a neutral in-line position.
    3. Use the tongue-jaw lift to move the tongue out of the way.
    4. Insert the device into the patient's mouth along the midline. Advance the tube until the flange rests against the patient's teeth.
    5. Loop the white strap around the patient's head, and secure it in place.
    6. Once in place, inflate both distal cuffs simultaneously by taking a deep breath and blowing into the inflation valve.
    7. Connect a ventilatory device to the green tube (oropharyngeal tube), and deliver a breath. If the chest rises, the longer tube is in the esophagus and ventilations should be continued through the green tube.
    8. If the chest does not rise, the longer tube is in the trachea. The stylet must then be removed from the longer tube and assisted breathing provided through it.
    9. Continue delivering ventilatory support, and reassess for proper placement on an ongoing basis.

207. b

208. c

209. Once the LMA is properly positioned into a patient's hypopharynx, an inflation line is used to inflate the cuff of the mask. This seals the larynx and situates the distal opening of the tube just above the glottis, thus providing an open, secure airway. At the proximal end of the tube there is a standard 15-mm adapter that is attached to a bag-mask device for the provision of ventilatory support.

210. **True**

211. **False:** The LMA does *not* ensure absolute protection against aspiration, but regurgitation is less likely with the LMA than with the bag-mask device.

212. LMA sizes for various-sized patients

Size of Patient	Size
Neonates/infants up to 6.5 kg	1
Babies and children up to 20 kg	2
Children between 20 and 30 kg	2½
Children and small adults more than 30 kg	3
Average-sized and large adults	4

213. Cuff inflation volumes for various-sized LMAs

LMA Size	Cuff Inflation Volumes
Size 1	2 to 4 mL
Size 2	Up to 10 mL
Size 2½	Up to 15 mL
Size 3	20 mL
Size 4	30 mL

214. **a:** The source of upper airway obstruction caused by a foreign body in the adult is usually **food.** Common factors associated with choking on food include large, poorly chewed pieces of meat; alcohol consumption; laughing, talking, or exercising while eating; or dentures. *In children* the obstruction is usually caused by *food or other objects such as bubble gum, balloons, marbles, beads, coins, or small toy parts.*

215. **d: Stridor,** or crowing (noisy airflow during inspiration); cyanosis; and suprasternal, supraclavicular, and/or intercostal retraction in the spontaneously breathing patient are indicative of partial upper airway obstruction. These signs suggest poor air exchange.

Airway obstruction is complete when the patient is unable to speak, breathe, or cough; airflow is not felt or heard from the nose and mouth; spontaneous breathing efforts result in retraction of the supraclavicular and intercostal areas; and there is tracheal tugging as well as an absence of chest expansion.

216. **c**

217. To use direct laryngoscopy to remove a foreign body, **begin by inserting the laryngoscope blade into the patient's mouth as you would during orotracheal intubation. If the foreign body is visualized, carefully and deliberately remove the foreign body with Magill forceps.**

218. Vomitus that is regurgitated from the stomach into the oropharynx during states of decreased consciousness contains partially dissolved food, protein-dissolving enzymes, and hydrochloric acid. **If aspirated into the lungs, this combination can lead to increased interstitial fluid, pulmonary edema, and destruction of the alveoli. This seriously impairs gas exchange and leads to hypoxemia and hypercarbia. Furthermore, food particles can obstruct the bronchiolar airways, thus compromising airflow.**

219. **a:** Gurgling sounds heard on inspiration and/or expiration indicate **the accumulation of fluids or vomitus in the upper airway,** prompting the EMT-I to quickly suction the upper airway.

220. **c:** Suctioning is used to remove vomitus, blood, fluids, and secretions from the airway. The primary complication of suctioning is hypoxia, so each attempt at suctioning should be limited to 15 seconds. **Suction units are capable of generating vacuum levels of at least 300 mm Hg when the distal end is occluded and allow a flow rate of at least 30 L/min when the tube is open.** After inserting the catheter into the oropharynx, suction is applied while rotating the catheter as it is removed. This prevents the catheter tip from adhering to the pharyngeal wall.

221. Types of suction catheters with characteristics: **a. Tonsil tip:** also referred to as the Yankauer suction; is a rigid tube that has a ball-like tip with multiple holes at its distal end; is designed to remove larger particles and voluminous secretions; vigorous insertion can cause lacerations or other injuries; **b. Whistle tip:** is ineffective in removing large volumes of secretions rapidly; can be inserted through the nares, into the oropharynx or nasopharynx, through a nasopharyngeal airway, along an oropharyngeal airway, or through an endotracheal tube; is a small, easy to use, flexible tube that is long enough to extend into the lower respiratory tract.

222. **b:** When fluids are voluminous or thick, **the catheter can be removed, and the thick-walled, wide-bore suction tubing can be used alone.** In addition, water can be suctioned through the tubing between suctioning attempts to help dilute the secretions and facilitate flow through the tubing.

223. Answers to crossword puzzle

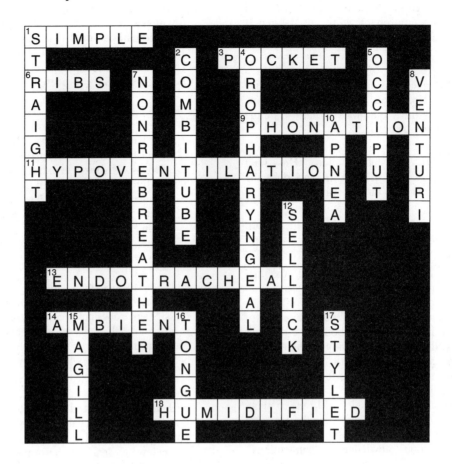

CHAPTER 10

1. **False:** When doing a patient assessment, historical information often comes from a *variety of sources.* These may include the patient, the family, friends, police officers, and other observers.

2. **True:** Weighing the reliability of the history in a nonjudgmental manner at the end of the evaluation, not the beginning, helps to avoid the trap of "first impressions" clouding your objectivity.

3. **True**

4. Four factors that affect the quality of historical data include **mental status, memory, trust,** and **motivation.**

5. History-taking terms with descriptions: **a. Chief complaint:** identifies, in the patient's own words, the symptoms for which the patient is seeking medical care; **b. History of the present illness:** should include a full, clear, and chronological account of the patient's symptoms; **c. Past medical history:** includes any significant past injuries, hospitalizations, operations, or diseases; **d. Current health status:** focuses on the patient's present state of health.

6. Factors related to patient's current health status include **current medications; allergies; alcohol; drugs and related substances; diet; screening tests; immunizations; sleep patterns; exercise and leisure activities; environmental hazards; use of safety measures; family history; home situation (including pets, spouse, or significant others); daily life; important experiences; religious beliefs;** and **patient's general outlook on life.**

7. **d**

8. **b**

9. **d**

10. **c**

11. Note-taking is generally well accepted by patients and essential for proper documentation. Although most patients are comfortable with note-taking, **if concerns arise, address them and explain to the patient your reasons for taking notes.**

12. **b:** Open-ended questions **tend to yield far more helpful information than close-ended questions.** Closed-ended or direct questions require a simple answer, such as yes or no.

13. Questions that are open ended include "How long have you been feeling ill?" "Can you describe your pain?" "How did you feel earlier today?"

14. Closed-ended questions may be better **in certain nonverbal patients.**

15. Terms with descriptions: **a. Facilitation:** combination of verbal and nonverbal actions that are used to encourage the patient to say more; **b. Reflection:** repeating the patient's words (or your summary of them) back to make certain you both are communicating; **c. Clarification:** interrupting or asking additional questions to clarify points; **d. Empathetic responses:** identifying with one's feelings or symptoms; **e. Confrontation:** more direct but potentially disruptive to your relationship with the patient; **f. Interpretation:** requires you to synthesize what the patient has told you (verbally and body language) with your own knowledge and "gut feelings."

16. **d**

17. **a**

18. **c**

19. **True**

20. **True**

21. **False:** Empathy is *very different* from sympathy (feeling sorry for someone). Although sympathy may be appropriate at some times, your job in history taking is to be professional, kind, and empathetic.

22. **False:** Whether you share your interpretation with the patient depends on the circumstances.

23. The easiest way to quantify the severity of a symptom is to **use a scale of 0 to 10, with 0 being symptom-free and 10 the worst pain (or other symptom) imaginable.**

24. SAMPLE stands for:
    S: **signs and symptoms**
    A: **allergies**
    M: **medications (prescription or over-the-counter)**
    P: **past pertinent medical history**
    L: **last oral intake—fluid or solid**
    E: **events leading to present event**

25. OPQRST stands for:
    O: **onset; when did the problem begin?**
    P: **provocation; what makes the problem worse?**
    Q: **quality; what is the problem (usually pain) like—is it sharp, crushing, viselike?**
    R: **radiation; does the pain go (move) anywhere?**
    S: **severity; on a scale of 0 to 10 (0 = no pain, 10 = the worst pain imaginable), how bad is the pain?**
    T: **time; does the symptom come and go, or is it always there?**

26. **c:** The best way to deal with a silent patient is to **show patience and remain alert for nonverbal clues of distress.** Silence does not necessarily show that the patient is hostile, problematic, or uncooperative. Patients may use silence as a way to collect their thoughts, remember details, or decide whether they trust you.

27. To cope with a talkative patient, **acknowledge that the patient is nervous and scared; lower your expectations—accept a less comprehensive history; give the patient free reign for the first few minutes of the interview if feasible; summarize frequently—politely interrupt and summarize, point by point, as best you can; and ask directed questions.**

28. When dealing with a patient who has multiple complaints, the crucial thing to do **is deal with appropriate priorities first.** Remember any disease or injury that threatens airway, breathing, or circulation (the ABCs) must be identified rapidly and cared for.

29. **d**

30. **False:** Everyone is usually anxious, to at least some extent, when sick or injured. Sometimes people talk fast as a response. Others *talk much slower or even become silent.*

31. **False:** Use caution with reassurance—it is tempting to be too reassuring, which may erode a patient's trust in you.

32. **True**

33. **True:** This simple act of kindness goes a long way to improve patient rapport.

34. **False:** Depression ranges in severity from a temporary response to a situation to a severe psychiatric illness that may result in violent behavior.

35. Six signs of depression are **sad appearance; crying; inappropriate responses, especially crying, with minimal stimuli; sleep disturbance; abnormal appetite (decreased or increased);** and **suicidal actions or gestures.**

36. **d:** Angry and hostile patients **are best handled when the EMT-I remains calm in response to the patient.** This can be very challenging at times. If there are perceived physical dangers, of course, get appropriate assistance immediately. Do not place yourself in or allow yourself to remain in a potentially volatile situation. This rule goes for *any* patient encounter as a basic rule of on-scene safety.

37. **c:** Intoxicated patients are best handled by **talking calmly and avoiding sudden moves.** Further, be respectful of patients and avoid challenging them. Often attempts to have the patient lower the voice or stop cursing simply aggravate them further. Many intoxicated patients also require more than usual personal space—avoid approaching them in a small area that may make them feel trapped.

38. If a patient becomes seductive or makes sexual advances, **make it clear that your relationship is professional, not personal. If the patient persists, remove yourself from the situation if possible. Sometimes, having another person as a "chaperone" is helpful.**

39. Consider confusing or unusual behavior to be caused by a potentially serious medical problem until proven otherwise because **hypoglycemia and hypoxia, and a myriad other conditions, can mimic mental illness or dementia.**

40. Challenge with method for managing: **a. Patient with limited intelligence:** speak clearly but normally; although it may not be the case, expect more time than usual for the patient to respond to your question. Getting additional information from family or friends is always helpful. If patients are capable of communicating, direct your interview toward them first. Remember to be patient and professional. **b. EMT-I–patient language barrier:** try to find a translator, including the dial-up services for language translation offered by several phone companies. Be aware of your local resources. **c. Patient with a hearing problem:** Find a translator if the patient can sign. Ask patients if they read lips by looking them in the eyes, pointing to your mouth, and saying, "Do you read lips?" If the answer is yes, speak slowly and avoid unusual terms and idiomatic language. **d. Blind patient:** Announce yourself and explain why you are there. Tell patient before touching him or her, even if just to obtain vital signs.

41. **False:** With the patient who has a hearing problem, communication will be lost if you turn your head out of the patient's line of vision.

42. **True**

43. **True**

44. **False:** As with any patient encounter, remember that any medical information is considered confidential.

45. Answers to crossword puzzle

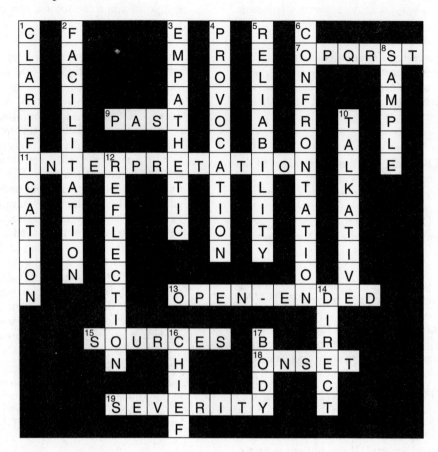

CHAPTER 11

1. **a. Inspection:** act of visually evaluating the patient; **b. Auscultation:** act of listening for sounds within the body to evaluate the condition of the heart, lungs, pleura, intestines, or other organs or to detect fetal heart sounds; **c. Percussion:** technique involving gently striking or tapping a part of the body to evaluate the size, borders, and consistency of internal organs and to discover the presence of fluid in body cavities; **d. Palpation:** process in which the examiner feels the texture, size, consistency, and location of certain parts of the body with the hands.

2. **d**

3. Four vital signs are **pulse, respirations, blood pressure, and temperature.**

4. **False:** Recheck vital signs every *5 to 10 minutes* or sooner if the patient's condition changes.

5. **True**

6. **True**

7. Examination experiments with descriptions

Examination Equipment	Description
ECG monitor	An electronic device for the continuous observation of cardiac function; it may include electrocardiograph and oscilloscope readings, recording devices, and a visual or an audible record of heart function and rhythm
Pulse oximeter	An electronic device attached to the patient's finger, ear, or foot to determine the amount of oxygen in the blood, measured as percent saturation of hemoglobin
Peak flow meter	A handheld mechanical device that measures the volume of a rapidly exhaled breath
Capnometer	An electronic device that measures how much carbon dioxide is exhaled during breathing
Glucose meter	An electronic device that determines the blood glucose level from a drop of blood

8. **b**

9. **d**

10. Normal mentation means **the patient is alert and responsive. The patient seems to understand questions and responds appropriately within a reasonable period.**

11. Levels of consciousness with descriptions: **a. Stupor:** state of lethargy and unresponsiveness in which a person seems unaware of the surroundings; **b. Obtundation:** reduced level of consciousness resulting in insensitivity to unpleasant or painful stimuli; often caused by an anesthetic or analgesic (pain) medication; **c. Coma:** state of profound unconsciousness; the patient cannot be aroused by any stimulation; **d. Drowsy:** sleepy, but otherwise normal; **e. Lethargic:** patients are drowsy, but open their eyes to look at you, respond, then fall back to sleep.

12. **Top figure represents decorticate posturing, whereas bottom figure represents decerebrate posturing.**

13. **c**

14. Postures and motor behaviors: **a. Opisthotonic posturing:** results from severe muscle spasms, such as during a seizure or from tetanus; **b. Motor tics:** spasmodic muscular contractions most commonly involving the face, mouth, eyes, head, neck, or shoulders; **c. Decerebrate posturing:** severe injury to the brain at the level of the brainstem is the usual cause; **d. Rigidity:** hardness, stiffness, or inflexibility, usually of the extremities; a sign of neurological disease, such as Parkinson's disease; **e. Tremor:** involuntary alternating contraction and relaxation of opposing groups of skeletal muscles.

15. **True**

16. **False:** Patients with altered mental status often *do not pay close attention* to hygiene, changing clothes, and other aspects of personal grooming. Without being judgmental, observe and record any of these findings.

17. **c:** Patients are said to have **a flat affect** if they appear emotionally unresponsive (e.g., no smiling or other facial expressions, quiet, simple answers with no variation in voice tone).

18. Four things regarding speech that the EMT-I should assess: **quantity, rate, loudness, and fluency.**

19. **a**

20. Three things a person's orientation centers around are **time** (date, year); **place** (where are we now?); and **person** (who are you?).

21. A & O × 3 means **"alert and oriented to time, place, and person."**

22. Answers to crossword puzzle.

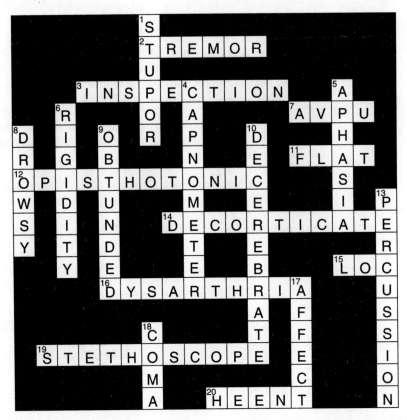

23. **b**

24. Components of the general survey:
    - **Assess the patient's level of consciousness.**
    - **Observe the patient for signs of distress.**
    - **Classify the patient's apparent state of health.**
    - **Assess the skin color and observe for obvious lesions.**
    - **Determine the patient's general weight.**
    - **Evaluate the patient's posture, gait, and motor activity.**
    - **Note the patient's dress, grooming habits, and state of personal hygiene.**
    - **Gauge if any unusual breath odors are present.**
    - **Observe the patient's facial expression.**
    - **Obtain a set of vital signs.**
    - **Perform additional assessment techniques as necessary.**

25. **Inspect and palpate the skin, and inspect the fingernails.**

26. Things to pay attention to while evaluating the skin and fingernails are **color, moisture, temperature, texture, mobility and turgor, and lesions.**

27. **b:** Decreased skin turgor is said to be present when the skin stays tented up after it has been pinched. This indicates that *dehydration* may be present.

28. **a:** Cyanosis is caused by **an excess of deoxygenated hemoglobin in the blood.** Jaundice is caused by greater than normal amounts of bilirubin in the blood. Bruising is caused by the leakage of blood into the subcutaneous tissues because of trauma to the underlying blood vessels or by fragility of the vessel walls. Flushing is caused by vasodilation of the peripheral blood vessels.

29. To assess the head, **inspect and palpate the head, ears, eyes, nose, and throat area for evidence of trauma, tenderness, or deformity. Observe the face for obvious deformities, swelling, or discoloration. Gently palpate the maxilla and mandible for possible fractures.**

30. To check the eyes, **inspect and palpate the eyes, orbits, and eyelids for evidence of trauma; check for conjugate gaze; and check the size, shape, symmetry, and reactivity of the pupils.**

31. **c:** *Conjugate gaze* means **the eyes move in the same direction.** If you were to draw a line from each pupil straight toward the examiner, both should remain parallel throughout all directions of gaze. The reason is the movement of each eye is controlled by the coordinated action of six muscles. These are often called the extraocular movements or EOMs.

32. **a**

33. Injury to either the muscles or nerves of the eye will result in paralysis of one or more muscles. **Here the eye deviates from its normal position, and the eyes no longer appear conjugate or parallel in that direction of gaze.**

34. The pupils shown are **unequal.**

35. Unequal pupils in any patient with an altered level of consciousness may **be a sign of head injury or brain dysfunction.**

36. Steps for checking a patient's pupils are:
    - **Briefly direct your light at one eye.**
    - **Observe for pupil constriction.**
    - **Remove the light and observe for dilation.**
    - **Repeat for the opposite eye, and compare the responses.**

37. **b**

38. **c**

39. **d:** Visual acuity is a measure of the accuracy of a patient's vision. You should note any blurring, double vision, or blindness.

40. To examine a patient's ears: **Examine the outer ear for lacerations, bleeding, or other evidence of soft tissue trauma. Visually inspect the ear canals.**

41. **a:** A basilar skull fracture is indicated by the presence of **blood or cerebrospinal fluid in the ear canal.** CSF may be mixed with blood. Bruising of the area *behind* the ear (Battle's sign) may also suggest a basilar skull fracture.

42. **In the unresponsive patient, gently separate the lips, and inspect the mouth for foreign material, broken teeth, or dentures. Note soft tissue injuries within the mouth. Lacerations on the floor of the mouth, the inner surface of the cheek, and the base of the tongue are often overlooked. While assessing the mouth, note the patient's breath odor.**

43. **a:** Dentures should be *left in place unless they are loose;* airway compromise *should* lead to the patient being reclassified to "priority" status; and alcohol ingestion *usually* gives off a distinct odor, whereas a fruity odor may indicate diabetes mellitus.

    Bleeding into the mouth can obstruct the upper airway. Suction may be required to keep the airway open and get a clear view. If you do not suspect spinal injury, position the patient to allow for drainage of blood.

44. **b:** Nuchal rigidity is stiffness of the neck with decreased range of motion. **It may indicate infection, such as meningitis, or may be caused by muscle spasm from a whiplash type of injury.** You should assume that a patient with nuchal rigidity has a potentially life-threatening problem until proven otherwise.

45. **False:** The trachea *should be midline.* Deviation of the trachea to either side may indicate the presence of a tension pneumothorax.

46. **True:** Blood flow to the brain could be disrupted if you palpate both sides of the neck simultaneously.

47. **False:** The extrication collar *should be left* if it is already in place.

48. **True**

49. **False:** JVD evaluation is best done with the patient sitting at a *45-degree* angle.

50. **False:** An open wound to the anterior neck, even if it appears minor, *is an emergency.* If swelling develops, pressure on the trachea may obstruct the airway.

51. **c:** Neck vein distention **indicates conditions such as congestive heart failure and cardiac tamponade.** It is said to be present when veins are bulging outward.

52. **b:** Subcutaneous emphysema **occurs when air leaks into the subcutaneous tissue.** It feels like a crunching or crackling below the skin.

53. Answers to crossword puzzle

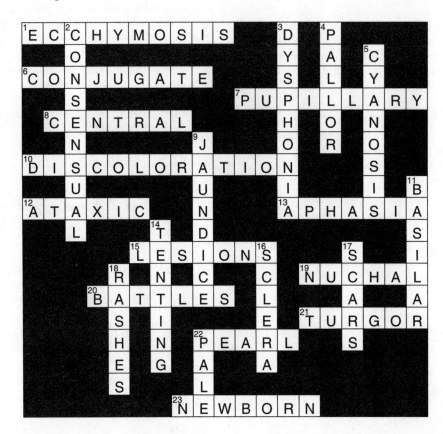

54. **Assess the chest by exposing and observing for symmetrical breathing, equal expansion, obvious injuries, open wounds, or scars. Observe the rate, rhythm, depth, and effort of breathing; always check for cyanosis.**

55. Average respiratory rates for:
    - Newly born   **30-50**
    - Infant   **20-30**
    - Toddler   **24-40**
    - Preschool   **22-34**
    - School age   **18-30**
    - Adolescent   **12-16**
    - Adult   12-20

56. **Bradypnea** is a respiratory rate that is too slow, and **tachypnea** is a respiratory rate that is too fast.

57. Seven indicators of respiratory distress are **nasal flaring; paradoxical or asymmetrical chest movements; use of accessory muscles; pursed lip breathing; noisy breathing; obvious difficulty in inhalation or exhalation;** and **cyanosis.**

58. Breathing patterns with descriptions: **a. Bradypnea:** slow respirations; **b. Cheyne Stokes:** series of rapid then slow respirations followed by periods of apnea; **c. Tachypnea:** rapid and usually shallow respirations; **d. Kussmaul:** rapid and deep respirations usually found in diabetic patients or others with imbalances of the acid content in their bodies; **e. Apnea:** absence of breathing.

59. To palpate a patient's chest, begin with the **clavicles,** and then palpate the **rib cage.** Note pain, **tenderness,** possible fractures, or **subcutaneous emphysema.** After palpation, **auscultate** the chest to verify **breath sounds.**

60. Three things to check the chest for are **deformities or asymmetry, impairment of respiratory movement,** and **abnormal retractions.**

61. **True**

62. **False:** It involves striking one finger against a *knuckle* of the other hand, which is *spread over* the chest. This "tapping" sends out vibrations, producing sound.

63. **True:** Some prefer to do one side (left or right) in its entirety.

64. **c**

65. **d:** Hyperresonance is **heard when the chest contains more air than usual** such as in the face of pneumothorax or COPD.

66. **b:** Auscultation of the chest **involves listening to the sounds generated by breathing and checking for symmetry.** It is used to assess *airflow* through the airways and to *identify* whether additional abnormal sounds (adventitious sounds) are present.

67. Locations on the posterior chest where the EMT-I should auscultate

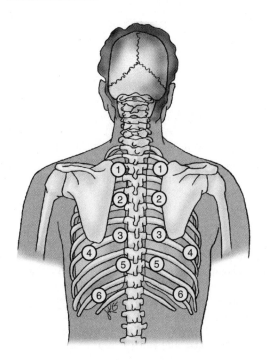

68. Sounds that may be heard during auscultation and their descriptions: *a. Tracheal*: normal breath sound heard during auscultation over the trachea; *b. Vesicular*: normal sound of rustling or swishing heard with the stethoscope over the lung periphery; usually higher pitched during inspiration and fading rapidly during expiration; *c. Bronchial*: normal if heard over the anterior sternum; otherwise, an abnormal sound heard with a stethoscope over the lungs, indicating consolidation or compression of normal lung; *d. Bronchovesicular*: sounds intermediate between tracheal sounds and vesicular sounds. These may be normal in the first and second interspaces anteriorly and between the scapulae, but otherwise suggest fluid in the lungs.

69. **a:** Discontinuous adventitious lung sounds include **rales.** These are sounds that are, by definition, not present for the entire respiratory cycle (full inspiration to full exhalation).

70. **d:** Rhonchi **are coarser gurgling-like sounds that are often present over the larger airways only and may be heard on both inspiration and expiration.** They indicate mucus or other type of material in the larynx, trachea, or bronchi—they are often present in *upper respiratory infections* such as bronchitis.

71. Diminished or absent lung sounds suggest **pleural effusion (fluid), consolidation (fluid in the lungs for any reason), collapsed lung, or surgically removed lung.**

72. A heart rate that is greater than 100 BPM is called **tachycardia,** whereas a heart rate less than 60 BPM is referred to as **bradycardia.** The normal adult pulse rate is 60 to 100 BPM.

73. **c:** The average pulse rate for the preschooler (4 to 5 years old) can range from a resting rate of **80** to a high activity rate of **140** BPM.

74. Four pulses that are used to assess vital signs are **radial, carotid, brachial, and femoral.**

75. In patients with shock or poor circulation, **the radial pulse may be either absent or difficult to assess.** In these patients you should palpate the carotid or femoral pulse.

76. Three important characteristics to evaluate when checking the pulse: **rate, regularity (rhythm), and character (amplitude).**

77. Average pulse rates for various age groups:

	BPM
Newly born (birth to 4 wk)	120–160
Infant (1 to 12 mo)	100–160
Toddler (1 to 3 yr)	90–150
Preschooler (4 to 5 yr)	80–140
School age (6 to 12 yr)	70–120
Adolescent (12 to 18 yr)	60–100
Adults (>18 yr)	60–100

78. **a**

79. Three factors that affect a patient's blood pressure: **age, sex, and body size.**

80. **c**

81. **b:** In some individuals, the blood pressure *decreases* suddenly *when the person stands up*. This is called *orthostatic hypotension*. It is said to be present when there is an increase in the pulse rate of 10 to 20 BPM or greater with a change in position along with a decrease in the systolic blood pressure of 10 to 20 mm Hg or greater.

82. **a:** The difference between systolic blood pressure and diastolic blood pressure is the **pulse pressure**. The normal value is 40 mm Hg. During early shock, cardiac tamponade, or tension pneumothorax, the resistance to flow in the blood vessels goes up—this is reflected as an increase in diastolic blood pressure and a *narrowing (decrease)* in the pulse pressure. As shock progresses and the body's compensatory mechanisms fail, this finding is no longer reliable.

83. **c**

84. **d:** The normal systolic blood pressure range for an adult at rest is 100 to 140 mm Hg. Diastolic pressure ranges from 60 to 90 mm Hg. Blood pressure greater than 140/90 in an adult is considered high. Continuous high blood pressure is defined as **hypertension**. Blood pressure that is less than 90/60 in an adult is considered low. Continual low blood pressure is known as *hypotension*.

85. **b:** Venous pulsations **are eliminated by light pressure on the vein just above the sternal end of the clavicle.** They are *rarely* palpable, and the level of venous pulsations changes with position, *decreasing* as the patient becomes more upright.

86. The illustration of the chest below shows the area that represents the point of maximum impulse.

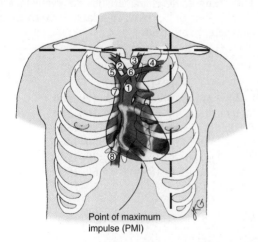

Point of maximum impulse (PMI)

87. **c:** The point of maximal impulse is **where the apical beat of the heart is observed.** It is located in the *fifth* intercostal space of the thorax, *medial* to the left midclavicular line, and where a stethoscope is placed to obtain an apical heart rate and to listen for heart tones.

88. **b:** The first heart sound **is called S_1**. It is the "lub" of the "lub-*dub*." The intensity of heart tones *varies* from person to person.

89. **False:** Examine with the patient in a *supine* position, if possible.

90. **False:** Ask patients to point out tender areas first, and examine these *last*.

91. Inspect the abdomen for signs of obvious injury, **ecchymosis,** or **swelling.**

92. **b**

93. **a**

94. **c**

95. **a**

96. It is preferable to auscultate the abdomen before palpating the bowel **because it may be jarred and alter the ability to listen to bowel sounds properly.**

97. **c**

98. **d**

99. **a:** There is a significant difference between the total *absence* of bowel sounds and *decreased* bowel sounds. Because of this, all four quadrants must be listened to for a period, before concluding that bowel sounds are absent. Absent bowel sounds often indicate an acute surgical condition (e.g., peritonitis).

100. **c**

101. Locations of bruits and what they suggest

Location	Suggests
Upper abdominal quadrant	**Renal artery stenosis caused by atherosclerosis, uncommon but surgically treatable cause of hypertension (high blood pressure)**
Lower abdomen or back	**Aortic aneurysm**
Over the groin	**Potentially significant arterial occlusion when heard through both systole and diastole**

102. **Gently palpate the entire abdomen, keeping your hand and forearm horizontal to the abdomen, fingers together, and flat on the abdominal surface. Barely raise your hand off the skin when you move it around.**

103. When palpating the abdomen you note tenderness, **guarding,** muscular **rigidity,** and any masses or lesions. Observe the patient's face for any **painful** response or **grimace.**

104. **Guarding occurs when the patient moves or deliberately tenses the abdominal muscles to avoid pressure from the palpating hand. Guarding that persists despite your best efforts to calm the patient indicates peritoneal irritation (peritonitis),** especially if bowel sounds are also absent.

105. **Sometimes peritoneal irritation is so extensive that the abdominal muscles become rock hard. This degree of spasm has been likened to feeling a hard board on the abdomen.**

106. **b:** The CVA is located **at the junction of the twelfth rib and the twelfth thoracic vertebra.** It is *palpated* as part of the abdominal assessment. CVA tenderness may indicate a kidney disorder.

107. **d**

108. **c**

109. Patients found to have abdominal discoloration, rigidity, exposed intestines (evisceration), or severe pain should be classified as **priority.**

110. **It may be beneficial for a male examiner of a female patient to have a female attendant present. This is for both patient comfort and legal protection. Some female examiners work alone with female patients, although a chaperone may be helpful, if available, for patients and examiners of both sexes.**

111. **In both men and women, note any inflammation, discharge, bleeding, or swelling.**

112. Answers to crossword puzzle

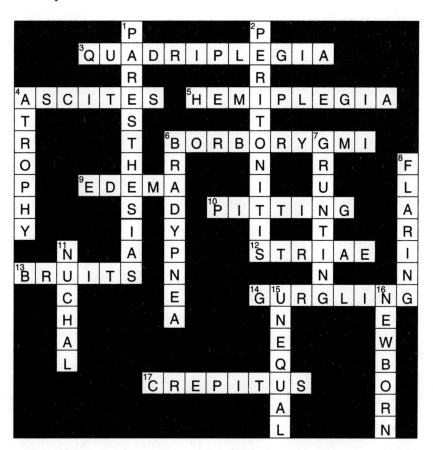

113. To assess the extremities, consider the functional implications of any **illness** or **injury** and the underlying **anatomy**. Assess the patient's general **appearance**, body proportions, and ease of **movement**. Be certain to note any **limitations** in the range of motion or any unusual **increase** in the **mobility** of a joint.

114. Decreased range of motion is common in arthritis, **inflammation**, or **fibrosis**.

115. Things to evaluate as part of an examination of the extremities are **signs of inflammation, crepitus, deformities, muscular strength, symmetry, atrophy, pain, tenderness, peripheral pulses, motor function,** and **sensory function.**

116. Pulses with correct locations: **a. Dorsalis pedis:** on the dorsum of the foot, lateral to the great toe extensor tendon; **b. Femoral:** in the inguinal region, about halfway between the anterior superior iliac spine and the symphysis pubis; **c: Popliteal:** in the back of the knee joint; **d: Posterior tibial:** posterior to the medial malleolus of the ankle.

117. **b**

118. Four-point scale for identifying degree of edema present:
    One-plus: **slight edema**
    Two-plus: **more edema**
    Three-plus: **moderate edema**
    Four-plus: **marked edema**

119. **True**

120. **False:** From *the side*, the EMT-I should assess that the normal cervical, thoracic, and lumbar curves are visible.

121. **False:** From behind, an imaginary line drawn from the spinous process of *T1* should run perpendicular to the ground and between the gluteal cleft.

122. **The EMT-I should gently palpate the spine over the spinous processes and the muscles of the neck and back for symmetry, tenderness, and spasm. Also, the costovertebral angle should be examined for deformities and pain.**

123. **d**

CHAPTER 12

1. **Patient assessment** is a structured method of evaluating a patient's physical condition. It is the process of knowing what to look for, knowing what to ask, and recognizing when an abnormal condition is found. Patient assessment is a process that continues throughout your time with the patient. A patient's condition can change quickly. There is a need for continual assessment that allows you to recognize critical situations early and positively alter patient outcome.

2. A **symptom** is a subjective indication of a disease or condition as perceived by the patient.

3. A **sign** is an objective finding detected by you, such as a rash or deformed arm.

4. Six phases of assessment are **scene size-up; initial assessment; resuscitation; focused history and physical of the medical and/or trauma patient; detailed assessment; and ongoing field management.**

5. Four pieces of information the emergency medical dispatch can usually provide to the responding EMS crew: **scene conditions, number of patients, patient conditions, and medical history.**

6. Five observations that the EMT-I should make at the scene are: **Is the scene safe? Should body substance isolation precautions be taken? Is this a medical or trauma patient? How many patients are involved? Is additional help required?**

7. **c:** The first phase of patient assessment is the **scene size-up.** This is where you evaluate the whole picture of the call. It allows you to ensure a reasonably safe environment for yourself, your partner, and your patient; anticipate potentially hazardous situations; and call for appropriate resources.

8. **d:** Potentially hazardous situations include calls to **high-risk parts of your response area, known unsafe situations, scenes involving domestic violence, and sometimes just your gut feeling based on the EMD's information.**

9. **Body substance isolation** is a set of guidelines for prehospital care providers to follow that minimizes one's exposure to contagious diseases.

10. **a:** Latex, nitrile, or vinyl gloves **should be worn whenever the EMT-I is likely to come in contact with blood or other body fluids, mucous mem-**

branes, or nonintact skin of any patient. For those incidents in which large amounts of blood or body fluids are present, wear thicker gloves or use two pairs of gloves. Although medical gloves provide good barriers, they may not protect you when there are sharp objects such as wood, metal, or glass. Work-type gloves, with latex or vinyl gloves underneath, are appropriate until the hazard has been removed.

11. **True:** A mask provides protection against splash exposure to the mouth and nose, as well as against airborne pathogens.

12. **True**

13. **b:** Assessing safety at the scene serves two basic objectives: preventing illness or injury to the rescuer or bystanders and preventing further illness or injury to patients. Look for things like collapsed structures, chemical spills, fire, weapons, and violent people. If you feel the scene is unsafe, **DO NOT ENTER.** No matter how critically ill or injured the patient is, a dead or injured EMT-I will not be of help. Instruct the EMD to notify the appropriate agencies for emergency assistance.

14. **d:** Call for additional help **immediately on arriving on the scene** (if not sooner). It is better to have additional help en route as soon as possible and to cancel their response than to have not requested necessary assistance in the first place.

15. **a**

16. **b:** The force that causes an injury and how it is applied to the body is referred to as **the mechanism of injury.** It provides the EMT-I with valuable information. For example, suppose you are called to treat a patient who was struck by a car but is up and walking around. Some people may think that because the patient is walking around, a significant injury must not be present. The fact that the patient was struck by a car is reason alone to immobilize him or her for a possible spinal injury. This precautionary treatment is based on the mechanism of injury and not necessarily the patient's outward appearance. As you assess the mechanism of injury, determine how many patients are present, and decide whether you will require additional help.

17. **a:** The *initial assessment* of a patient includes **obtaining a general impression;** quickly determining the nature of the illness or the mechanism of injury; providing spinal stabilization if indicated; assessing the level of consciousness (determine the degree of responsiveness), airway status, breathing, and circulation (including determining the pulse rate); evaluating the skin for color, temperature, and moisture; checking for major hemorrhage; and identifying priority (unstable) patients. In children younger than 6 years of age, the EMT-I should also determine adequacy of capillary refill.

18. **c**

19. **d**

20. The general impression of the patient is formed by your immediate **sensory** assessment and the patient's **chief** complaint.

21. If you suspect **trauma** and potential **injury** to the cervical spine, stabilize the spine.

22. Life-threatening conditions include an **obstructed airway, marked breathing difficulty,** and **severe bleeding**—treat these immediately. Your general impression of the patient's condition forms the basis for the rest of your care. If the patient looks bad, consider him or her unstable (priority), and treat according to local protocol.

23. AVPU stands for:
    A: **patient is awake and alert**
    V: **patient responds to verbal stimulus**
    P: **patient responds to painful stimulus**
    U: **patient is unconscious**

24. **c:** Conscious and speaking patients have an **open airway.** For these patients the initial survey can continue. For patients who are unresponsive, you must open the airway.

25. **a:** For trauma patients or those with unknown nature of illness, **stabilize the cervical spine and perform the jaw-thrust maneuver.** While one rescuer provides airway and spine protection, the other rescuer continues the initial survey. If a second rescuer is not available, the first rescuer must maintain the airway and protect the spine. Once the jaw thrust is performed, the rescuer stabilizes the neck until it is properly immobilized. For semiconscious or unconscious medical patients, perform the head-tilt/chin-lift maneuver. If the airway is not clear, clear it.

26. Three steps for determining the effectiveness of ventilation are: **look** for rise and fall of the chest; **listen** for air moving in and out of the patient's nose or mouth; and **feel** exhaled air against your chin, face, or palm of your hand with the rise and fall of the chest.

27. **a:** You should **ventilate the patient either by mouth to mask or by an adjunct device** supplied with high-concentration oxygen in any case in which inadequate air exchange is suspected, including:

- Patients who are not breathing
- Patients whose respiratory rate is less than 12 breaths/min or greater than 20 breaths/min
- Patients who have a decreased level of consciousness

In all cases, supplemental oxygen should be used. In the presence of a perfusing rhythm, ventilate the patient with a tidal volume of 500 to 600 mL (approximately 6 to 7 mL/kg) over 1 second (enough to make the chest rise clearly). Breaths should be delivered at a rate of at least 10 to 12 times per minute (1 breath every 6 to 7 seconds). Any patient with difficulty breathing should be treated as a "priority" patient.

28. Things to check to determine whether you are performing effective ventilatory support:
    - **Check for rise and fall of the chest wall.**
    - **Auscultate the chest to determine the adequacy of lung sounds.**
    - **Assess the skin color**—as the patient becomes better oxygenated, skin color should improve.
    - **Monitor the heart rate**—typically, persons with respiratory compromise develop tachycardia, then bradycardia. With proper ventilation you should see a change in the heart rate toward normal.
    - **Assess the pulse oximetry**—if a person is not being effectively ventilated, the pulse oximetry reading may be low.

29. **All patients with a serious illness or injury should receive high-concentration oxygen. If the patient is unresponsive and the respirations are adequate, the patient should receive high-concentration oxygen.**

30. **False:** If the patient is responsive, quickly check for a *radial* pulse. In a *child younger than 1 year old*, palpate the brachial pulse. If no radial pulse is present, palpate the carotid pulse. If the patient is unresponsive, feel for the carotid pulse first.

31. **True:** For children 1 to 8 years of age, when available, use a **pediatric dose-attenuating system**. A conventional AED (without pediatric attenuator system) should be used for children about 8 years of age and older (larger than about 25 kg or 55 pounds in weight or about 127 cm or 50 inches in length) and for adults.

32. Pulse locations with approximate systolic pressures: **a. Carotid artery:** 60 mm Hg; **b. Femoral artery:** 70 mm Hg; **c. Radial artery:** 80 mm Hg.

33. d

34. **c:** Jaundiced skin is indicative of **liver disease**, *gallbladder disease*, and *kidney disease*.

35. **b:** Pallor is seen with **shock**, stress, heart attack, anemia, and hypothermia. The face, lips, nail beds, mouth, earlobes, and eyelids are all places in which the patient's color may be assessed. On dark-pigmented patients, look for color changes in the nail beds, under the tongue, and in the conjunctiva.

36. **a:** Capillary refill **is checked by pressing on the nail bed of the patient's finger or toe, releasing the pressure, and determining the time it takes for the nail bed to return to its initial color.** Capillary refill that is slow (greater than 2 seconds) indicates *poor* tissue perfusion, whereas capillary refill that is fast (less than 2 seconds) indicates a state of *adequate* perfusion.

37. **b:** Use of capillary refill as an assessment tool has been reported to be effective only in children (under 6 years) and infants.

38. **d: Priority patients are unstable and require more advanced level care as soon as possible. They should be promptly transported to the nearest appropriate medical facility.** In certain cases, you may call for paramedic backup at the scene or en route. In some EMS systems, you may activate an aeromedical helicopter service.

39. Patient conditions that would be considered priorities: **patients receiving CPR, in respiratory arrest, or being provided life-sustaining ventilatory/circulatory support, poor general impression; altered mental status, unresponsive patients, especially if there is no gag reflex; responsive patients who are unable to follow simple commands; difficulty breathing; pale skin or other signs of shock (hypoperfusion); complicated childbirth; chest pain with suspected cardiac origin; hypoxia that fails to rapidly correct (within 1 to 2 minutes) of field intervention; multiple trauma (including severe burns); severe hypertension; uncontrolled bleeding; and severe pain anywhere, inability to move any part of the body.**

40. **a:** A patient who is experiencing congestive heart failure and has *labored respirations* should be regarded as **unstable (a priority patient).**

41. **a: Splinting fractures** is not part of the resuscitation phase. The resuscitation phase of patient assessment includes initiating airway management (such as relief of airway obstruction), artificial respiration, control of hemorrhage, CPR, defibrillation of cardiac arrest victims, initiation of shock management (e.g., administration of epinephrine in anaphylactic shock), and giving glucose (sugar) to those with

severe hypoglycemia. The resuscitation phase is performed concurrently with the initial survey. Thus if an obstructed airway is noted during the initial survey, you should stop at this point and immediately take steps to relieve the obstruction.

42. Acronym OPQRST with descriptions: **a. O:** (onset) When did the problem begin? **b. P:** (provocation) What makes the problem worse? **c. Q:** (quality) What is the pain like—is it sharp, crushing, or viselike? **d. R:** (radiation) Does the pain go anywhere? **e. S:** (severity) on a scale of 1 to 10, how bad is the pain? **f. T:** (time) Does the symptom come and go, or is it always there?

43. **d**

44. Seven areas of the body that are examined as part of the Rapid Trauma Assessment: **head, neck, chest, abdomen, pelvis, extremities, and posterior aspect of the body.**

45. Meaning of the acronym DCAP-BTLS:
    D: **deformity**
    C: **contusions**
    A: **abrasions**
    P: **punctures/penetrations**
    B: **burns**
    T: **tenderness**
    L: **lacerations**
    S: **swelling**

46. If a cervical spine injury is present or suspected, **apply a rigid extrication collar. A second EMT should continue to stabilize the head until the patient is secured to a long backboard.** In some cases a second rescuer or an extrication collar may not be immediately available. You should continue with the initial assessment by stabilizing the patient's head between your knees until additional assistance is obtained.

47. The detailed assessment includes **determining the chief complaint; examining the neck, chest, and abdomen; palpating the pelvis and lower extremities; checking pupillary response; having the patient grasp your hands;** and **obtaining the patient history.**

48. **False:** A simple cut finger would *not* require a detailed assessment, but a victim of multiple trauma would.

49. **False:** A detailed assessment should be performed on "priority" patients (if indicated) while *en route to the hospital*. In some cases, the time required to care for life-threatening conditions does not allow for completion of the detailed assessment.

50. **b**

51. Things that are part of the ongoing assessment: **reassess mental status; monitor the airway; monitor breathing—rate and quality; reassess pulse—rate and quality; monitor skin color, temperature, and condition; realign patient priorities as needed; reassess vital signs; repeat focused exam regarding complaint or injuries; and check efficacy of interventions.**

52. **True**

53. **d:** Patients should be directly transported to the most appropriate facility for their condition. If possible, and if allowed by local protocol, the EMT-I may consider also the patient's wishes to be taken to a certain hospital.

54. **a:** Helicopter transport should *not* be used for transporting combative patients, patients contaminated by hazardous materials, and patients whose size prohibits proper securing inside the aircraft. Helicopter transport *should also be avoided* during lightning or high winds, during heavy cloud periods (unless the helicopter can fly on instruments), and when ground transport is faster, including waiting time for the helicopter to reach the scene.

55. Six pieces of information that should be communicated to medical direction or the receiving hospital are **nature of the incident; number of patients to be transported; life-threatening problems; care being rendered; results of that care; and estimated time of arrival (ETA) to the facility.**

56. **A well-documented report is essential for proper transfer of care to the receiving facility, as well as for your defense if you ever have to justify your care in a hearing or negligence suit.**

57. Answers to crossword puzzle

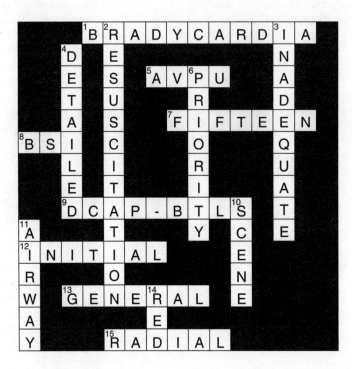

CHAPTER 13

1. A tremendous number of variables can affect almost every aspect of the prehospital environment, including weather, patient position, contamination, hostile animals, locked entrances, bystanders, and environmental factors. Emergency departments are well lit, seldom bounce around, and are absent of extremes of temperature and weather.

2. Patients experiencing a life-threatening emergency include **61-year-old with a gunshot wound to the head; 32-year-old who has severe wounds to his chest, abdomen, and extremities from an explosion; 75-year-old who has a history of COPD and is in extreme respiratory distress; and 81-year-old patient with cancer who is emaciated, obtunded, and has minimal respirations.**

3. **True**

4. **True**

5. **False:** Chronic medical conditions *may* affect a patient's response to new illnesses or injuries.

6. **c**

7. **a**

8. Disadvantages of protocols: **unusual presentations may not fit into one specific protocol; patients with multiple complaints or conditions may generate the need to follow multiple protocols concurrently; integration of multiple protocols can be difficult; and reliance on pure memorization of protocols without understanding the physiology of how the protocol is intended to affect the patient.**

9. The mechanism of collecting, integrating, and synthesizing information takes part largely at the **subconscious** level.

10. The product of critical thinking is an understanding of the patient's **illness** or **injury** and development of a **treatment** plan.

11. Components of thinking process with definitions: **a. Concept formation:** pattern of understanding based on initial information gathered; **b. Data interpretation:** comparing current information with past education and experience to draw conclusions; **c. Application of principle:** formulating an initial impression of what disease processes or injuries are affecting the patient; **d. Evaluation:** constantly reassessing the patient; and **e. Reflection on action:** critiquing the actions and interventions performed on each individual call.

12. **b**

13. General patient **affect** can provide clues to the patient's mental status.

14. Mental status directly relates to **perfusion** of the central nervous system (CNS), electrolyte disturbances, intoxication, **head** trauma, and **psychological** disorders.

15. Initial interventions are selected based on the **cumulative** interpretation of all the **data** the EMT-I has received with the current patient and with **similar** patients who have been cared for in the past.

16. The EMT-I should routinely reevaluate the **vital** signs and physical state of the patient to determine the response to **therapies** or progression of the physiological insult.

17. **False:** As new information is learned, the working diagnosis *may be expanded or changed*. This may necessitate modifications in the current treatment protocols and planned therapies.

18. **True**

19. Eight elements that form the foundation of critical thinking for the EMT-I: **adequate fund of knowledge; focusing on specific and multiple elements of data; gathering information, organizing data, forming concepts; identifying and dealing with medical ambiguity; differentiating between relevant and irrelevant data; analyzing and comparing similar situations; recalling contrary situations;** and **articulating assessment-based decisions and constructing arguments.**

20. **d**

21. **b**

22. **d**

23. The **sympathetic** nervous system releases **adrenaline**, which is responsible for the "fight or flight" response.

24. The useful aspects of this **adrenaline** surge are heightened senses of vision and **hearing.**

25. **The key to quality performance under pressure is to develop habits of evaluation and management that are applied to every patient encountered. First, stay calm. Do each patient assessment in a systematic manner so that it can be followed reflexively under stressful situations. Try to anticipate potential changes in the patient's condition. This enables you to mentally prepare for additional therapies or procedures and avoid hesitation in the face of a sudden unexpected finding.**

26. Five key points for effective thinking during each patient encounter: **stop and think; scan the situation; decide and act; maintain clear, concise control; and perform regular and continual reevaluation of the patient.**

27. Two key questions to address while assessing a patient experiencing an acute event: "What is my current working diagnosis and best treatment plan?" and "What additional problems could my patient potentially develop, and how would I treat them?"

28. Six "R's" used during each patient encounter: **Read the patient; Read the scene; React; Reevaluate; Revise the management plan; and Review performance at run critique.**

29. Five critical questions to keep in mind while approaching the patient:
    - **What is the level of consciousness?**
    - **Is the patient interacting with bystanders or family?**
    - **Is there any obvious respiratory distress?**
    - **Is there obvious deformity or bleeding?**
    - **Is the skin pale or cyanotic?**

30. **a**

31. **b**

32. Answers to crossword puzzle

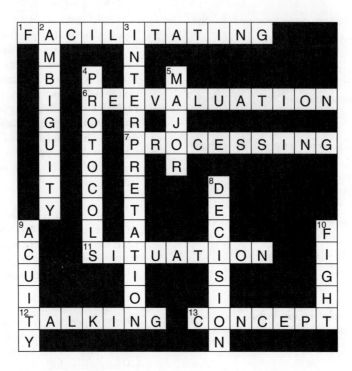

CHAPTER 14

1. Effective **communication** is essential to the smooth and **efficient** operation of the EMS team.

2. There must be a coordinated **communication** system that allows information to flow internally and **externally** in both routine and **emergency** modes.

3. Communications that take place as part of providing EMS are done verbally, through **written** means, or **electronically**.

4. Correct order for the basic communication model:
   1. You form an idea or message you wish to pass along.
   2. You encode the message in a language that can be understood by the person who will receive the message or in a manner that is appropriate for the situation.
   3. You select the medium for sending your message, such as speaking to someone face to face or over the radio or telephone, leaving a voice mail, writing a note or letter, or sending a fax or electronic mail.
   4. Your message arrives at its destination, and the receiver decodes it.
   5. The receiver provides feedback to you that the message has been received and understood.

5. Components of the basic communication model

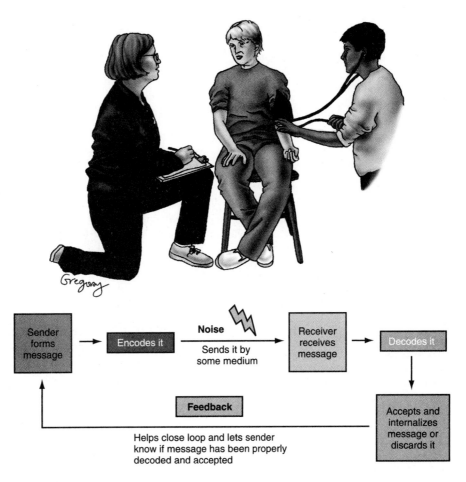

6. **b**

7. **Feedback is critical to closing the communication loop or circle. Without feedback, the message may remain out there, and the sender may have no idea that it has not been received, decoded, and accepted.**

8. **False:** Verbal communication is a **good way but not the only way** to exchange system and patient information with other members of the EMS team. Some communication is effective, whereas other communication fails to achieve its intent.

9. **False:** Semantic and technical factors can **either** boost or hinder communications.

10. **False:** To improve your communications, make sure they are unambiguous, to the point, and *avoid* technical or semantic jargon that cannot be clearly understood by all parties.

11. **True**

12. Factors that lead to noise in communication model include: **People have a tendency to listen to only part of the message and block out other information. New information may conflict with established values, beliefs, or expectations. Uncomfortable environmental conditions can also distract the receiver. Several messages may be delivered to the receiver all at once, and he or she cannot effectively decode your message. Perceptions and cultural differences can also interfere with the message being decoded and interpreted in the intended manner. In face-to-face communication, the facial expressions and body language of the sender can also influence how a message is received. Voice inflection, tone, pitch, and the words used also play a role in verbal communication.**

13. Two techniques that can be used to overcome noise in emergency communications: **Get feedback from the receiver to ensure he or she understands and accepts the message, and look for the best time to deliver the message. If your message must be communicated promptly, you should first try to get the**

receiver's attention—then deliver your message. Follow that up by asking the receiver to repeat back to you the information you provided.

14. **b:** An automatic vehicle-locating system is a beneficial tool for an EMS system, but it is not considered part of a typical communication system for EMS. The typical configuration would include **telephones, radios, pagers,** repeater systems, and recording equipment.

15. **True**

16. **False:** The recommended telephone number for accessing EMS is 9-1-1.

17. **True:** Enhanced 9-1-1 is the emergency telephone number that includes a visual system that displays the caller's telephone number and address. The benefit of E 9-1-1 is that the dispatcher has the needed information immediately available. In cases where the victim is unsure of his or her location, E 9-1-1 is invaluable and can prove to be lifesaving.

18. **b:** Dedicated land lines **may be used by dispatchers to notify EMS personnel of emergency calls;** are telephone lines with an continuous connection from one geographical location to another; are a reliable method of communicating with receiving hospitals, medical control facilities, remote radio communication receivers, communication consoles, and police and fire dispatch centers; and offer the advantage of not requiring the dispatcher to go through a switchboard, dial a telephone number, or be confronted with a busy signal, thus saving time.

19. **d:** This is often the case in disaster situations where cellular communication systems are largely ineffective because of so many other users (such as the news media and private citizens) overloading the available cells.

20. Radio system components with characteristics: **a. Base station:** typical power output of 45 to 275 W; most powerful radio in the system; usually located in a dispatch center that serves as the communication network for the EMS system; may be controlled by a remote console; **b. Mobile radios:** mounted in vehicles such as ambulances, rescue units, or supervisory vehicles; typical power output of 40 to 100 W; characteristic transmission range is 10 to 15 miles over average terrain; **c. Portable radios:** typical power output of 1 to 5 W; allow communications to take place while EMT-Is are away from the ambulance; handheld devices; will maximize coverage when they are held in a vertical and elevated position.

21. **d**

22. **c:** Radio transmissions over flatlands or **water** will increase the range, whereas transmissions over mountains, through dense foliage, or in urban areas with large buildings will decrease the range.

23. **c**

24. MHz ranges with bands: **b. 30 to 50 MHz:** VHF (very high frequency) low band; **e. 150 to 170 MHz:** VHF high band; **d. 450 to 470 MHz:** UHF (ultra high frequency).

25. **True**

26. **False:** Medical channels 9 and 10 are used for dispatch purposes, whereas medical channels 1 through 8 are used for EMT-I–to–physician communications.

27. **True**

28. **True**

29. **b:** VHF high band **signals are transmitted in a straight line and do not follow the curvature of the earth,** are better for communications in metropolitan areas than VHF low band, and provide reliable coverage for dispatcher-to-unit and EMT-I–to–hospital communication over a relatively large area. Base station antennas are usually located on high sites to increase the area of coverage, and VHF is less susceptible to electrical disturbances or skip phenomenon.

30. **a:** Radios that operate on the 800 MHz frequency **permit more effective utilization of the assigned frequencies and can permit interagency communications;** have excellent penetration of buildings, minimal interference, and reduced channel noise; require only a short channel; and have characteristics that make them ideal for use in major metropolitan operations.

31. **a**

32. **Repeater systems are devices that receive transmissions from relatively low wattage transmitters on one frequency and retransmit them at a higher power on another frequency. This increases the range of the transmissions.**

33. **False:** A repeater system receives a transmission from a low-power portable or mobile radio on one frequency and then retransmits it at a higher power on another frequency.

34. **False:** Repeaters can be situated in permanent locations or mounted in the vehicles.

35. **b**

36. Modes with characteristics: **a. Simplex:** least complicated type of communication; the EMT-I must avoid starting any communication until all other communications have ended; communication can occur in only one direction at a time; **b. Duplex:** two separate frequencies are paired together to allow simultaneous transmission and reception to take place; **c. Multiplex:** most complicated type of communication; used by many base station hospitals that provide on-line medical direction; has the ability to simultaneously transmit two or more different types of information (e.g., voice and telemetry) in either or both directions over the same frequency.

37. **d**

38. **False:** Cellular communications are becoming a cost-effective way to transmit essential patient information to medical control.

39. **False:** The Federal Communications Commission (FCC) does not deal with the dispatching of ambulances across state borders.

40. Proper documentation during an EMS event **provides a written, legal record of each case. It conveys important clinical information from the EMS team to the emergency department staff. After delivery of the patient to the hospital, the documentation becomes a part of the medical record. Medical direction uses patient documentation to perform quality improvement audits to monitor a system's compliance with existing patient care protocols. The EMS run report may also be used to gather important system data such as patient billing information and data for research.**

41. **When completing documentation, remember that all patient information is confidential and can only be shared with the nurse or physician continuing the care of the patient in the emergency department.**

42. **c:** Electronic information gathering can allow for real-time capturing of information; medical diagnostic technology can be integrated into it; and it facilitates data collection for quality improvement, research activities, and patient billing. **However, electronic documentation carries with it the same responsibility of ensuring patient confidentiality as hand-written documentation.** This may require additional equipment or software to prevent others from accessing patient information that is being sent electronically.

43. Terms with definitions: biotelemetry: **process of transmitting physiological data such as an ECG over distance, usually by radio**; computer: **desktop, laptop, notebook, handheld and palm electronic devices used to gather, manipulate, store, and send data**; facsimile: **scan of printed information, digitized line by line, and then transmitted over normal telephone lines to another fax machine that then decodes and prints it, or a document that is generated and sent or received through computers or cellular technology.**

44. Causes of biotelemetry interference include **loose ECG electrodes, muscle tremors, 60-MHz noise, fluctuations in transmitter power, and interference of the radio transmission.**

45. **Encrypting is scrambling a message to prevent illicit access to the information. With its use, faxes (as well as other digital transmissions) sent via cellular technology cannot be viewed or retrieved by anyone other than those who were intended to receive them.**

46. **The fax must be received in a secure location rather than one that serves as the general emergency department fax machine. This may require the hospital emergency department to maintain a dedicated telephone line and fax machine for receiving EMS run reports. Also, steps should be in place to ensure that only authorized personnel handle EMS run reports. Last, the EMS communications should be encrypted (as described above).**

47. Answers to crossword puzzle

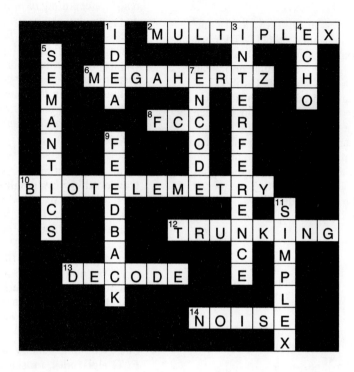

48. Progression of a typical EMS run:
    - Occurrence
    - Detection
    - Notification and response
    - Treatment and preparation for transport
    - Transport and delivery
    - Preparation for the next event

49. **a: EMDs do not give medical direction to EMT-Is working in the field.** Responsibilities of the EMD include obtaining, in a rapid and controlled manner, as much information about the emergency from the caller as possible; directing the appropriate emergency response unit(s) to the scene; monitoring and overseeing communications between EMS and other public safety personnel; providing prearrival medical instructions by telephone for the caller to follow until emergency care arrives; assisting with safeguarding of the providers on scene (e.g., calling for police, fire, hazardous materials team, additional EMS units); assisting with resolution of communication difficulties; and securing and maintaining written records.

50. **False:** The first information the EMD must gather from the caller includes the location and nature of the emergency. (The ambulance can be dispatched as soon as these are known.)

51. **True**

52. **True:** The provision of these instructions may continue throughout the time the ambulance is being dispatched and responding to the scene. This allows for the delivery of emergency care until the first responding unit arrives.

53. Reasons for medical communications include **to obtain orders for patient care in the field; to obtain advice when the EMS team is uncertain of what course of action to take with a given patient; to provide the hospital with information regarding the patient's condition so they can begin preparing for care; to help convince obviously ill patients who are refusing treatment/transport of the need to be treated and seen at the hospital; to resolve uncertainty as to the continuation or termination of resuscitation (i.e., questionable "do not resuscitate" cases); to assist in resolving difficulty with non-EMS physicians who are interfering at the scene; and EMT-Is may find it useful to consult with a physician when patient transport is deemed unnecessary.**

54. **Using a standard format allows efficient use of the communication system by limiting radio time and allows the physician to quickly receive and assimilate information regarding the patient's condition.**

55. **b:** The **patient's name** *should not* be conveyed over the radio. Useful elements of the report, in the order they should be given, include:
    - Identification number and level of the provider
    - Description of the scene
    - Patient's age and sex

- Chief complaint
- Associated signs and symptoms
- Brief, pertinent history of the present illness
- Pertinent past medical history, medications, and allergies
- Physical exam findings, including:
  - Level of consciousness
  - Vital signs
  - General appearance and degree of distress
  - Trauma index or Glasgow Coma Scale (if applicable)
  - Pertinent findings of the physical exam
- Treatment given so far
- Response to treatment
- Advanced life support given on standing orders
- Orders being requested
- Name of private physician
- Estimated time of arrival at the hospital

56. **False:** To help ensure that correct information has been provided, the EMT-I *should* repeat, or "echo," back orders given by the physician.

57. **False:** When the orders from medical command are not clear or seem inappropriate for the patient's condition, the EMT-I *should* question the physician.

58. **True:** Additionally, the EMT-I should report back to the physician when orders have been carried out, and he or she should report the patient's response to those treatments. Further, repeat vital signs should be taken and reported to the medical direction physician with each medication administration.

59. An example of a report to medical direction or the receiving hospital, based on the case history, is as follows:

    Methodist Hospital, this is Andover Rescue 3, Paramedic Andrews, on-line number 261 . . . we are en route to your hospital with a 21-year-old, 120-pound female who is complaining of shortness of breath following a bee sting.

    We found her sitting bolt upright on the couch. She was in obvious respiratory distress with intercostal retraction and accessory muscle usage. Auscultation of her chest revealed bilateral wheezing. We also noted swelling about the patient's face, particularly around the eyes.

    Initial vital signs were as follows: respiratory rate was 24, pulse rate was 132, blood pressure was 164/82, skin was cool and moist, and the pulse oximetry showed an Sao_2 of 88%. ECG shows sinus tachycardia without ectopy.

    The mother states the daughter was mowing the lawn when she was stung by a bee and immediately started itching all over. Then patient said she could not catch her breath. The mother reports the patient is allergic to bee stings.

    We started her on 15 L/min via nonrebreather mask and placed an IV line in her right forearm with an 18-gauge catheter-over-needle. We are delivering 1000 cc of NS with a macrodrip administration at a TKO rate. We administered one albuterol breathing treatment and 0.3 cc of 1:1000 epinephrine subcutaneously. She has responded favorably to the treatment. Reassessment shows the patient has a respiratory rate of 18, a pulse rate of 116, a blood pressure of 130/84, and warm, dry skin. Auscultation of her chest reveals a marked decrease in the bilateral wheezing, and she is moving air much better. The ECG monitor continues to show sinus tachycardia without ectopy, and the pulse oximetry reveals an Sao_2 of 94%.

    Do you have any further orders for us?

60. Reasons for verbally communicating patient information to the hospital are **it makes the staff aware of the patient's problem before his or her arrival at the hospital, and allows them to mobilize resources, determine bed availability, and prepare teams within the hospital to deal with the patient's problems.**

61. **c:** When speaking into the radio, **use words like "affirmative" and "negative."** Avoid words that are difficult to hear like "yes" or "no."

62. **a:** Proper radio communication techniques include listening to the channel before transmitting to ensure that it is not in use, **pressing the transmit button for approximately 1 second before beginning to speak,** speaking at a close range (2 to 3 inches) directly into the microphone, speaking slowly and clearly and in a normal pitch, avoiding use of superfluous phrases, and "echoing" back information to the dispatcher or physician.

63. **False:** Avoid using codes and abbreviations unless they are part of your system and everyone understands them.

64. **True**

65. **False:** Keep your transmissions brief. If longer transmissions are needed, pause for a few seconds after every 30 seconds or so to allow other units to transmit information if needed.

66. **True**

67. **True**

68. **False:** Hold portable radios in an upright (vertical) position to achieve maximum radio coverage.

69. **c:** Appropriate handling and maintenance of portable radio equipment includes **placing a fresh, recharged battery in the unit every day**. Regular cleaning of the radio equipment will improve its physical appearance. Exterior surfaces should be wiped with a moist cloth and mild detergent. Avoid harsh cleaning agents. Additionally, the radio should be carried in an appropriate holster.

70. Factors that limit communication capabilities during a disaster include **incompatible frequencies between agencies; overloading of radio frequencies; damage to the communication system infrastructure;** and **general equipment failure**.

CHAPTER 15

1. Patient care documentation **facilitates a continuation of care by supplying vital information to the emergency department staff. It serves as a legal record of each case. Quality improvement audits performed by medical control can be used to monitor appropriate compliance to standing orders.**

2. **EMS run reports serve as a key source for data collection that can be used to guide system improvements, training programs, research, and revenue collection.** Operational statistics, when properly linked to geographical and definitive care resources, can help determine appropriate locations for stationing ambulances and other equipment. Patient care statistics can show which EMT-Is need additional training. Run reports can also be used to demonstrate good documentation, as well as how to handle unusual cases.

3. **b**

4. **d: The EMT-I must be as objective as possible** when documenting information on the run report. Also, avoid concluding or making assumptions about what has taken place; be specific rather than general, and printing is preferred to cursive.

5. **c:** A **ballpoint pen** creates a permanent record, making it difficult to tamper with or erase information. Additionally, the second and third copies of the report are more legible when a ballpoint pen is used.

6. **a:** The use of abbreviations as part of prehospital documentation **allows more information to be included in narrative sections of the run report** and allows quicker documentation of information. However, abbreviations can have multiple meanings, so only those approved by the EMS system should be used.

7. Answers to crossword puzzle

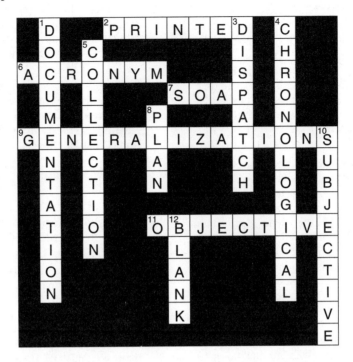

8. **False:** The EMT-I should avoid filling out the run report while still wearing gloves that were used to provide patient care. This helps prevent the run report from being contaminated with blood or bodily fluids.

9. **False:** Avoid filling out the run report close to where patient care is occurring because blood or bodily fluids can be splashed onto the run report.

10. **False:** Patient care should not be delayed or compromised to fill out the run report.

11. Extraneous or nonprofessional information with alternatives

Extraneous or Nonprofessional Information	Alternatives
"The patient says he was already seen in the emergency department five times for the same problem but they didn't do anything to help him."	"The patient reports he was seen in emergency department five same problem."
"The patient is stinking drunk."	"The patient is confused and agitated and is having trouble with his coordination."
"There was a significant delay in response time due to the emergency department not moving patients through triage fast enough."	"There was a dealy in response time due to our being unable to transfer the patient over to the emergency department staff."

12. **False:** Run reports can be scrutinized by a variety of individuals, including hospital personnel, quality assurance personnel, supervisors, the court system, and the news media. Additionally, the patient or patient's family may request a copy of the run report. As such, the EMT-I must avoid making entries on the run report using "street slang" or flippant or derogatory remarks such as the patient is "faking it" or is "a drunk." These types of remarks can prove embarrassing to the EMT-I and the EMS service and may be construed as libelous.

13. **True:** Refining a few basic abilities such as grammar, spelling, and conciseness can help to avoid pitfalls, enhance the delivery of patient care, reduce the risk of litigation, and promote the image of the EMT-I. It is helpful to solicit feedback on the thoroughness and appearance of the run report from other EMS team members before it is turned in.

14. Meaning of the mnemonic SOAP: S: **subjective;** O: **objective;** A: **assessment;** and P: **plan.**

15. Subjective is **what the patient feels or tells you**; objective is **what you observe**.

16. Subjective and objective statements: **S:** "I can't feel my toes"; **S:** "My head hurts"; **O:** The steering wheel was bent, and the patient's chest was bruised; **S:** The patient says he felt nauseous at the same time as his chest started to hurt and he became sweaty; **O:** Skin is cool, pale, and diaphoretic; **O:** Patient has decreased grip on right side.

17. Assessment methods with descriptions: **a. Chronological method:** documentation follows the care of the patient by identifying the steps taken in the order in which they were performed. It begins with the time of arrival on the scene. Each entry starts with a time notation followed by the pertinent information for that time period; **b. Head-to-toe method:** documents the assessment the same way you performed it—head to toe. Start by noting the patient's age, sex, and level of consciousness, and how the patient was initially found. Then list the results of your initial assessment and focused history and examination. Describe your assessment findings of the head, chest, abdomen, pelvis, genitalia, lower extremities, upper extremities, and then the back. Conclude by describing the interventions and care delivered to the patient; **c. Body systems approach:** uses a comprehensive review of the primary body systems. It includes a detailed review of the skin, skeletal, head, endocrine, respiratory, cardiac, hematological, lymph nodes, gastrointestinal, genitourinary, neurological, and psychiatric systems. Because it is time-consuming, the body systems approach is better suited for nursing than the prehospital setting.

18. Information that should be included on the run report: **dispatch information; care being provided before arrival; important observations; demographic and billing information; chief complaint; present history; past medical history; physical assessment findings; treatments provided; run times; run disposition; and signatures.**

19. **a:** The chief complaint **is the reason why the patient (or family member, friend, or bystander) called for EMS assistance,** should be stated in the patient's own words, and in cases where the patient is unconscious or in cardiac arrest, the chief complaint should be reported as that.

20. **a:** The past medical history includes **surgeries and hospitalizations,** illnesses and injuries, current medications the patient is taking, allergies, last meal the patient ingested, and the name of the patient's physician.

21. Elements of the vital signs that should be documented on the run report: **level of consciousness; respiratory rate and character; pulse rate and character; blood pressure; skin color and temperature; and capillary refill.**

22. **b:** Repeat vital signs **provide important information regarding changes in the patient's condition over time**, are important in situations where the patient is seriously ill or injured or his or her condition is changing for the better or worse, and are usually recorded in the vital signs section along with the time each was taken.

23. Treatment documentation should include **what was done, who performed the procedure,** and **time the treatment was provided.**

24. The following treatments are described in appropriate detail: **"Proventil, 0.25 mL, by inhalation, administered at 08:04 per medical command," "IV of D5W, 18-gauge needle to right antecubital fossa, microdrip administration set, run TKO, established at 18:05 according to standing orders,"** and **"15 L of oxygen administered via nonrebreather mask, started at 10:15 pm."** "Placed an endotracheal tube" may be expanded in the following way: "Placed a 7.0 i.d. endotracheal tube, 2:20 pm, bilateral lung sounds and chest rise are present."

25. Elements with examples: **a. Chief complaint:** Patient says he "is having a hard time breathing." **b. Past medical history:** Patient takes Diabinese for diabetes. **c. Physical assessment:** BP 190/110, pulse 110 and regular, labored respirations at a rate of 20 per minute; patient has deformity and swelling to his left upper leg. **d. Pertinent positives or negatives:** Patient denies shortness of breath and nausea. **e. Patient's response or lack of response to treatment:** Cyanosis subsided after oxygen administration; chest pain subsided after the patient took a nitroglycerin tablet; patient's blood pressure decreased to 110/86 after infusion of 500 mL of normal saline. **f. Present history:** Patient was found sitting at kitchen table on arrival. **g. Treatment:** Administered 15 L of oxygen via nonrebreather mask.

26. **c**

27. As part of documentation, the EMT-I should collect demographic information such as name, **age**, sex, date of birth, **address**, and **telephone number**. In some systems you also may be required to obtain **billing information,** such as type of medical insurance.

28. **False:** Corrections can be made to the run report even after it has been completed and signed.

29. **False:** If an entry is made after a run report has been completed, the time and date of the entry should be added, and an explanation of the reason for the late entry should be written next to it. No attempt should be made to cover up the fact that it is a late entry.

30. **b:** Mistakes on run reports can be corrected by: **indicating that they are errors, initialing and dating them,** drawing a single, horizontal line through the inaccurate section so that the previous entry is still legible, and writing the correct information beside it. It is acceptable to state on the report why the correction was made or to have the correction witnessed.

31. Example of corrected mistake:

    Lopressor, BA, 4/16/96

    > Patient takes Lasix ~~and Digitalis~~ for hypertension and heart failure.

32. Items that should be listed if normal protocol or standard of care is not followed: **the reason why; what steps were taken (if any) to correct the situation; and whether medical command was notified of the problem.**

33. Falsification of information on the run report may lead to **suspension or revocation of the EMT-I's certification/license and poor patient care because other health care providers have a false impression of which assessment findings were discovered or what treatment was given.**

34. **c**

35. **d:** When a patient refuses care, **assessment findings and emergency medical care given should be documented, and the patient should be asked to sign a refusal form.** Also, a police officer or bystander should sign the form as a witness, and if no other witnesses are available, a family member may be asked to sign as a witness.

36. **d:** At multiple casualty incidents, the EMT-I **must document the best he or she can with the limited information available.** Just like when dealing with a critically ill or injured patient, documentation may need to be done after delivering the patients to the hospital. The standard for completing the form in a multiple casualty incident is not the same as for a typical call.

37. **True:** Documentation of invasive or advanced treatments should include a brief notation as to whether they were done with permission of on-line or off-line medical direction.

38. **True:** This documentation should include a brief description of the problem and the EMT-I's identification number or initials.

39. **False:** All personnel responsible for the run should sign the run report (or at least their names or identification numbers should be clearly printed).

40. Answers to crossword puzzle

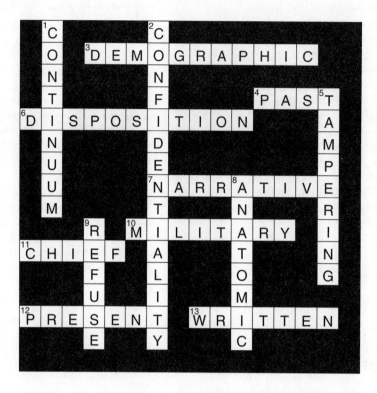

CHAPTER 16

1. **c:** Trauma is the leading cause of death in people ages **1** to **44** years.

2. **a:** Trauma is linked to alcohol in many fatal motor vehicle crashes.

3. The top five causes of unintentional trauma deaths (in 2003) were **motor vehicle accidents; falls; poisoning; choking; drowning; and tied with drowning fire, flames, and smoke; and suffocation.**

4. **False:** In the *preincident* phase, the focus is prevention of intentional and unintentional trauma deaths.

5. **False:** Properly preparing the patient for transportation to an appropriate medical facility is considered part of the *postincident* phase.

6. Activities that health care providers can do to reduce trauma include **conduct public education (i.e., use of automobile occupant restraint systems and helmets, promotion of nonviolent conflict resolution, and the appropriate use of the 9-1-1 system) and promote legislation that supports injury prevention programs.**

7. **b**

8. Definitive intervention provided to the trauma patient within the Golden Hour can enhance **survival** and reduce **complications.**

9. The EMT-I must recognize critically injured patients and ensure that prehospital **care** activities do not unnecessarily delay patient **transportation.**

10. The EMT-I can best serve severely injured trauma patients through **performance of lifesaving procedures; properly preparing the patient for transport to an appropriate medical facility; and promptly transporting the patient to an appropriate medical facility.**

11. Components of a sophisticated trauma system: **injury prevention; prehospital care to include treatment, transportation, and trauma triage; emergency department care; interfacility transportation as necessary; definitive care; trauma critical care; rehabilitation; and data collection/trauma registry.**

12. **a**

13. **d**

14. Trauma centers are categorized based on the **resources** and **programs** available at the facility.

15. This categorization identifies those hospitals capable of handling trauma patients and enables EMS providers to **rapidly** transport patients to the most **appropriate** medical facilities.

16. Trauma center levels with capabilities: **a. Level I:** provides a full spectrum of services from prevention programs to patient rehabilitation and serves as the leader in trauma care for a geographic area; **b. Level II:** usually provides initial definitive patient care; research is not an essential component; **c. Level III:** usually a community hospital that provides evaluation, resuscitation, and operative intervention for stabilization; **d. Level IV:** may not be a hospital but rather it can be a clinic-type facility; provides initial stabilization and then transfers the patient.

17. Structure of a trauma care system

Environments	Components	Providers
Urban Rural	• Medical direction • Prevention • Communication • Training • Triage • Prehospital care • Transportation • Hospital care • Public education • Rehabilitation • Medical evaluation	• System management • Prehospital providers • Acute care facilities • Rehabilitation/reconstructive services

18. **The patient's needs and condition, as well as the advice of medical direction, determine the appropriate level of care and hospital destination.**

19. Air transport should be considered **when the time needed to transport a patient by ground to an appropriate facility poses a threat to the patient's survival and recovery; when weather, road, or traffic conditions would seriously delay the patient's access to definitive care;** and **when critical care personnel and equipment not available from ground crews are needed to adequately care for the patient during transport.**

20. **d:** Seriously injured patients should be **promptly** transported to a definitive care facility. Therefore none of the answers is correct. Ideally, the patient should be initially assessed, provided with lifesaving interventions, packaged, and moved to the ambulance for transport all within 10 minutes of the EMT-Is reaching his or her side. Begin transport as soon as the patient is placed in the ambulance. IV attempts and a detailed ongoing assessment should be done en route. Depending on local protocol, communicate with the receiving facility as early as possible. If the patient is critically injured, every effort should be made to transport the patient to a trauma center.

21. *Kinematics* is defined as **the process of predicting injury patterns that may result from the forces and motions of energy.**

22. Newton's first law of motion states that a body in motion will remain in motion unless acted on by an **outside force.** Furthermore, a body at rest will remain at rest until acted on by an outside force.

23. The second principle of physics is that energy cannot be **created** or **destroyed.** It can, however, change its form. For example, when the car crashes into a telephone pole, the energy is spread out over the frame of the car, the fenders, and other parts of the vehicle (mechanical). The more energy that is present, the greater the changes or damage will be to the structure of the car, as well as to the patient.

24. **False:** In trauma, the weight of a patient has a *significant effect* on the amount of injury. So, too, does the speed at which the person is traveling.

25. **True**

26. Terms with descriptions: **a. Motion:** the process of changing place; movement; **b. Inertia:** the tendency of an object to remain at rest or to remain in motion unless acted on by an external force; **c. Kinetic energy:** the energy an object has while it is in motion; it is related to the object's velocity and mass; **d. Acceleration:** the rate at which speed or velocity increases; **e. Impact:** forceful contact or collision; **f. Mass:** weight; **g. Deceleration:** the rate at which speed decreases.

27. **a:** Blunt trauma: **results from change of speed and compression,** most often fails to break the skin yet causes injuries beneath it, and generally produces an injury that extends into the tissue beneath the impact site, trapping consecutive layers of tissue between others that are either accelerating or decelerating.

28. **True**

29. Motor vehicle collisions are classified by type of impact, including **head on, lateral, rear end, rotational,** and **rollover**.

30. In a head-on car crash, an automobile hits a second vehicle, resulting in damage to the front of the car. As the vehicle abruptly stops, the occupant continues to move at the speed of the automobile before impact. **The front seat occupant continues forward into the restraint system, steering column, or dashboard, resulting in the second collision.**

31. **b**

32. **d**

33. Injuries that are predictable when the abdomen strikes the steering wheel of a vehicle: **liver laceration, spleen rupture, internal hemorrhage,** and **abdominal organ movement into the thorax (ruptured diaphragm).**

34. **d**

35. **b**

36. **a**

37. **a**

38. Restraints available in the United States: **lap belts, diagonal shoulder straps, air bags,** and **child safety seats.**

39. **True**

40. **False:** The injuries sustained in small motor vehicle crashes usually are *more* severe than those received from automobile crashes.

41. **a**

42. **The midshaft of the femur absorbs the rider's forward motion, which can result in bilateral fractures to the femur and lower leg.**

43. Common injury mechanisms to riders of ATVs include the following: **The rear tire runs over the rider's foot, catching the leg, and throwing the rider forward off the vehicle and onto his or her shoulder or crushing the rider beneath the ATV. Wires not easily visible catch the driver across the neck or chest. The rider is thrown from the vehicle, or the vehicle lands on top of the rider.**

44. **c**

45. **c:** Children tend to face the oncoming vehicle, resulting in frontal impact injuries. Because children are smaller than most adults, the initial impact of the automobile occurs higher on the body, usually above the knees or pelvis. The second impact occurs as the front of the vehicle's hood continues forward, making contact with the victim's thorax. The victim immediately is thrown backward, forcing the head and neck to flex forward. Depending on the position of the child in relation to the automobile, the head and neck may contact the vehicle's hood. The third impact occurs as the child is thrown downward. Because of a child's smaller size and weight, he or she can fall under the vehicle and be dragged for some distance or fall to the side of the vehicle and be run over by the front or rear wheels.

46. **a**

47. **d**

48. **b**

49. **a**

50. **b**

51. **True:** With penetrating trauma, there is a temporary cavity created (as happens with blunt trauma), as well as a permanent cavity when the skin is broken (opening in the chest wall, for example, from a gunshot wound).

52. **c**

53. **b**

54. **a**

55. Answers to crossword puzzle

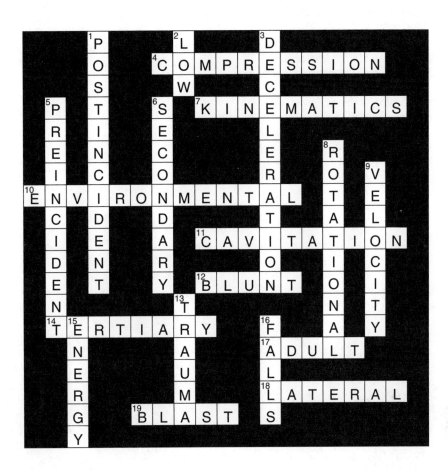

CHAPTER 17

1. Perfusion is important because **it results in the delivery of oxygenated blood to the tissues.** All cells require oxygen to survive. Shock results when perfusion falls below the needed level.

2. Four elements necessary for tissue oxygenation to occur (Fick principle) include **adequate cardiac function, an adequate volume of blood flow and proper routing of blood through the vasculature (blood vessels), close approximation of the tissue cells to the capillaries to allow for diffusion of oxygen, and ideal conditions of pH and temperature.** On reaching the capillary circulation, blood interfaces with the tissues. The tissues are composed of cells that are oxygen deficient as a result of normal metabolism. Because the concentration of oxygen is greater in the bloodstream, oxygen diffuses from the red blood cells into the tissues and cells.

3. **d**

4. Elements necessary for off-loading of oxygen from the red blood cells at the tissue level: **close proximity of the tissue cells to the capillaries to allow for diffusion of oxygen,** and **ideal conditions of pH and temperature.**

5. The body's cells require a continuous supply of **oxygen** and **nutrients** to live. Without one or the other, the cells become depressed and eventually die.

6. **d**

7. **c:** The first step of cellular respiration occurs after the glucose molecule enters the cell and splits into the **pyruvic acid** molecules. This process is called glycolysis.

8. Types of metabolism with characteristics: **a. Aerobic:** produces carbon dioxide, water, and acid as waste products; occurs in the mitochondria of the cell; yields a great deal of energy; is the primary source of energy production in the body; **b. Anaerobic:** occurs without oxygen; yields a very small amount of energy; some small and primitive organisms such as certain bacteria can survive using this type of metabolism alone; is the first part of cellular metabolism.

9.

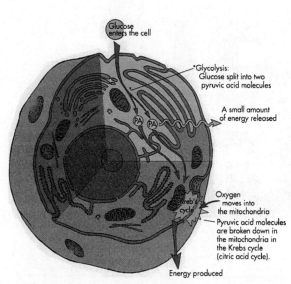

10. **d:** Stroke volume is the amount of blood pumped out of the heart during each contraction and **is affected by circulatory volume, preload, afterload, and myocardial contractility.**

11. Terms with descriptions: **a. Preload:** passive stretching force exerted on the ventricular muscle at the end of diastole; **b. Contractility:** extent and velocity (quickness) of muscle fiber shortening; **c. Afterload:** the resistance against which the heart must pump; d. Perfusion: blood passing through an organ or part of the body; **e. Cardiac output:** the amount of blood pumped through the circulatory system over 1 minute.

12. **Blood is ejected out of the heart when ventricular pressure, resulting from ventricular contraction, exceeds the pressure in the aorta and pulmonary artery.** c: *Calcium* triggers the action that causes muscle filaments to slide together, producing a shortening of the muscle fibers and subsequent myocardial contraction. The ventricular walls squeeze in on the blood contained in the chamber at the onset of contraction, resulting in the same amount of blood occupying a *smaller* space with the pressure in the ventricle increasing quickly and dramatically. Contractility is the extent and velocity or quickness of muscle fiber *shortening*.

13. **b**

14.

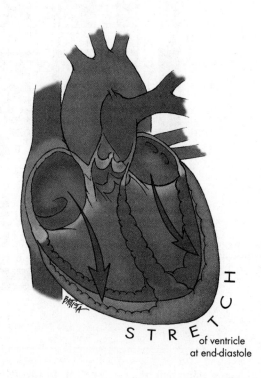

15. Preload is influenced by the **volume** of blood returning to the heart. More blood returning **increases** preload, whereas less blood returning **decreases** preload.

16. The greater the afterload, the **harder** it is for the ventricles to eject blood into the arteries.

17. **a**

18. **d**

19. **c: Increased myocardial contractility** does not reduce the blood pressure. Severe damage to the myocardium, decreased heart rate, and an excessive heart rate can all lead to a decreased blood pressure.

20. **False:** An abnormally low or high blood pressure *will likely have an adverse effect* on perfusion.

21. **True**

22. **b:** Increased blood pressure may be caused by **increases in the heart rate,** *vasoconstriction, increased* myocardial contractility, and increased afterload.

23. **c**

24. **d**

25. **b:** The blood vessels are *elastic, that is, they change in size and adjust the size of the container* in which the blood is held. **The vascular system size is changed by either the dilation or constriction of the blood vessels.** The volume of the container is *directly* related to the diameter of the blood vessels. *Any change* in the diameter of the blood vessels will change the size of the container. This change in size affects the amount of blood returning to the heart and the amount of tissue oxygenation.

26. **b**

27. Two regulatory mechanisms used to control blood flow to the tissues are **local stimulation and sympathetic nervous system stimulation.** The blood vessels in the capillary network adjust their diameter to permit the microcirculation to selectively supply undernourished tissue while temporarily bypassing tissues with no immediate need. The sympathetic nervous system also directly stimulates the blood vessels to constrict or dilate, thereby redistributing blood to organs in need.

28. **a**

29. Elements of blood with descriptions: **a. Plasma:** watery, salty fluid that makes up more than half the volume of blood; **b. Platelets:** tiny formed elements that when ruptured release chemical factors needed to form blood clots; **c. White blood cells:** also called leukocytes; involved in destroying germs and producing substances called antibodies that help the body resist infection; **d. Red blood cells:** also called erythrocytes; are the most abundant of the blood cells; carry oxygen to the tissues and carbon dioxide away from tissues.

30. **a:** Hemoglobin **is a protein that contains iron and bonds the oxygen.** This oxygen-hemoglobin complex makes it possible for the blood to efficiently transport large quantities of oxygen to the body cells. It carries *oxygen* from the lungs to the tissues and *carbon dioxide* from the tissues to the lungs. Under normal situations, *between 97% and 100%* of the hemoglobin is saturated with oxygen. It turns *bright red* when combined with oxygen.

31. **b:** Hematocrit is a term used to identify the volume percentage of red blood cells in whole blood. For example, a hematocrit of 45 means that every 100 mL of whole blood has 45 mL of red cells and 55 mL of plasma. On average, the hematocrit **is 42 for a woman and 45 for a man.**

32. **d:** Blood **viscosity is determined by the ratio of plasma cells and formed elements.** Also, blood *is a viscous fluid, thicker and more adhesive than water.* Because of this, it flows more slowly than water. The *lesser* the ratio of plasma to cells and formed elements, the *greater* the viscosity. Viscosity *affects* peripheral resistance; the greater the viscosity, the greater the resistance.

33. Closed wounds with characteristics: **a. Contusions and hematomas:** with these injuries the blood vessels are torn beneath the dermis; bruising may result. The blood also may leak into deeper tissues and lead to swelling. **b. Crush injuries:** usually involve the extremities, torso, or pelvis; can result in blood vessel injury and internal organ rupture. **c. Compartment syndrome:** caused by blunt trauma or compressive forces to areas with a minimal ability to stretch; it develops as bleeding and swelling increase pressure in a closed area, which compromises circulation and leads to ischemia of the tissues. **d. Crush syndrome:** life-threatening condition caused by prolonged compression or immobilization (beyond 4 to 6 hours). This condition is rare, and the exact mechanism is unknown.

34. Open wounds with mechanisms, signs and symptoms, and treatments

	Mechanism	Signs and Symptoms	Treatment
Abrasions	Occurs when the outermost layer of skin is rubbed away by friction with a hard object or surface	Pain and minimal bleeding. Abrasions may involve loss of body fluids and/or blood depending on the size, depth, and location of the injury.	Cleaning the surface and removing any contaminants
Lacerations	Caused by a tear, split, or incision into the skin. Blunt or penetrating forces can cause it.	Pain and bleeding. Amount of bleeding may be minimal or major depending on the site and mechanism.	Directed at controlling hemorrhage and monitoring for signs and symptoms of hemorrhagic shock
Punctures	Caused by contact with sharp, pointed objects. Because of their nature, they may involve underlying tissues, and internal bleeding may be severe.	Pain and bleeding (the amount will depend on the mechanism).	Controlling hemorrhage and monitoring for signs and symptoms of hemorrhagic shock. If an object is impaled, the EMT-I SHOULD NOT REMOVE IT. He or she should control bleeding and stabilize the object. The object should only be removed if there is interference with airway management, ventilation, or chest compressions if needed.
Avulsions	Tearing away of a part or structure	Pain and bleeding	If the tissue is still attached, the EMT-I should cleanse the area, return the skin to its normal position as much as possible, control bleeding, and apply a bulky dressing. If the tissue is separated, it should be treated as an amputation.
Amputation	Involves partial or complete loss of a limb as a result of some type of mechanical force	Pain, bleeding, and associated injuries dependent on the mechanism	Control the bleeding, and save the amputated part.

35. Hemorrhage (bleeding) occurs **when there is a break in the body's vascular system.** Hemorrhage may be external, from obvious cuts, punctures, or other wounds, or it can occur internally, in which case no obvious signs of hemorrhage will be evident. Internal bleeding, even when not apparent, may still be critical, leading to shock or death.

36. Type of bleeding with characteristics: **a. Arterial:** blood is bright red, and if the artery is exposed, the blood may escape in spurts synchronized with the pulse; this type of bleeding is the least frequent but the most serious; **b. Venous:** blood is dark red and flows slowly and steadily; this is the type of bleeding associated with deeper cuts; **c. Capillary:** blood is medium red and oozes slowly; this type of bleeding is associated with minor scrapes and cuts.

37. **False:** The application of direct pressure *can usually control external bleeding* from an ordinary cut or puncture.

38. **False:** Whenever tissue is cut, the body releases *chemicals that interact with blood components to promote clotting (coagulation) while constricting or narrowing the blood vessels.* This will not be sufficient to stop all types of bleeding.

39. **False:** Internal bleeding *often is not readily apparent*, although in some cases there may be coughing or vomiting of blood or bleeding from the rectum, urethra, or vagina, depending on the location and nature of the injury or medical condition.

40. An adult can lose **500 mL** of blood without any harm, but the loss of **300 mL** may cause death in an infant.

41. Stages of hemorrhage with characteristics: **a. Stage 1:** blood pressure maintained; normal pulse pressure, respiratory rate, and renal output; skin pallor; anxiety; up to 15% intravascular loss; compensated for by constriction of vascular bed; **b. Stage 2:** up to 15% to 25% intravascular loss; cardiac output cannot be maintained by arteriolar constriction; reflex tachycardia, increased respiratory rate, blood pressure maintained; catecholamines increase peripheral resistance; narrow pulse pressure; diaphoresis from sympathetic stimulation; **c. Stage 3:** up to 25% to 35% intravascular loss; classic signs of hypovolemic shock; **d. Stage 4:** loss of greater than 35%; extreme tachycardia; pronounced tachypnea; significantly decreased systolic blood pressure; confusion, lethargy, and unconsciousness; skin is diaphoretic, cool, and extremely pale.

42. **False:** Serious injuries *do not always bleed heavily*, whereas some relatively minor injuries bleed profusely.

43. **True**

44. **False:** Puncture wounds *usually do not bleed much* but carry a high risk of infection.

45. The body's first response to bleeding is to stop it by chemical means (hemostasis). **This vascular reaction involves local vasoconstriction, formation of a platelet plug, coagulation, and the growth of fibrous tissue into the blood clot that permanently closes and seals the injured vessel.**

46. **c**

47. Correct order of steps used to control bleeding:
    1. **Use body substance isolation precautions.**
    2. **Apply direct pressure to the wound with sterile dressings and a gloved hand.**
    3. **If the bleeding is uncontrolled, elevate the wound (if it is on an extremity).**
    4. **Apply additional dressings if the wound continues to bleed.**
    5. **If the bleeding continues, apply a pressure dressing and bandage to the wound.**
    6. **Locate and apply pressure to the appropriate arterial pressure point if the wound continues to bleed. These pressure points are found on the main artery above the wound.**

48. Signs of internal bleeding include **coughing up red, frothy blood; vomiting blood the color of coffee grounds or bright red; passing of feces with a black, tarry appearance; passing urine that has a red appearance; pain; tenderness; rigidity of abdominal muscles; faintness or dizziness; restlessness; nausea; thirst; weak, rapid pulse; cold, clammy skin; rapid, gasping breathing;** and **sweating.**

49. **A lack of tissue perfusion results in the cells being deprived of essential nutrients, most importantly oxygen. Eventually this leads to anaerobic metabolism and toxic waste products building up in the cells. If not corrected, the cells become depressed and die.**

50. **c:** Shock **is a lack of oxygen delivered to the tissues.** It cannot be defined by measuring the blood pressure, pulse rate, and respiration or by identifying whether the patient's skin is cool and clammy. These are signs and symptoms of shock and do not indicate what is happening on the cellular level.

51. **hypo**perfusion

52. **a:** Baroreceptors **detect changes in the blood pressure.** They are found in the walls of the atria of the

heart, vena cava, aortic arch, and carotid sinus. When hypotension occurs, it is detected, and the information is passed along to the brain, which sends a signal to the sympathetic nervous system. Norepinephrine is then released, and there is a constriction of the smooth muscles in the peripheral arterioles and venules. This results in blood being shunted from the peripheral vasculature to the internal organs. The heart rate also increases, as does the strength of cardiac contractions. The result is improved circulation to the vital organs and decreased circulation to the rest of the body.

53. Initially in shock, compensatory adjustments begin with the **baroreceptors** detecting a decrease in arterial blood pressure. Messages are sent to a regulatory center in the brain that activates the **sympathetic** nervous system. The **sympathetic** nervous system stimulates the heart to beat **faster** and more **forcefully** in an effort to compensate for the decreased blood flow.

54. Stimulation of the sympathetic nervous system also causes a release of **norepinephrine** from sympathetic nerve endings and **epinephrine** (also called adrenalin) from the adrenal glands.

55. **d:** Chemoreceptors are **located in the walls of the atria of the heart, vena cava, aortic arch, and carotid sinus.** They detect changes in the concentration of oxygen, carbon dioxide, and pH and activate the sympathetic nervous system. Increases in carbon dioxide and/or decreases in oxygen typically initiate a sympathetic response that increases the rate and depth of respirations. The increased respiratory volume brings in more oxygen and removes more carbon dioxide. Initially this compensatory hyperventilation helps to maintain acid-base balance in early shock by creating a respiratory alkalosis that acts to offset the metabolic acidosis, resulting in a shift of the pH back toward normal.

56. **a:** Specifically, with sustained anaerobic metabolism there is an *increase* in hydrogen ions, a *decrease* in the pH, and metabolic *acidosis*.

57. a

58. c

59. c

60. **a:** During compensatory shock the **signs and symptoms can be hidden by activation of the sympathetic nervous system.** Signs and symptoms commonly seen at this stage include altered mental status, usually restlessness, increased pulse rate, increased respiratory rate, and pale, cool skin.

61. **c:** This occurs as blood is shunted away from the skin and to the vital organs. This vasoconstriction leads to **pale, cool skin** and an increase in blood pressure (by increasing peripheral vascular resistance).

62. If blood volume decreases more than **15% to 25%,** the shock becomes steadily worse because **compensatory** mechanisms are no longer able to maintain **perfusion.**

63. As the cardiovascular system progressively deteriorates, cardiac output **decreases** dramatically. This condition can lead to further reductions in **blood pressure** and **cardiac function.**

64. d

65. **Hypo**tension is an abnormal condition in which the blood pressure is too low for normal perfusion and oxygenation of the tissues. Eventually patients in the decompensated (progressive) stage of shock will develop hypotension, which is a late sign of shock. By the time hypotension develops, the body's compensatory mechanisms have failed.

66. **b:** The sensation of thirst **helps regulate fluid intake.** It occurs when body fluids become *decreased*, stimulating the person to take in more fluids. Conversely, when too many fluids enter the body, the kidneys are activated and more urine is excreted, thus eliminating the excess fluid. The body also maintains fluid balance by shifting water from one compartment to another.

67. b

68. **c:** With irreversible shock, **the liver, kidneys, and lungs become progressively ischemic and begin to falter, eventually becoming ineffective.** Even if the cause of shock is then to be treated and reversed, the damage to the vital organs cannot be repaired, and the person eventually dies. Some signs and symptoms of pending irreversible shock include marked decrease in level of consciousness, decreased respiratory rate and effort, profound hypotension and inability to palpate a pulse (even in a conscious patient), decrease in the pulse rate from too fast to too slow, and the patient communicating a feeling of impending doom.

69. Phases of shock with characteristics: **a. Compensatory:** earliest phase of shock; body recognizes the catastrophic event that is occurring and triggers corrective action in an attempt to return cardiac output and arterial blood pressure to normal; **b. Decompensated:** includes signs and symptoms such as sweating, cold and clammy skin, narrowing

pulse pressure, hypotension, nausea, and vomiting; the cells in the tissues become hypoxic, leading to anaerobic metabolism and the production of harmful acids, eventually bringing about metabolic acidosis; arteries that are deprived of their blood supply cannot remain constricted and begin to dilate, resulting in decreased venous return, which in turn decreases cardiac output; **c. Irreversible:** the heart deteriorates to the point that it can no longer effectively pump blood, and there are life-threatening reductions in cardiac output, blood pressure, and tissue perfusion; adult respiratory distress syndrome (ARDS), renal failure, liver failure, and sepsis may develop; vital organs begin to die because of inadequate perfusion.

70. **b:** Hypovolemic shock may be caused by the loss of blood from the body such as internal or external hemorrhage resulting from trauma or medical conditions such as gastrointestinal bleeding or ruptured aortic aneurysm. Hypovolemic shock also results from other conditions associated with fluid volume loss without bleeding, such as **profuse sweating,** burns, and severe dehydration. Burns cause the loss of plasma through the damaged skin. Dehydration can occur following severe vomiting, diarrhea, diabetic ketoacidosis, or inadequate fluid intake.

71. **False:** *Hypovolemic* shock is the most common type of shock seen in the prehospital setting.

72. **True:** Cardiogenic shock is caused by profound failure of the heart, primarily the left ventricle. When greater than 40% of the left ventricle is nonfunctional, the heart loses its ability to efficiently pump blood into the circulatory system. Hence, blood will not be adequately circulated to the body.

73. **a**

74. **b: Blood pools in the blood vessels in certain areas of the body.** In neurogenic shock the nervous system is no longer able to control the diameter of the blood. This causes venous return to the heart to decrease and shock to result.

75. **d:** With neurogenic shock, the patient will likely experience **hypotension and abnormal mental status.** Because of decreased epinephrine secretion, the patient may not exhibit tachycardia, sweating, or pale skin.

76. **d: The reaction between antigen and antibody** causes anaphylactic shock. It occurs as a result of the release of chemicals from a specialized type of white blood cell known as a mast cell. The antibody triggers the release of these chemicals after it has reacted with the foreign antigen. The most important substance released from mast cells during anaphylactic shock is histamine.

77. **b:** Antibodies function to destroy foreign substances that enter the body. In the event of anaphylaxis, however, the antibody does not destroy the antigen. Instead, the reaction between the antigen and the antibody triggers a series of events in the patient's body that leads to shock.

78. **b:** The release of histamine during anaphylaxis causes the following responses: intense vasodilatation; sudden, severe bronchoconstriction, which can cause airway compromise; and leaking of fluid from the blood vessels as a result of a change in permeability. Responses can range from mild to extreme, sometimes causing death. **Blood loss** is not caused by histamine release.

79. **a:** Septic shock **is caused by an overwhelming infection** (usually bacterial) that leads to massive vasodilatation. The blood vessels dilate because of toxins released into the bloodstream. This leads to ineffective circulation because blood is pooled or trapped in dilated veins. In addition, blood plasma is lost through blood vessel walls, resulting in a loss of blood volume. With expanded long-term care facilities and increased utilization of EMS by elderly persons, EMS personnel more commonly see septic shock.

80. **b: Fever** is seen with septic shock. The trunk of the body is often warm, but the extremities are cold because of shunting of blood from the skin of the arms and legs. As septic shock progresses, the entire body becomes cool; this is an ominous sign.

81. **b**

82. **c:** Treatment of a patient experiencing hypovolemic shock includes **administering one or two IVs of lactated Ringer's or normal saline solution** with macrodrip administration sets and infusing them according to local protocol, administering 100% oxygen, placing the patient in a supine position with the legs elevated 10 to 12 inches, and preserving warmth by covering the patient with a blanket. The patient's vital signs should be monitored frequently, at least every 5 minutes. The patient should be transported to an appropriate medical facility as soon as possible. In addition, some protocols may call for the application and inflation of the PASG (follow your local protocol).

83. **d:** Because of the high energy requirements of the brain, any reduction in cerebral blood flow may be manifested by restlessness, agitation, disorientation,

confusion, an inability to respond to questions or commands appropriately, belligerence or combative behavior, and unconsciousness.

84. **b:** Compensatory hyperventilation acts to **reduce the carbon dioxide and compensate for metabolic acidosis.** It tends to occur early in shock and produces respiratory alkalosis.

85. **c:** Any indication of hypoventilation should prompt the EMT-I to **assist the patient's breathing with a bag-mask device** or another ventilatory device supplied with 100% oxygen.

86. **False:** Compensatory mechanisms can maintain a normal pulse rate even in the presence of a *10% to 15%* volume deficit.

87. **True**

88. **False:** Initially in shock, the skin appears *normal*. As compensatory mechanisms such as vasoconstriction take effect and blood is routed to the central circulation, the skin becomes pale (decreased perfusion), cyanotic (a bluish discoloration caused by stagnant pooling of blood with inadequate oxygenation), mottled (combination of pale and cyanotic skin, late sign of shock), cool to the touch, and diaphoretic (sweaty).

89. **a:** Capillary refill that is slow (greater than 2 seconds) indicates poor tissue perfusion, whereas capillary refill that is fast (less than 2 seconds) indicates a state of adequate perfusion; it is a *reliable vital sign in children but not adults*.

90. **d**

91. **a:** Fluid replacement in hypovolemic shock is **guided by medical direction and protocol.** The patient should be continually monitored for signs of circulatory overload.

92. **True**

93. **False:** Normal saline is an electrolyte solution containing sodium chloride in water that is *isotonic* with the extracellular fluid.

94. **False:** Lactated Ringer's solution is an *isotonic electrolyte solution*. It contains sodium chloride, potassium chloride, calcium chloride, and sodium lactate in water. The lactate of this solution, when metabolized by the liver, is broken down to bicarbonate, a buffer.

95. **False:** *Lactated Ringer's solution and normal saline* are used to replace fluid volume in patients experiencing shock because their administration causes an immediate expansion of the circulatory volume. The other solution, 5% dextrose in water, is a hypotonic glucose solution used to keep a vein open and to supply calories necessary for cell metabolism.

96. **c:** Red blood cells have no substitutes. Therefore once the oxygen-carrying capacity is diminished by a massive loss of red blood cells, only the infusion of additional red blood cells replenishes the oxygen supply to the body. Packed red blood cells and **whole blood** both have oxygen-carrying capacity.

97. IV solutions with the conditions they are used to treat: **a. 5% Dextrose in water (D_5W):** 45-year-old man who is complaining of chest pain and has a blood pressure of 170/96; **b. Lactated Ringer's or normal saline (0.9%):** 17-year-old girl experiencing vaginal hemorrhage with a blood pressure of 80/60; 41-year-old man with a gunshot wound to the head and a blood pressure of 240/110; 33-year-old man who has been stabbed four times in the chest and has a blood pressure of 70 by palpation; 65-year-old man with severe diarrhea for the past week and a blood pressure of 100/78.

98. **b:** The PASG may be used by some EMS systems for the care of hypotension and shock. Another indication for its use is stabilization of fractures of the femur, lower leg, and pelvis. Recent studies suggest that the "autotransfusion effect" is minimal, less than 250 mL. The criteria for use of the PASG include a systolic blood pressure less than 90 mm Hg when obvious signs and symptoms of shock are present.

99. **b:** Use of the PASG is contraindicated in **pulmonary edema.** Increased venous return (preload) and/or an increase in afterload (arterial resistance) is bad for the failing heart. Inflation of the abdominal compartment is contraindicated in pregnancy, respiratory distress of any nature, evisceration, and when there is an impaled object in the abdomen.

100. **a:** The PASG should be **positioned so the garment top is just below the rib cage.** If placed too high, it will interfere with respirations.

101. **b:** When inflating the PASG, the EMT-I should quickly compress the foot pump until **crackling sounds are heard from the Velcro,** the vents on the stopcocks start to leak, and/or the systolic blood pressure increases to 100 to 110 mm Hg systolic.

102. **a:** The PASG should only be removed **with a physician's order.** Typically, this is done only after the patient's volume loss has been corrected through IV fluid administration; there is monitoring and recording of vital signs; and the availability of an operating room has been ensured.

103. **d:** When deflating the PASG, **the patient's vital signs should be reassessed every 5 minutes.** The abdomen should be deflated first; stopcock(s) should be opened slightly to allow a small amount of air to escape; and deflation should be discontinued if the blood pressure decreases by more than 5 mm Hg systolic (or the patient's condition deteriorates).

104. **d**

105. **b:** Treatment for this patient includes using direct pressure to control the bleeding from his wrists; administering 100% (at least 15 L) oxygen via nonrebreather mask; **establishing one or two IV lines with macrodrip administration sets, 14- to 16-gauge catheters, and normal saline (0.9%) or lactated Ringer's solution;** placing him in a supine position with legs elevated 10 to 12 inches; and promptly transporting him to an appropriate medical facility. The EMT-I also may consider the application and inflation of the PASG.

106. **a**

107. **c:** Treatment includes **administering epinephrine, 1:1000 solution, subcutaneously.** In addition, administer 100% (at least 15 L) oxygen via nonrebreather mask; establish one or two IV lines with macrodrip administration sets, 14- to 16-gauge catheters, and normal saline (0.9%) or lactated Ringer's solution; place her in a sitting position; and provide prompt transport to an appropriate medical facility.

108. **d**

109. **b:** The next treatment is to **establish one or two IV lines with macrodrip administration sets with normal saline or lactated Ringer's solution.** In addition, consider the application of the PASG (if called for by local protocol), and transport him to the most appropriate medical facility (preferably a trauma center).

110. **b**

111. **c: Administering 100% oxygen via nonrebreather mask** is indicated. In addition, establish an IV line with a microdrip administration set, 18- to 20-gauge catheters, and normal saline (0.9%) or 5% dextrose in water; place him in a supine position with legs elevated 10 to 12 inches (if he can tolerate a supine position); and promptly transport him to an appropriate medical facility. If shortness of breath occurs when the patient is in a supine position, he should be moved into a semisitting position.

Some local protocol may call for initiating a fluid challenge of 100 to 200 mL of volume-expanding fluid. If the patient's condition improves, fluid therapy should continue until the blood pressure stabilizes and the pulse decreases. Lung sounds should be assessed frequently. If the patient shows signs of increased lung congestion, the rate of infusion should be adjusted to keep the vein open.

112. **c**

113. **a:** Treatment of this patient includes **establishing two lines with macrodrip administration sets and normal saline and running them wide open.** Additional treatment should include assisting the patient's breathing with a bag-mask device supplied with 15 L of oxygen per minute, and establishing one or two IV lines with macrodrip administration sets and normal saline (0.9%). Some local protocols may also call for the application and inflation of the PASG.

114. **a**

115. **b:** Treatment of this patient includes **placing her in a supine position with legs elevated 10 to 12 inches.** Additional treatment for this patient would include administering 100% (at least 15 L) oxygen via nonrebreather mask, establishing one or two IV lines with macrodrip administration sets and normal saline (0.9%) and running them wide open (however, caution must be taken to avoid circulatory overload), and promptly transporting her to an appropriate medical facility.

CHAPTER 18

1. Fires rank **fifth** among unintentional injuries following motor vehicle–related crashes, poisonings, falls, and drowning.

2. Morbidity and mortality rates from burn injuries depend on **age, gender,** and **socioeconomic status.**

3. a

4. **True**

5. **False:** Children playing with ignition sources such as matches or cigarette lighters cause approximately 2% of the burn fatalities.

6. **True**

7. **True**

8. **False:** The exposure and length of contact with the substance or flame *determine* the extent of the burn injury.

9. Factors that influence the body's ability to resist burn injury include **water content of the skin tissue; thickness and pigmentation of the skin; presence or absence of insulating substances such as skin oils or hair;** and **peripheral circulation of the skin that affects dissipation of the heat.**

10. Major burns have **three** distinct zones of injury that usually appear in a **bull's** eye pattern.

11. **c:** The central area of the burn wound **sustains the most intense contact with the thermal source.** It is called the zone of *coagulation*. In this area necrosis of the cells has occurred, and the tissue is no longer viable.

12. **a:** Tissues in the zone of hyperemia **recover in 7 to 10 days if infection or profound shock does not develop.** These tissues are located at the periphery of the zone of stasis and have increased blood flow as a result of the normal inflammatory response.

13. The zone of **stasis** surrounds the critically injured area and consists of potentially viable tissue despite the serious thermal injury. In this area, cells are **ischemic** because of clotting and **vasoconstriction.** These cells die within **24** to **48** hours after injury if no supportive measures are taken.

14. A large thermal injury can cause **hypovolemic** shock with a decrease in venous return, **decreased** cardiac output, and **increased** vascular resistance except in the hyperemic zone.

15. Depths of burn with characteristics: **a. Superficial:** heals in 3 to 6 days; skin is red; **b. Partial thickness:** there are blisters with weeping; **c. Full thickness:** Appears very dry and leathery or white, dark brown, or charred; there is no sensation in the skin.

16. Elements used to categorize the severity of a burn: **depth or degree of the burn; percentage of body surface affected; locations on the body that affect function such as the face and upper airway, hands, feet, and genitalia;** and **preexisting medical conditions.**

17. The "rule of nines" is as follows: **a. 9%, b. 18%, c. 9%, d. 1%, e. 18%.**

18. **d**

19. **c**

20. **d:** Treatment for this patient includes maintaining a patent airway (possibly including endotracheal intubation), administering humidified 100% oxygen, removing any smoldering clothing, placing one or two IV lines (if permitted by protocol), and administering IV morphine or meperidine (Demerol) as per local protocol and medical direction.

21. Answers to crossword puzzle

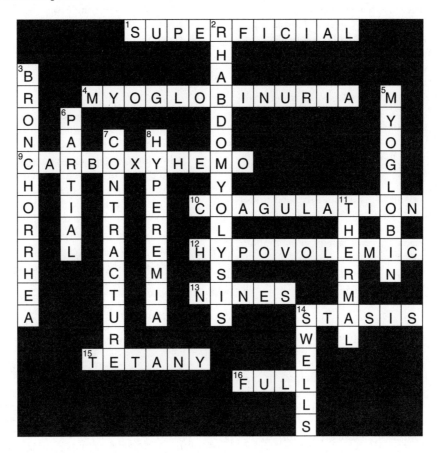

CHAPTER 19

1. **A. trachea; B. heart; C. diaphragm; D. rib cage; E. right lung.**

2. a. **Visceral pleura:** fine lining covering the lungs; b. **Pleural space:** the potential space between the parietal pleura and the visceral pleura; c. **Trachea:** windpipe, the main conduit for air passing to and from the lungs; d. **Parietal pleura:** fine fibrous sheath covering the interior of the thorax; e. **Alveoli:** microscopic chambers within the lungs where the gases of respiration are exchanged; f. **Lobes:** regions of the lung; g. **Alveolar-capillary membrane:** provides interface between the respiratory and circulatory systems.

3. Chest injuries account for about **16,000** deaths per year in the United States and are directly responsible for more than **20%** of all traumatic deaths, regardless of the mechanism of **injury.**

4. **b**

5. **d:** Fractured ribs are more likely in adults than in children because children have more cartilage than bone in the chest.

6. **c:** Even though sternal fractures are not common, when they do occur they are serious.

7. Three causes of sternal fractures include **a direct blow to the chest as in a massive crush injury; line-drive baseball to the middle of the chest; and when the chest strikes the steering wheel of a motor vehicle during a head-on crash.**

8. Three significant injuries that can be associated with sternal fractures include **an unstable chest wall, myocardial injury, and cardiac tamponade.**

9. **c:** Decreased ventilation caused by paradoxical movement of the involved segment of the thoracic wall is seen with flail chest. In addition, there are *two or more* fractured ribs in two or more places; the trachea will usually be in a *normal, midline* position; and lung sounds tend to be *diminished* on the affected side. There may also be a serious injury (pulmonary contusion) to the lung under the area of the broken ribs. This condition hinders the patient's breathing and produces hypoxia and hypercarbia.

10. In the field setting, **flail segments of the chest can be splinted in the inward position with simple hand pressure or bulky dressings or towels taped to the chest wall.** Alternatively, intubation and positive-pressure ventilation can be used. This strategy is usually reserved for those patients in respiratory distress from a flail chest.

    Additional treatment includes providing high-concentration oxygen, immobilizing the patient's cervical spine, securing him or her to a long backboard, and placing one or two large-bore IV lines of normal saline or lactated Ringer's solution once en route to the hospital.

11. **b:** A pulmonary contusion **is frequently seen under a flail chest.** It can be described as bleeding that occurs in the *interstitial* and *alveolar* areas of the lung. It usually occurs as a result of *blunt* trauma. Because the contused area of the lung is not able to function properly after an injury, *profound hypoxemia* may develop. The degree of respiratory complication is directly related to the size of the contused area.

12. **c:** A simple pneumothorax occurs when air enters the *pleural* space through an opening in the lung and **can cause the affected lung to collapse.** It *may become* life threatening if it develops into a tension pneumothorax, occupies more than 40% of the hemithorax, or occurs in a patient with shock or preexisting pulmonary or cardiovascular disease.

13. **a:** An open pneumothorax occurs when an opening **(caused by penetrating trauma)** is created between the *intrathoracic cavity* and the outside of the body. The wound allows air to freely enter *and* exit the pleural cavity. It may result in severe ventilatory dysfunction, hypoxemia, and death unless it is rapidly recognized and corrected.

14. **d**

15. **True:** This can occur when an internal or external wound (or deficit) allows air, blood, or fluid to enter the space between the pleural tissues. The lung begins to collapse as the pressure in the pleural space increases.

16. **False:** With pneumothorax, auscultation of the chest will typically reveal *diminished lung sounds on the affected side.*

17. **False:** A closed pneumothorax is associated with *the internal introduction of air, blood, or fluid into the pleural space.* Causes of closed pneumothorax include a torn bronchus, bronchiole, or alveolus resulting from penetrating or blunt trauma, COPD, or congenital defect.

18. An open pneumothorax that has a bubbling sound is referred to as a **sucking** chest wound. This open injury to the chest is caused by penetrating trauma. It creates an opening between the intrathoracic cavity and the outside of the body. The wound allows air to freely enter and exit the pleural cavity.

19. To treat an open pneumothorax, it should be covered with an **occlusive** dressing. This may include petroleum gauze, self-adhering defibrillator pads, aluminum foil, or the inside of a plastic wrapper. To allow air to escape during expiration, only three sides of the dressing should be taped down. It does not allow air back into the wound. Frequently reassess the patient. It is critical to monitor these patients for the development of a tension pneumothorax.

20. **b:** When air enters the pleural space but does not exit, pressure builds inside the chest. This is a tension pneumothorax and is considered to be life threatening. With this condition, cardiac output is *decreased* because of the kinking of the vena cava and increased intrapleural pressure; there is *collapse* of the involved lung and *decreased* ventilation in the opposite lung.

21. Signs and symptoms characteristic of tension pneumothorax include **tachycardia, hypotension; tracheal deviation** (late sign), **severe dyspnea** (late sign); **increasing cyanosis; apprehension, agitation; external jugular vein distention** (late sign), *normal* heart sounds; *cold, clammy, diaphoretic* skin; and *diminished or absent* breath sounds. Additional late signs associated with tension pneumothorax are signs of acute hypoxia, tympany, and narrowing pulse pressure.

22. **b:** When a tension pneumothorax is present, the patient can deteriorate quickly unless immediate intervention is accomplished. Provide high-concentration oxygen to maximize whatever oxygen exchange is still occurring. To relieve the tension pneumothorax, perform a **needle thoracentesis** (emergency chest decompression) if properly trained.

23. **b**

24. Locations for needle decompression of the chest are the second and third intercostal spaces on the midclavicular line on the affected side.

25. Severe blunt trauma to the abdomen may rupture the **diaphragm,** permitting the abdominal contents to enter the thoracic cavity.

26. Four signs of diaphragmatic rupture are *abdominal* **pain; dyspnea; decreased breath sounds; and presence of bowel sounds in the affected hemitho-**

rax (caused by abdominal contents displaced into the chest).

27. **d**

28. Three signs of traumatic asphyxia are **reddish purple discoloration of the face and neck (skin below the area remains pink); jugular vein distention; and swelling or hemorrhage of the conjunctiva.**

29. When bleeding into the thoracic cavity occurs, it is referred to as **hemothorax.** Causes include bleeding from the lung or from blood vessels within the chest. Most critical is the loss of blood and associated hypotension.

30. The type of shock that results from hemothorax is **hypovolemia.**

31. **False:** Bruising of the myocardium is referred to as *myocardial contusion*. It often presents similarly to acute myocardial infarction (e.g., chest pain, dysrhythmias). It occurs when the heart is compressed between the sternum and the thoracic vertebrae. Injuries can involve a disturbance to the cardiac electrical system, bruising to the cardiac wall, or a complete rupture of the myocardium. Treatment of myocardial contusion is similar to that of acute myocardial infarction (e.g., oxygen, lidocaine, and atropine).

32. **False:** Cardiac tamponade may occur as a result of *penetrating or blunt trauma*. It occurs when the pericardial sac fills with blood or fluid, compromising the ability of the heart to fill, contract, and pump blood. Cardiac output is decreased, which leads to hypotension. This occurs despite the fact that the patient may have an adequate circulating blood volume (normovolemia).

33. Signs of cardiac tamponade

	Signs Seen with Cardiac Tamponade
Jugular veins	**Distended**
Tracheal position	**Normal, midline**
Lung sounds	**Equal bilaterally**
Pulse	**Reflex tachycardia; also the pulse may be stronger during inspiration (pulsus paradoxus)**
Blood pressure	**Hypotension, narrowed pulse pressure**
Heart sounds	**Muffled**

34. **Because of the potential for life-threatening injury, patients with chest trauma require rapid transport to an appropriate facility (preferably a trauma center).** Rapid transport means that no more than 10 minutes (or less whenever possible) should be spent in the field with these patients.

35. **c**

36. **b**

37. **d:** Treatment of this patient includes **covering the wound with an occlusive dressing** (taping just three sides of the dressing down while leaving the fourth side free), administering *15 L via a nonrebreather mask,* placing him on the *injured* side on a long backboard, and rapidly transporting him to the hospital. One or two large-bore IV lines of normal saline or lactated Ringer's solution should be placed once en route with the patient.

38. **a**

39. **a**

40. **b**

41. **a:** *Because there is a need for rapid transport, the placement of the IV should be performed while en route to the hospital.*

Additional prehospital treatments may include securing the patient to a long backboard. The definitive treatment for cardiac tamponade is needle pericardiocentesis. Given the difficulty of the skill and the potential complications associated with its use, needle pericardiocentesis is generally not performed in the field setting.

42. **c**

43. **a**

44. **a**

45. **b:** This patient's **ECG must be monitored** because cardiac dysrhythmias may occur. Additional treatment includes administering 15 L of oxygen via nonrebreather mask, placing him in the most comfortable position, and rapidly transporting him to the hospital. An IV line of normal saline or lactated Ringer's solution should be placed once en route with the patient.

46. Answers to crossword puzzle

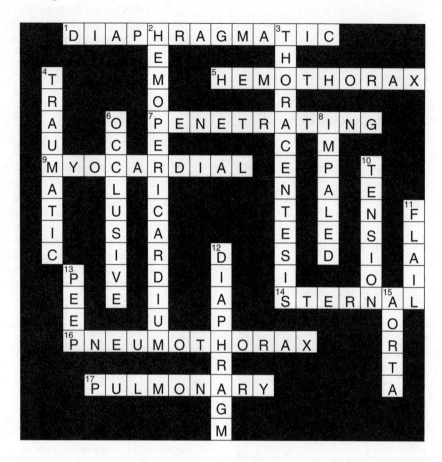

CHAPTER 20

1. **d:** An unresponsive patient is unable to provide a past medical history or details surrounding the incident.

2. The two age groups at highest risk for traumatic brain injury are *0* to *4* years of age and *15* to *19* years of age.

3. **d: Hypotension** is generally not seen with head injury. Look for other injuries to explain any decrease in blood pressure. Suspect a skull fracture if the patient has history of trauma to the head with or without unconsciousness, altered level of consciousness, pupils sluggish to react or dilated, obvious penetrating or impalement injury, deformity of the skull, blood or cerebrospinal fluid draining from the nose or ears, raccoon eyes (may be a late sign), or Battle's sign (may be a late sign).

4. **d**

5. If the meninges are disrupted, cerebrospinal fluid may leak and drain into the nostrils or ear canal. CSF is normally clear and watery in appearance. Because bleeding can occur from a bone fracture, blood may mix with the CSF. Thus drainage may appear watery or bloody. Consider any type of clear or bloody drainage from the nostrils or ears following head trauma an indication of a possible skull fracture.

6. **c:** The term for **raccoon eyes** is bilateral periorbital ecchymosis. *Battle's sign* is a discoloration of the skin at the mastoid region behind the ear. Both signs are caused by an accumulation of blood after a basilar skull fracture that may not occur until 12 hours or more after the injury.

7. **False:** Unequal pupils are *indicative* of brain injury.

8. **True**

9. **b**

10. **a. Cheyne-Stokes respirations:** a repetitive pattern of slow, shallow breathing to rapid, deep ventilations back to slow, shallow breaths followed by a period of apnea (early sign of increased ICP); **b. Cushing**

reflex or triad: progressive increase in the blood pressure (especially the systolic reading), an increase in the respiratory rate or a changing pattern, and a decreasing pulse rate (late sign of increased ICP); **c. Hemiplegia:** paralysis on one side of the body; **d. Quadriplegia:** paralysis of all four extremities; **e. Decorticate posturing:** position of a patient in which the upper extremities are flexed at the elbows and at the wrists; **f. Decerebrate posturing:** position in which the arms are extended and internally rotated and the legs are extended with the feet in forced plantar flexion; **g. Paraplegia:** paralysis of the lower extremities.

11. **False:** The goal of treatment is to maintain cerebral oxygenation and perfusion while protecting the cervical spine. An oropharyngeal airway or endotracheal tube may be inserted if the patient is unconscious and has no gag reflex. *One hundred percent oxygen should be delivered* (15 L/min via nonrebreather mask or with assisted ventilations, e.g., bag-mask device supplied with a reservoir and 15 L/min of oxygen).

12. **True:** Both are contraindicated because the tube may inadvertently pass through the fracture(s) and into the brain.

13. **c:** Treatment of this patient includes **applying cervical immobilization and placing him on a long backboard,** assisting his breathing with a bag-mask device supplied with 15 L/min of oxygen (or other type of ventilatory device), and establishing an IV of *lactated Ringer's or normal saline with a macrodrip administration set* and running it at a TKO rate.

    If fluid or blood is coming from the nose or ears, loosely cover the nostrils and/or ears with a clean dressing. Allow slight leaking to occur because this will prevent a complete tamponade of the fluid. If the fluid is not permitted to drain, the intracranial pressure may increase. Repeated vital sign determinations and frequent reassessments help to detect signs of increased intracranial pressure as they occur. Any changes that suggest a progressive increase in intracranial pressure should be immediately reported to medical direction and/or the receiving hospital.

    Whenever possible, raise the long backboard so that the head is elevated. This may help to decrease intracranial pressure. In addition, this type of patient should be transported immediately.

14. **True:** Head, face, and neck injuries are closely related. Trauma to one area is likely to involve injury to several areas. A force to the scalp can also injure the brain and neck.

15. **True**

16. **False:** The patient with an extensive open scalp injury may bleed significantly because the scalp has a very rich blood supply. To control this bleeding, the EMT-I should avoid *using his or her fingers* to stop the bleeding. If the skull is fractured, this may drive bone fragments into the brain. Instead, *apply pressure over a broad area with the palm of a gloved hand.*

17. **a. Mandibular:** malocclusion, numbness in the chin, and inability to open the mouth. The patient also may have difficulty swallowing and excessive salivation. **b. Orbital:** periorbital edema, subconjunctival ecchymosis, double vision, recessed globe, epistaxis, and anesthesia in the region of the anterior cheek. Impaired extraocular movements may also be present. **c. Zygomatic:** flatness of a usually rounded cheek area; numbness of the cheek, nose, and upper lip; and epistaxis. Altered vision may also be present. **d. Nasal:** injuries to the nose may depress the nose or displace it to one side. In some instances, nasal fractures may result only in epistaxis and swelling without apparent skeletal deformity.

18. Common mechanisms of anterior neck injury: **motor vehicle crashes; neck striking dashboard or steering column; hyperextension and hyperflexion injuries; sport and recreational activities; contact sports (boxing, karate, basketball, football, hockey); all-terrain vehicles (ATVs) and other small motor vehicles ("clothesline" injuries to the neck from running into wires, ropes, and fences); water sports (jet-skiing and water skiing); snow skiing; horseback riding; industrial accidents; "strangulation" injuries (from clothing, jewelry, or personal equipment getting caught in machinery); violent altercations; stab wounds (knives, screwdrivers, and ice picks); missile injury from firearms; blows to the neck; and hangings.**

19. **c**

20. **a:** Treatment of this patient includes applying direct pressure to control the bleeding, covering the injury with an occlusive (nonporous) dressing, administering high-concentration oxygen via a nonrebreather face mask, stabilizing the head and neck, and immobilizing him to a long backboard. If a venous injury is suspected, keep the patient supine or in a slight Trendelenburg position to prevent air embolism. If this lethal complication is suspected, tilt the long backboard so that the patient is on his left side. Keep the head lower than the feet to try to trap the air embolus in the right ventricle. Consider fluid replacement using large-bore catheters and isotonic crystalloids if signs of shock are present. **Removing the knife** is contraindicated—instead it should be stabilized in place.

21. **a. Extension:** tear of the ligaments and vertebral instability that occur with hyperextension. **b. Flexion:** occurs when the spinal structures are violently bent forward such as when hitting one's head while diving. **c. Rotation:** seldom occurs as an isolated event, occurring instead as a combination with rotation of the spine that causes dislocation of the intervertebral joints. **d. Vertical compression:** occurs when a force is directed along the axis of the spine. The intervertebral disk is compacted into the body of the vertebra, leading to spinal cord damage.

22. **b:** Spinal shock is a form of *neurogenic* shock that results from *complete transection of the spinal cord.* There is complete loss of sensation and voluntary movement beyond the injury. As a rule, the patient will *not* have an elevated pulse rate. The patient's skin will be pink, warm, and *dry* and possibly even flushed because of vasodilation, especially below the level of the injury. Hypotension from spinal shock is difficult to treat.

23. Manual stabilization of the cervical spine **helps establish and maintain the patient's airway; places the head and neck into neutral alignment, which is the splinting position for the spine; and minimizes the risk of additional damage to the cervical spine.**

24. **c:** For the supine patient, the EMT-I should grasp the corner of the jaw and provide stabilization of the neck by wrapping his or her hands around the posterior portion of the neck. The patient's head should be placed in the *neutral* position in alignment of the spine.

25. **False:** A rigid cervical collar reduces movement of the cervical spine and helps maintain neutral alignment of the head and neck. However, *the rigid collar does not completely immobilize, and movement of the head can still occur.* Always combine it with an appropriate body immobilization device, such as a long backboard, and some type of head immobilization to prevent lateral movement. A commercial head immobilization device may be used in conjunction with the rigid cervical collar to immobilize the patient's head to the long backboard.

26. **True:** Soft cervical collars are not strong enough to support the head nor do they prevent movement of the neck. Do not use soft collars.

27. **b:** When using a short spine board or vest-type device, several important rules must be followed. First, use the device only if the patient's condition is stable and rapid transport is not indicated. When the device is to be used, as soon as you are at the patient's side, immediately provide manual immobilization. Ensure manual immobilization of the head in a neutral in-line position until it is maintained with the immobilization device. **Apply a rigid cervical collar if the head is in a neutral position.** Secure the patient's head to the immobilization device *only after the device has been secured to the torso.* Be sure the apparatus used to secure the head does not obstruct the airway. During use of the device, continually maintain neutral alignment. *Tightly secure the device while allowing for sufficient* chest expansion. Avoid moving the patient excessively while applying the device, and do not pull on it to move the patient.

28. **a**

29. To immobilize the patient's head in preparation to apply a short spine board or vest-type device, the EMT-I should **move behind the patient, place one hand on each side of the head, fingers spread wide, with the thumbs on the occipital area, and place/maintain the patient's head in a neutral, in-line position.**

30. **False:** In stable patients the EMT-I should assess motor, sensory, and distal circulation in *all four* of the patient's extremities before and after application of a short spine board or vest-type device.

31. **False:** Gaps between the patient and the device *must be padded* to ensure neutral alignment.

32. **False:** Secure the immobilization device to the patient's torso so that it cannot move up or down, left or right. When using the KED, *be sure that it is snug against the axillae (armpits).*

33. **True**

34. **False:** When applying the KED, *the chest straps are applied first and then the groin straps.* As you tighten the torso straps, be careful not to jerk or move the patient unnecessarily. Secure the leg straps so that the legs are not pulled upward.

35. **a**

36. **c**

37. **a:** Patients with known or suspected spinal injuries present challenges for airway management. *Do not move or hyperextend the head of a patient with a possible spinal injury.* To open the airway, perform a jaw-thrust (trauma) *without* head-tilt maneuver. Administer high-concentration oxygen, and assist breathing as necessary. In this case, assisted ventilation with 100% oxygen is indicated. Insert one or two large-bore IV lines of normal saline or lactated Ringer's solution once en route with the patient.

38. **b:** To logroll a patient who is in a supine position onto a long backboard, four people are ideal, but *two or three people can accomplish the task.* **Approach the patient from the side of his or her head to limit the patient's motion before you begin cervical immobilization, and then carefully move the patient's head into neutral in-line alignment.** Select an appropriately sized, rigid cervical collar, and apply it without moving the patient. Position a long backboard alongside the patient. Kneel next to the patient's midthorax. Direct your second partner or EMT assistant to kneel next to the patient's knees. Each rescuer should kneel within 1 inch of the patient. Straighten the patient's arms so that they are in a "palm-in" position next to the torso, and direct your second partner or EMT assistant to bring the legs together into neutral alignment. *Do not raise the patient's arm to assist with the logroll.* Grasp the far side of the patient by the shoulder and wrist. Direct your second partner or EMT assistant to grasp the patient's hip with his or her left hand just distal to the wrist, and tightly grasp both pant cuffs at the ankles with the right hand. Usually the rescuer *at the head* decides when the patient is logrolled. Instruct your partner or EMT assistant to follow the directions of the person at the patient's head. With the patient's arms locked firmly at his or her sides, slowly roll the patient to the side (toward you) only until there is enough room to insert the long backboard. Elevate the ankles as necessary to maintain lateral alignment. This must be done without compromising the integrity of the spine. Slide the backboard close to the patient, and instruct your EMT assistant as to when the patient will be rolled back down. On command, roll the patient back onto the board. This must be done without compromising integrity of the spine. Keeping the patient in neutral alignment, adjust the patient's position so that he or she is centered on the board and proper space exists between the top of the board and the patient's head. Ensure alignment by padding gaps or voids between the long backboard and the patient's body. Carefully place padding under the head to assist with alignment or to reduce patient discomfort. Immobilize the patient's torso to the long backboard so that it cannot move up or down or laterally.

39. **c**

40. **Immobilize the patient's head to a long backboard in a neutral, in-line position by placing pads or rolled blankets on each side of the patient's head and fastening a strap tightly over the pads and patient's lower forehead. Place a second strap over the pads and rigid cervical collar, and secure it to the long backboard.**

41. Patients found in a prone position require a special technique to be used to maintain the airway and provide in-line support as the patient is being logrolled. **The EMT-I stabilizing the head places his or her hands right over left, twisted about the head. This allows the hands to be in the correct position after the roll. Roll the prone patient into a supine position while carefully immobilizing his (or her) head, neck, and body.**

42. Rapid extrication techniques are used in two instances: an **unsafe** scene or patients with **life-threatening** injuries.

43. **d:** The presence or threat of fire, rising water, danger of explosion, and danger of structure collapse are examples of conditions that justify rapid extrication.

44. Life-threatening injuries that may require rapid removal: **patients in cardiac or respiratory arrest, whose airways cannot be maintained while in a sitting position, in whom bleeding cannot be controlled, who exhibit severe shock, and whose mechanism of injury indicates the potential for rapid decompensation.**

45. For the EMT-I to properly manage the airway and cervical spine, access to the head is essential. Three things that would give the EMT-I reason not to remove a football helmet include: **the patient is obviously dead, the helmet is entangled into the patient's head, or an impaled object penetrates the helmet and head.**

46. Answers to crossword puzzle

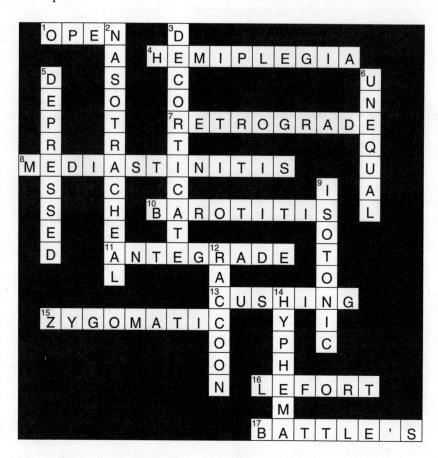

CHAPTER 21

1. **False:** The abdomen is a region of the body *where it is most difficult to correctly identify* traumatic injuries that require surgical repair.

2. **False:** There are *multiple organs* that may be injured in the abdomen, and physical findings may be exaggerated or absent.

3. **True:** It is also the second leading cause of preventable trauma deaths.

4. With abdominal injuries the EMT-I must have a high degree of suspicion based on the **mechanism** of injury because death usually results from continuing **hemorrhage** and/or delay of **surgical** repair.

5. **b**

6. Peritonitis is defined **as inflammation of the peritoneum. It is caused by the release of acids, enzymes, or bacteria from the gastrointestinal tract into the peritoneal cavity.**

7. **a**

8. **d:** The degree of injury caused by blunt forces is related to the **type of abdominal structure injured** (i.e., fluid filled, gas filled, solid, or hollow), as well as the **quantity and duration of force applied.**

9. **False:** Multiple organ damage can occur with any penetrating trauma, although it is *less likely with a stab wound* than with a gunshot wound.

10. **True**

11. Injury to the **solid** abdominal organs usually results in rapid and significant blood loss. The two solid organs commonly injured are the **liver** and **spleen**. Both of these are primary sources of **exsanguinations.**

12. Injury to the **liver** should be suspected in any patient with a steering wheel injury, lap belt injury, or history of epigastric trauma.

608

Answer Keys and Rationales

13. **a: Kehr's sign** is thought to be caused by referred pain secondary to irritation of the adjacent diaphragm from splenic hematoma or hemoperitoneum (blood in the peritoneum).

14. In contrast to **solid organ injury, in which hemorrhage is the major cause of symptoms, injury to the hollow organs results in symptoms from spillage of their contents, resulting in peritonitis.**

15. **True**

16. **True**

17. **c**

18. Hemorrhage within the retroperitoneal space may be massive and usually results from **pelvic** and/or **lumbar** fractures.

19. Injuries to the kidneys involve **contusion** fractures and **lacerations,** resulting in hemorrhage, urine extravasation, or both.

20. **b**

21. Indicators for establishing the index of suspicion for abdominal injury include **mechanism of injury or damage to the passenger compartment of a motor vehicle (e.g., bent steering wheel); outward signs of trauma; shock with unexplained cause; level of shock greater than explained by other injuries; and presence of abdominal rigidity, guarding, or distention (a rare finding).**

22. **False:** Once the pregnant patient has been immobilized to the long backboard, the board *should be tilted to the left approximately 10 to 15 degrees*. This will take pressure off of the inferior vena cava and assist with blood return to the heart.

23. **b:** With this type of injury, organ(s) protrude through the wound.

24. **d:** Treatment for this patient includes **administering 100% oxygen via a nonrebreather mask,** covering the organs with a *moist,* sterile dressing (or an occlusive dressing large enough to cover all the organs), keeping his legs *flexed,* and promptly transporting him to an appropriate hospital (preferably a trauma center). The EMT-I also should establish one or two IV lines using large-bore catheters (14 to 16 gauge) and lactated Ringer's or normal saline (0.9%) solution.

25. **a**

26. **a:** Treatment includes **administering 15 L/min oxygen via nonrebreather mask.** Additional treatment includes placing one or two IV lines with *macrodrip* administration sets, 14- to 16-gauge catheter-over-needles, and normal saline and prompt transport to an appropriate treatment facility (e.g., trauma center). If the pneumatic antishock garment (PASG) is used, *all three sections* should be inflated.

27. **b**

28. **c**

29. **d:** This patient should be **promptly transported to a trauma center.** Additional treatment includes administering *high-concentration* oxygen and placing one or two IV lines with *macrodrip* administration sets, 14- to 16-gauge catheter-over-needles, and normal saline. If the pneumatic antishock garment (PASG) is used, all three sections should be inflated.

30. Answers to crossword puzzle

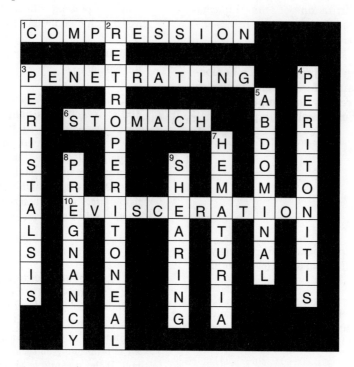

31. **False:** Extremity trauma involves injury to muscles and bones and can occur by a variety of mechanisms. Violence, sports, and other recreational activities—as well as daily routines—can cause damage to muscles, bones, and the related tissues. Extremity or musculoskeletal trauma *can be a single injury* or can occur with other injuries.

32. **False:** Fractures occur when there is *any* break in the continuity of bone or cartilage.

33. **True**

34. **True**

35. **d:** There are two types of bone injuries. An **open** injury occurs when there is a break in the continuity of the skin. A *closed* injury is present when there is no break in the continuity of the skin.

36. A **dislocation** occurs when there is a separation of two bones at the joint. It can cause an area of **instability** that may produce a large amount of pain. It may be difficult to distinguish between a fracture and a dislocation.

37. Complications that can occur from extremity trauma: **damage to muscles, nerves, or blood vessels caused by broken bones; conversion of a closed fracture to an open fracture; restriction of blood flow as a result of bone ends compressing blood vessels; excessive bleeding resulting from tissue damage caused by bone ends; increased pain associated with movement of bone ends; and paralysis of extremities caused by damage to the spine.**

38. **b: Crepitus** is a grating sound heard when broken bone ends rub together. Other signs and symptoms of a bone or joint injury include deformity or abnormal position of an extremity, pain and tenderness, swelling, bruising or discoloration, guarding, exposed bone ends, and a joint that is locked into position.

39. **a:** When immobilizing a fracture **immobilize the joints above and below the injury site.** Assess distal neurovascular function *before and after* application of the splinting device and periodically thereafter. Rings or other pieces of jewelry should be *removed*. Handle the injured extremity carefully—do not allow gross movement. Avoid applying the splint too tightly or too loosely.

40. **a**

41. **Rigid splints:** board splints (wood [includes LBB], plastic, metal); inflatable "air splints"; **Formable splints:** vacuum splints; pillows; blankets; cardboard splints; wire ladder splints; foam-covered moldable metal splints; **Traction splints:** Hare traction splint; Sager splint.

42. **b:** When applying a Hare traction splint, **the patient should be placed on a long backboard.** Distal pulses also should be assessed both before and after application of the splint.

43. **d**

44. Complications of splinting include **compression of nerves, tissues, and blood vessels if the splint is too tight; distal circulation can be compromised, and the bone or joint injury can become worse because of improper treatment; and surrounding tissue, nerves, blood vessels, or muscles can be damaged from excessive movement.** If the patient complains of numbness or tingling of the extremity or you notice the feet or fingers to be cool and/or mottled, loosen the splint. Reapply the splint, and reassess the extremity.

45. Answers to crossword puzzle

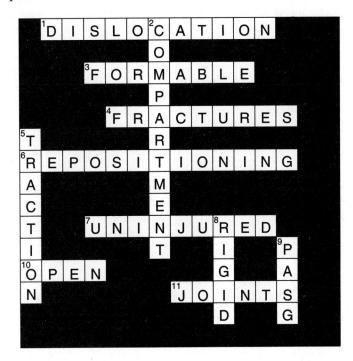

CHAPTER 22

1. The respiratory system is responsible for **filtering, warming, humidifying,** and **exchanging** more than 10,000 L of air per day in an adult.

2. Upper respiratory system components include the **mouth, nasal cavity, oral cavity, larynx,** and **vocal cords.** The lower respiratory system components include the **trachea, bronchi, bronchioles,** and **alveoli.**

3. a. **Respiration:** involves inspiring oxygen-containing air and exhaling carbon dioxide; b. **Ventilation:** refers specifically to exchange of carbon dioxide; c. **Oxygenation:** refers only to the exchange of oxygen; d. **Diffusion:** movement of oxygen and carbon dioxide from areas of greater concentration to areas of lesser concentration; e. **Perfusion:** the process in which oxygenated blood is pumped to the tissues and waste products returned to the lungs.

4.

Function	Respiratory Abnormality Affecting Function	Specific Condition
Ventilation	Upper airway obstruction	Trauma, epiglottitis, foreign body obstruction, tonsillitis
	Lower airway obstruction	Trauma, obstructive lung disease, mucus accumulation, bronchospasm, airway edema
	Impairment of chest wall movement	Trauma, hemothorax, pneumothorax, empyema, pleural inflammation, neuromuscular diseases such as multiple sclerosis or muscular dystrophy
	Problems in neurological control, involving either the central nervous system or the peripheral nervous system	CNS depressant drugs, stroke, other medical condition, trauma, phrenic or spinal nerve dysfunction caused by trauma or neuromuscular diseases
Diffusion	Alveolar pathology	Asbestosis, blebs from COPD, inhalation injuries
	Interstitial space pathology either caused by elevations of hydrostatic pressure in the pulmonary circulation or secondary to abnormal permeability of the pulmonary vessels	Pulmonary edema, pulmonary hypertension, adult respiratory distress syndrome (ARDS), environmental lung diseases, near-drowning, hypoxia, inhalation injuries
Perfusion	Inadequate blood volume or hemoglobin levels	Hypovolemia, anemia
	Impaired circulatory blood flow	Pulmonary embolus, cardiac tamponade
	Chest wall pathology	Trauma

5. Signs of potentially life-threatening respiratory distress: **alterations in mental status; severe cyanosis; absent breath sounds; audible stridor; 1- or 2-word dyspnea; tachycardia of greater than 130 BPM; pallor and diaphoresis; and presence of retractions or the use of accessory muscles of respiration.**

6. **b**

7. **False:** Diaphoresis is a *nonspecific* finding but typically indicates that the patient is in more distress than someone who is not diaphoretic.

8. **False:** Cyanosis, either peripherally or centrally, is *always* worrisome.

9. **False:** Bradycardia is *an ominous sign of severe hypoxemia and suggests imminent cardiac arrest, especially in pediatric patients.* Tachycardia is a sign of hypoxemia and fear. It may also occur because of sympathomimetic medication use, such as inhaled bronchodilators.

10. **d**

11. **b**

12. **Kussmaul respirations** are abnormally deep, very rapid sighing respirations often caused by the presence of metabolic acidosis such as diabetic ketoacidosis.

13. **Biot's respiration** is a type of breathing characterized by a series of several short inspirations followed by regular or irregular periods of apnea.

14. Air trapping **is increasing difficulty getting breath out.**

15. **a**

16. **True**

17. **False:** Thick green or brown sputum suggests *infection, possibly pneumonia*. Yellow or pale gray sputum may be caused by allergy or inflammation.

18. **True**

19. Barrel chest deformity suggests **the presence of long-standing chronic obstructive lung disease (COPD).**

20. Capnometry provides **ongoing assessment of endotracheal tube position; the end-tidal CO_2 decreases almost immediately when the tube is displaced from the trachea.** It can also be used in the nonintubated patient. An easy-to-use, one-piece sample line can be used. Normal levels vary between 30 and 40 torr. When the amount of CO_2 coming from the lungs is abnormally high or low, the capnography monitor alerts you of a potential problem with the patient and prompts further investigation.

21. a. **Asthma:** chronic disease that involves the lower airway, beyond the level of the trachea and mainstem bronchi; it occurs when the bronchial airways narrow and make breathing difficult; b. **Hyperventilation:** the result of an increased frequency of breathing, an increased volume of air moved, or both; it causes excessive elimination of carbon dioxide; c. **Spontaneous pneumothorax:** sudden accumulation of air in the pleural space caused by rupture of a weak area on the lung surface; as the air enters the pleural space, the lung on the involved side collapses; d. **Emphysema:** destruction of the walls of the alveoli that leads to a decrease in elastic recoil and creates resistance to expiratory airflow; air is then trapped within the lungs, resulting in poor air exchange; e. **Pulmonary embolism:** blockage of a pulmonary artery by foreign matter; in most cases, the obstruction is caused by a piece of a blood clot that has broken away from a pelvic or deep leg vein; f. **Pulmonary edema:** refers to filling of the lungs with fluid in the interstitial spaces, the alveoli, or both; it is not a disease in itself, but rather a pathophysiological condition resulting from many possible causes.

22. **False:** The *major* cause of COPD is *cigarette smoking*. Industrial inhalants (such as asbestos and coal dust), air pollution, and tuberculosis also contribute to the condition.

23. The underlying pathophysiology of all forms of obstructive lung disease is decreased **expiratory** airflow and air **trapping** primarily caused by obstruction in the small bronchioles.

24. Factors that exacerbate underlying conditions in COPD include **stress, infection,** and **exercise.**

25. External factors that exacerbate COPD include **tobacco smoke, allergens, drugs,** and **occupational hazards.**

26. Things that happen when bronchial airways of an asthma patient are irritated include **bronchospasm, increased mucus production, swelling and edema,** and **inflammatory cell.**

27. **False:** Asthma *can begin at any age, but it is most common in children and young adults.*

28. **True:** Acute **asthma** is a chronic inflammatory pulmonary disorder that is characterized by reversible obstruction of the airways.

29. **False:** About one third of the children who have asthma outgrow it before they reach adulthood. Adult asthma, however, is usually *persistent*. One fourth of all asthma cases *begin* after age 50.

30. **False:** There are two kinds of asthma. *Extrinsic* asthma is when some specific outside substance such as pollen causes the air tubes to narrow. The onset of extrinsic asthma is more common in childhood. With intrinsic asthma, *no specific substance can be identified as causing the air tubes to narrow*. Intrinsic asthma more commonly has adult onset.

31. Common asthma triggers include **respiratory infections, allergens, irritants, exercise, emotions, chemicals,** and **changes in environmental conditions.**

32. **c: Wheezing** is commonly seen with an acute asthma attack. Signs and symptoms also may include tachycardia, diaphoresis, pallor, shortness of breath, extreme difficulty moving air in and out of the lungs, hyperinflated chest, coughing (may or may not be productive of sputum), hypertension, tachypnea, mild cyanosis, decreased oxygen saturation on pulse oximetry, anxiety, agitation, anxiousness, diaphoresis, and pallor. The patient may also be unable to complete a phrase or sentence without having to stop to breathe. If the asthma attack is so severe that the patient cannot speak, the Pao_2 is probably less than 40 torr (normal range at sea level is 80 to 100 torr).

33. **b: Status asthmaticus is a severe prolonged asthma attack that does not respond to standard medications.** Its onset may be sudden or insidious and is frequently precipitated by a viral respiratory infection. Out-of-hospital treatment is the same as for acute asthma; however, *rapid transport* is more important. Patients should be closely monitored, and the EMT-I should anticipate the need for intubation and aggressive ventilatory support.

34. **Chronic obstructive pulmonary disease (COPD)** is a progressive and irreversible disease of the airway marked by decreased inspiratory and expiratory

capacity of the lungs. It may result from **chronic bronchitis** (excess mucus production) or **emphysema** (lung tissue damage with loss of elastic recoil of the lungs).

35. After a period of time, the right side of the heart may develop failure because of the effort required to move blood through diseased lungs. This condition is known as chronic **cor pulmonale** and indicates severe COPD.

36. **b:** Patients with chronic lung disease **are typically cigarette smokers.** In chronic lung disease patients, the chest often takes on a *barrel-shaped appearance,* and individuals demonstrate progressive limitation of activity because they easily tire.

37. Signs of cor pulmonale include **marked neck vein distention (although this finding may occur from COPD alone), abdominal bloating (from fluid in the abdominal cavity),** and **leg edema.**

38. **a:** Albuterol **is used to treat bronchospasm.** It should be used with caution in patients who have a history of cardiac disorders.

39. **d:** Treatment of obstructive lung disease includes **administering an aerosolized bronchodilator.** Additional treatment includes calming and reassuring the patient, placing an IV line of normal saline or lactated Ringer's solution or 5% dextrose in water, providing *high-concentration* oxygen using a nonrebreather mask, placing him or her in the *most comfortable position (typically sitting upright if having trouble breathing),* providing timely transport with treatment en route, monitoring vital signs (including pulse oximetry), frequently monitoring the ECG for cardiac rhythm disturbances, and identifying priority patients and making transport/backup decisions. Also, the EMT-I may be directed to administer epinephrine (Adrenalin), at a dose of *0.1 to 0.5 mL (mg), of a 1:1000* solution, subcutaneously, and/or terbutaline (Brethine), 0.25 mL subcutaneously.

40. **True**

41. **False:** Pneumonia is an acute inflammatory condition of the lungs, usually caused by *either bacterial or viral infection.* It is the fifth leading cause of death in the United States.

42. Risk factors that make persons susceptible to pneumonia include **cigarette smoking, alcoholism, cold exposure, extremes of age,** and **abnormal immune systems.**

43. The "typical" picture of bacterial pneumonia is heralded by acute onset of **fever** and **chills.** Cough productive of **purulent** (rust-colored or green) sputum soon follows. Depending on the location of the infection, the patient may have **pleuritic** chest pain—pain that worsens with deep **breathing** or **moving** (caused by inflammation near the external lung surface).

44. With bacterial pneumonia **bronchial and/or decreased breath sounds are often present.**

45. **a:** Additional treatment includes administering a high-concentration oxygen (at times, either assisted ventilation or intubation may be required), administering IV fluids (according to local protocol), using inhaled beta-2 agonists (e.g., albuterol) when applicable, and monitoring patients appropriately and transporting them to the correct facility. Generally antibiotics are *not* given by EMTs (any level) in the field. The EMT-I should also provide psychological support because fear and anxiety are usually present.

46. **a. High pressure:** the inability of the ventricle to pump blood adequately results in an increase in ventricular pressure. The increased ventricular pressure is back-transmitted to the left atrium, then the pulmonary vessels, causing an increase in the pulmonary venous pressure; most commonly results from acute myocardial ischemia but may also be caused by heart valve disease, chronic hypertension, or myocarditis; **b. High permeability:** may be caused by acute hypoxemia, near-drowning, cardiac arrest, shock, high altitude exposure, inhalation of pulmonary irritants (e.g., chlorine gas), and adult respiratory distress syndrome (ARDS); the alveolar-capillary membrane is disrupted, and fluid leaks into the interstitial space. Widening of the interstitial space by fluid impairs diffusion; symptoms may develop over a longer period, but an acute onset is still common.

47. **b**

48. **c**

49. **c**

50. **d:** Risks for pulmonary embolism include *thrombophlebitis, oral contraceptives, fracture of a long bone,* pregnancy, sedentary lifestyle, obesity, surgery, and blood diseases.

51. **b:** Patients with massive pulmonary emboli often suffer cardiac **arrest** or **syncopal** spell as the first symptom of the illness.

52. **True**

53. **False:** Spontaneous pneumothorax is *more common in men* than in women.

54. **False:** The most frequent cause of spontaneous pneumothorax is *rupture of a congenital defect on the surface of the lung*. A congenital bleb is an air-filled sac that has been present since birth. Young, tall, thin male smokers are most likely to develop pneumothorax from rupture of a congenital bleb.

55. Signs of spontaneous pneumothorax include **increasing respiratory distress, cyanosis, decreased breath sounds on the affected side, subcutaneous emphysema,** weak pulse, hypotension, distended neck veins, and tracheal deviation away from the side of the injury (a late sign).

    Patients with spontaneous pneumothorax often complain of the sudden onset of sharp chest pain accompanied by shortness of breath. The pain is often localized to the side of the lung involved. The patient may be coughing and be anxious or agitated.

56. **a**

57. **d:** Hyperventilation leads to excessive excretion (blowing off) of carbon dioxide, resulting in a decreased **Paco$_2$**.

58. **b:** Excessive excretion (blowing off) of carbon dioxide results in low blood levels (hypocapnia)—this disturbs the normal blood acid-base balance by increasing the pH. This leads to **respiratory alkalosis.** These pH changes can interfere with the normal function of other body systems. While the patient is hyperventilating, she is blowing off carbon dioxide and hence depleting the carbonic acid (H_2CO_3) levels of the body. Because carbonic acid has a direct effect on the pH, its removal causes the pH to move toward alkalosis. Because it is respiratory in nature, it is referred to as "respiratory alkalosis."

59. Conditions that can result in hyperventilation include **asthma attack, COPD, myocardial infarction, pulmonary embolism, spontaneous pneumothorax, congestive heart failure, increased metabolism (exercise, fever, hyperthyroidism, infection), central nervous system lesions (stroke, encephalitis, head injury, meningitis), hypoxia, accumulation of metabolic acids in the body (kidney failure, diabetic ketoacidosis, alcohol poisoning), drugs (cocaine, amphetamines, aspirin, epinephrine),** and **psychogenic factors (acute anxiety or pain).**

60. **c**

61. **d:** Having a hyperventilating patient rebreathe into a paper sack **is no longer considered appropriate.** Many patients who appear to have simple hyperventilation have serious illness. Having the patient breathe into a paper bag causes a marked decrease in the available oxygen, and dangerous hypoxia can result.

62. **c**

63. **d:** Treatment for a patient experiencing an acute asthma attack includes **administering an aerosolized bronchodilator.** Additional treatment includes administering *humidified* oxygen, 10 to 15 L/min via nonrebreather mask, and *placing an IV line*.

64. **d**

65. **c:** Additional treatment includes maintaining an open airway, giving oxygen *as per local protocol,* keeping the patient warm but not overheated, transporting the patient in a *semisitting position,* encouraging the patient to cough up secretions (do not force the patient to cough if it provokes nonstop spasms), placing an IV of normal saline at a TKO rate or using a heparin lock, administering a nebulized bronchodilator as per local protocol, and transporting her as soon as possible.

66. **d**

67. **b:** Treatment for this patient includes **administering high-concentration oxygen, via nonrebreather mask.** Additional treatment for this patient includes *placing an IV line,* placing the patient on a cardiac monitor, and transporting the patient in a position of comfort.

68. Answers to crossword puzzle

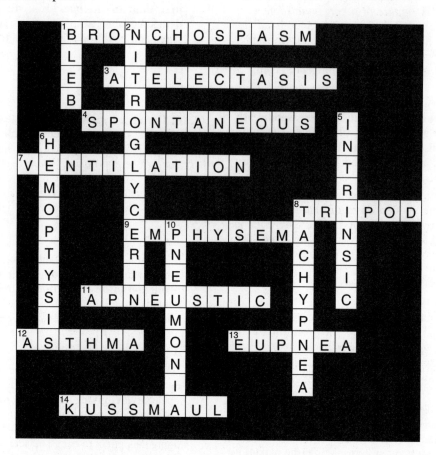

CHAPTER 23

1. **a:** The heart **is divided into right and left sides, separated by a thick wall.** The thick wall is the interventricular septum. It consists of two upper chambers, the *atria,* and two lower chambers, the *ventricles,* and it is about the size of a *closed fist.*

2. **c**

3. Order blood returning from the systemic venous circulation flows through the heart:
   1. **Deoxygenated blood returns to the right atrium via the superior and inferior venae cavae.**
   2. **Blood passes through the tricuspid valve into the right ventricle.**
   3. **Blood flows from the right ventricle through the pulmonary (semilunar) valve into the main pulmonary artery. This vessel branches off, taking blood to both the left and right lungs.**
   4. **Blood that was oxygenated in the lungs is returned to the left atrium via the pulmonary veins.**
   5. **Blood traverses the mitral (bicuspid) valve into the left ventricle.**
   6. **Blood is pumped through the aortic (semilunar) valve into the aorta.**

4. **a**

5. **a:** Contraction of the atria and ventricles, with concomitant pumping of blood vessels, is known as systole. Diastole is the relaxation phase. It is during this time that the heart receives most of its blood supply from the coronary arteries.

6. **d**

7. **d**

8. **b**

9. a. **Afterload:** resistance to blood flow out of the ventricle; b. **Stroke volume:** the amount of blood pumped out of the ventricle during each contraction; c. **Ejection fraction:** the amount of blood returning to the right atrium, which varies somewhat from minute

to minute, yet the normal heart continues to pump out the same *percentage* of blood returned; **d. Cardiac output:** the amount of blood pumped by the heart in 1 minute.

10. **Arteries** are blood vessels that carry blood away from the heart to the body. **Veins** transport blood from the body back to the heart. **Arteries** decrease in size as they move away from the heart, branching into many small **arterioles.** Arterioles then divide many times until they form **capillaries,** microscopic thin-walled vessels through which oxygen, carbon dioxide, and other nutrients and waste products are exchanged.

11.

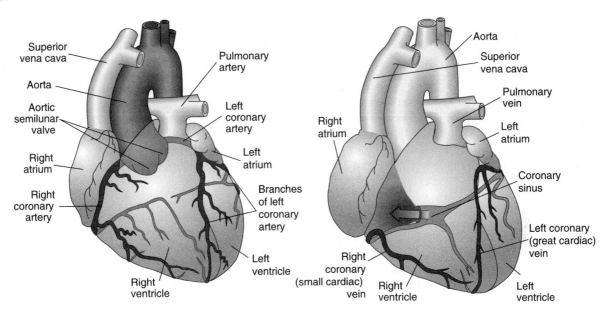

12. The heart muscle (myocardium) has the ability to generate and conduct electrical impulses. **Normally, electrical signals begin in the right atrium and pass via specialized tissue (the cardiac conduction system) throughout the heart.** As the electrical signal reaches various portions of the myocardium, it causes them to contract. The electrical conduction system of the heart allows electrical impulses to spread through the heart six times faster than muscle alone.

13. The conduction system of the heart.

Name	Function
A. **Sinoatrial (SA) node** • Intraatrial pathways • Internodal pathways	Dominant pacemaker of the heart Spread impulses from the SA node through the atria Carry impulses between the SA node and AV node
B. **Atrioventricular (AV) node**	Responsible for creating a slight delay in conduction of the impulse before sending it to the ventricles; this allows atrial contraction to finish filling the ventricles
C. **Bundle of His**	Makes electrical connection between atria and ventricles
D. **Bundle branches**	Carry electrical impulses at high velocity to the interventricular septum and each ventricle simultaneously
E. **Purkinje fibers**	Network of fibers that help to spread the impulse throughout the ventricular walls

14. The SA node has an intrinsic rate of **60 to 100** BPM.

15. The AV junctional tissue has an intrinsic rate of **40 to 60** BPM.

16. The ventricles have an intrinsic rate of **20 to 40** BPM.

17. Sequence an impulse is initiated and travels through the heart:
    1. **SA node**
    2. **Interatrial and internodal tracts**
    3. **AV node**
    4. **Bundle of His**
    5. **Bundle branches**
    6. **Purkinje fibers**

18. **d:** The Purkinje fibers **supply a conduction pathway to the individual cells of the ventricles.** They have an inherent rate of *20 to 40* BPM.

19. **a. Automaticity:** the ability to self-generate electrical activity (action potential) without the need for extraneous nerve stimulation; **b. Excitability:** the ability to respond to an appropriate electrical stimulus; **c. Conductivity:** the ability to transmit an appropriate electrical stimulus from cell to cell throughout the myocardium; **d. Contractility:** the ability of the myocardial cell to contract when stimulated by an appropriate electrical stimulus

20. The interior of the heart cell (myocyte) is **negatively** charged (–90 mV) during the resting (nondepolarized) phase. This is referred to as the **resting membrane potential** (RMP).

21. When depolarization begins, **sodium, calcium,** and **potassium** ions move from their "resting" locations in and out of the cell. The net result is that the interior of the myocyte becomes more **positively** charged.

22. When a certain level or **threshold** is reached, **depolarization** of the entire cell occurs.

23. After a period of time, each cell returns back to the **resting** state (repolarizes), again because of the movement of **sodium, calcium,** and **potassium,** waiting for the next stimulus.

24. **d**

25. **As one cell is depolarized, it chemically passes the signal to the next one, causing similar changes to occur, and the "wave of depolarization" (followed by repolarization) progresses through the heart.**

26. **True:** Also called automaticity.

27. **True**

28. **c: No stimulus will depolarize the myocyte** during the absolute refractory period. A sufficiently strong stimulus, however, *will* depolarize the myocardium during the *relative* refractory period.

29. **c**

30. **c**

31. Influences on the chronotropic, dromotropic, and inotropic states of the heart come partially from the **brain, via the autonomic nervous system, from hormones of the endocrine system, and from the heart tissue.** Receptors in the blood vessels, kidneys, brain, and heart constantly monitor body homeostasis.

32. **a**

33. **d**

34. **b**

35. **a**

36. **c:** The baroreceptors **sense changes in the blood pressure.** If abnormalities are sensed, nerve signals are transmitted to appropriate target organs, leading to release of hormones or neurotransmitters to rectify the situation. Once conditions normalize, the receptors stop firing, and the signals cease. The *chemoreceptors* sense changes in the CO_2 and O_2 concentrations and pH of the arterial blood.

37. **False:** The ECG is a record of the electrical activity of the heart as sensed by electrodes on the body surface. It is sometimes called an EKG. The ECG tells the EMT-I little about the pumping action of the heart. Checking the pulse and blood pressure assesses pumping effectiveness.

38. The ECG is a **tracing or graphic** representation of the electrical activity of the heart, which is picked up by **electrodes** that are placed on the patient's skin in at least *two* different locations. Electrode sites can vary depending on which lead or view of the heart's activity is being monitored. Different leads may be used for different purposes. Some monitors have multiple lead capabilities. Electrocardiographs are widely used in the prehospital setting to permit continuous monitoring of the electrical activity of the heart.

    However, the EMT-I can never depend solely on the cardiac monitor. Patient assessment and subjective reports by the patient are very important to detect conditions such as heart failure or pulmonary complications.

39. The electrodes are attached to the cardiac monitor by means of a **cable.** The monitor transforms the electrical activity of the heart into a waveform that can be interpreted.

40. **c:** A monitoring lead or rhythm strip will provide the following information: how fast the heart is beating, how long the conduction is taking to occur in different parts of the heart, and the regularity of the heartbeat. It will *not* show the EMT-I the presence or location of myocardial infarction, axis deviation and chamber enlargement, or quality of pumping action.

41. When stimulated by the electrical impulse of the conduction system, the heart muscle cell becomes **depolarized** and contracts in response.

42. **a. P wave:** electrical depolarization of the atria; **b. PR interval:** electrical depolarization of the atria and delay at the AV junction; **c. QRS complex:** electrical depolarization of the ventricles; **d. ST segment:** period between ventricular electrical depolarization and repolarization; **e. T wave:** electrical repolarization of ventricles; **f. R-to-R interval:** time between two ventricular depolarizations.

43.

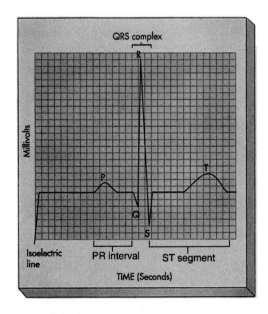

44. **c**

45. Elements that should be evaluated when analyzing an ECG strip include **rate, rhythm, QRS complexes, P waves,** and **PR intervals.** Five steps for analyzing ECG dysrhythmias are described below.

Step 1: Determine the rate. Is it within normal limits (60 to 100 BPM), or is it fast or slow?
Step 2: Evaluate the rhythm. Compare the R-to-R intervals to determine whether the ventricular rhythm is regular or irregular and whether all or some QRS complexes are related to preceding atrial depolarizations (represented by P waves).
Step 3: Measure the QRS duration. Is it within the normal limit (less than 0.12 second)? QRS complexes of less than 0.12 second represent impulses that travel through the ventricles in a normal fashion. QRS complexes of greater than 0.12 second indicate abnormal conduction through the ventricles or impulses that originate from the ventricles.
Step 4: Look for P waves. Note their size and shape. Where do they occur? Does a QRS complex follow each one? If so, the cardiac cycle is being initiated in the SA node or the atria. Look at the atrial rhythm. Compare the P-P intervals to determine whether the atrial rhythm is regular or irregular.
Step 5: Measure the PR intervals. Are they between 0.12 and 0.20 second? Longer PR intervals indicate a delay in conduction of the impulse to the ventricles. Are they constant, or do they vary in length? Varying PR intervals indicate certain dysrhythmias.

The information gained from this analysis, together with knowledge of dysrhythmias, will help to identify the particular rhythm that a patient is experiencing.

46. **c:** To count the heart rate per minute, the 3-second marks at the top of ECG paper can be used. Two complete sections represent **6 seconds.** The number of R waves that occur within this time (the 6-second interval) is counted and the number multiplied by **10** to obtain the patient's heart rate.

47. **In this example, six waves appear in the 6-second interval. Multiply this number by 10. The heart rate is 90 BPM.**

48. The heart rate of the dysrhythmia is 60 beats per minute.

Another method for determining the heart rate is to count the number of small squares that are between two consecutive waves. Because each small square represents 0.04 second, then 1500 small squares are equal to 1 minute. These may be between R waves to determine the ventricular rate, or between P waves to determine the atrial rate. The number of small squares counted is then divided into 1500 to determine the heart rate.

49. If the distance between consecutive R waves remains constant, the ventricular rhythm is considered to be **regular.** If the interval varies, the rhythm is **irregular.**

50. An upright, rounded P wave usually indicates an impulse originating from the **SA node.**

51. If each P wave on the ECG is followed by a **QRS** complex, it indicates that the impulses are being transmitted to the ventricles.

52. In the healthy adult, the PR interval is between **three** and **five** small squares, or **0.12** to **0.20** second in duration. To measure the PR interval, count the number of small squares between the beginning of the P wave and the beginning of the QRS complex. Multiply the number of small squares in the PR interval by 0.04 second to find the value of the interval. Example: If the number of squares is four, multiply by 0.04 for a PR interval of 0.16 second.

53. Normal QRS duration is less than **three** small squares, or less than **0.12** second. A duration of **three** small squares or more indicates a delay in the conduction of the impulse through the **ventricles** (or an impulse that originates in the ventricles).

    The QRS duration is measured in the same manner as the PR interval. Count the number of small squares from the beginning of the Q wave to the end of the QRS complex. This value is multiplied by 0.04 second. Normal QRS duration is less than three small squares, or less than 0.12 second.

54. Dysrhythmia is **any deviation from the normal electrical rhythm of the heart.** Dysrhythmias can occur in patients with both normal and diseased hearts. Often their occurrence indicates the need for rapid intervention on the part of the EMT-I. Alterations in cardiac function caused by dysrhythmias can precipitate conditions such as angina pectoris, myocardial infarction, acute heart failure, or pulmonary edema. Dysrhythmias can also affect cardiac output, resulting in decreased perfusion in other areas of the body. Whenever dysrhythmias are detected, responsibilities of the EMT-I include observing the patient's tolerance of the dysrhythmia; assessing the patient's cardiovascular status; analyzing the findings; intervening appropriately; and evaluating the results and closely monitoring the patient's electrocardiogram. The EMT-I should be particularly alert for signs of decreased cardiac output such as cool, clammy skin; weak, thready peripheral pulses; hypotension; tachycardia; decreased urine output; hyperventilation; and alterations in sensorium.

55. Causes of dysrhythmias include **myocardial ischemia or necrosis; autonomic nervous system imbalance; distention of heart chambers; acid-base abnormalities; hypoxemia; electrolyte imbalance; drug effects or toxicity; electrical injury; hypothermia; and central nervous system injury.**

56. **b:** Characteristics of sinus rhythm include **a rate of between 60 and 100 BPM,** a *regular* rhythm, an *upright* P wave that precedes each QRS complex, and PR intervals that are *constant*.

57. **a**

58. **c**

59. Sinus tachycardia is a regular sinus rhythm with a rate greater than **100 BPM.** Usually the rate does not exceed **160 BPM.**

60. In sinus tachycardia, the P waves, PR intervals, and QRS intervals are **normal.**

61. Sinus rhythm, sinus bradycardia, sinus tachycardia, and sinus dysrhythmia originate in the SA node.

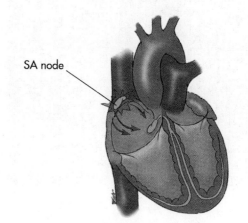

62. Sinus rhythms

	Rate	Rhythm	QRS Complex	P Wave	PR Interval
Sinus rhythm	60 to 100 BPM (atrial and ventricular rates are equal)	Regular (R-to-R intervals and P-P intervals are constant)	Within normal limits (<0.12 sec in duration)	Upright and uniform, precede each QRS complex	Within normal limits (0.12-0.20 sec in duration) and constant
Sinus tachycardia	Between 100 and 150 BPM	Regular (R-to-R intervals and P-P intervals are constant)	Within normal limits (<0.12 sec)	Upright and uniform, precede each QRS complex	Within normal limits (0.12-0.20 sec) and constant
Sinus bradycardia	<60 BPM	Regular (R-to-R intervals and P-P intervals are constant)	Within normal limits (<0.12 sec)	Upright and uniform, precede each QRS complex	Within normal limits (0.12-0.20 sec) and constant
Sinus dysrhythmia	Between 60 and 100 BPM	Rhythm is irregular (patterned)	Within normal limits (<0.12 sec)	Upright and uniform, precede each QRS complex	Within normal limits (0.12-0.20 sec) and constant

63. **c**

64. **a**

65. Origin of atrial dysrhythmias is in the atria (as denoted by the shaded area on the heart below).

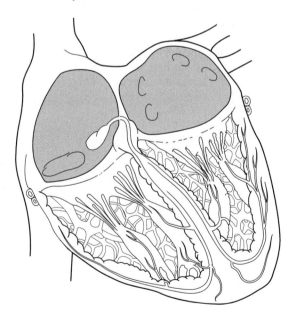

66. With atrial rhythms the QRS complexes are typically **less** than **0.12** second in duration.

67. **a. Wandering pacemaker:** morphology of P wave changes from beat to beat; **b. Premature atrial contraction (PAC):** early beat causes the underlying rhythm to be irregular; **c. Supraventricular tachycardia (SVT):** atrial and ventricular rate is 150 to 250 BPM; **d. Atrial flutter:** atrial rate is 250 to 350 BPM; normal P waves absent; "sawtooth" flutter waves present; **e. Atrial fibrillation:** the baseline is chaotic because the atrial activity is represented by "fibrillatory waves" or "f" waves; atrial rate is between 350 and 700 BPM; rhythm is totally (grossly) irregular.

68. **a**

69. **d**

70. **b**

71. Atrial rhythms

	Rate	Rhythm	QRS Complex	P Wave	PR Interval
Wandering atrial pacemaker	Usually normal, 60 to 100 BPM.	Rhythm is slightly irregular.	Usually <0.12 sec.	Change in P wave morphology from beat to beat.	PR interval often varies.
Premature atrial contraction (PAC)	Rate will depend on underlying rhythm	Early beat causes the underlying rhythm to be irregular.	QRS complex accompanying the premature beat is usually <0.12 sec.	P wave, often with different morphology (appearance) than normal, occurs early.	PR interval accompanying the premature beat is within normal limits of 0.12 to 0.20 sec.
Supraventricular tachycardia (SVT)	Atrial and ventricular rate is 150 to 250 BPM.	Rhythm is regular (except if there is an onset and termination as seen with PSVT).	QRS are narrow (<0.12 sec) (provided no ventricular conduction disturbance is present).	There is one P wave preceding each QRS complex. The P wave is typically buried in the T wave of the preceding beat. If present, the P waves may be flattened or notched.	Because the P waves tend to be buried, the PR intervals are typically indeterminable. If visible, the PR interval is often shortened but may be normal or rarely prolonged.
Atrial flutter	Atrial rate 250 to 350 BPM. Ventricular rate depends on ventricular response; may be normal, slow, or fast.	Atrial rhythm is regular. Depending on conduction ratio, ventricular rhythm may be regular or irregular.	QRS complexes are usually normal (<0.12 sec), unless ventricular conduction disturbance (aberrancy) is present.	Normal P waves absent; "sawtooth" flutter waves present. 1:1 atrioventricular conduction rare; usually 2:1, 3:1, or 4:1. Conduction ratios may be constant or variable.	PR interval usually constant.
Atrial fibrillation	Atrial rate too rapid to be counted (350 to 700 BPM). Ventricular rate depends on AV conduction; may be normal, slow or fast.	Rhythm is totally (grossly) irregular. Also referred to as irregularly irregular.	QRS complexes are usually normal (<0.12 sec).	There are no discernible P waves; the baseline is chaotic as the atrial activity is represented by "fibrillatory waves" or "f" waves.	No PR intervals are present.

72. With atrial dysrhythmias the P waves (if present) differ in appearance from normal sinus P waves **because they originate from a site outside the SA node. P waves originating from the atria may appear upright, notched, inverted, rounded, biphasic, or buried in the QRS.**

73. Origin of junctional dysrhythmias

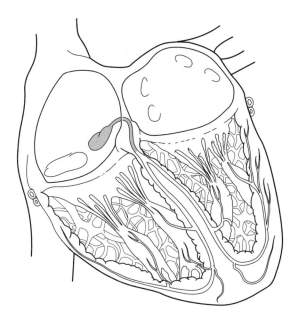

74. **b:** The impulse that depolarizes the atria travels in a backward or retrograde direction, resulting in **inverted P waves in lead II with a short PR interval, absent P waves (as they are buried by the QRS complex), or P waves that follow the QRS complex.**

75. **b**

76. In junctional rhythms, **electrical impulses travel in a normal pathway from the AV junction through the bundle of His and bundle branches to the Purkinje fibers, ending in the ventricular muscle. Because conduction through the ventricles proceeds normally, the QRS complex is usually within normal limits of 0.04 to 0.12 second.**

77.

	Rate	Rhythm	QRS Complex	P Wave	PR Interval
Premature junctional contraction (PJC)	Rate is dependent on the rate of the underlying rhythm.	Rhythm is irregular (underlying rhythm is disrupted by presence of early beats).	QRS complexes are within normal limits (<0.12 sec).	P waves may precede, be lost in (absent), or follow the QRS complex. When present, the P wave will be inverted.	PR interval, if present, will be <0.12 sec.
Junctional escape rhythm	Rate is between 40 and 60 BPM.	Rhythm is regular if it is an escape rhythm but irregular if it is an isolated escape complex.	QRS complexes are within normal limits (<0.12 sec).	P waves may precede, be lost in (absent), or follow the QRS complex. When present, the P wave will be inverted.	PR interval, if present, will be <0.12 sec.
Accelerated junctional rhythm	Rate is between 60 and 100 BPM.	Rhythm is regular.	QRS complexes are within normal limits (<0.12 sec).	P waves may precede, be lost in (absent), or follow the QRS complex. When present, the P wave will be inverted.	PR interval, if present, will be <0.12 sec.
Junctional tachycardia	Rate is between 100 and 180 BPM.	Rhythm is regular (except if there is an onset and termination as seen with PSVT).	QRS complexes are within normal limits (<0.12 sec).	P waves may precede, be lost in (absent), or follow the QRS complex. When present, the P wave will be inverted.	PR interval, if present, will be <0.12 sec.

78. Origin of ventricular dysrhythmias

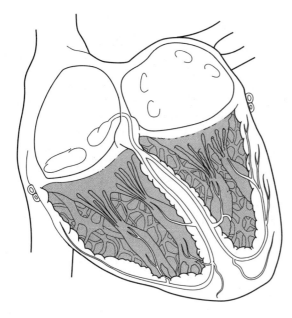

79. **False:** A PVC is a single irritable focus within the *ventricles* that fires prematurely to initiate an ectopic complex.

80. **True**

81. **b:** The PVC is an extra heartbeat initiated by an ectopic site in one of the ventricles. It has a QRS complex that appears *wide and bizarre* (greater than the normal 0.12 second) and is *often* followed by a compensatory pause.

82. Types of PVCs considered malignant include **frequent PVCs (usually more than five per minute), runs of PVCs (three or more in a row), multiform PVCs, the R-on-T phenomenon, and PVCs associated with chest pain.** These types of PVCs represent added risk of more dangerous dysrhythmias occurring and are referred to as malignant.

83. **a.** *Trigeminal:* PVCs that occur every third beat; **b. Multiformed:** PVCs that appear different from each other; **c. Bigeminal:** PVCs that occur every other beat; **d. Couplets:** two PVCs that occur together without a normal complex between; **e. Uniform:** PVCs that have the same morphology (appearance); **f. R-on-T phenomenon:** occurs when the PVC wave falls on the T wave, interrupting the rhythm; **g. A run of PVCs:** three or more PVCs in a row.

84. **b**

85. **d:** Ventricular tachycardia has **wide and bizzare QRS complexes.** It also has a *regular rhythm (usually),* a rate of between *100 and 250* BPM, and *no* P waves preceding the QRS complexes.

86. **a**

87. **a**

88. Those dysrhythmias considered life threatening include **ventricular fibrillation, asystole, pulseless electrical activity (PEA),** and ventricular tachycardia.

89. **c**

90. **b**

91. Reversible causes of PEA include **hypovolemia (most common), tension pneumothorax, hypoxia,** and **pericardial tamponade.**

92. Ventricular dysrhythmias

	Rate	Rhythm	QRS Complex	P Wave	PR Interval
Premature ventricular contraction (PVC)	Rate is dependent on rate of underlying rhythm.	Rhythm is irregular because underlying rhythm is disrupted by presence of the early beat(s).	Wide (>0.12 sec), usually bizarre looking QRS complex is seen, which is NOT preceded by a P wave. It appears earlier in the cycle than the normal set of complexes would be expected to occur. The QRS complexes of the PVCs differ from QRS complexes of the underlying rhythm. T waves of the premature beats take an opposite direction to the R waves. Following each PVC is a pause called a compensatory pause.	P waves are typically present with the underlying rhythm but not the premature beats.	PR intervals are typically present with the underlying rhythm but not the premature beats.
Ventricular escape rhythm	Rate is usually 0 to 40 BPM; 2 may be slower.	Rhythm is usually regular (becomes irregular as the heart dies).	QRS complexes are wide (>0.12 s) and bizarre; the T wave typically takes the opposite direction of the R wave.	P waves present or absent; if present, there is no predictable relationship between P waves and QRS complexes (AV dissociation).	PR interval, if present, is variable and irregular.
Ventricular tachycardia	Ventricular rate is between 150 and 250 BPM. If the rate is between 100 and 150 BPM, it is referred to as slow VT. If the rate is > 250 BPM, it is referred to as ventricular flutter.	Rhythm is typically regular.	Rhythm consists of frequent wide (>0.12 sec) and bizarre QRS complexes. T waves may or may not be present and typically are of the opposite direction of the R waves.	Typically, P waves are not discernible (if seen, they are dissociated).	PR interval is absent.

Continued

	Rate	Rhythm	QRS Complex	P Wave	PR Interval
Ventricular fibrillation	No coordinated ventricular contractions are present. The unsynchronized ventricular impulses occur at rates from 300 to 500 BPM.	Rhythm is totally chaotic.	There are no discernible QRS complexes.	There are no discernible P waves.	PR intervals.
Asystole			There is no electrical activity, only a flat line.		

93. **d:** It is the erratic quivering of the heart that results in ineffective pumping action and is said to be the mechanism of sudden death in approximately 60% of cases.

94. Origin of heart block

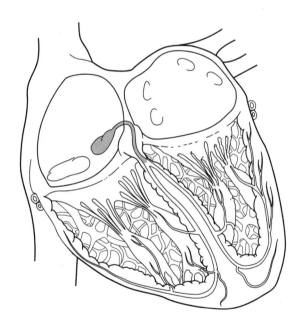

95. **a**

96. **b**

97. **a**

98. **a. First-degree AV block:** not a true block; there is a delay at the AV node; each impulse is eventually conducted; **b. Second-degree AV block, Wenckebach:** PR interval gets progressively longer until a P wave fails to conduct, resulting in a "dropped" QRS complex. After the blocked beat, the cycle starts all over again; **c. Second-degree AV block, Mobitz II:** some beats are conducted and others are blocked; **d. Third-degree AV block:** there is a complete block at or below the AV node; there is no relationship between the P waves and QRS complexes.

99. **c**

100. **d**

101. **c**

102. **False:** With third-degree AV heart block, the ventricular rate is usually *less than* 60 BPM.

103. **False:** With second-degree AV heart block, Mobitz II, the PR interval *remains constant on those beats that are conducted.*

104. **False:** With third-degree AV heart block, the R-to-R waves are *regular.*

105. **True:** It will be irregular if the conduction ratio (number of P waves to each QRS complex) varies.

106. **True**

107. AV heart blocks

	Rate	Rhythm	QRS Complex	P Wave	PR Interval
First-degree AV block	Rate is that of the underlying rhythm.	Rhythm is usually regular, depends on the underlying rhythm.	QRS complexes are within normal limits (<0.12 sec).	P waves normal; one precedes each QRS complex.	PR interval is constant and >0.20 sec.
Second-degree AV block, Wenckebach	Atrial rate is that of the underlying rhythm; ventricular rate slightly less than atrial rate (slower than normal).	Ventricular rhythm is irregular with "grouped beating." It appears as a pattern (cycle seems to occur over and over again). P-P interval is constant; R-R interval a QRS.	QRS complexes are within normal limits (<0.12 sec).	P waves are upright and uniform; there are more P waves than QRS complexes because some of the QRS complexes are blocked.	PR interval gets progressively longer until a P wave fails to conduct, resulting in a "dropped" QRS complex. After the blocked beat, the cycle starts all over again.
Second-degree AV block, Mobitz II	Atrial rate is that of underlying rhythm; ventricular rate is less than atrial rate.	Rhythm is typically regular. It will be irregular if the conduction ratio (number of P waves to each QRS complex) varies.	QRS complexes may be within normal limits (<0.12 sec) or wide.	P waves are upright and uniform; some are not followed by QRS complexes (there are more P waves than QRS complexes).	PR interval constant for conducted beats; may be normal or prolonged.
Third-degree AV block	Atrial rate is that of the underlying rhythm; ventricular rate depends on the escape focus (40 to 60 BPM junctional, <40 BPM ventricular).	Atrial and ventricular rhythms regular but independent of each other.	QRS complexes are normal if escape focus is junctional, widened if escape focus is ventricular.	P waves are present and normal, unrelated to QRS complexes. There are more P waves than QRS complexes.	There is no relationship between the P waves and QRS complexes; "the P waves seem to march right through the QRS complexes."

108. **d**

109. **c**

110. **d**

111. **b**

112. **c**

113. **a**

114. **a:** With normal pacer function, a *wide* QRS should follow each pacing spike. P waves *may be present or absent* and are *unrelated to pacing spikes and paced QRS complexes*. The PR intervals *depend on the underlying rhythm*.

115. **True**

116. **False:** With pacemaker failure the EMT-I should consider immediate *transcutaneous pacing (TCP)*.

117. **False:** Ventricular conduction disturbances involve *delays* in electrical conduction through either the bundle branches (right or left) or the fascicles (anterior, posterior).

118. **True**

119. The hemiblocks (LAHB, LPHB) involve a block of conduction in one of the **left fascicles. Left anterior** hemiblock is far more common.

120. With hemiblock the normal conduction pathway is **blocked.** The affected myocardium receives its electrical innervation "**retrograde**" from the remaining intact parts of the **conduction** system.

121. Patients with any type of **ventricular** conduction block, and especially those with a combination, are at high risk of developing **complete** heart block. Consider standby **transcutaneous pacing (TCP)** for these individuals, especially in the face of acute myocardial ischemia.

122. Preexcitation syndromes **involve the presence of abnormal conduction pathways (called accessory conduction pathways) between the atria and ventricles. These pathways bypass the AV node and bundle of His, allowing atrial impulses to depolarize the ventricles earlier than usual.**

123. The ECG features of Wolff-Parkinson-White (WPW) syndrome include **normal rate; regular rhythm; QRS widened with slurring of the initial portion (delta wave); P waves are normal; and PR interval is usually shorter than normal (greater than 0.12 second).**

124.

Rate:	50 BPM
Rhythm:	Regular
P waves:	Upright and round; each is followed by a QRS complex
QRS complexes:	0.06
PR intervals:	0.16
Interpretation:	Sinus bradycardia

125.

Rate:	88 BPM (underlying rhythm)
Rhythm:	Irregular
P waves:	Upright and round (preceding sinus beat), absent (ectopic beats)
QRS complexes:	0.08 (sinus beats), wide and bizarre (ectopic beats)
PR intervals:	0.20 (sinus beats), none (ectopic beats)
Interpretation:	Sinus rhythm with a run of VT and a PVC

126.

Rate:	80 BPM
Rhythm:	Regular
P waves:	Upright and round; each is followed by a QRS complex
QRS complexes:	0.06
PR intervals:	0.16
Interpretation:	Sinus rhythm; ST segment elevation

127.

Rate:	83 BPM (underlying rhythm)
Rhythm:	Irregular
P waves:	Upright and round; each is followed by a QRS complex (sinus beats); the P wave preceding the premature beat differs from the underlying rhythm
QRS complexes:	0.08
PR intervals:	0.16
Interpretation:	Sinus rhythm with a PAC (the fifth complex from the left is the PAC)

128.

Rate:	75 BPM
Rhythm:	Regular
P waves:	Upright and round; each is followed by a QRS complex
QRS complexes:	0.06
PR intervals:	0.28
Interpretation:	Sinus rhythm with first-degree AV block

129.

Rate:	70 BPM (ventricular), 100 BPM (atrial)
Rhythm:	Irregular (patterned)
P waves:	Upright and round, but not all are followed by a QRS complex
QRS complexes:	0.06
PR intervals:	Gets progressively longer until a QRS complex is dropped and then it starts all over; the cycle repeats itself
Interpretation:	Second-degree AV block, Wenckebach

130.

Rate:	150 BPM
Rhythm:	Regular
P waves:	Unable to determine
QRS complexes:	0.16
PR intervals:	Unable to determine
Interpretation:	Ventricular tachycardia

131.

Rate:	80 BPM
Rhythm:	Regular
P waves:	Absent (or buried in QRS complexes)
QRS complexes:	0.06
PR intervals:	Unable to determine
Interpretation:	Accelerated junctional rhythm

132.

Rate:	180 BPM
Rhythm:	Regular
P waves:	Unable to determine
QRS complexes:	0.06
PR intervals:	Unable to determine
Interpretation:	Supraventricular tachycardia

133.

Rate:	Unable to determine
Rhythm:	Chaotically irregular
P waves:	Unable to determine
QRS complexes:	Unable to determine
PR intervals:	Unable to determine
Interpretation:	Ventricular fibrillation (coarse)

134.

Rate:	56 BPM
Rhythm:	Regular
P waves:	None
QRS complexes:	0.16
PR intervals:	None
Interpretation:	Idioventricular rhythm (accelerated)

135.

Rate:	170 BPM
Rhythm:	Irregular (totally)
P waves:	Absent; "f" waves present
QRS complexes:	0.06
PR intervals:	Unable to determine
Interpretation:	Atrial fibrillation with an uncontrolled ventricular response

136.

Rate:	100 BPM
Rhythm:	Irregular (slightly because of the ectopic beat)
P waves:	Upright, and each is followed by a QRS complex (sinus beats), inverted (ectopic beat)
QRS complexes:	0.08
PR intervals:	0.16 (sinus beats), 0.10 (ectopic beat)
Interpretation:	Sinus rhythm (borderline sinus tachycardia) with one PJC

137.

Rate:	80 BPM
Rhythm:	Irregular, patterned
P waves:	Upright, and each is followed by a QRS complex
QRS complexes:	0.04
PR intervals:	0.16
Interpretation:	Sinus dysrhythmia

138.

Rate:	100 BPM
Rhythm:	Irregular
P waves:	Upright, and each is followed by a QRS complex (sinus beats); unable to determine (ectopic beats)
QRS complexes:	0.06 (sinus beats) wide and bizarre (ectopic beats)
PR intervals:	0.12
Interpretation:	Sinus rhythm with two PVCs (fourth and eighth complexes are the PVCs)

139.

Rate:	150 BPM
Rhythm:	Regular
P waves:	Upright; each followed by a QRS complex
QRS complexes:	0.12
PR intervals:	0.12
Interpretation:	Sinus tachycardia (with significant Q waves)

140.

Rate:	40 BPM
Rhythm:	Regular
P waves:	Upright and round; each is followed by a QRS complex
QRS complexes:	0.08
PR intervals:	0.16
Interpretation:	Sinus bradycardia (with ST segment elevation)

141.

Rate:	80 BPM
Rhythm:	Regular
P waves:	Atrial pacing
QRS complexes:	Ventricular pacing
PR intervals:	Unable to determine
Interpretation:	Normal functioning AC sequential pacemaker

142.

Rate:	56 BPM (ventricular), 107 BPM (atrial)
Rhythm:	Regular
P waves:	Upright and rounded, but every other P wave is not followed by a QRS complex (2:1 conduction ratio)
QRS complexes:	0.08
PR intervals:	0.16 and constant (for the conducted beats)
Interpretation:	Second-degree AV heart block, Mobitz II

143.

Rate:	60 BPM
Rhythm:	Regular
P waves:	Upright and round; precede each QRS complex
QRS complexes:	0.08
PR intervals:	0.16
Interpretation:	Sinus rhythm (with inverted T waves)

144.

Rate:	160 BPM
Rhythm:	Regular
P waves:	Upright; each is followed by a QRS complex
QRS complexes:	0.04
PR intervals:	0.10
Interpretation:	Sinus tachycardia

145.

Rate:	54 BPM (ventricular), 83 BPM (atrial)
Rhythm:	Regular
P waves:	Upright and round; appear to "march through the QRS complexes"
QRS complexes:	0.16
PR intervals:	There is no relationship
Interpretation:	Third-degree AV heart block

146.

Rate:	214 BPM
Rhythm:	Regular
P waves:	Unable to determine
QRS complexes:	0.16
PR intervals:	Unable to determine
Interpretation:	Ventricular tachycardia

147.

Rate:	60 BPM
Rhythm:	Regular
P waves:	Upright and round; each is followed by a QRS complex
QRS complexes:	0.06
PR intervals:	0.32
Interpretation:	Sinus rhythm (borderline sinus bradycardia) with first-degree AV block

148.

Rate:	36 BPM
Rhythm:	Regular
P waves:	Unable to determine
QRS complexes:	0.12
PR intervals:	Unable to determine
Interpretation:	Idioventricular rhythm

149.

Rate:	96 BPM (underlying rhythm), 214 BPM (PSVT)
Rhythm:	Irregular (because of a run of PSVT)
P waves:	Upright and each followed by a QRS complex
QRS complexes:	0.08
PR intervals:	0.16 (sinus beats)
Interpretation:	Sinus rhythm with a run of PSVT

150.

Rate:	80 BPM
Rhythm:	Regular
P waves:	Upright and round; each is followed by a QRS complex
QRS complexes:	0.06
PR intervals:	0.16
Interpretation:	Sinus rhythm

151.

Rate:	20 to 60 BPM (ventricular), 60 BPM (atrial)
Rhythm:	Irregular
P waves:	Upright and round, but not all are followed by a QRS complex
QRS complexes:	0.12
PR intervals:	0.16 (for the conducted beats)
Interpretation:	Second-degree AV heart block, Mobitz II

152.

Rate:	110 BPM
Rhythm:	Irregular (totally)
P waves:	Unable to determine
QRS complexes:	0.06
PR intervals:	Unable to determine
Interpretation:	Atrial fibrillation with uncontrolled ventricular response

153.

Rate:	40 BPM (ventricular), 80 BPM (atrial)
Rhythm:	Regular
P waves:	Upright and rounded; not all followed by a QRS complex (2:1 ratio of P waves to each QRS complex)
QRS complexes:	0.06
PR intervals:	0.24 (and constant on the conducted beats)
Interpretation:	Second-degree AV heart block, Mobitz II

154.

Rate:	65 BPM (ventricular), 100 BPM (atrial)
Rhythm:	Regular
P waves:	Upright and round; appear to "march through the QRS complexes"
QRS complexes:	0.08
PR intervals:	No relationship
Interpretation:	Third-degree AV heart block

155.

Rate:	50 BPM according to visible P waves; true sinus rate is probably 100 BPM
Rhythm:	Irregular
P waves:	Upright and round; each is followed by a QRS complex (sinus beats); none (ectopic beats)
QRS complexes:	0.06 (sinus beats)
PR intervals:	0.12
Interpretation:	Sinus rhythm with bigeminal PVCs (unifocal)

156.

Rate:	30 BPM
Rhythm:	Regular
P waves:	Upright and round; each is followed by a QRS complex
QRS complexes:	0.06
PR intervals:	0.12
Interpretation:	Sinus bradycardia

157.

Rate:	75 BPM (ventricular), 300 BPM (atrial)
Rhythm:	Regular
P waves:	Flutter waves (4:1 conduction ratio)
QRS complexes:	0.08
PR intervals:	Unable to determine
Interpretation:	Atrial flutter

158.

Rate:	80 BPM (underlying rhythm)
Rhythm:	Irregular
P waves:	Upright and round; each is followed by a QRS complex (underlying rhythm); none (ectopic beats)
QRS complexes:	0.08 (underlying rhythm), wide and bizarre (ectopic beats)
PR intervals:	0.16 (underlying rhythm), none (ectopic beats)
Interpretation:	Sinus rhythm with frequent uniform PVCs

159.

Rate:	50 BPM
Rhythm:	Regular
P waves:	Inverted; each is followed by a QRS complex
QRS complexes:	0.06
PR intervals:	0.10
Interpretation:	Junctional escape rhythm

160.

Rate:	60 BPM (ventricular), 70 BPM (atrial)
Rhythm:	Irregular (patterned)
P waves:	Upright and round; not all are followed by a QRS complex
QRS complexes:	0.08
PR intervals:	Gets progressively longer until a QRS complex is dropped, and then it starts all over; the cycle repeats itself
Interpretation:	Second-degree AV block, Wenckebach

161.

Rate:	80 BPM
Rhythm:	Irregular (slightly)
P waves:	Upright, each is followed by a QRS complex (underlying rhythm); P wave of the ectopic beat differs from underlying rhythm
QRS complexes:	0.08
PR intervals:	0.16
Interpretation:	Sinus rhythm with one PAC (beat 6 is a PAC)

162.

Rate:	90 BPM (ventricular), greater than 350 BPM (atrial)
Rhythm:	Irregular (totally)
P waves:	Fibrillatory waves
QRS complexes:	0.08
PR intervals:	None
Interpretation:	Atrial fibrillation

163.

Rate:	80 BPM
Rhythm:	Irregular (totally)
P waves:	Absent "f" waves present
QRS complexes:	0.08
PR intervals:	Unable to determine
Interpretation:	Atrial fibrillation with controlled ventricular response

164.

Rate:	80 BPM
Rhythm:	Irregular
P waves:	Upright and round (sinus beats) undetermined (PVCs)
QRS complexes:	0.06 (sinus beats), wide and bizarre (PVCs)
PR intervals:	0.16 (sinus beats); unable to determine (PVCs)
Interpretation:	Sinus rhythm with frequent episodes of paired PVCs (couplets)

165.

Rate:	65 BPM
Rhythm:	Irregular
P waves:	Upright and round; each is followed by a QRS complex (underlying rhythm), inverted and follow the QRS complexes (ectopic beats)
QRS complexes:	0.08
PR intervals:	0.16
Interpretation:	Sinus rhythm with 2 PJCs (the third and sixth beats from the left are the PJCs)

166.

Rate:	180 BPM
Rhythm:	Regular
P waves:	Upright; each is followed by a QRS complex
QRS complexes:	0.06
PR intervals:	0.08
Interpretation:	Atrial tachycardia (SVT)

167.

Rate:	70 BPM (ventricular), 300 BPM (atrial)
Rhythm:	Regular
P waves:	Flutter waves
QRS complexes:	0.06
PR intervals:	Unable to determine
Interpretation:	Atrial flutter

168.

Rate:	100 BPM
Rhythm:	Regular
P waves:	Upright and round; each is followed by a QRS complex
QRS complexes:	0.14
PR intervals:	0.16
Interpretation:	Sinus rhythm (borderline sinus tachycardia) with wide QRS complexes and inverted T waves

169.

Rate:	80 BPM
Rhythm:	Regular
P waves:	None
QRS complexes:	0.08
PR intervals:	None
Interpretation:	Accelerated junctional rhythm

170.

Rate:	80 BPM
Rhythm:	Irregular (patterned)
P waves:	Upright and round; each is followed by a QRS complex (sinus beats); appears as a point on the T wave of the preceding beat (ectopic beats)
QRS complexes:	0.04 (sinus beats), 0.08 (ectopic beats)
PR intervals:	0.16
Interpretation:	Sinus rhythm with bigeminal PACs

171.

Rate:	50 beats per minute
Rhythm:	Regular
P waves:	Inverted; each is followed by a QRS complex
QRS complexes:	0.06
PR intervals:	0.08
Interpretation:	Junctional escape rhythm

172.

Rate:	110 BPM
Rhythm:	Regular
P waves:	Upright and round; each is followed by a QRS complex
QRS complexes:	0.08
PR intervals:	0.12
Interpretation:	Sinus tachycardia

CHAPTER 24

1. **b**

2. **c**

3. Ischemic heart disease (IHD) includes **coronary artery disease, myocardial infarction, angina pectoris,** and congestive heart failure.

4. Reasons for decrease in ischemic heart disease death rate in United States: **increased prevention efforts—dietary changes, decreased cigarette smoking, control of hypertension; improved methods of treatment (e.g., thrombolytic therapy for acute myocardial infarction); improved public education with earlier recognition of symptoms;** and **prevention of recurrences in patients with previous cardiac ischemic events.**

5. **a**

6. Risk factors that predispose to ischemic heart disease include **age, family history, hypertension, sex, hypercholesterolemia, smoking,** and **diabetes mellitus.**

7. The presence of pink-tinged frothy sputum may suggest acute **pulmonary edema.**

8. The most common symptom of cardiac problems is **chest pain.**

9. **True:** Quite commonly, persons with angina or myocardial infarction have discomfort in the epigastrium (pit of the stomach), jaw, arm, or shoulder. They may complain of indigestion as the first symptom of a heart attack. Any person with pain in the anterior portion of the body from the umbilicus (navel) to the jaw should be assumed to have cardiac problems until proven otherwise. Persons with diabetes and elderly patients often present with atypical cardiac pain.

10. **True**

11. **False:** The sudden onset of profuse sweating *without preceding heavy activity* can indicate a cardiac problem.

12. **True**

13. Findings suggestive of acute myocardial ischemia include **diaphoresis; dyspnea; anxiety and irritability; nausea and vomiting; feeling of impending doom; abnormal heart rate or rhythm;** and **abnormal blood pressure.**

14. The past medical history of a cardiac patient may include **coronary artery disease; previous cardiac surgery; elevated cholesterol levels; congenital heart disease; hypertension; valvular or inflammatory heart disease; aneurysm; lung disease; kidney disease; diabetes;** and **vascular disease.**

15. Most patients complain of **"feeling their heartbeat,"** or palpitations, rather than of an **"abnormal pulse rate."**

16. Patients who are uncomfortable for any reason, especially those who are hypoxic, will feel **anxious.**

17. **b**

18. Management of sinus tachycardia focuses on treating the **underlying cause** of the tachycardia.

19. Algorithm for bradycardia

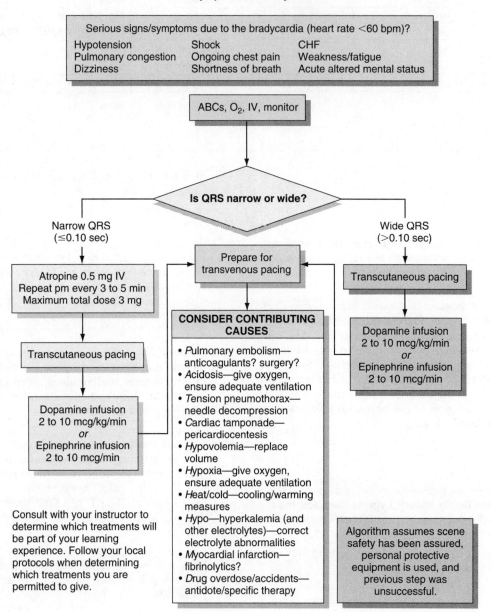

20. Algorithm for supraventricular tachycardia

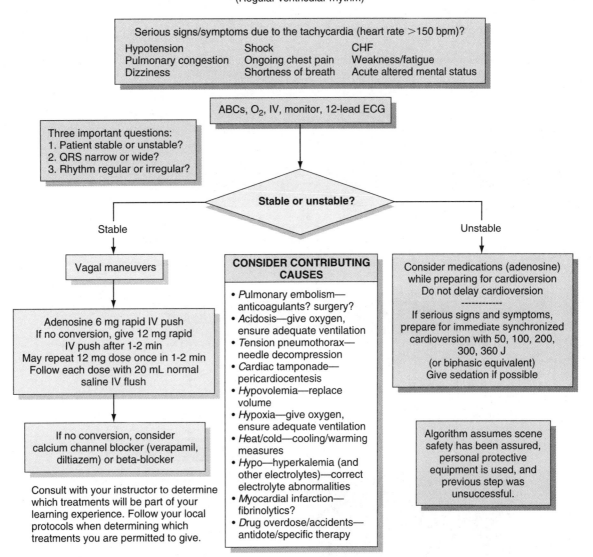

21. **c:** Treatment for stable ventricular tachycardia includes **oxygen,** IV line, and amiodarone.

22. Algorithm for universal cardiac treatment

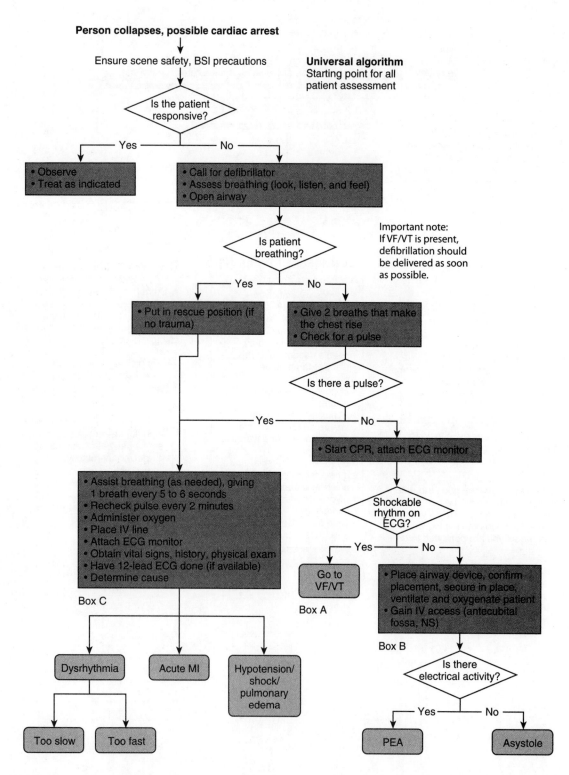

23. **d:** Oxygen, epinephrine (and/or vasopressin), and lidocaine (or amiodarone, procainamide), as well as other medications, may also be used.

24. **b:** Lidocaine (or amiodarone) and 100% oxygen, as well as several other drugs, can also be used to treat this condition.

25. **c**

26. **b:** Atropine, 1 mg, IV push may also be given in PEA when the heart rate is slow.

27. **d**

28. Treatment algorithm

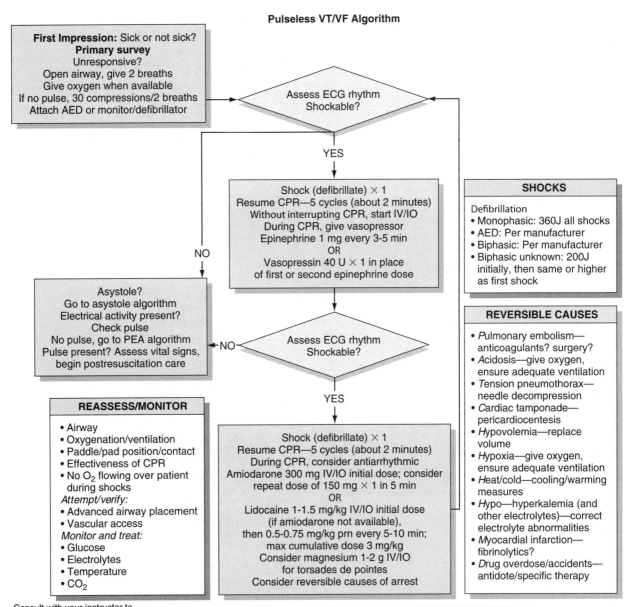

29. Treatment algorithm

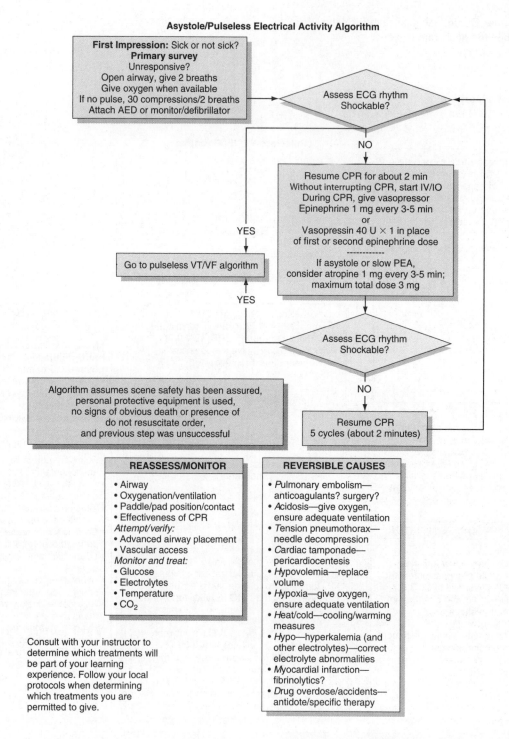

30. **c:** Vagal maneuver **should be preceded by the placement of an IV line and ECG monitoring.** Vagal maneuvers also stimulate the *parasympathetic* nervous system and may be used to terminate PSVT in *hemodynamically stable* patients. The EMT-I should only attempt vagal maneuvers with *medical direction authorization*.

31. **a. Valsalva maneuver:** involves having the patient take in a deep breath and "bear down" as if to have a bowel movement; results in forced expiration against a closed glottis and vagal nerve stimulation; **b. Ice water maneuver:** should not be performed if ischemic heart disease is present or suspected; involves having the patient hold his or her breath and then immersing the face briefly into ice water;

stimulates the vagus nerve because of the mammalian diving reflex; **c. Unilateral carotid sinus pressure:** should be done only after auscultating both carotid arteries for a bruit (pulse-related "whooshing" sound); is done using your index and middle fingers placed over the carotid artery on the neck, just below the angle of the jaw.

32. **If a bruit is present, if the carotid pulses are not equal bilaterally, or if the patient has a history of cerebral vascular disease,** unilateral carotid sinus pressure should not be performed.

33. **c:** Also compress the carotid artery *gently* while massaging the area; maintain pressure for no longer than *5 to 10 seconds;* and compress *only one side at a time*.

34. **d**

35. Adenosine is effective in terminating **PSVT** (and SVT).

36. The initial dose of adenosine is a **6**-mg rapid IV bolus followed by a 20-mL normal saline flush. If there is no response in **1 to 2** minutes, a **12**-mg dose should be administered in the same manner. A third dose at 12 mg can be administered if there is no response to the second dose.

37. Side effects of adenosine include **flushing, bradycardia,** and, rarely, **cardiac arrest caused by asystole.**

38. Atropine **blocks** discharge from the **parasympathetic** nervous system, leading to an **increase** in the heart rate.

39. Indications for atropine include hemodynamically significant **bradycardias, asystole,** and bradycardic pulseless electrical activity (PEA).

40. **b:** Atropine is administered at a dose of **1.0 mg IV push in cardiac arrest,** *0.5* mg IV push in symptomatic bradycardia, and *2.0 to 2.5* mg when delivered endotracheally.

41. Doses of atropine may be repeated **every 3 to 5 minutes to a maximum dose of 3 mg.**

42. **Because atropine may cause paradoxical** *slowing* **of the heart rate in second-degree AV heart block, type II and third-degree AV block with new wide QRS complexes, it should be used just as a temporizing treatment until TCP can be established.**

43. Effects of epinephrine include **increased aortic diastolic pressure and increased coronary perfusion pressure.** It also produces increased contractility, increased myocardial oxygen consumption, peripheral vasoconstriction, increased heart rate, and increased coarseness of fibrillation.

44. Epinephrine is indicated in all types of arrest, including **VF, pulseless VT, asystole, and PEA.**

45. **c**

46. **a**

47. **True**

48. **a:** Lidocaine is also acceptable for control of hemodynamically compromising PVCs. It may also be delivered as a maintenance infusion at a dose of 1 to 4 mg/min following successful conversion of VF or pulseless VT (follow your local protocols).

49. **b**

50. **b:** Amiodarone is a complex drug with *multiple* effects and is *preferred to other antiarrhythmic agents* in patients with severely impaired heart function.

51. Indications for the use of amiodarone include **ventricular rate control of rapid atrial arrhythmias when digitalis has proved ineffective; after defibrillation and epinephrine in cardiac arrest with persistent VT or VF; hemodynamically stable VT and wide QRS tachycardia of uncertain origin; and control of rapid ventricular rate caused by accessory pathway conduction in preexcitation syndromes.**

52. Vasopressin is the **naturally** occurring **antidiuretic** hormone. In high doses it acts as a powerful **vasoconstrictor** by direct stimulation of specific **nonautonomic** receptors.

53. The primary condition vasopressin is used to treat is **adult shock–refractory VF (as an alternative to the first or second dose of epinephrine).**

54. If there is no response to vasopressin administration in the treatment of cardiac arrest, **resume the use of epinephrine at recommended doses.**

55. **a. Vasopressin:** given as a one-time dose of 40 units, IV; **b. Amiodarone:** in nonarrest situations, give 150 mg IV over 10 minutes, followed by 1 mg/min infusion for 6 hours; in cardiac arrest caused by pulseless VT or VF, give 300 mg, IV push (diluted in a volume of 20 to 30 mL of saline); can repeat at dose of 150 mg (diluted in a volume of 10 to 15 mL of saline) if VF/VT recurs.

56. Five mechanical interventions used to treat cardiac emergencies that require no special equipment are **vagal maneuvers, stimulation, precordial thump, cough, and CPR**.

57. **b**

58. **b**

59. **d**

60. With synchronized cardioversion, **the EMT-I activates a specific switch on the defibrillator that allows the shock to be automatically delivered during a portion of the cardiac cycle when the heart is not susceptible to development of worse ventricular dysrhythmias (pulseless VT or VF). It is typically used to treat unstable tachycardia in which a pulse is still present.**

61. **a**

62. **False:** The *earlier* that defibrillation is applied following the onset of VF, *the more likely it is to be successful*. Survival rates after VF cardiac arrest decrease 7% to 10% with every minute of delay to defibrillation.

63. **True**

64. **False:** The greater the transthoracic resistance, the *less* energy delivered to the heart.

65. Factors that influence transthoracic resistance to defibrillation include **delivered energy; electrode size; interface between the chest wall and the electrodes; the number and time interval between previous shocks; pressure applied to the electrodes; the phase of the patient's ventilation; and the distance between electrodes.**

66. **d**

67. Basic steps for using an automated external defibrillator are:
    - **Recognize that the patient is in cardiac arrest.**
    - **Prepare and attach the defibrillator pads or electrodes.**
    - **Turn on the automated defibrillator.**
    - **Push the "analyze" button on the automated defibrillator.**
    - **Deliver the shock if indicated. The device will either automatically deliver a shock or instruct the operator (via audible and visible signals) to "SHOCK."**

68. **a:** Resistance is very high if the metal electrodes are bare. For this reason, **defibrillation pads should be placed on the patient's chest or conductive gel should be applied to the paddles.** *All* surfaces of the paddles should be touching the patient's skin. The EMT-I should push down with *20 to 25 lb* of firm arm pressure. Resistance is also lower when the patient's phase of ventilation is at *full expiration*.

69. **On an ongoing basis, check the batteries and defibrillator unit for proper operation; ensure the electrode pads, if used, have not expired; ensure that the paddles are clean from the last use; if using conductive gel or paste, make certain that the paddles are adequately coated; ensure everyone is clear of the patient, including the operator, before delivering the countershock; use extreme caution when defibrillating patients who are wet or in contact with metal; double-check the rhythm before delivering a countershock to ensure that the patient has not reverted to another rhythm; make sure the synchronized mode is turned off when defibrillating VF; and if the rhythm changes, or following three sequential shocks, check the carotid pulse.**

70. **c:** Transcutaneous pacing **may resolve symptomatic bradycardia and heart block that is not responsive to atropine.** It is *unlikely* that transcutaneous pacing will resolve most cases of asystole or pulseless electrical activity. It also is *contraindicated* in patients with open wounds or burns on the chest and in patients who are in a wet environment.

71. **d**

72. **b:** Atherosclerosis is a *progressive, degenerative* disease of the medium and larger arteries (aorta and its branches, cerebral arteries, coronary arteries) that *interferes with blood flow* and occurs *throughout a person's lifetime*.

    Atherosclerosis results from the deposition of lipids and cholesterol under the tunica intima layer of the blood vessels. After lipids are deposited, an injury response occurs in the vessel wall, which subsequently damages the tunica media as well. Over time, the deposition of calcium occurs with resultant plaque formation. Small hemorrhages into the plaque can occur, followed by more scarring and fibrosis, further enlarging the plaques. The involved arteries can become completely blocked, either by additional plaque or by a blood clot.

73. **a**

74. **d**

75. **c:** Stable angina can be of a relatively short duration, 3 to 5 minutes, or prolonged, lasting 15 minutes or more; is chest pain that **is brought on by stress or exertion** (when the oxygen demands of the heart are increased); and can be relieved by rest, nitroglycerin, or oxygen administration.

76. **Unstable angina is angina that is either new in onset or differs from a patient's typical stable angina pattern.** For example, a patient may now be awakened at night with pain, which has never happened previously. Or pain now comes on at rest. Either way, a change in previously stable angina is often a warning sign of an impending myocardial infarction (heart attack).

77. **d:** With patients experiencing chest pain, nitroglycerin administration may result in **dilation of peripheral blood vessels. This reduces the preload and afterload and decreases the myocardial workload.** There is also improvement of myocardial perfusion through *dilation* of the coronary arteries.

78. **True:** The area of myocardium supplied by the artery receives little or no oxygen, and dies.

    Research has shown that certain factors increase the chances of a person experiencing a heart attack. The presence of any of these in a patient with chest pain should increase your suspicion of a heart attack.
    - Cigarette smoking; cigarettes double the risk for heart attack
    - Family history of heart attack or sudden death
    - Male sex; men have a greater risk for heart attack than women. Women who take birth control pills or who are postmenopausal are at a higher risk than other women.
    - Diabetes mellitus
    - Hypertension
    - Elevated blood cholesterol levels (hypercholesterolemia)
    - Obesity
    - Sedentary lifestyle—failure to get sufficient aerobic exercise
    - Stress

78. **True**

79. **False:** A patient experiencing acute myocardial infarction *may not always have chest pain.* This is more common in elderly patients and is referred to as "silent heart attack."

80. **b**

81. **d:** Coronary artery trauma, coronary artery spasm, inflammation of the blood vessels, and *coronary* thrombosis are precipitating factors of acute myocardial infarction.

82. **c: Cardiac dysrhythmia (sudden death)** is the most common cause of death in acute myocardial infarction. If death results with this problem, it will usually occur within 1 to 2 hours of onset. This is why it is so important for patients to recognize the signs and symptoms of a heart attack and seek medical help right away. When treating patients suffering from an acute myocardial infarction, EMTs should remove any factors that will increase the patient's anxiety and potentially lead to sudden death.

    Two other complications of acute myocardial infarction are congestive heart failure—mild heart failure occurs far more frequently than severe heart failure or pulmonary edema—and cardiogenic shock—MI patients who present in cardiogenic shock usually have suffered a massive heart attack.

83. **False:** Supplemental oxygen *increases* the oxygen in the blood flowing to ischemic tissue in the patient experiencing acute myocardial infarction (AMI). Always use oxygen when AMI is suspected.

84. **b: Severe tearing-like chest pain** is seen with aortic dissection. Other signs include hypotension, tachycardia, pallor, and mild to moderate midabdominal or lumbar pain. The pain often becomes severe and is experienced over the entire abdomen, chest, or lumbar area.

85. **d:** Signs and symptoms of pulmonary emboli include **sudden, unexplained onset of chest pain that increases in intensity with a deep breath** (pain may be localized to the area of the chest overlying the involved lung tissue), respiratory distress, shortness of breath, increased respiratory rate (patient may hyperventilate), wheezing, coughing up of blood (hemoptysis), anxiety, shock, and hypotension.

86. **a:** Congestive heart failure (CHF) is circulatory congestion caused by inadequate flow of blood. It is caused by heart muscle damage that reduces the heart's ability to function as a pump. As a result of inadequate pumping, blood backs up in the tissues. CHF varies from mild to severe and may be chronic or acute in onset. It **is characterized by tachycardia, dyspnea, deviated blood pressure, rales, and edema to the lower extremities.**

87. **d**

88. **a. Paroxysmal nocturnal dyspnea:** shortness of breath at night—the patient may wake up unable to breathe; **b. Orthopnea:** worsening of shortness of breath when lying down; **c. Ascites:** abdominal swelling; and **d. Pedal edema:** fluid collects in the feet and legs.

89. **c:** With left-sided CHF, the pumping capability of the *left* ventricle is decreased; fluid backs up into the *lungs, causing pulmonary congestion and edema;* and signs and symptoms include shortness of breath (dyspnea in patients with CHF is often worsened by lying down), audible abnormal breath sounds (rales and wheezes), **and the patient often displays pink, frothy sputum.**

In *right*-sided CHF, the pumping capacity of the right ventricle is impaired. Blood draining into the right heart backs up into the vascular system, resulting in swelling (edema) of the extremities and lower back, abdominal swelling (ascites), swelling of the liver and spleen, and distention of the neck veins.

Other signs and symptoms of heart failure include:
- Weakness, fatigue
- Tachycardia
- Chest pain (if CHF occurs with acute myocardial infarction)
- Cyanosis
- Increased systolic blood pressure (most patients with acute CHF have *elevated* blood pressure)

90. **False:** Patients with hypertensive emergency have markedly elevated blood pressure. *Generally*, in hypertensive crisis, the patient's systolic pressure is greater than 200 mm Hg, and the diastolic pressure is greater than 120 mm Hg. However, these are not rigid criteria. *Patients may have significant symptoms at lower readings.*

91. **False:** Treatment of hypertensive crisis includes maintaining a patent airway and administering a high concentration of oxygen, starting an IV line of normal saline at a TKO rate, monitoring the cardiac rhythm (if permitted by your local protocol), and monitoring the vital signs and pulse oximetry frequently—at least every 5 minutes.

92. Signs that are characteristic of cardiogenic shock include **a systolic blood pressure of less than 80 mm Hg, cold and clammy skin, tachypnea (rapid and shallow respirations),** abnormal mental status because of decreased flow of blood and oxygen to the brain, collapse of peripheral veins, rapid and thready pulse, and lowered oxygen saturation on pulse oximetry.

93. **b:** Additional treatment includes administering a high concentration of oxygen.

94. **d**

95.
    1. **Defibrillate at 360 J.**
    2. **Defibrillate a second time at 360 J.**
    3. **Place an endotracheal tube**
    4. **Establish an IV line.**
    5. **Administer epinephrine, 1 mg, IV push.**
    6. **Deliver the third defibrillation at 360 J.**
    7. **Administer lidocaine or amiodarone.**
    8. **Deliver the fourth defibrillation at 360 J.**

96. **d: With left-sided CHF,** the pumping capability of the left ventricle is decreased. Fluid backs up into the lungs, causing pulmonary congestion. In its worst form, the lungs fill with large amounts of fluid, resulting in pulmonary edema. The treatment priority in this case is to ensure an adequate airway and breathing.

97. **d:** Treatment for this patient includes administering **furosemide, 20 to 80 mg IV push;** placing the patient in a *semisitting* position, with the legs dependent (below the level of the heart) if possible; administering *100% oxygen via nonrebreather mask* (be prepared to assist ventilation and possibly intubate if necessary); starting an IV line of *normal saline* at a KVO drip rate; monitoring the ECG rhythm (dysrhythmias are especially likely in the face of acute pulmonary edema); and monitoring the vital signs, including pulse oximetry if available, at least every 5 minutes. Some protocol may call for the EMT-I to administer nitroglycerin, morphine sulfate, and other drugs if the patient's systolic BP is greater than 100 mm Hg.

Furosemide acts initially as a vasodilator, decreasing the preload. In addition to this and its action as a diuretic, the drug has been shown to increase lymphatic flow from the lungs (efferent lymphatic flow), thus *reducing* the amount of pulmonary edema fluid.

Morphine is a narcotic agent with many unique beneficial effects in acute pulmonary edema. It acts on the central nervous system to reduce patients' anxiety. This leads to a decrease in epinephrine release, decreasing the workload on the failing heart. In addition, morphine also causes vasodilation (mostly via a central effect on the brain), leading to decreased preload and increased cardiac output.

Some EMS protocols include the use of inhaled bronchodilators, such as albuterol, in persons with either APE or a possible combination of APE and COPD.

98. **c**

99. **d:** Additional treatment for this patient includes administering *100% oxygen via nonrebreather,* monitoring the ECG rhythm and vital signs, and including pulse oximetry, if available, at least every 5 minutes. Because the chest pain has subsided and the patient has already taken three nitroglycerin tablets, *no more should be administered.*

100. **b**

101. **c:** Additional treatment for this patient includes starting an IV line of *normal saline* at a KVO drip rate, and monitoring the vital signs, including pulse oximetry, if available, at least every 5 minutes. Some protocols may call for administering *lidocaine,* IV push, followed by an appropriate maintenance dose or other antidysrhythmics such as amiodarone or procainamide.

102. **d**

103. **a:** Atropine blocks discharge from the parasympathetic nervous system, leading to an increase in the heart rate. By blocking parasympathetic (vagal) action on the heart, atropine enhances conduction through the AV junction and accelerates the heart rate, thereby improving cardiac output.

104. **a:** Atropine administration may be repeated every 3 to 5 minutes to a total of 3.0 mg.

105. **b:** It is caused by profound failure of the cardiac muscle, primarily the left ventricle. When greater than 40% of the left ventricle is nonfunctional, the heart loses its ability to efficiently pump blood into the systemic circulation.

106. **a:** Additional treatment for this patient includes starting an IV line of normal saline at a KVO rate, giving a 250 to 500 cc fluid challenge if called for by medical direction or local protocol, and transporting him to the hospital without delay.

107. **b**

108. **a:** Treatment of this patient should include maintaining a patent airway; giving oxygen at 15 L/min by nonrebreather mask (if the patient's condition deteriorates or he develops significant respiratory distress, intubate according to local protocol); starting an IV line, saline via a microdrip at a KVO rate; regularly monitoring the vital signs, including pulse oximetry, if available; **monitoring the ECG rhythm;** minimizing patient motion (do not allow him to move, especially if he is still having pain); loosening restrictive clothing and, if local protocol permits, administering nitroglycerin, 0.3 to 0.4 mg, SL, or if permitted by local protocol, administering chewable aspirin. In addition, morphine sulfate may be administered.

109. Answers to crossword puzzle

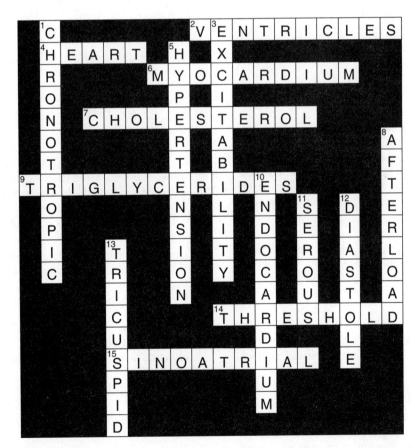

CHAPTER 25

1. **a:** Diabetes mellitus is a chronic disease of the **endocrine** system caused by a **decrease** in the secretion or activity of the hormone **insulin.**

2. **a:** Insulin **is released from the beta cells of the pancreas.** It *blocks* the breakdown of fat tissue in the body and *decreases* the blood sugar.

3. Glucagon, secreted by the alpha cells of the pancreas, and epinephrine, secreted by the adrenal gland, **both help to regulate the blood glucose level by increasing it.** This is opposite the effect of insulin. They are often called counterregulatory hormones.

4. **False:** Persons with diabetes *do not produce enough insulin to regulate the blood glucose level.* As a result, the blood sugar level may become too high (hyperglycemia) or too low (hypoglycemia). Either condition can result in life-threatening problems.

5. **False:** *Hypoglycemia* is an abnormally low blood sugar level. This condition is sometimes called insulin shock.

6. **True**

7. **b**

8. Glucose is the sole source of oxidative metabolism (nutrition) for the central nervous system. **When the blood sugar level decreases significantly, altered states of consciousness or loss of consciousness may occur. Prolonged hypoglycemia (greater than 20 to 30 minutes) may lead to permanent brain cell damage.**

9. **a. Type 1:** insulin dependent; patients typically have disease onset at a younger age; prone to diabetic ketoacidosis; **b. Type 2:** non–insulin dependent; usually onset is after the teenage years; less prone to diabetic ketoacidosis.

10. Complications of diabetes include **eye disease, kidney disease, nerve disease,** and **increased risk of cardiovascular disease.**

11. Causes of hypoglycemia include **medications (insulin, oral diabetic medications), excessive exercise (causes too rapid absorption of insulin), endocrine diseases, alcohol consumption, poor diet, hypothermia,** and **liver disease.**

12. The most common causes of hypoglycemia in a diabetic patient are when he or she takes his or her insulin and does not eat enough **food.**

13. Hypoglycemia generally develops **rapidly** (over a few minutes to a few hours).

14. **True**

15. **True**

16. **False:** Differentiating hypoglycemia from a stroke *may be impossible* because hypoglycemia can cause paralysis and altered levels of consciousness.

17. **a. Hypoglycemia:** diaphoresis; slurred speech; seizures; shakiness, weakness; **b. Hyperglycemia:** frequent urination; thirst; fruity, acetone-like odor to the breath; nausea and vomiting; Kussmaul respirations.

18. Two questions to ask the diabetic patient: "Did you eat today?" "Did you take your insulin [or other diabetic medication] today?"

19. **d**

20. **b: Helping the patient take insulin** is not part of managing a hypoglycemic patient. Treatment for this patient includes administering high-concentration oxygen via nonrebreather mask; administering 50% dextrose, 50 mL, IV push; and establishing an IV line of normal saline.

21. **d:** 50% dextrose **can cause tissue necrosis if it is allowed to leak from the vein.** It is *contraindicated* in the presence of cerebral ischemia or stroke administration and should be *preceded* by thiamine in the patient who has a history of alcoholism.

22. Diabetic ketoacidosis (DKA) occurs **when a diabetic person has inadequate insulin circulating in the blood to properly control the blood sugar level. The patient's blood sugar increases significantly, and the fatty tissues break down. The body forms compounds called ketones and ketoacids from the fat tissue. These substances change the acid-base balance in the body, harming the patient.** The elevated blood sugar level makes the patient urinate more frequently than usual, leading to dehydration and loss of body chemicals (particularly potassium).

23. The most common reason a diabetic patient develops DKA is **infection.** This stress results in an increased insulin requirement in the body. Diabetic ketoacidosis has a relatively *slow* onset. Patients with DKA have symptoms that become worse over a matter of hours to days.

24. **a:** Diabetic ketoacidosis (sometimes called diabetic coma) is a metabolic condition consisting of hyperglycemia, dehydration, and the accumulation of abnormal compounds, called ketones and ketoacids, in the body.

25. **d:** With diabetic ketoacidosis, fats are used as the primary energy source because glucose is unavailable for metabolism (because the glucose molecules cannot penetrate the cell membrane without insulin). Because fats are extremely inefficient energy sources, producing many acids and ketones as waste products, *metabolic acidosis* results. The body, attempting to keep the pH at a tolerable level, enlists the help of the respiratory system. The patient experiences Kussmaul respirations (compensatory hyperventilation) and subsequently blows off carbon dioxide, decreasing the carbonic acid level. This results in a *respiratory alkalosis*. This patient has metabolic acidosis that is partially offset by respiratory alkalosis.

26. **True:** Patients with DKA have symptoms that become worse over a matter of hours to days.

27. **False:** The patient with diabetic ketoacidosis usually has *rapid, deep, sighing respirations (Kussmaul respirations)*.

28. Treatment of diabetic ketoacidosis includes **maintaining the airway; assisting breathing as necessary; giving a high concentration of oxygen; monitoring the ECG; establishing an IV line and giving a fluid bolus according to your local protocol (many systems use 500 to 1000 cc of normal saline or Ringer's lactate solution as rapidly as possible); watching carefully for shock and caring for the patient accordingly; and giving nothing by mouth.**

29. **a:** Persons with hyperosmolar hyperglycemic nonketotic coma (HHNC) **have poor underlying health,** are typically *older* than 60 years of age, and experience *gradual* deterioration in mental status over 4 or 5 days. HHNC is precipitated by infection, extreme cold, or dehydration. Other signs and symptoms include altered mental status; the patient may be unconscious or may appear to have had a stroke; evidence of dehydration; poor skin turgor; and furrowed tongue. Kussmaul respirations and fruity breath odor, present in diabetic ketoacidosis, are conspicuously *absent* in HHNC.

30. Answers to crossword puzzle

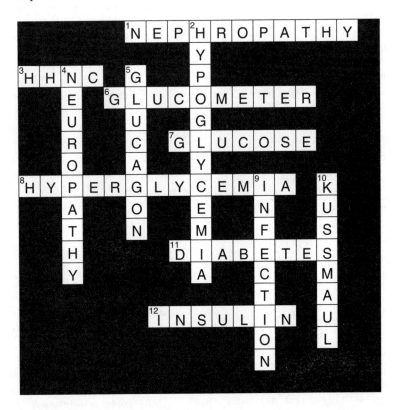

CHAPTER 26

1. Allergic reactions **result from exposure to *any* substance to which an individual is sensitive.** It can be an extremely severe allergic reaction, including airway edema, difficulty breathing, and/or vascular collapse leading to shock. This condition can occur quickly and may lead to serious illness or death if not cared for immediately.

2. *Anaphylaxis* is a **specific type of allergic reaction caused by the interaction of an allergen called an antigen, and one kind of antibody.**

3. When an **antigen** to which one is sensitive enters the body, it is attacked by a substance known as an **antibody.** Antibodies function to destroy foreign substances.

4. Five types of antibodies are formed by the immune system and reside on the surface of **mast** cells, a type of **white** blood cell.

5. Antibodies are also called **immunoglobulins** and are abbreviated as **Ig,** followed by a letter.

6. The **IgE** antibody is the only one involved in an anaphylactic reaction.

7. The release of histamine may cause **sudden, severe bronchoconstriction/spasm,** which can lead to airway compromise; **intense vasodilation,** which can lead to neurogenic shock; and **leaking of fluid from vessels** caused by a change in permeability.

8. Four primary ways allergens enter the body:

Skin contact	Poison ivy, skin creams, cosmetics, and detergents
Injections	Medications such as penicillin, insect bites, and stings
Inhalation	Molds, pollen, and perfumes
Ingestion	Foods, chocolate, shellfish, and peanuts

9. **True**

10. **False:** Stridor indicates *upper* airway constriction.

11. **a: Urticaria** is described as raised lesions on the skin (also known as hives). It is not a life-threatening condition.

12. **c:** Diphenhydramine **blocks the effects of histamine.** It is administered slow IV push or intramuscularly (follow local protocol).

13. **c**

14. **a:** Care of an allergic reaction is generally supportive in nature. Diphenhydramine administration is appropriate if local protocol permits and if vital signs are normal, there are no respiratory symptoms, and the only manifestations of the reaction are itching, rash, and/or swelling on the outside of the body. The ECG rhythm also should be monitored, and high-concentration oxygen should be administered via nonrebreather mask.

15. **b:** With anaphylaxis **the progression to death can be extremely rapid, sometimes within minutes.** It may be necessary to place an endotracheal tube to secure the airway. When the airway is patent, administer high-concentration oxygen, *10 to 15 L/min (85% to 100%)* by nonrebreather mask, and place the patient in a position of comfort based on his or her physiological needs (usually *sitting* if respiratory distress is present). Identify priority patients, and make transport/backup decisions. Epinephrine is nearly always administered under these circumstances. Nebulized bronchodilators may be helpful as well. Rapidly transport the patient to the *nearest appropriate medical facility.* Continue to reassess the patient's vital signs and response to treatment. Apply ECG electrodes, and provide continuous monitoring if protocol permits.

16. **c:** IV lines used in the management of anaphylaxis should be established using a *large-bore* catheter, consist of either *normal saline* or lactated Ringer's solution, and include a *macro*drip administration set.

17. **d:** Epinephrine (1:1000) **is used in the treatment of anaphylaxis.**

18. **In cases of bee stings, examine the sting site. If the stinger is still present, do not grasp it between your fingers or with a hemostat, tweezers, or any kind of grasping device. Instead, take a flat object, such as a tongue depressor, and scrape flat along the skin to remove the venom sac with or without the stinger.**

19. If wheezing or stridor is present, **administer a nebulized bronchodilator treatment with medications such as albuterol (Proventil, Ventolin) or isoetharine (Bronkosol) by nebulizer** if permitted by your local protocol. Both albuterol and isoetharine reverse bronchospasm.

CHAPTER 27

1. **False:** About *one half* of poisonings involve prescription drugs.

2. **False:** Poisoning is most common among children younger than *10* years.

3. **True**

4. *Overdose* **suggests excessive exposure to a substance that has normal treatment uses (e.g., aspirin). In excess, harm results.**

5. Three generic types of toxicological emergencies include **unintentional poisoning; drug and alcohol abuse (substance abuse); and intentional poisoning or overdose.**

6. **a. Dosage errors:** may occur by the prescribing physician, treating EMS provider, nurse, physician assistant, or pharmacist. Patients or their families may also be responsible for mistakes; **b. Idiosyncratic reactions:** untoward side effects that are unpredictable and different from that common to any particular drug; **c. Childhood poisoning:** most childhood poisonings are the result of caregiver inattention and innate childhood curiosity; **d. Environmental exposures:** examples include carbon monoxide in a school with inadequate ventilation, chemical exposure when driving near a freshly sprayed crop field, or smoke inhalation in persons living downwind from a large fire in progress; **e. Occupational exposures:** usually the result of an unforeseen leak or explosion, resulting in the widespread distribution of toxic materials absorbed by unprotected workers.

7. When responding to a call where poisons may be present, the EMT-I should immediately assess the need for personal protective equipment (PPE). This may include airway protection (respirators, SCBA packs), hooded chemical barrier suit or appropriate PPE, isolation, thick butyl rubber protective gloves, boots, and other specialized equipment. Do not enter the scene until doing so is safe for you. As in any toxic exposure, it may be necessary to enlist assistance of special hazardous materials teams to extricate, remove, and detoxify the patient before your care.

8. **c**

9. Exposure to a poison can occur through **ingestion, inhalation, absorption,** or **injection.**

10. **Ingestion** is the most common poisoning route.

11. Examples of exposure potentials that are geographically specific include **venomous snakes, spiders, marine animals, manufacturing industries,** and **transportation industries.**

12. Items of information that should be acquired when caring for a patient who has been poisoned: **What was taken? How much was ingested? When did the poisoning occur? What, if anything, has been done for the patient?**

13. Physical findings that may help identify the poison involved:
    - **Pulse—tachycardia suggests stimulant ingestion; bradycardia may be caused by various heart medications, as well as by pesticide poisoning.**
    - **Respiratory rate—isolated increases in the respiratory rate, especially in children, suggest the possibility of aspirin toxicity (which causes hyperventilation). Depressed respirations occur from narcotics, sedatives, and carbon monoxide poisoning.**
    - **Temperature—elevated from aspirin and stimulants; lowered (hypothermia) with alcohol, sedatives, narcotics, and pesticides.**
    - **Blood pressure—may be decreased if the patient took depressant or narcotic agents. The BP is often elevated if the patient has taken cocaine or amphetamines.**

14. **c**

15. **b:** Cholinergic agents **prevent the breakdown of acetylcholine by acetylcholinesterase.** This leads to *overstimulation* of the parasympathetic nervous system.

16. **a:** Signs of exposure to cholinergic agents include bradycardia, wheezing, bronchoconstriction, myosis (small pupils), coma, and convulsions.

17. SLUDGE means:
    S: Salivation
    L: Lacrimation
    U: Urination
    D: Defecation
    G: GI cramping
    E: Emesis

18. **a**

19. **False:** Some cholinergic agents, such as nerve gas, are extremely toxic and penetrate the skin and respiratory system easily. The EMT-I must always ensure his or her own safety first before attempting

to provide patient care. *Appropriately trained and equipped EMT-Is (in appropriate levels of protection)* or hazardous materials teams must be used as necessary, especially to help in patient and rescuer decontamination.

20. **True**

21. With anticholinergic poisoning, **the skin is red because patients are warm (unable to sweat). Tachycardia and tachypnea are often present because of parasympathetic inhibition (unopposed sympathetic stimulation). Especially in larger doses, anticholinergics induce a temporary psychotic state (thus, "mad").**

22. **d**

23. **d**

24. **c**

25. **d:** The patient who has inhaled a toxic substance may be expected to display laryngeal edema, hoarseness, inspiratory stridor, and noncardiogenic pulmonary edema.

26. **a:** The first thing to do is to **remove the patient to fresh air.** Be certain to use necessary safety equipment to protect yourself.

27. **c:** Carbon monoxide (CO) is a colorless, odorless, flavorless, and nonirritating gas that is a common source of poisoning. Carbon monoxide is a product of incomplete combustion of carbon-containing substances.

28. **a:** The product that is produced when carbon monoxide binds with hemoglobin in red blood cells is called carboxyhemoglobin.

29. **d:** Pulse oximetry may give inaccurate readings in cases of carbon monoxide poisoning, with the oxygen saturation (Sao_2) readings being falsely high.

30. Physiological properties of snake venom include **neurotoxicity** (paresthesias, paralysis, neuromuscular transmission disturbances); **hemotoxicity** (coagulant, anticoagulant, hemolytic, platelet problems); and **cardiotoxicity** (decreased cardiac output and blood pressure); in addition, **enzymes in the venom lead to tissue destruction**.

31. **d**

32. Answers to crossword puzzle

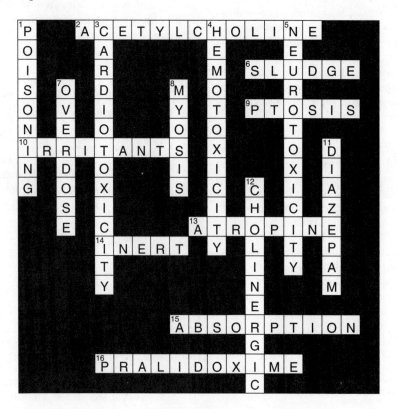

CHAPTER 28

1. **a**

2. A major goal of cerebral **homeostasis** is to maintain brain perfusion and oxygenation despite fluctuations in the mean arterial blood pressure.

3. **Within a wide range of mean arterial blood pressures, cerebral blood flow remains constant.** This is cerebral autoregulation. **It is caused by the opening and closing of prearteriolar and postarteriolar sphincters.**

4. **b:** Alterations in the motor control systems include **localized random movements,** generalized seizures, weakness, and generalized paralysis.

5. VINDICATE means:
   V: Vascular
   I: Infectious
   N: Neoplastic (tumor)
   D: Degenerative
   I: Inflammatory
   C: Congenital
   A: Allergic and autoimmune
   T: Traumatic
   E: Endocrine and metabolic

6. A **stroke** is a condition that results from a disruption of circulation to the brain, causing ischemia and damage to brain tissue.

7. There are two types of strokes, **occlusive** and **hemorrhagic.** About three of four strokes are occlusive, caused by a blockage in a blood vessel as a result of either an atherosclerotic plaque or an embolus. Hemorrhagic strokes are caused by bleeding into the brain tissue resulting from the rupture of a weakened blood vessel.

8. **a:** Stroke may present as **sudden onset of unilateral weakness, numbness, and an inability to walk.** There also may be paralysis of an arm or leg. Usually, one complete side of the body is affected. This is called hemiplegia. Because nerve fibers cross sides in the brainstem, damage to one side of the brain affects the opposite side of the body. You may also notice facial droop on one side of the face—sagging muscles beneath the eye and cheek and asymmetrical movement of the mouth. The victim may have other neurological deficits, such as impaired language or speech and decreased sensation. Assume that the acute onset of slurred speech or hemiplegia is caused by a stroke or cerebral hemorrhage. Patients with a stroke may have gradual or rapid onset of neurological symptoms. The patient may wake up in the morning with a deficit, or the symptoms may appear suddenly while he or she is awake.

   Other signs and symptoms of stroke include increased blood pressure, tachycardia, seizures, loss of consciousness, stiff neck, headache, altered level of consciousness, airway problems, hypoventilation, cardiac dysrhythmias, nausea, vomiting, and pupillary abnormalities.

9. **d**

10. **a**

11. **c**

12. Types of seizures include **generalized major motor seizures, focal motor seizures, behavioral seizures,** and **status epilepticus.**

13. Seizures are not a **disease,** but a symptom of an underlying **abnormality.**

14. Seizures may be **idiopathic** (no demonstrable cause) or **secondary** (caused by a brain lesion or metabolic abnormality).

15. Causes of central nervous system origin–seizures include **infection, fever, trauma, stroke,** and **tumor.**

16. **a**

17. **b:** Jerking movements of the entire body as the muscles rapidly contract and relax are called **tonic-clonic** seizure movements. An aura is a warning sign that a patient sees, hears, or smells before losing consciousness. Following a seizure, the patient is usually in a postictal state. This is a period of decreased level of consciousness after a generalized seizure.

18. **d:** To treat the convulsing patient, you should maintain the airway as best possible, be prepared to suction the patient during the seizure, avoid restraining the patient, start an IV line and run it at a TKO rate (this may be difficult during the seizure; in this case, wait until the seizure movements have lessened), **place the patient on an ECG monitor,** keep bystanders and nonessential EMS personnel back to avoid frightening or embarrassing the patient as he or she wakes up, check oxygen saturation via the pulse oximeter, and transport the patient in the coma position following the seizure.

19. c

20. d

21. b

22. c

23. Causes of coma that originate from within the brain include **intracranial bleeding, stroke, tumor, infection, meningitis, encephalitis,** and **seizure.**

24. Causes of coma arising outside the nervous system include **blood chemistry abnormalities (hypernatremia, hyponatremia, hypercalcemia, hypoglycemia, hyperglycemia); hypertensive crisis; kidney or liver failure; abnormalities of the endocrine glands (hypothyroidism, Addison's disease, pituitary gland failure); vitamin deficiencies; drugs (alcohol, narcotics, depressant drugs, antidepressants, tranquilizers);** and **psychiatric problems (catatonia).**

25. a

26. d

27. c

28. b

29. **Syncope is a partial or complete loss of consciousness, from which the patient has recovered.**

30. a

31. c

32. Causes of headache resulting from potentially serious conditions include **brain tumors, intracranial bleeding, hypertensive crisis, meningitis,** and **poisoning.**

33. d

34. a

35. Treatment for the patient complaining of headache includes **carefully monitoring the ABCs, preparing for vomiting, reducing bright lights, placing an ice pack to the head over the area of pain,** and **giving oxygen via nasal cannula.**

36. b

37. **a:** Treatment includes **administering high-concentration oxygen,** placing him into the *most comfortable position* and *promptly* transporting him to the hospital. Administration of 50% dextrose is *contraindicated* in the presence of possible stroke.

38. Answers to crossword puzzle

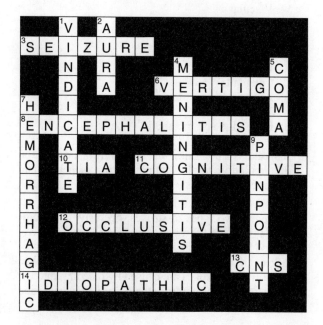

CHAPTER 29

1. a

2. **Right upper quadrant** (RUQ): liver, gallbladder, part of the large intestine, right kidney; **left upper quadrant** (LUQ): stomach, spleen, pancreas, part of the large intestine, left kidney; **right lower quadrant** (RLQ): appendix, part of the large intestine, right ovary, right ureter, uterus, urinary bladder; **left lower quadrant** (LLQ): part of the large intestine, left ovary, left ureter, uterus, urinary bladder.

3. Common causes of acute abdominal pain include **bacterial contamination, chemical irritation, peritoneal inflammation, bleeding,** and **obstruction.**

4. d

5. *a. Acute myocardial infarction:* the pain of AMI may occur anywhere from the umbilicus upward; **b. Ruptured abdominal aortic aneurysm:** an outpouching of the abdominal portion of the aorta caused by atherosclerosis. Severe abdominal and back pain, as well as shock, results. The patient may easily bleed to death. **c. Ruptured ectopic pregnancy:** occurs when the fertilized egg implants outside the uterus. Internal structures may rupture, causing severe internal bleeding. **d. Ruptured viscus:** rupture of any hollow organ; produces sudden onset of sharp epigastric pain and shock; the abdomen is rigid.

6. c

7. a

8. d

9. **a. Appendicitis:** results from obstruction of the lumen of the appendix. The patient initially has pain around the umbilicus that then localizes to the right lower quadrant. Loss of appetite (anorexia) is common; **b. Cholecystitis:** occlusion of the gallbladder duct, leading to inflammation and pain. The pain is usually intermittent, located in the right upper quadrant, and accompanied by nausea. Pain may radiate to the posterior scapula or right shoulder; **c. Pyelonephritis:** kidney infection that leads to flank pain, which may radiate to the abdomen, discomfort with urination, nausea, and vomiting; **d. Diverticulitis:** infection of small, saclike outpouchings in the intestine that causes cramplike abdominal pain in the left lower quadrant. May be accompanied by fever, diarrhea, or constipation; **e. Bowel obstruction:** blockage of the intestinal tract that produces cramping pain, vomiting, abdominal tenderness, and distention of the abdomen.

10. **False:** The abdominal organs *have nerve receptors for pressure, but not for pain*. For this reason, patients with an acute abdominal condition complain of localized or diffuse pain.

11. **True**

12. **False:** The EMT-I should *always* ask the patient about recent weight loss and *when his or her last meal was.*

13. Patients with acute abdominal conditions **may be lying extremely still or writhing in pain.**

14. The abdomen may be soft, **rigid,** or **distended.** There may be localized or diffuse **tenderness** to palpation. **Rigidity** means that the abdomen feels rigid to palpation. **Guarding** is voluntary or involuntary resistance to your touch.

15. **False:** Allow the patient to lie in a comfortable position. Many times the best position is *flat on the back or on the side with the knees drawn up*. Patients experiencing abdominal pain should not be given anything by mouth.

16. **True**

17. **True**

18. **a**

19. Common causes of upper GI bleeding include **peptic ulcer disease, gastritis,** and **esophagitis.**

20. Common causes of lower GI bleeding include **diverticulosis, tumors, hemorrhoids,** and **polyps.**

21. The common cause of upper GI bleeding in alcoholic patients is esophageal **varices.**

22. **a:** The new medication, indomethacin (Indocin), has GI bleeding as a side effect and is the likely cause of the problem.

23. **a:** Other treatments include starting an IV line of *normal saline or lactated Ringer's solution,* giving a fluid bolus as per local protocol, anticipating vomiting and being prepared to suction the patient, and giving nothing by mouth. Placing the patient into a semisitting position on the cot is *contraindicated because the blood flow to the brain would be decreased.* The preferred position for this patient is a *supine* position with the legs elevated. Having the patient breathe into

a paper sack is contraindicated because the patient is hyperventilating as a result of shock. In shock, the cells are deprived of necessary oxygen, and cellular depression and cellular death may result. The treatment of choice is to **administer high-concentration oxygen**. *Some* protocols may call for applying and inflating the pneumatic antishock garment.

24. **d:** Keeping the nonrebreather mask in place may lead to aspiration of the vomitus.

25. **d**

26. **Hematochezia** is the presence of bright red blood in the stool. **Melena** is black, tarry stool caused by digested blood passing slowly through the GI tract. **Hematemesis** is the vomiting of blood. Coffee ground vomitus is the vomiting of liquid resembling coffee grounds. The appearance is caused by digestion of the blood by stomach acid.

27. Answers to crossword puzzle

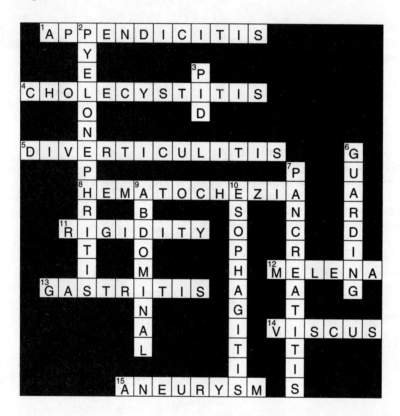

CHAPTER 30

1. An environmental emergency is **a medical condition caused or exacerbated by weather, terrain, atmospheric pressure, or other local factors.**

2. Preexisting risk factors that make environmental emergencies dangerous include **climate, season, weather, atmosphere,** and **terrain**.

3. **Extremes of age (small children, geriatric patients); poor health; fatigue; predisposing medical conditions; and certain medications.**

4. Environmental illnesses can be divided into two categories, **systemic** and **localized.** Regarding emergency care, **systemic** problems are more potentially harmful than are **localized** ones.

5. **d**

6. **True**

7. **False:** A *rectal* temperature most accurately measures core temperature.

8. **Thermolysis** refers to normal body means of heat loss and gain. Heat is generated by muscular **activity** and through **metabolic** reactions in the body.

9. **a. Radiation:** transmission of heat through space; **b. Conduction:** transmission of heat from warmer to cooler objects in direct contact; examples are touching a cold surface or lying on a cold floor; **c. Convection:** examples are wind chill, cold water exposure; **d. Evaporation:** loss of heat at the surface from vaporization of liquid; examples are sweating, spraying water mist on the body to keep cool while sunbathing.

10. Heat is lost **during respiration; the majority is thought to be caused by evaporation.**

11. **b**

12. **False:** As the ambient temperature approaches body temperature, *radiation is no longer effective to dissipate heat*. The body may pick up heat by conduction and convection.

13. **False:** At high temperatures, evaporation becomes the only effective method of heat dissipation. *High humidity seriously impairs heat dissipation because evaporation occurs slowly.*

14. Heat illness is defined as **increased** core body temperature caused by inadequate **thermolysis.**

15. **Extremes of age markedly increase a person's sensitivity to both heat and cold. Underlying diabetes often leads to autonomic neuropathy. This interferes with heat regulation by affecting vasodilation and perspiration. Medications, especially antihistamines, also impair the body's ability to sweat and eliminate heat.**

16. **d**

17. Signs and symptoms associated with heat cramps include **muscle twitching, followed by painful spasms, especially involving the lower extremities and abdomen, nausea and vomiting, weakness,** and **diaphoresis.**

18. **c:** Signs and symptoms of heat exhaustion include **diaphoresis;** the skin is usually *cold and clammy and the face gray*. The patient may complain of feeling dizzy, weak, or faint with accompanying nausea or headache. The vital signs may be normal, although the pulse is often rapid. The body temperature is usually *normal or slightly elevated.*

19. **a**

20. **b:** Heatstroke or sunstroke, a failure of the body's temperature regulation mechanisms, is an extreme medical emergency. Heatstroke develops when the body is no longer able to get rid of heat. Unlike the heat exhaustion victim, the person in heatstroke sweats very little or not at all. Usually, the skin is hot, red, and dry. As heat accumulates, body temperature can reach a dangerously high level.

21. **c:** An oxygen flow rate of **6 L/min via nonrebreather mask** is too low. Treatment includes having her rest, moving her to a cool environment (such as an air-conditioned ambulance), removing her clothing, and misting her with tepid water and fanning her. Rapid cooling is vital for the victim of heatstroke. Time is extremely important. If the victim's body temperature is not quickly lowered, permanent brain damage may result. Also give high-concentration oxygen by mask; start one or two IV lines (normal saline or lactated Ringer's solution); monitor the ECG; and wrap the patient with wet sheets if there is good ambient airflow present. Do not postpone transport to cool the patient in the field; transport the patient to the hospital as soon as possible. Use the air conditioner in your ambulance, as well as any available fans, to cool the patient.

22. Generalized hypothermia is a condition in which the core or internal body temperature is less than **95° F** as a result of either decreased production of **heat** or increased heat **loss** from the body.

23. Primary causes of hypothermia include **cold water immersion, cold weather exposure,** and **"urban hypothermia."**

24. **False:** *Cold water immersion* is the principal cause of death following boating accidents.

25. **True**

26. **True**

27. **c**

28. Predisposing factors of hypothermia include **any elderly person living alone, especially one with chronic disease or who has suffered a stroke; people who are intoxicated with alcohol; children younger than 1 year; victims of submersion injury, especially in cold water; patients suffering head trauma, especially if the accident occurred outdoors; any patient with a history of trauma and subsequent blood loss with shock; and getting lost or immobilized in cold weather, especially if the individual is wet.**

29. **True**

30. **False:** Victims of hypothermia stop shivering when the body temperature is below *90° F.*

31. a

32. a

33. b

34. a

35. d

36. **c:** Hypothermia is a condition in which the core or internal body temperature is less than 95° F as a result of either decreased production of heat or increased heat loss from the body. In severe hypothermia, the body functions slow dramatically, even to the point where the heartbeat is less than 10 BPM. Severe hypothermia is a life-threatening condition that requires specialized care (preferably in an appropriate definitive care setting).

37. **d:** Treatment for this patient includes **assisting respirations** with 100% oxygen. Oxygen and assisted ventilations are important because the body cells need oxygen and waste products of metabolism (CO_2) need to be removed. Rewarming the patient is generally *contraindicated* as a treatment of hypothermia (in the prehospital setting) unless the transport time to the hospital is longer than 1 hour. Check the pulse for 30 to 45 seconds before beginning chest compressions. CPR is *used only if the patient is in cardiac arrest*. Handle these patients gently. Rough handling (as well as intubation attempts) may precipitate cardiac dysrhythmias, including ventricular fibrillation. Start an IV line because hypothermic persons tend to be dehydrated. Consider a fluid bolus of normal saline or lactated Ringer's solution as rapidly as possible, if allowed by local protocol.

38. Cold may affect the **potency** of first-line **cardiac** drugs. There is no increased risk of inducing ventricular fibrillation (VF) from **orotracheal** or **nasotracheal** intubation as long as the patient is **preoxygenated** adequately. **Rough** handling, however, *can* induce VF.

39. **False:** The most common dysrhythmias in hypothermia-associated cardiac arrest are *VF* and asystole.

40. **True:** The risks of VF are related to both the depth and duration of hypothermia. It is generally impossible to electrically defibrillate a hypothermic heart that is colder than 86° F.

41. **False:** The use of lidocaine and procainamide should be avoided in patients with hypothermia because they *paradoxically decrease the VF threshold, increasing the resistance to defibrillation.*

42. **True**

43. **If down time is greater than 4 to 5 minutes (which is typical for hypothermic patients), consider performing 2 minutes (5 cycles of 30:2 compressions to ventilations) before defibrillation attempt for VF/pulseless VT. After defibrillation, perform 2 minutes of CPR, and then perform a pulse check. Administer a vasopressor (like epinephrine) after the first shock and an antidysrhythmic (like amiodarone) after the second shock.**

44. Drowning is defined as **death caused by asphyxiation during an immersion episode**. Near-drowning **occurs when the process of drowning is interrupted or reversed—a submersion episode with at least transient recovery.**

45. **d**

46. **a. Dry:** these victims have the best chance of survival; asphyxiation is caused by anoxia as a result of laryngeal spasm that prevents the entrance of water, as well as air, into the lungs. This leads to cerebral anoxia, edema, and unconsciousness; **b. Wet:** involves 80% to 90% of cases; victim makes a violent respiratory effort, and fluid fills the lungs; **c. Secondary:** recurrence of respiratory distress (usually in the form of pulmonary edema or aspiration pneumonia) after successful recovery from the initial incident.

47. **b:** With saltwater drowning, **the presence of a concentrated fluid in the lung causes an influx of hypotonic serum into the alveoli, leading to pulmonary edema.** This fills the alveoli and leads to a large shunt with profound hypoxemia (i.e., blood cannot exchange oxygen and carbon dioxide with filled alveoli, and they are bypassed).

48. Signs of near-drowning include **progressive dyspnea; wheezing or other extraneous lung sounds; tachycardia; cyanosis; high, low, or normal temperature; chest pains; and mental confusion.** Coma and respiratory or cardiac arrest can also occur.

49. **c**

50. **a:** If there is any possibility of neck injury (e.g., diving accident), stabilize the neck before removing the patient from the water. Also monitoring the ECG, placing an IV of *normal saline or lactated Ringer's* solution TKO, maintaining body temperature, and transporting to an appropriate medical facility all are indicated.

51. **All submersion victims must be transported to the hospital. Even if patients initially appear to be**

fine, they can deteriorate rapidly. **Pulmonary edema is especially likely.** Late deterioration occurs in about 1 of 20 near-drowning victims. It usually occurs within 4 hours, but with saltwater immersion, latent periods of up to 46 hours have been reported.

52. **a**

53. **b:** Treatment includes **immediately performing emergency needle thoracostomy,** administering high-concentration oxygen via *nonrebreather mask,* placing her in a *Trendelenburg position (feet elevated) or on her left side (left lateral decubitus position),* and promptly transporting her to an appropriate treatment facility.

54. Acute mountain sickness (AMS) **occurs after rapid ascent by an unacclimatized person to elevations in excess of 8000 feet.** Symptoms usually develop within 4 to 6 hours of reaching elevation and may last 3 to 4 days.

55. Signs and symptoms of AMS include **dizziness, headache, irritability, breathlessness,** and **euphoria.** Older persons and those with underlying cardiac or respiratory disorders may suffer pulmonary edema or heart failure. If AMS becomes severe, the victim may experience an altered level of consciousness and impaired judgment. Coma often follows.

56. **b:** HAPE **is caused by increased pulmonary artery pressure that develops in response to hypoxia.** This leads to the *release of various vasoactive substances that increase alveolar permeability; fluid then leaks into the alveoli, and pulmonary edema occurs.* Symptoms often begin *24 to 72* hours after exposure.

57. **a:** HACE **is the most severe form of high-altitude illness.** Patients have signs of AMS and a progressively worsening level of consciousness. Progression from mild AMS to HACE and unconsciousness usually takes 1 to 3 days. It may occur, however, within hours of altitude exposure. HACE rapidly progresses to coma and death without treatment. Thus the patient must be transported to an appropriate facility as soon as possible.

58. **a:** Frostbite is the formation of ice crystals within the tissues. These crystals damage the blood vessels and other tissues. Eventually, frostbitten tissues may die. Initially with frostbite, the affected area **appears waxy, yellowish white, or bluish white.** Whether the skin of a frostbite victim feels soft or firm to frozen *depends on the severity of injury*. In severe frostbite, the area is hard to the touch, cold, and insensitive to pain.

59. **d:** Do *not* allow the patient to smoke. This constricts blood vessels and aggravates hypoxemia to the involved area. Do *not* rewarm frostbite in the field. An exception is if a limb is frozen to an object that cannot be moved. In this case, warm the area just enough to move the patient. Rubbing the affected area is *contraindicated* because the ice crystals that have formed beneath the skin (in the interstitial spaces) may severely damage cells of the tissues when rubbed back and forth.

60. Answers to crossword puzzle

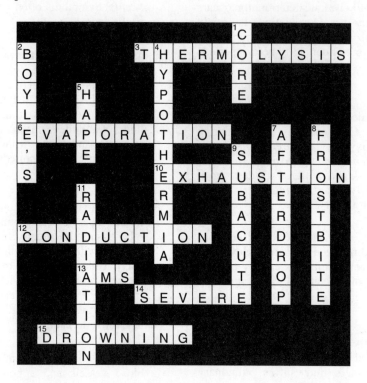

CHAPTER 31

1. *Behavior* is defined as **how a person acts.**

2. **b**

3. **A behavioral emergency is a situation in which the patient feels he or she has, in some way, lost control of his or her life.**

4. Causes of behavioral emergencies can be **biological/organic, psychosocial, or sociocultural.**

5. **c**

6. **False:** Management of behavioral emergencies consists of *first* building good rapport with the patient. You must speak in a calm, even voice and exhibit a willingness to listen to the patient. Be honest. Describe everything you intend to do step by step to the patient. Avoid any sudden moves.

7. **False:** Allow the patient to express anger and frustration *verbally instead of physically.*

8. **True:** Looking someone directly in the eye is often taken as a challenge or threat.

9. Clues that the patient may develop violent behavior include:
   - **Pacing back and forth; unable to keep one position for more than a couple of seconds**
   - **Appearing to get more and more angry as he or she speaks**
   - **Starting to act out, such as thrashing out with the arms, hitting the wall, throwing things**
   - **Bragging about how tough he or she is**
   - **Any domestic violence–related situation, particularly when the alleged perpetrator is still present**
   - **Any patient who is intoxicated or on drugs of abuse**
   - **If the patient persistently complains about your EMS system or the service received in the past by the patient or his or her family**
   - **Males are more likely than females to exhibit violent behavior**

10. **a**

11. Things the EMT-I should pay attention to while assessing the behavioral emergency patient include **general appearance, hygiene and dress, motor activity, physical complaints, intellectual function, thought content, language,** and **mood.**

12. **Neurosis** is an abnormal anxiety reaction to a perceived fear. There is no basis in reality for that fear. **Psychosis** is when the patient has no concept whatsoever of reality. The person truly believes his or her situation or condition is real—often the person hears voices.

13. In drug-induced **psychosis**, hallucinogens or stimulant agents cause the patient to lose touch with reality.

14. Signs and symptoms of depression include **an unkempt appearance, speech that is different from usual, frequent crying bouts, abnormally increased or decreased appetite,** and **sleep disturbances.**

15. **c:** This is when the patient has a true desire to die. Often the person has planned the event—purchased a gun, driven far out of town, or gotten a double refill of a prescription medication.

16. **d:** Treatment includes **inserting an oropharyngeal airway** and assisting his ventilations with a *bag-mask device and 100% oxygen*. Also watch for vomiting, be prepared to suction, monitor the ECG, place an IV line and monitor for shock, and provide care as appropriate. Give naloxone if directed by medical direction (to rule out other drugs that may have been taken). Last, notify law enforcement officials as required by local protocol.

17. **a**

18. **False:** Alcohol abuse is defined as medical, behavioral, or social problems related to excessive alcohol consumption. Alcohol abuse is not the same as alcoholism, which is a chronic condition characterized by dependence on alcohol and a pattern of abnormal behavior.

19. **True:** Alcohol tends to potentiate, or increase the strength of many drugs, especially sleeping pills and other depressants.

20. **c:** Signs and symptoms of alcohol intoxication include **slurred, loud, and inappropriate speech;** *unsteady* gait; *flushed* face; odor of alcohol on the breath; nausea; vomiting; altered level of consciousness; abnormal behavior that ranges from elation to violence; and injuries, often from unexplained sources.

21. **d:** Serious conditions that mimic alcohol intoxication include head injury, drug abuse, brain tumor, hypoglycemia, meningitis, stroke, postictal state, and diabetic ketoacidosis.

22. Severely intoxicated patients should be transported to the hospital because **it is possible that another illness may be present. Severely intoxicated patients are a danger to themselves and to others. These patients should be evaluated medically and observed for a period of time in the emergency department.**

23. **b**

24. **Drug addiction** is a condition characterized by an overwhelming desire to continue taking a drug to which one has become "hooked" through repeated consumption because it produces a particular effect.

25. **Drug dependence** is a psychological craving for, or a psychological reliance on, a chemical agent, resulting from abuse or addiction.

26. **Drug withdrawal** is a set of signs and symptoms that develop in a person following abrupt cessation of taking a drug.

27. **a. Stimulants (uppers):** include cocaine, amphetamines, and "ice." Symptoms include hyperactivity, euphoria, tachycardia, hypertension, dilated pupils, diaphoresis, sleeplessness, seizures, and disorientation. Cocaine causes hypertensive crises, seizures, myocardial infarction, and stroke; **b. Narcotics:** include heroin, morphine, methadone, meperidine (Demerol), hydromorphone (Dilaudid), pentazocine (Talwin), codeine, hydrocodone (Vicodin), and propoxyphene (Darvon). Symptoms include drowsiness, coma, impaired coordination, sweating, respiratory depression, constricted pupils, shock, convulsions, and coma. Respiratory and cardiac arrest is possible; **c: Hallucinogens:** lysergic acid diethylamide (LSD), mescaline, psilocybin, and phencyclidine (PCP or angel dust). Symptoms include hallucinations, unpredictable behavior, tachypnea, nausea, dilated pupils, and increased pulse and blood pressure; **d. Depressants (downers):** include marijuana, barbiturates, sleeping pills, tranquilizers, and antidepressant pills. Symptoms include sluggishness, poor coordination, slurred speech, decreased respiration or respiratory arrest, and impaired memory and judgment.

28. **c**

29. **b:** Treatment includes assisting the patient's breathing with a bag-mask device and 100% supplemental oxygen, establishing an IV line, and **administering 0.4 to 2.0 mg of naloxone, IV push.** In addition, give D_{50} if indicated by blood glucose assessment.

30. Answers to crossword puzzle

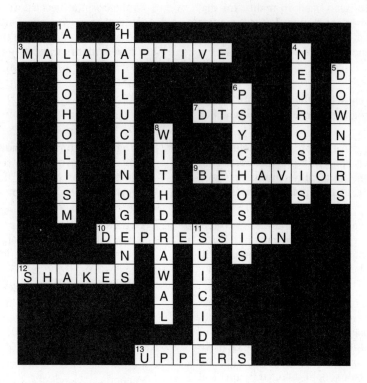

CHAPTER 32

1. **A.** ovary
   B. fallopian tube
   C. vagina
   D. cervix
   E. uterus

2. **b:** The menstrual cycle **is vaginal bleeding that typically occurs every 28 days** when an egg *does not implant* in the uterus.

3. **c:** Menarche **is the first menstrual cycle that the woman experiences.** It typically occurs at age 12 but can occur anywhere from the age of 8 to 14.

4. **If an egg is fertilized by sperm and implants within the endometrium, the pregnancy begins, and the woman typically has no further menses.**

5. **False:** Although not typically associated with the high acuity of critical trauma or cardiac patients, *women experiencing acute gynecological emergencies can have significant hemorrhage or overwhelming infection that can cause shock and be life threatening.*

6. **True**

7. **True**

8. Questions asked of patients experiencing gynecological emergencies include: **Is there any pain or cramping? Is there any radiation of the pain? When did the pain or cramping start? Is there any vaginal bleeding or vaginal discharge? Is there any nausea, vomiting, or change in appetite? Is there any fever? Is there any diaphoresis or sweating? Has the patient experienced any change in her normal bowel habits, including diarrhea or constipation? Is there any frequency of urination, pain with urination, or blood noted during urination?**

9. **d**

10. **d**

11. Causes of tachycardia in patients with acute gynecological emergencies include **dehydration, blood loss with anemia, infection (including sepsis), pain,** and **anxiety**.

12. **True**

13. **False:** Guarding may be present when the patient either has voluntary or involuntary tightening of the abdominal wall muscles. This is in response to *significant irritation and inflammation* within the abdominal cavity.

14. **False:** If the patient has significant pain *following the release of pressure on the abdomen (during deep palpation)*, it is considered a positive rebound tenderness test.

15. Rebound tenderness is elicited by **slowly pressing down at a specific point on the abdomen and then quickly releasing. If the patient has significant pain following the release of pressure, this is considered a positive rebound tenderness test.** It is a sign of significant intraabdominal inflammation.

16. **d**

17. **a**

18. **During the menstrual cycle, hormonal stimulation causes follicles on the ovaries to enlarge during the midcycle phase. Large follicles are generally considered cysts, and the presence of the cyst itself may cause pain. Rupture of an ovarian cyst can cause severe intense lower abdominal pain that is typically located on one side of the abdomen. Some ruptured cysts are associated with significant hemorrhage into the pelvis, and the patient may become hypotensive.**

19. **c**

20. **a:** Ectopic pregnancy occurs when a fertilized egg implants itself anywhere outside the uterus, usually in the fallopian tube. This implantation can also occur anywhere, including in an ovary, the cervix, or the abdominal cavity. The developing embryo cannot grow in the limited space available within the fallopian tube and will eventually stretch the tube to the point of rupture.

21. **a:** Treatment for this patient includes maintaining ABCs, **administering 100% oxygen via nonrebreather mask,** suspecting shock and treating it accordingly, considering the application of the PASG if shock is present, keeping the patient warm, helping the patient assume a comfortable position, and reassessing vital signs every 5 to 10 minutes.

22. **c:** Note that *14- to 16-gauge* needles should be used; *macro*drip administration sets are preferred; and the IVs should be infused at a *wide-open* rate.

23. **a**

24. **c:** Treatment of the female with vaginal bleeding includes **establishing a second IV line if shock is present.** Additionally, placing the patient in the *Trendelenburg position* with the head down and feet elevated facilitates blood flow to the CNS and vital organs. A count of the number of sanitary pads the patient has used, as well as other towels or clothing that are soaked in blood, may help determine the volume and rate of bleeding. The EMT-I *should not pack any dressing in the vagina* in an attempt to tamponade or slow the bleeding. *A high concentration of oxygen* should be administered in the presence of shock.

25. **d**

26. Answers to crossword puzzle

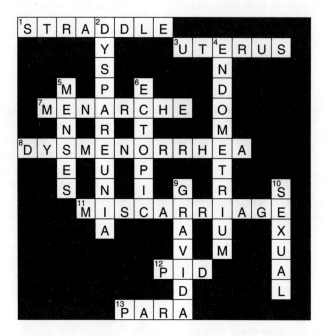

CHAPTER 33

1. **a. Ovaries:** walnut-sized pair of glands located on each side of the uterus in the upper pelvic cavity; produce mature eggs and secrete primarily female sexual hormones; **b. Fallopian tubes:** pair of muscular tubes that extend from the uterus to the pelvic cavity; provide a passageway for the transport of sperm to the egg (ova) and transport of the ova back to the uterus by wavelike, muscular contractions; **c. Uterus:** hollow, muscular organ shaped like an inverted pear located in the pelvic cavity; **d. Cervix:** inferior narrow portion of the uterus where it opens into the vagina; dilates to allow the baby and placenta to pass into the birth canal or vagina during labor; **e. Vagina:** The birth canal or passageway between the uterus and the external opening in a female; **f. Perineum:** external female genital region between the urinary opening (urethra) and the anus or rectal opening.

2. **b:** The placenta **provides for the exchange of respiratory gases and transport of nutrients from the mother to the fetus,** produces several important hormones, plays a role in the excretion of waste products or the transfer of heat, and is attached to the developing fetus by the *umbilical cord*.

3. **c**

4. **a:** The amniotic sac **consists of membranes that surround and protect the developing fetus,** contains approximately *500 to 1000* mL of amniotic fluid, and normally ruptures by the *second stage of labor* if not before.

5. **c**

6. A. **umbilical cord**
   B. **placenta**
   C. **fetus**
   D. **amniotic sac**
   E. **cervix**
   F. **anus**

7. **a. Postpartum:** the time after delivery of the infant; **b. Primipara:** a woman who has delivered her first child; **c. Gravidity:** the number of times a woman has been pregnant; **d. Natal:** means birth; **e. Multipara:** a woman who has had two or more deliveries.

8. **b**

9. **a: Missed or late menstrual period** is a sign of early pregnancy. Other signs and symptoms include nausea and vomiting (which may occur *at any time of the day*), breast *tenderness and enlargement,* and *increased* urinary frequency.

10. **b:** During pregnancy, **uterine blood flow increases from 2% to 20% of cardiac output.** Other cardiovascular changes are that maternal blood volume and

cardiac output are increased up to *50%*, pulmonary functional residual capacity is *decreased,* and maternal heart rate, minute volume, and oxygen consumption are *increased.*

Pregnant patients also develop increased respiratory rate and depth. The reason is that during the fourth to fifth month, the fetus begins to take up increased space in the abdominal cavity and compromises the ability of the diaphragm to flatten completely. The expectant mother may become tachypneic to compensate for this decreased volume of the thoracic cavity. Respiratory alkalosis can develop as a result of the increased respiratory rate.

11. There tends to be **decreased motility of the gastrointestinal (GI) organs and upward displacement of the diaphragm during pregnancy. This results in a decrease in movement of foodstuffs through the GI tract.** For this reason, there is an increased risk of vomiting and aspiration in the later stages of pregnancy, and heartburn is common.

12. At approximately 20 weeks' gestation, the **weight of the pregnant uterus may compress the inferior vena cava when the mother is in a supine position. This results in hypotension and a restriction of blood flow to the placenta.** Although easily relieved, this situation can be fatal to the fetus if uncorrected.

13. **c:** To prevent supine hypotensive syndrome from occurring, the pregnant patient should be positioned **on her left side** rather than in a supine position. In pregnant trauma victims, apply immobilizing devices as you normally would, using caution to not compress the uterus with the straps. Once the patient is immobilized, the backboard should be tilted to 15 degrees to the left, placing the patient with her left side down.

14. **c:** Appendicitis **is more difficult to assess during pregnancy** (especially in the last two trimesters) and occurs in 1 of every *1000* pregnancies. The appendix is two to three times more likely to rupture in the pregnant patient. Care for the pregnant patient experiencing appendicitis includes giving her nothing by mouth, administering oxygen, considering an IV line, and transporting her left side down.

15. **d:** Eclampsia is present when a pregnant patient experiences **coma and convulsions.** Signs and symptoms of preeclampsia (the condition that can lead to eclampsia) include visual disturbances and headache, fluid retention (edema), excessive weight gain, epigastric abdominal pain, and decreased urine output. The vital signs include an elevated blood pressure and irritability or change in mental status.

16. **d:** Treatment of a patient experiencing eclampsia includes ensuring that the ABCs are secured, administering a *high concentration of oxygen,* starting an IV line and running it at a *keep open* rate, placing the patient on her left side, and providing seizure care as needed (protecting the airway and patient from injury, using medications to stop the seizure and control the blood pressure if local protocol allows). To avoid precipitating seizures in these patients, the **emergency lights or sirens should not be used during transport.** Notify the receiving hospital of your patient's status and your ETA.

17. **c:** If the placenta implants low in the uterus, it will be the presenting part. At the onset of labor with the dilation of the cervix, the placenta will begin to detach. Once the placenta delivers or begins to separate, the fetus will not receive oxygen or nutrients. This will prove life threatening to the fetus.

18. Factors that predispose patients to placenta previa include **multiple pregnancies, rapid succession of pregnancies, mothers older than age 35,** and **previous history of placenta previa.**

19. Typically, the placenta previa patient presents with **profuse painless bright red bleeding from the vagina.** The uterus may be soft or may develop contractions.

20. **c:** This condition is **abruptio placentae.** It is the premature detachment of a normally situated placenta. The detachment may be complete or partial and can occur in any stage of pregnancy, but it is usually a third trimester complication.

21. **a:** Treatment for this patient includes **administering high-concentration oxygen via nonrebreather mask;** starting one or two IVs of lactated Ringer's solution; continuously monitoring her vital signs; placing her on the left side; considering PASG application but inflating *the legs only*; rapid, gentle transport to the closest appropriate hospital with OB neonatal care; notifying the receiving hospital to alert the obstetrics staff; and reassuring the patient.

22. Indications of labor include **ruptured membranes, contractions, bloody "show," pain, transition, urge to push,** and **crowning.**

23. **b**

24. **a. Crowning:** occurs when the presenting part of the baby first bulges from the vaginal opening; **b. Breech birth:** situation in which the buttocks or both feet of the baby deliver first; **c. Cephalic delivery:** head-first delivery of the newly born; **d. Third stage of labor:** the time from the delivery of the baby to the delivery of the placenta; **e. Contraction time:** the time from the beginning of contraction to when the uterus relaxes.

25. Delivery is imminent when a woman with her first pregnancy **has the urge to move her bowels, the "bag of waters" has broken, and crowning is present.**

26. **b**

27. **c:** Treatment includes **placing her in a breathing position and waiting at the scene until the baby is born.** Oxygen also should be administered to the expectant mother and an IV placed according to local protocol.

28. **a**

29. **d:** When the umbilical cord is wrapped around the baby's neck during delivery, you should avoid applying excessive tension on the cord, slip the cord over the baby's head, and clamp the cord in two places and cut it between the clamps. You should not **apply steady pressure on the infant's head to delay delivery until after arrival at the hospital.**

30. **d**

31. **b**

32. **d:** Meconium is a fetal waste substance. **Its presence during delivery indicates fetal respiratory distress.** If aspirated, the baby may suffer severe respiratory damage. Thick, dark meconium is associated with more severe aspiration. To prevent aspiration the baby's airway must be suctioned *before* the first breath. After deep suctioning of the baby, encourage the mother to push and deliver the shoulders. Avoid excessive stimulation of the nares until thorough suctioning is complete. To remove thick meconium from the airway, the EMT-I may need to perform direct laryngoscopy and suction below the vocal cords. This should be done before the baby's first breath.

33. **d:** This will reduce the bleeding by constricting the uterus. The EMT-I also can massage the mother's *lower* abdomen. This will also stimulate uterine contractions and reduce bleeding following delivery of the placenta. Apply a maternity sanitary napkin and cold pack to the mother's perineal area. If heavy bleeding continues, establish a second IV line, and administer a fluid bolus.

34. **c**

35. **True:** If the baby starts breathing on his or her own, assess the respiratory rate and depth and heart rate. If the heart rate remains less than 100 BPM, continue to ventilate with 100% oxygen. If the baby's pulse is absent, is less than 60 BPM, or is between 60 and 80 BPM and does not increase even with 30 seconds of positive-pressure ventilation, initiate CPR.

36. **False:** During insertion of an oropharyngeal airway in an infant, it *should not be rotated* at a 180-degree angle as is done for adults. This may cause damage to the mouth and tongue. Instead, use a tongue depressor to hold the tongue in place while inserting the airway.

37. **d:** Using a sterile knife or scissors (provided in commercial obstetric kits), cut the cord between the clamps.

38. **b:** The rubbing action taken to dry the baby provides stimulation. Any wet towels should be discarded. In addition, the EMT-I should use a stockinette, blanket, or towel to cover the baby's head, wrap the infant in an infant swaddler and a warmed blanket or towel, and let the mother hold the infant on her abdomen.

39. **c**

40. **d**

41. **c:** A breech birth is identified by the *buttocks or lower extremities* being the presenting part, *can be delivered* in the field setting, **is treated by placing the mother in a head-down position and administering a high concentration of oxygen,** and requires immediate transport to the hospital.

42. **a. Breech delivery:** gloved hand is placed into the vagina with the palm toward the infant's face, a "V" is formed with the index and middle fingers on either side of the infant's nose, and the vaginal wall is pushed away from the infant's face to allow unrestricted respiration; **b. Prolapsed cord:** two fingers of a gloved hand are inserted into the vagina to raise the presenting part of the fetus off the cord, the cord is checked for pulsations, and the mother is placed in a knee-chest position; **c. Abruptio placentae:** premature detachment of a normally situated placenta; **d. Placenta previa:** the attachment of the placenta very low in the uterus so that it partially or completely covers the internal cervical opening; most common sign associated with condition is painless, bright red vaginal bleeding; **e. Preeclampsia:** disorder of pregnancy marked by hypertension, abnormal weight gain, edema, headache, protein in urine, epigastric pain, and occasionally visual disturbances.

43. Cephalopelvic disproportion **occurs when the relative size of the fetus in respect to the pelvis may compromise a normal delivery.** The fetus may be abnormally large, as in a woman with diabetes, or a past due delivery. The pelvis may also be unusually small, most often seen in primiparous women.

44. Things that may cause postpartum hemorrhage include **vaginal or cervical tears and lacerations, retained placenta,** and **bleeding or clotting disorders.**

45. Answers to crossword puzzle

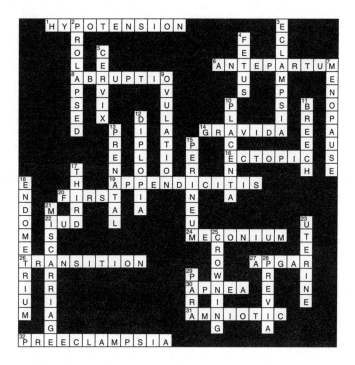

CHAPTER 34

1. **b:** A baby is considered a *newborn* or newly born during the first few hours of life. A neonate is a **baby during the first 28 days of life.** *After that time,* the baby is referred to as an infant.

2. **c:** Infants who **are born at low birth weight** are 20 times more likely to die within the first month of life than are newly borns who have weights greater than 2500 g.

3. The younger the newly born's gestational age at birth, the **greater** the mortality risk, especially if the infant is less than **32** weeks of gestation.

4. Intrauterine events that result in low birth weight include **decreased placental perfusion; infection; maternal complications of pregnancy; lack of prenatal care; and complications involving the placenta, cord, and membranes.**

5. The higher incidence of prematurity and low birth weight in infants born to teenagers is **a result of the developmental stage of the mother or a reflection of multiple factors associated with teenage pregnancies, including poor nutrition, lower socioeconomic status, ongoing disease, and late or no prenatal care (or perhaps both).**

6. **a**

7. **c**

8. **a:** The primary stimuli that help initiate respiration in the neonate after delivery are **low oxygen and high carbon dioxide levels, and a low pH,** as well as the excitation of sensory impulses in the skin that occurs with the abrupt change in temperature when the fetus moves from a *warm* environment to the *cooler* atmosphere—these impulses are transmitted to the respiratory center.

9. During delivery **the pulmonary capillaries and lymphatic vessels remove fetal lung fluid. Some fluid is also removed during the normal forces of labor and delivery. As the chest emerges from the birth canal, fluid is squeezed from the lungs through the nose and mouth. Following complete emergence of the neonate's chest, a brisk recoil of the thorax occurs. Air enters the upper airway to replace the lost fluid.**

10. **d**

11. The transition from fetal circulation to postnatal circulation involves the functional closure of the **foramen ovale** and ductus **arteriosus.**

12. The most important factor controlling ductal closure is the increased **oxygen** concentration of the blood.

13. Next to establishing respiration, **heat** regulation is most critical to the newly born's survival.

14. **False:** A full-term newly born has a blood volume of about 80 to 85 mL/kg of body weight. Immediately after birth, the total blood volume averages *300* mL.

15. **True**

16. **True**

17. **a**

18. **a**

19. **b:** The rubbing action taken to dry the baby provides stimulation. It also allows the baby to be kept warm until arrival at the hospital.

20. To keep the newly born warm, **wrap it in a different towel than the one that was used to wipe off the newly born. Then cover the head with a blanket, towel, or hat to prevent heat loss.**

21. **d**

22. **Touching, drying, and suctioning can stimulate breathing in the newly born experiencing primary apnea. Secondary apnea will not reverse with simple stimulation techniques and requires assisted ventilation.**

23. If the baby does not respond within 30 seconds to stimulation techniques described earlier, **it should be positioned with its head in a sniffing position. A rolled towel can be placed under the baby's shoulders** to promote good positioning, but the EMT-I should avoid hyperextending the head because this action may cause airway collapse.

24. **a**

25. **False:** During insertion of an oropharyngeal airway in the newly born, the airway *should not be rotated at a 180-degree angle* as is done for adults because it may cause damage to the baby's mouth and tongue. Instead, use a tongue depressor to hold the tongue in place while inserting the airway.

26. **True**

27. **False:** If the heart rate is below 100 BPM, ventilate with a *bag-mask device supplied with 100% oxygen* even if breathing is already present.

28. **b**

29. **b:** Acrocyanosis is **a bluish color to the hands and feet.** Many newly borns will have acrocyanosis for *up to 48 hours* after birth. This condition *does not require any additional therapy.*

30. Cyanosis may be present until the baby has begun to breathe air. This color is normal immediately after birth. If central cyanosis (bluish color to the trunk and face) persists after stimulation and breathing has started, it requires treatment with 100% oxygen. Hypoxia is present in this case and will not resolve without additional oxygen.

31. **c: Hypoxia** is the most common cause of cardiopulmonary arrest in the newly born. For this reason, initial therapy consists of ventilation and oxygenation.

32. a. Position, suction, tactile stimulation
    b. Oxygen
    c. Bag-mask ventilation
    d. Chest compressions
    e. Intubation
    f. Medications

33. **c: Verapamil** is not used to treat the newly born who is in cardiac arrest. Medications including atropine, epinephrine, lidocaine, and naloxone *may* be administered to treat the newly born who is in cardiac arrest.

34. The delivery of IV fluid therapy in the newly born should consist of **10 mL/kg of saline or lactated Ringer's solution given by syringe over a 5- to 10-minute period.**

35. Meconium aspiration syndrome (MAS) occurs when the newly born **inhales thick, sticky meconium. Once the meconium is swallowed or inhaled by the fetus, any gasping activity may cause the sticky and tenacious material to be aspirated into the lower airways. This can lead to partial airway obstruction, air trapping, and hyperinflation of the lungs distal to the obstruction. As the infant struggles to take in more air (air hunger), even more meconium may be aspirated. Hyperinflation, hypoxemia, and acidemia result in increased pulmonary vascular resistance.**

36. **True:** Those with more recent meconium passage may not be stained.

37. **False:** *Tachypnea, hypoxia, and a depressed mental state may be present at birth* in newly borns experiencing severe meconium aspiration. They develop expiratory grunting, nasal flaring, and retractions similar to those experienced by infants with respiratory distress syndrome.

Severe meconium aspiration progresses very rapidly to respiratory failure. These infants exhibit profound respiratory distress with gasping, ineffective ventilations, marked cyanosis and pallor, and hypotonia.

38. **a**

39. **b**

40. Answers to crossword puzzle

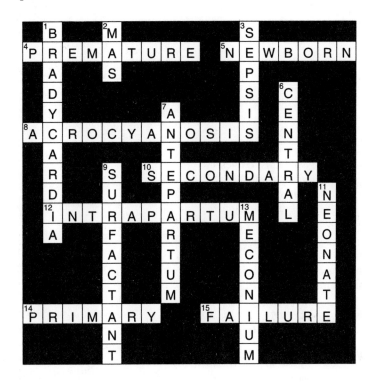

CHAPTER 35

1. **b**

2. **c:** A child is between **ages 1 and 8.** The term *infant* is used to refer to those individuals under the age of 1 year.

3. **False:** The key to determining medication dosages and providing treatment in pediatric cases is the *patient's weight*.

4. **c: The airway of a child younger than 8 years has a large and floppy epiglottis** and is narrowest at the *cricoid cartilage*. The overall size of the airway also is *smaller* in infants and children and is more likely to become occluded with foreign bodies, blood, vomit, or loose teeth.

5. The vocal cords of a child sit more **superior** and **anterior** on the cervical spine than in an adult. In infants the cords are located at approximately the **first** (or second) cervical vertebra. As the child grows, the cords begin to move **downward,** closer to the level of the third vertebra.

6. A. Tongue
   B. Palate
   C. Epiglottis
   D. Vocal cords
   E. Cricoid cartilage
   F. Trachea

7. **Many childhood accidents involve a head injury because the head of an infant and young child is**

so large. Cervical injuries also are more likely because the head is large and heavy and exerts more pressure on the cervical spine.

8. **c:** Fontanelles, or soft spots, on the *tops* of infants' heads are spaces between the bones of the cranium that are covered by a *tough membrane*. These fontanelles will bulge with any *increase* in intracranial pressure and be *depressed* when dehydration is present. The EMT-I should gently palpate the fontanelles during the infant's assessment.

9. **True:** This is because children's bones are softer and have less calcium and fewer other minerals as compared with an adult.

10. **False:** Because of the pliability of the *ribs, the underlying lung can be injured* without an overlying rib fracture.

11. **False:** An infant or child *does not know how to move out of the way* when an object suddenly comes at him or her. This is because the child's control of the nervous system is immature. Their nerves are not well insulated, and their reflexes are less developed.

12. **c:** The parents of an injured child **often require psychological assistance in dealing with their injured or ill child.** They *must be considered* part of the child's environment and must know what is happening. Further, *they may feel responsible* for the child receiving the injuries or that there was something they did or did not do to cause the injury.

13. **If the parents are calm, the EMT-I should make eye contact and have them assist with the care of their child. However, if the parents are not able to control their emotions, others should be sought at the scene to assist with the parents. The EMT-I should always keep the parents informed.**

14. The pediatric assessment triangle includes **appearance (mental status and muscle tone); work of breathing (respiratory rate and effort); and circulation (skin signs and color).**

15. **c:** The first sign of respiratory distress in an infant is usually **tachypnea.** Other signs of respiratory distress that may be present in infants or children are increased respiratory rate and/or effort, diminished breath sounds, decreased level of consciousness or response to parents or pain, poor skeletal muscle tone, and/or cyanosis.

16. **If an infant or child is acutely ill, a slow or irregular respiratory rate is a dismal sign. This usually indicates that the child's status is declining because of fatigue, central nervous system depression, or hypothermia.** Many times the child will be tachypneic for a period, become fatigued from working so hard, and slow his or her rate of breathing. Do not be fooled into thinking the child is improving because the respiratory rate decreases. In reality, the child may progress to respiratory arrest and possibly cardiac arrest if not treated aggressively.

17. **b:** Many of the usual heart rates for infants and children show *normal tachycardia*. Bradycardia usually occurs when the child *can no longer maintain adequate tissue oxygenation*. This is usually a precursor to cardiopulmonary arrest and should be treated quickly. Many times, proper oxygenation will cause the heart rate to *increase,* thus *increasing* the child's cardiac output.

18. **d:** Infants have short, chubby necks, which makes it extremely difficult to palpate the carotid artery. For this reason, rescuers should palpate the **brachial** artery on the inside of the upper arm between the infant's elbow and shoulder to determine the presence of a pulse. The carotid artery can be used for children older than 1 year of age.

19. **True**

20. **False:** The *tongue* is the primary cause of airway obstruction in the infant or child. Two other potential causes are foreign objects and swelling from infections. If the tongue is the culprit, reposition the head.

21. **c:** Suspect **foreign-body upper airway obstruction** in infants and children experiencing sudden onset respiratory distress with associated coughing, gagging, or stridor. Children often put everything they can into their mouths (e.g., small objects such as balloons, marbles, peanuts, coins, and small toys).

    A foreign body obstruction in the child can lead to a partial or complete airway obstruction. Partial airway obstruction may be associated with adequate air exchange or poor air exchange. The child with adequate air exchange can cough forcefully and has good color. Poor air exchange is characterized by an ineffective cough, high-pitched noises on inspiration, increased respiratory distress, and cyanosis. In complete airway obstruction, there is no air exchange.

22. The initial management of a child experiencing upper airway obstruction caused by a foreign body includes **administering subdiaphragmatic abdominal thrusts** (Heimlich maneuver).
    Remember, the EMT-I should only relieve an obstructed airway if:
    - The cough is (or becomes) ineffective
    - There is increased respiratory difficulty
    - The patient loses consciousness

First determine that poor air exchange or complete airway obstruction is present. Then make a fist by grasping your thumb with your right hand. Stand behind the patient, placing your fist on the midline just above the umbilicus. Reach around and place your left hand on top of your fisted right hand. Deliver quick upward and inward thrusts. Each thrust is delivered as a separate and distinct movement with the intent of relieving the obstruction.

Remember, there can be a rapid downhill progression from respiratory distress to respiratory failure and finally to cardiopulmonary arrest. Treatment decisions must be made quickly to avoid deterioration of the child's condition to cardiopulmonary arrest.

23. Indications for intubating a child include **inadequate central nervous system control of ventilation; functional or anatomical airway obstruction; excessive work of breathing leading to fatigue;** and **the need for high peak inspiratory pressure or positive end-expiratory pressure to maintain effective alveolar gas exchange.**

24. **d**

25. **b:** At this age their "natural cuffs" are at the level of the cricoid cartilage. A cuffed endotracheal tube should be used in children 8 to 10 years of age or older.

26. **c:** The ventilation rate for infants and children is 12 to 20 breaths/min in the patient with a perfusing rhythm but absent or inadequate respiratory effort. If an advanced airway is in place during CPR (e.g., ET, Combitube, LMA), ventilate at a rate of 8 to 10 breaths/min. Be sure that the oxygen is attached to the bag-mask device and is set to at least *15* L/min. It is best to use a bag-mask device that provides at least *450* cc of volume on pediatric patients. The infant bag-mask device only provides about 250 cc and should *not* be used because it cannot deliver enough tidal volume.

27. **False:** Keeping the head in a *neutral, sniffing position without hyperextension is usually adequate for infants and toddlers.* Hyperextension can occlude the infant's soft airway. Children older than 2 years of age do well with padding behind the head to displace the cervical spine anteriorly.

28. **False:** When using a nasal cannula to administer oxygen to a child, a flow rate of *between 2 and 4 L/min* should be used. Higher rates irritate the nasopharynx and do not substantially improve the child's oxygenation. If more oxygen is needed, switch to a face mask.

29. **a:** With intraosseous infusion a needle is inserted into the long bone of the leg; **intravenous fluids are infused into the marrow cavity of the bone;** the amount of fluid resuscitation is *comparable with* IV therapy; both fluids *and* drugs may be administered; and a *boring or twisting* motion is used to advance the needle through the bone.

This procedure should be used only in children who are unconscious and *only* after all other attempts at peripheral cannulation have failed (e.g., situations like cardiopulmonary arrest, shock from trauma, burns, and sepsis that leads to peripheral vascular collapse). Typically, local protocol dictates when an IO infusion can be attempted.

30. **c:** When administering fluid resuscitation therapy, *20*-mL/kg boluses of an *isotonic, crystalloid* solution should be administered, and **frequent reassessments are necessary to determine the need for additional fluid boluses.** Many times these boluses are given through a 35- to 50-mL syringe to facilitate rapid administration. Lactated Ringer's or normal saline solution can be used for this purpose. Do not use large volumes of dextrose-containing solutions because the child may become hyperglycemic.

31. **c**

32. **d:** As compared with adults, in whom ventricular fibrillation is the most common cause of cardiac arrest, children most often experience cardiopulmonary arrest secondary to hypoxemia, hypotension, and acidosis. These conditions interfere with normal function of the SA node and AV nodes and slow conduction through the normal conduction pathways. This leads to dysrhythmias such as sinus bradycardia, sinus node arrest with a slow junctional or ventricular escape, and asystole.

Asystole is characterized as a flat line on the ECG monitor; occasionally P waves are seen. Clinically, there is no pulse, absent spontaneous respirations, and poor perfusion.

33. Treatment for asystole includes:
    - **Continuing CPR**
    - **Ventilating her with a bag-mask device equipped with a reservoir and supplied with 10 to 15 L/min of oxygen**
    - **Performing endotracheal intubation using a number 3.5 to 4.0 ID uncuffed tube**
    - **Establishing an IV line using normal saline (or lactated Ringer's) solution**
    - **Administering epinephrine at an initial dose of 0.01 mg/kg (1:10,000) for the IV/IO routes and 0.1 mg/kg (1:1000) for the ET route**
    - **Repeating epinephrine at a dose of 0.01 to 0.1 mg/kg (1:1000) for the IV/IO/ET routes (doses up to 0.2 mg/kg of 1:1000 may be effective) every 3 to 5 minutes**

34. **c:** Treatment of this child includes:
    - Continuing CPR
    - Ventilating him with a bag-mask device equipped with a reservoir and supplied with 10 to 15 L/min of oxygen

- Defibrillating one time 2 J/kg (maximum of 200 J), immediately resuming CPR (give five cycles of CPR)
- Defibrillating at 4 J/kg, immediately resuming CPR
- Performing endotracheal intubation using a number 6.0 or 6.5 ID cuffed or uncuffed tube
- **Placing an IV line using normal saline (or lactated Ringer's) solution**
- Administering epinephrine at an initial dose of 0.01 mg/kg (1:10,000) for the IV/IO routes and 0.1 mg/kg (1:1000) ET (maximum dose: 1 mg IV/IO; 10 mg ET). Repeat epinephrine administration every 3 to 5 minutes.
- Repeating defibrillation at 4 J/kg (maximum of 360 J), immediately resume CPR
- Considering administration of antidysrhythmics such as amiodarone, 5 mg/kg bolus IV/IO (maximum dose: 300 mg) or lidocaine, 1 mg/kg IV/IO (maximum dose: 100 mg), and 2 to 5 mg ET
- Identify and treat causes such as hypoxemia, hypovolemia, hypothermia, hyper/hypokalemia and metabolic disorders, tamponade, tension pneumothorax, toxins/poisons/drugs, and/or thrombosis, trauma
- Repeating defibrillation at 4 J/kg (maximum of 360 J), immediately resume CPR

35. **a**

36. **a**

37. **c**

38. **d:** Respiratory failure is common in infants and children, with a rapid downhill progression from respiratory distress, to respiratory failure, and finally to cardiopulmonary arrest. Treatment decisions must be made quickly to avoid progression to cardiopulmonary arrest.

Respiratory failure results from prolonged impairment of gas exchange in which there is inadequate oxygenation of the blood and inadequate elimination of carbon dioxide. It may occur because of intrinsic lung or airway disease or because of inadequate respiratory effort. Respiratory failure is often preceded by a compensated state in which the patient is able to maintain the work of breathing. This compensated state is characterized by respiratory distress, the use of accessory muscles of respiration, inspiratory retractions, tachypnea, and tachycardia.

39. **b:** Treatment of this child includes positioning his head in a neutral or sniffing position using the head-tilt/chin-lift maneuver, and **assisting his breathing with a bag-mask device** equipped with a reservoir device and supplied with high-concentration oxygen per minute. Hyperextending the neck of the infant is contraindicated because it may obstruct the airway by kinking the soft cartilaginous trachea. When ventilating with a bag-mask device, the rescuer should auscultate the patient's chest to ensure the presence of equal bilateral lung sounds. If the baby requires continuous bagging to maintain his color, endotracheal intubation is indicated. As in other cases, when endotracheal intubation is performed, the tube must be properly secured in place to prevent accidental displacement or advancement into the right or left bronchus. Lung sounds should be frequently reassessed to ensure proper placement. It is important to remember that the majority of cardiac arrest cases in children are of respiratory and not cardiac origin. Bradycardia often responds to airway management, ventilatory support, and oxygenation.

If time permits, an IV line of normal saline or lactated Ringer's solution should be placed en route to the hospital.

40. Table regarding epiglottitis and croup

	Epiglottitis	**Croup**
Cause	**Usually caused by bacterial infection**	**Usually caused by viral infection**
When it occurs	**No seasonal preference**	**Usually occurs during late fall and early winter**
Age groups seen in	**Occurs in ages 3 to 7 years**	**Occurs in ages 3 months to 3 years**
Type of onset	**Rapid onset**	**Slow onset**
How the patient presents	**Patient will sit upright in a "tripod" position**	**Patient will either lie down or sit up**
Type of cough	**No barking cough**	**"Barking" cough present**
Presence of drooling	**Pain on swallowing causing drooling**	**No drooling**
Temperature	**Temperature >104° F**	**Temperature >104° F**

41. **d: Epiglottitis** is a bacteria-caused inflammation of the epiglottis that most often occurs in children who are ages 3 to 7 years. It is a true emergency because the child can progress to complete airway obstruction and respiratory arrest if the epiglottis swells over the opening of the trachea.

    Epiglottitis tends to occur abruptly, often with the sudden onset of a severe sore throat—so sore that the child refuses to swallow (explaining the drooling associated with this condition). The child with epiglottitis usually has a muffled voice, inspiratory stridor, a fever, and appears quite ill. The child will sit upright and lean slightly forward on his or her hands with the neck extended forward (tripod position). The child typically resists any attempt to be placed in a supine position. In addition, the child will usually show signs of respiratory distress and, in severe cases, hypoxia.

42. **b:** Patients who have indications of epiglottitis should be treated as having a life-threatening condition. Treatment includes **administering humidified oxygen,** placing him or her into the most comfortable position, and providing expeditious transport to the hospital. If possible, sit the child on a parent's lap. Handle the child gently. Rough handling and stress could lead to total airway obstruction.

    Examination of the child's oropharynx with a tongue blade and penlight *is contraindicated* in epiglottitis. Give high-concentration, humidified oxygen via either a mask or blow-by method, depending on what the child will tolerate. Do not delay administration of oxygen, however, while waiting for humidification. Monitor the child's vital signs, cardiac rhythm, and pulse oximeter if doing so does not further agitate the child. If respiratory arrest occurs, bag-mask ventilation with 100% oxygen should precede any attempt to intubate the patient. Typically, ventilatory support with the bag-mask device is sufficient to maintain effective oxygenation and carbon dioxide removal.

43. **b:** Children can have **an acute asthma attack,** as well as status asthmaticus, exhibiting the same signs and symptoms as adults including wheezing. Status asthmaticus is a life-threatening situation in which an asthma attack is severe, prolonged, and cannot be broken with traditional bronchodilators. Asthma is a recurrent lower airway disease producing moderate to severe respiratory distress. Acute asthma attacks are brought on by overreaction of the trachea and bronchi to various stimuli. This gives rise to reversible spasm and constriction of the airways. Mucosal edema and hypersecretion of mucus (that forms tenacious plugs) act to further block the air passages. As a result, expiratory airflow decreases and air becomes trapped in the airways, causing alveolar hyperinflation. If allowed to progress, ventilation is progressively impaired, with increasing hypoxia, hypercarbia, acidosis, and dehydration.

    A child experiencing an acute asthma attack will often have shortness of breath, tachypnea, tachycardia, noticeable expiratory wheezing, intercostal retractions, nasal flaring, coughing, pallor or mottled skin, and apprehension and restlessness. Sometimes the attack can be so bad that there is no wheezing because the child is not able to move air adequately. As with adult patients with asthma or status asthmaticus, this condition should be considered life threatening.

44. **a:** Treatment of this child includes assessing and monitoring her ABCs, administering *high-concentration oxygen* by nonrebreather mask (humidified if possible—do not wait for humidifier if not immediately available), **establishing an IV of lactated Ringer's or normal saline solution,** and administering an aerosolized bronchodilator such as albuterol (Ventolin). Orotracheal intubation should be performed if airway management becomes difficult or ventilatory failure occurs.

    Also monitor the child's vital signs, cardiac rhythm, and pulse oximeter. Communicate with medical control.

    In severe cases, respiratory failure can occur. If the child has been struggling for awhile, he or she may finally tire and stop breathing altogether. Have equipment available to assist the child's ventilations and intubate if necessary. Circulatory support may also be necessary if the ventilatory support is not adequate.

45. **b:** Provide high-concentration, humidified oxygen (again, do not wait for humidifier if not readily available), **nebulized bronchodilator,** and transport to the hospital for further evaluation. These patients must be seen at a medical facility. Monitor the respiratory and cardiac status, as well as vital signs and pulse oximeter. Keep the child as calm as possible to maximize respiratory effort.

    If the respiratory distress increases, provide ventilatory support to include intubation if necessary. Medical control should be contacted with an update.

46.

	Asthma	Bronchiolitis
Age affected	Occurs at any age	Occurs between 6 and 18 months
Time occurs	Occurs in winter and spring	Can occur at any time
Caused by	Response to allergy, exercise, or infection	Caused by a virus
Family history	Family history of asthma	Usually no history of asthma
Effect of medications	Drugs reverse bronchospasm	Drugs may not always be effective

47. **b:** Shock is a clinical state characterized by inadequate delivery of oxygen and metabolic substrates to meet the metabolic demands of the tissues. Failure to deliver critical substrates and remove metabolites leads to anaerobic metabolism, accumulation of acid, and irreversible cellular damage. The presence of decompensated shock (hypotension, faint or absent central pulses, and obtundation) requires prompt intervention to prevent cardiac arrest.

In this case, shock was precipitated by dehydration. Vomiting, diarrhea, fever, burns, and poor fluid intake can contribute to a loss of body fluids. Children are more vulnerable to dehydration than adults because more of their body is water and their fluid maintenance needs are greater.

48. **b:** Initial treatment of this child includes conducting an initial assessment (checking the airway, breathing, and circulation), administering *100% oxygen*, establishing an IV line using *lactated Ringer's solution or normal saline* (avoid using dextrose-containing solutions unless the patient is hypoglycemic), and **delivering a fluid bolus of 20 mL/kg.** Repeat this procedure in 5 minutes if the child's vital signs do not improve. Further boluses may be necessary to restore an adequate blood pressure and subsequent tissue perfusion.

Monitor the child's vital signs and cardiac status. Assist ventilations if necessary. Prepare for immediate transport, and maintain contact with medical control. CPR may be required.

49. **a:** In many children seizures are a complication of fever, often occurring in those under the age of 5 years. Children frequently have febrile seizures in response to illnesses, with a temperature range between 101° F and 105° F. Neurological damage does not occur until the temperature reaches 107° F. These seizures are triggered by how quickly the temperature rises rather than how high the temperature goes.

50. **a:** Treatment of this patient includes monitoring her ABCs and vital signs. *If clinically indicated,* an IV of normal saline solution should be started and supplemental oxygen provided.

If a seizure is witnessed, the child should be gently assisted to a lying position with the head turned to the side. In addition, the area should be cleared of hazardous items that might cause injury during the seizure activity. *Do not insert anything into the mouth* if the teeth are clenched. A nasal airway is an appropriate alternative adjunct for this situation. The airway should be maintained and suctioned *only* as necessary.

51. **a:** This is referred to as **status epilepticus.** If this condition occurs, immediate intervention is necessary. Complications include aspiration of blood or vomit, hypoxia resulting in brain damage, long bone and spinal fractures, and severe dehydration.

52. **False:** Meningitis is defined as an inflammation of the *membranes that surround the brain and spinal cord*. It is caused by viruses, bacteria, or other microorganisms and may develop concurrently with viral illnesses such as mumps or chickenpox or a bacterial illness such as that seen with an ear infection. As the bacteria or virus spreads, the child will become increasingly more ill. In bacterial meningitis, cerebral edema can occur, which can lead to increased intracranial pressure with brainstem herniation.

53. **True:** This, along with fever in children older than 3 months, may be the only presenting sign of the disease.

54. Signs and symptoms of meningitis include fever; **vomiting;** dehydration; disorientation; **lethargy and irritability** (infant or child does not want to be touched or held); headache (in children older than 2 years); **stiff neck (in children older than 2 years);** tachycardia and tachypnea; **bulging fontanelle (in infants younger than 1 year);** photophobia (sensitivity to light); convulsion; loss of appetite; poor feeding (may be a sign in young infants); respiratory distress; cyanosis; rash; altered sleep pattern; vomiting and decreased oral intake (in children younger than 3 months); and Kernig's sign (pain when extending the legs).

55. Types of poisons ingested by children include **household products (i.e., petroleum-based agents, cleaning agents and cosmetics, lawn and garden

supplies); medications (prescription and nonprescription); toxic plants (i.e., poinsettia plants during the Christmas season); and **contaminated foods (i.e., potato salad left out all day at a summer picnic).**

56. **Blunt trauma continues to be the most common pediatric mechanism of injury.** However, penetrating injuries have increased to almost 15%. Causes of pediatric injuries categorized from most to least common are as follows:
    1. **Falls (most frequent in children less than 5 years of age)**
    2. **Vehicular-related trauma**
    3. **Accidental injury**
    4. **Sports-related injury**
    5. **Assaults**

57. **d:** Typically, during the initial stages of brain tissue injury the cerebral blood vessels dilate to increase cerebral blood flow to the injured areas. This is followed by an increase in cerebral water (which tends to occur after several hours). Because the brain tissue is enclosed in a "closed box," there is no room for the brain to expand. This increase in volume within the skull leads to an increase in pressure (referred to as increased intracranial pressure). As pressure builds in the closed compartment of the skull, the brain is squeezed and cerebral blood flow is reduced. Because the brain is extremely dependent on adequate oxygenation to meet its energy needs, severe brain damage can result from oxygen deprivation (and source of energy). Another possible consequence of increased intracranial pressure is herniation. Herniation occurs when the pressure within the skull is so great that it forces parts of the brain downward, against the tentorium or foramen magnum, causing severe damage to the brain structures that are being squeezed against the skull.

58. **b:** Treatment for this preschooler includes ensuring the ABCs, stabilizing her cervical spine by using manual in-line stabilization, opening the airway using the jaw-thrust (rather than the head-tilt/chin-lift) maneuver, **ventilating her with a bag-mask device** (supplied with 100% oxygen and equipped with a reservoir), placing an endotracheal tube, applying a cervical immobilization device and securing her to a full backboard, and establishing an IV line using *normal saline (or lactated Ringer's)* solution and running it at a keep-open rate (TKO).

    To avoid extending the neck, trauma intubation should be used in the head-injured patient. However, nasotracheal intubation and nasopharyngeal suctioning are contraindicated if basilar skull fracture is suspected (as indicated by the presence of cerebrospinal fluid leak, raccoon eyes, or Battle's sign). Rapid transport is indicated in the management of this child.

59. **c:** A **tension pneumothorax** occurs when air leaks into the pleural space through a hole in the lung or chest wall. This hole acts as a one-way valve, allowing air to enter the pleural space during inhalation but preventing its escape during exhalation. As air accumulates, pressure on the affected side builds to the point where there is a shift of the trachea, heart, and esophagus toward the unaffected lung. This squeezes the unaffected lung, thereby compromising ventilations. Shifting of the heart causes "kinking" of the major blood vessels, resulting in decreased cardiac output. Signs and symptoms of tension pneumothorax include extreme dyspnea, restlessness, anxiety, rapid and weak pulse, diminished or absent lung sounds on the affected side, and/or signs of cardiovascular collapse.

60. **c:** Additionally, you should ensure the ABCs, stabilizing his spine by using manual in-line stabilization, opening the airway using the jaw-thrust (rather than the head-tilt/chin-lift) maneuver, applying a cervical immobilization device and securing him to a full backboard, covering the wound with a nonporous dressing, performing emergency needle decompression of the chest, administering *100%* oxygen, and establishing one or two IV lines with *normal saline or lactated Ringer's solution*. Medical direction may order a bolus of 20 mL/kg initially, and repeat this procedure in 5 minutes if the child's vital signs do not improve. Further boluses may be necessary to restore an adequate blood pressure and subsequent tissue perfusion.

61. Signs of blunt trauma to the abdomen include **bruising (e.g., from a lap belt in a motor vehicle); unstable pelvis; abdominal distention, rigidity, or tenderness;** or **signs of unexplained levels of shock.** Children younger than 8 years of age also tend to be "belly breathers," so that respiratory distress may also be a sign of abdominal trauma.

62. **a:** This patient is suffering from **a fractured femur** and possible internal bleeding. The most common causes of hypovolemic shock in pediatric patients are blunt trauma to the liver or spleen. You should always maintain a high index of suspicion of significant intraabdominal injury in children.

63. **b:** Treatment for this child includes ensuring the ABCs, stabilizing her spine by using manual in-line stabilization, opening the airway using the jaw-thrust (rather than the head-tilt/chin-lift) maneuver, applying a cervical immobilization device and securing her to a full backboard, administering *100% oxygen via nonrebreather mask,* **immobilizing the injured leg with a pediatric traction splint,** and establishing one or two IV lines using normal saline (or lactated Ringer's) solution and large-bore catheters. Boluses of 20 mL/kg may be given rapid IV push, reassessing the patient after each bolus.

Aggressive fluid resuscitation should be instituted in patients with significant trauma when early signs and symptoms of blood loss are apparent or suspected, not just when the blood pressure is decreasing or absent.

A secondary exam should be performed on the child en route to the hospital.

64. **d:** In **severe hypothermia** the body functions slow down dramatically, even to the point where the heart beats less than 10 times per minute. Severe hypothermia is a life-threatening condition that requires specialized care (preferably in an appropriate definitive care setting).

65. **a:** Treatment for this patient includes moving him to a warmer environment as quickly as possible, **removing all of the wet clothes,** wrapping him in blankets (once the blankets become wet, apply new, dry blankets), assisting his breathing with a *child-sized bag-mask device supplied with 15 L/min of oxygen and a reservoir,* avoiding rough handling, and rapidly transporting him to the hospital. In addition, do not waste time attempting to start an IV. Removing wet clothes is important because the patient's body temperature will lower even more if clothes are wet and are allowed to remain. Oxygen and assisted ventilations with the appropriate size bag-mask device are important because the body cells need oxygen, and waste products of metabolism (CO_2) need to be removed. *Under no circumstances should you let anyone give the child any form of alcohol to increase warmth.*

66. **b:** Your partner suggests that the patient be placed on a full backboard. His rationale for doing this might be that **the patient may have a neck or back injury** and can be moved about more "gently" when on a backboard. Because it is undetermined how the patient got to the bottom of the ravine in the first place (i.e., he could have been hit on the head or could have fallen, striking his head), a backboard will provide needed spinal immobilization. The patient should remain on the backboard until adequate assessment for spinal injuries can be performed.

Hypothermia patients must be handled gently because rough handling may cause them to develop ventricular fibrillation (a chaotic quivering of the heart that results in ineffective pumping action). A backboard allows the patient to be moved from the ground to the cot and from the cot to the hospital bed with very little unwanted motion.

67. If a child dies within 24 hours of a submersion incident, it is called a **drowning-related death.**

68. **False:** Behaviors inflicted on the child that are degrading, terrorizing, isolating, or rejecting are referred to as *emotional or psychological abuse.*

69. **False:** Neglect is when there is a failure to meet a child's *basic needs (e.g., food, clothing, shelter, medical care, safety).*

70. Indicators of child abuse or maltreatment include **any obvious or suspected fractures in a child less than 2 years of age; injuries in various stages of healing, especially burns and bruises; more injuries than usually seen in other children of the same age; injuries scattered on many areas of the body; bruises or burns in patterns that suggest intentional infliction; suspected increased intracranial pressure in an infant; suspected intraabdominal trauma in a young child; any injury that does not fit the description of the cause given; an accusation that the child injured himself or herself intentionally; long-standing skin infections; extreme malnutrition; extreme lack of cleanliness; inappropriate clothing for the situation; child who withdraws from parent; and child who responds inappropriately to the situation (e.g., quiet, distant, withdrawn).**

71. To resolve an occluded tracheostomy tube in the child, **begin by suctioning the tube. Only about 4 or 5 seconds of suctioning is necessary because the length of the tube is so short. If you cannot remove the obstruction or insert the suction catheter, remove the entire tube. Suction the "stoma" or opening in the neck. Insert a new tube if it is available and you have been trained to do so. If another tracheostomy tube is not available, a standard infant endotracheal tube can be substituted.**

If you are unable to ventilate through the stoma and the upper airway is patent, manually occlude the stoma. Perform bag-mask ventilation over the nose and face until orotracheal intubation can be done or a replacement tracheostomy tube becomes available.

CHAPTER 36

1. **False:** Many geriatric patients are able to function independently, residing *in their own homes.*

2. **False:** There are *numerous types* of assisted living facilities that range from simply providing assistance with food or transportation to having multiple nursing, physical therapy, and pharmacy resources available to the patient 24 hours a day.

3. Resources for elderly patients include **emergency departments; hospital social services; government social service agencies; local law enforcement; local religious organizations; community agencies (e.g., United Way); and neighbors, local and distant family members.**

4. Some of the most significant problems that people face as they age involve difficulties with **general mobility.** Because of difficulties with ambulation, coordination, and strength, the incidence of **falls** is greatly increased.

5. Consequences that decreased mobility has on elderly persons include **difficulty preparing or eating food with subsequent poor nutrition; difficulty with elimination; skin abrasions, injuries, and circulatory compromise from falling; additional orthopedic or intracranial injuries from falling;** and **decreased medication compliance because of difficulties ambulating to where medications are stored.**

6. The patient who experiences decreased mobility **may feel a loss of independence. This can lead to episodes of depression, general loss of confidence in abilities, and concerns over feeling "old" in the eyes of society.**

7. **c:** You can also use this as an opportunity to do safety education—pointing out the dangers of loose rugs on slick floors, for example. Following this you can have her sign a refusal form and return to service.

8. Two significant changes in vision in persons more than 40 years of age are **cataracts** and **glaucoma.**

9. Problems that occur when older persons do not have their glasses include **impairment in their ability to recognize potential hazards, take medications,** and **prepare food.**

10. **False:** There is a *measurable* decay in hearing as the aging process progresses. This can be a significant barrier to proper communication.

11. **True**

12. **True**

13. **Decreased hearing impairs the elderly patient's ability to comprehend instructions and commands. It may also impair proper communications between the prehospital providers and the patient. Many patients experience extreme frustration when unable to adequately understand conversation directed to them.**

14. **a**

15. **Incontinence that is not cared for appropriately, leading to prolonged exposure to urinary or fecal matter on the skin, can cause tissue irritation, excoriation, and even infection.**

16. **d**

17. Communication strategies that can be used to provide psychological support to elderly patients include **recognizing that there may be barriers that can prohibit them from understanding the EMT-I; assisting with locating any hearing aids or eyeglasses; ensuring adequate lighting during assessment and treatment; respecting patients' requests; and making them a participant in their care.**

18. **a: Dentures or partial dentures may impair intubation attempts in elderly patients.** Adequate bag-mask ventilation of patients also may be difficult in certain patients *once dentures are removed.* Consideration may be needed to replace the dentures to allow adequate ventilation.

19. Many patients in the elderly population have **small** or **friable** veins. This may make venipuncture and intravenous access **difficult.**

20. Caution should be used in the **quantity** of intravenous fluid administered to patients who have any history of cardiac disease, especially **congestive heart** failure. This may precipitate acute respiratory failure and require additional ventilatory support.

21. The **EMT-I should monitor the patient for increased rales, respiratory effort, tachypnea, and difficulty with speaking.**

22. **b:** Medications administered to the elderly patient **may compete with the normal metabolic process,** are metabolized more *slowly* than in the middle-aged adult, have *significantly prolonged degradation,* and therefore may exhibit *prolonged* length of action and effect.

23.

Drug	Class
Ibuprofen	Analgesic/antiinflammatory
Morphine	Analgesic
Meperidine	Analgesic
Diltiazem	Cardiovascular agent
Lidocaine	Cardiovascular agent
Propranolol	Cardiovascular agent
Verapamil	Cardiovascular agent
Furosemide	Diuretic
Diazepam	Psychoactive

24. **False:** Elderly patients typically experience *more* adverse reactions to prescription medications than younger patients.

25. **True:** This is why lidocaine doses are typically reduced in the elderly population.

26. **True**

27. Significant changes in the patient's respiratory status that occur with the aging process include **decreased lung function because of chronic exposure to pollutants in the atmosphere; decreased efficiency in the alveolar capillary exchange; decreased tone of the respiratory muscles;** and **changes in the central nervous system's respiratory center.**

28. Common causes of respiratory disease in the elderly population include **pneumonia, pulmonary embolism,** and **obstructive lung disease.**

29. **b**

30. **d**

31. **b:** Treatment of this patient includes **administering bronchodilator therapy,** providing *supplemental* oxygen, establishing an IV line, and transporting her in a *position of comfort*. Because the patient is hypoxic, oxygen should be administered at a high concentration.

32. A high percentage of EMS calls relate to patients being evaluated for **chest** pain or **palpitations.** As individuals age, arteries tend to become more **rigid.** Patients with **hypertension** can further have cardiac and vascular damage as a result of the effects of the **elevated** blood pressure.

33. Things the EMT-I should do when gathering the present history from neurological emergency patients: **determine when the current neurological event started; maintain a calm demeanor and do not appear rushed; speak clearly and directly to the patient with very direct questions or commands;** and **allow the patient time to formulate answers and respond to questions.**

34. Prehospital management of most acute neurological events is **essentially limited to supportive care. Patients should be transported in a position of comfort, with the head elevated approximately 30 degrees on the cot. If the patient is a victim of trauma, or there is a concern for cervical spine injury, the patient should be fully supine with cervical spine immobilization and a long backboard. The patient should be placed on oxygen, and, if available, cardiac monitoring should be performed.**

35. **b**

36. **a**

37. **a:** Treatment includes **administering 100% oxygen,** establishing an IV line, and transporting the patient in a *position of comfort*.

38. **a. Alzheimer's disease:** progressive loss of cognitive function that has been associated with anatomical changes within the cerebral cortex; represents approximately 65% of all the dementias in the elderly population; typically has a subtle onset, with patients noticing diminished performance in normal tasks such as memory loss; episodes of depression, fear, and anxiety may occur; **b. Parkinson's disease:** slowly progressing degenerative disorder of the nervous system; typically distinguished by a tremor at rest, sluggish initiation of movements, and muscle rigidity; primary site of insult is an area of the brain known as the basal ganglia, which helps to initiate actions such as lifting an arm and other movements; some cases may be caused by infection or insults from drugs or toxins.

39. **False:** On average, the elderly patient may take *four or five* prescription medications routinely, as well as numerous over-the-counter medications.

40. **True:** Other physiological changes related to prescription medications within the elderly population include decreased elimination because of decreased kidney function, decreased metabolism in the liver, or inhibition from other drugs.

41. **False:** For any given drug, geriatric patients are typically *more likely* to have more significant side effects from the medication compared with the younger population. This is especially true with side effects involving the central nervous system.

42. **True**

43. **False:** *Smaller amounts* **of intoxicants may be responsible for significant levels of impairment in the geriatric patient.**

44. Signs of substance abuse in elderly patients include **mood swings, bouts of depression, anger, episodes of confusion, hallucinations,** and **falls.**

45. Patients with dementia or delirium **may wander outside in the colder climates without adequate thermal protection. These patients may have difficulty remembering where they live and getting back into a warm environment.**

46. Hyperthermia can result from inadequate **fluid** intake and **high** ambient temperatures. The **elderly** population represents the vast majority of fatalities that occur during heat waves. There are additional causes of hyperthermia in elderly persons that may be seen in response to infection, brain injury, or medication use.

47. **True**

48. **False:** *Less* **energy is needed to fracture a long bone, spinal bone, or pelvis in an elderly patient than in a young healthy adult. In some patients who have limited mobility, osteoporosis can be advanced, and fractures can occur with only trivial manipulation.**

49. **a: Cardiac function and cardiac output are reduced** in the elderly population. This leads to a *decreased* compensatory mechanism when shock or other blood loss occurs. In addition, many elderly patients take cardiac medications that may limit the heart's ability to mount the normal cardiac response to maintain adequate organ perfusion following a traumatic insult.

50. **True**

51. **True**

52. In elderly persons **preexisting diseases such as diabetes mellitus, lung disease, or malignancy can make it difficult for the body to tolerate and ultimately heal from a severe burn. Elderly burn patients are at specific risk for infection from the burn and may have a prolonged hospitalization while attempting to recover. There are additional stresses placed on the patient's heart during an acute burn that may place the patient at additional risk for a myocardial infarction as a secondary component of the injury.**

53. You **should support the patient by placing pads, sheets, or blankets in void areas between the patient and board.** Every attempt should be made to provide some padding before placing the patient on the board.

54. Answers to crossword puzzle

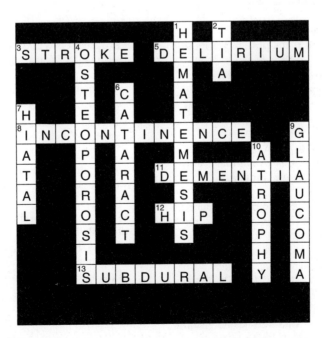

CHAPTER 37

1. With the increased usage of specialized technology, infants survive life-threatening illnesses and birth anomalies to become productive adult citizens. Children and adults also are successfully resuscitated from critical illness or injury only to require rehabilitation or special adaptive devices to function. This population is at a higher risk for emergencies. To properly treat this unique group, the EMT-I must develop the necessary knowledge and skill.

2. **Deafness** is a complete or partial inability to hear.

3. Type of hearing loss with the correct characteristics: **a. Conductive:** related to problems of the outer or middle ear, most common, interference with loudness of sound; **b. sensorineural:** Result of problems with inner ear or auditory nerve, also called perceptive or nerve deafness, distortion of sound and problems with discrimination of sound (identifying one sound from another); **c. Mixed:** combination of conductive and sensorineural, interference with transmission of sound in the middle ear and along the neural pathways.

4. c

5. Six things you can do to communicate with persons who are hearing impaired are:
   - If the patient reads lips, face the person whenever speaking.
   - Try not to use complicated language or large words.
   - Talk at a slow and even pace.
   - Provide paper and pencil if the patient wants to write a note.
   - If the patient uses sign language, ask for assistance from anyone present. Remember that an injury to the hands or upper extremities may greatly inhibit the patient's ability to communicate through sign language.
   - Consider using pictures to show basic medical procedures. Laminate pictures of routine treatments, and keep them in the ambulance.

6. Type of vision loss with the correct description: **a. Partially sighted:** refers to a patient who has some type of visual problem who may need assistance; **b. Low vision:** refers to individuals who are unable to read a newspaper at the usual viewing distance even if they use glasses or contact lenses; **c. Legally blind:** refers to a person who has less than 20/200 vision in at least one eye or has a very limited field of vision; **d. Totally blind:** refers to anyone who has no vision and uses nonvisual media or reads via Braille.

7. Five things you can do to assist persons who are visually impaired include:
   - Orient the patient to whatever care or treatment is being provided.
   - "Lead" ambulatory patients instead of "pushing" them.
   - Explain any movements in position (moving the stretcher from the home to the back of the ambulance).
   - Retrieve visual aids if necessary and take them to the hospital.
   - Notify staff at the hospital so that appropriate assistance can be available.

8. **True**

9. **False:** Aphasia can affect both children and adults and may affect their ability to speak and/or to comprehend written or spoken words.

10. **b**

11. Four things you can do to assist persons who have speech impairment are:
    - Provide extra time for the patient to respond to questions.
    - Avoid displays of impatience.
    - Provide a pen and paper if that will facilitate the communication.
    - Work with other people at the scene, if available, who know the person's style of communication.

12. **b**

13. **Paraplegia** is weakness or paralysis of both legs and possibly the trunk. **Quadriplegia** is weakness or paralysis affecting the level below the neck and chest area, involving all four extremities.

14. Paralysis is **complete** when there is no voluntary movement or sensation below the level of the injury.

15. **False:** Medical illnesses may also cause paralysis or weakness.

16. **a:** The head of the spina bifida patient is kept in the **neutral, in-line** position because of the possibility of an Arnold-Chiari malformation. Hyperextension of the head for this patient can cause apnea because of compression of the brainstem.

17. **d**

18. A person with spina bifida is prone to **latex** allergy. Latex-free equipment should be available in the ambulance to use in this instance, or the person may have a life-threatening allergic reaction.

CHAPTER 38

1. c

2. Failure to perform an adequate assessment may lead the EMT-I to **underestimate the severity of illness or injury, not discover acute life-threatening injuries or medical conditions, and not initiate the proper treatment for the condition that is truly affecting the patient.**

3. Effective assessment skills involve the continuous **gathering, evaluation,** and ongoing **synthesizing** of the information that the EMT-I learns from the **environment** and the patient.

4. Things an effective assessment will allow the EMT-I to do: **have a functional understanding of the patient's current medical crisis; make the appropriate determination of which actions are necessary; and initiate the appropriate treatment and transportation decisions.**

5. **a:** It is said that as much as 80% of medical diagnoses are based on history alone.

6. **b:** The history is most often gathered from **the patient.** It can also be gathered from friends, family members, or medical records at the patient's home.

7. An effective history-taking process involves asking **key** and **focused** questions regarding certain components of the patient's **signs** and **symptoms** throughout the history taking.

8. These **key** questions should be focused toward the **chief complaint** and **associated** problems that are learned during the history-taking process.

9. **False:** A *strong* knowledge of the disease or injury process *is required* for the EMT-I to determine which key questions are needed.

10. **False:** The EMT-I needs to be suspicious for different working diagnoses that may become apparent while obtaining the patient history.

11. c

12. The physical examination is utilized **to support diagnostic clues that are gained during the history of present illness, as well as to ensure that basic life functions are occurring appropriately.**

13. a

14. As information is gathered through the history of present illness and physical examination, this information is cognitively compared with information already in the EMT-I's knowledge base. Patterns within the information learned will prompt the EMT-I to suspect certain medical conditions or injuries. This is the basis of the working diagnosis.

15. The determination of the proper working diagnosis **allows the EMT-I to select the appropriate treatment protocol. Proper assessment not only allows the EMT-I to know how to apply the protocols but also helps identify situations in which deviations from protocol are necessary.**

16. Factors the EMT-I uses to form a proper attitude include **a knowledge base composed of understanding of traumatic injuries and medical emergencies, training and proper use of life-saving equipment,** and **an understanding of the responsibilities to the patient that the EMT-I assumes.**

17. **True**

18. **False:** *Any patient assessment will be flawed* if the EMT-I is judgmental at any time during the encounter.

19. A judgmental attitude may lead the EMT-I to **ignore critical information or neglect to ask important questions in the history gathering. Judging, or labeling, patients unfortunately causes the EMT-I to assume certain aspects of the patient's overall condition that may easily be false.**

20. Uncooperative patients, friends, or family members **can severely limit needed information sharing and may lead to critical treatment not being undertaken.**

21. Another component of the EMT-I's attitude in patient assessment is the **thoughtfulness** put into each component of the **decision-making** process.

22. "Locking on" to a specific working diagnosis early in the assessment process **may cause the EMT-I to overlook crucial pieces of information from the history or physical examination that may reveal a more life-threatening condition.**

23. Without an organized team approach to patient assessment and interventions **a member of the team may overlook critical pieces of information regarding the patient's current medical emergency, injury, or pertinent medical history when that information is needed.**

24. **True**

25. **False:** *Before the patient is even reached,* team members should have roles assigned so that job responsibilities are clear and can be immediately undertaken.

26. **False:** The EMS crew member should *avoid always performing the same duties* for each patient encounter. Rotating specific job duties, so that each team member gets exposed to history taking, assessment, and interventions, will allow the whole crew to maintain critical skills that are needed for optimal patient care.

27. The team leader **coordinates and ensures that a thorough history is obtained; ensures an appropriate patient assessment is performed; provides that interventions are undertaken and completed in their appropriate fashion; handles communications with medical control and hospital personnel; establishes personal contact with the patient and serves as the primary personnel obtaining the patient's history; designates tasks for other team members to perform, as well as coordinating interactions among providers for other patients; acts as the EMS on-scene commander during mass casualty situations until additional resources arrive; and oversees all advanced life support functions in clinical cases, including interpretation of the ECG, communications with medical direction, pharmaceutical intervention, and ensuring the proper record keeping takes place.**

28. **The EMT-I must assume that every patient encounter may be the worst possible situation. For critical patients, there is not enough time to go back and retrieve the critical equipment off the ambulance. For these patients, certain essential life-saving interventions may be initiated while the assessment process is still occurring. Not bringing key equipment to the patient can seriously compromise overall patient care.**

29. Management of the high-acuity patient requires an **oxygen tank and regulator, a laryngoscope and a selection of laryngoscope blades, suction devices including rigid and flexible suction catheters, a bag-mask device,** and **a cardiac monitor/defibrillator.**

30. The EMT-I should approach the patient appearing **calm** and **well organized.**

31. The EMT-I must portray a high degree of **confidence** and **skill** to the patient to establish and maintain a level of trust.

32. Patients who have concern over the abilities of their caregiver **frequently will comment on negative aspects of the encounter to providers once the patient is at the hospital and may require a more significant amount of time when obtaining consent to begin therapies.**

33. To ensure that the prehospital patient care team comes across as a strong, confident, highly skilled unit they must **have preestablished plans designating roles and assignments, identify one team member who will essentially function as team leader and carry on all dialog with the patient,** and **make sure that all necessary equipment is initially brought to the scene.**

34. The team member who is obtaining history and interacting with the patient should **maintain eye contact with the patient and speak at a level the patient can easily understand. Ask open-ended questions, and listen thoroughly for the patient's answers. The key to a successful history-gathering process is not only asking the right questions but also listening for the detailed answer.**

35. **a. Evacuation approach:** with the initial assessment, the EMT-I determines that critical life-saving interventions are needed that cannot be provided by on-scene caregivers; most commonly used in trauma patients with penetrating injuries to the thorax or abdomen; **b. Resuscitative approach:** initial assessment identifies that immediate interventions are needed and can be initiated by the EMT-I; typically involve patients who have cardiac or respiratory arrest, respiratory failure or distress, unstable cardiac dysrhythmias, and so on; **c. Uncomplicated approach:** patients typically do not need immediate intervention; a more "relaxed" patient history, physical assessment, and interventions can be undertaken.

36. **b**

37. Components of the systemic patient assessment include **rapidly identifying the chief complaint; assessing the degree of distress the patient is currently experiencing; performing an initial assessment; completing a complete set of vital signs; and then proceeding with a focused interview of the relevant history, as well as a focused physical examination.**

38. **a:** Until the EMT-I is comfortable doing both at the same time, the history should be obtained separately, with key findings of the history documented before the assessment is undertaken. In the rush to perform a thorough physical exam, the inexperienced EMT-I may not listen to key components of the patient history. This may lead the EMT-I to make the incorrect working diagnosis.

39. Failure to effectively **communicate** is often identified as one of the weakest links in the prehospital-to-hospital transition of patient care.

40. Utilizing effective communication skills will help the EMT-I gain more **trust** and **credibility** within the health care system.

41. Highlights of prehospital-to-hospital communications include **concise reports that typically last approximately 1 minute or less; following relatively standard reporting formats that are utilized by all EMS providers in the region; providing the working diagnosis as the first part of the medical report; reporting pertinent pieces of the history of present illness, past medical history, and physical findings;** and **reporting pertinent negative findings.**

42. Answers to crossword puzzle

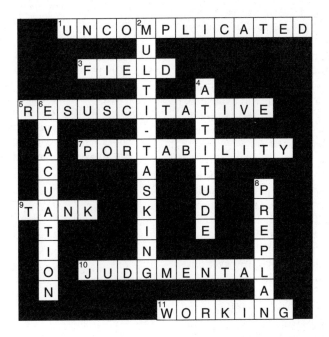

CHAPTER 39

1. **Terrorism is a crime directed toward the achievement of a political goal not achievable by normal means.**

2. Three classes of terrorists are **international groups, domestic issue groups, and loners**.

3. **The first warning sign of terrorism may be ill victims. These ill individuals must be differentiated from typical patients through careful assessment and consideration of all the pertinent information. For example, an outbreak with patients presenting with flulike symptoms at a time of year when flu would be unexpected should be closely scrutinized because it indicates the use of bioterrorism.**

4. Type of chemical agent with the correct description: **a. Organophosphate nerve agents:** produce an overload of acetylcholine by blocking acetylcholinesterase, the enzyme that breaks down acetylcholine in the body; **b. Vesicants:** inhibit deoxyribonucleic acid (DNA) replication; **c. Chemical asphyxiants:** interfere with the use and metabolism of oxygen in the body.

5. **d**

6. SLUDGE means: **Salivation, Lacrimation (tearing), Urinary incontinence, Defecation or fecal incontinence, Generalized weakness, Emesis.**

7. **c**

8. **Barrier protection refers to personal protective equipment (PPE). This involves the use of hazardous materials (HAZMAT) gear, consisting of heavy rubber gloves and chemical-resistant garments and respiratory protection through use of either air filtration or supplied air.**

9. Three medications that are used in the treatment of exposure to organophosphate nerve agents: **atropine, pralidoxime, and diazepam (Valium).**

10. The contents of a Mark I kit: **atropine (2 mg) and pralidoxime (600 mg)**

11. **b**

12. The medications used to treat exposure to organophosphate nerve agents are supplied in **autoinjectors** and delivered by **intramuscular** injection.

13. **a**

14. **a**

15. **Mustard is more sinister than Lewisite because it is painless until the blisters begin forming, 2 to 24 hours after exposure. This lag time between exposure and the emergence of symptoms means that victims will have moved from the site of exposure, making recognition more difficult, and contaminated victims may have unwittingly contaminated other areas and victims.**

16. **First, remove the person with cyanide poisoning from the scene of exposure. If the person remains symptomatic, a cyanide antidote kit may be used. The cyanide treatment kit contains amyl nitrite, sodium nitrite, and sodium thiosulfate. The amyl nitrite is in the form of a "pearl" or "popper" and is intended to be inhaled before intravenous administration of the sodium nitrite.**

17. **The most efficient way to spread biological weapons is aerosolization of disease-causing microbes or toxins, which results in the mist of particles being breathed in by the victim. A biological aerosol is invisible because the particles are very small (1 to 5 microns) and dustlike.**

18. **True**

19. Five conditions or types of diseases that may be caused by biological agents include **respiratory conditions, neurological conditions, hemorrhagic viral diseases, gastroenteritis-causing diseases, and infectious skin diseases.**

20. Eight biological agents that can be aerosolized are **anthrax (inhaled), ricin (inhaled), T-2 mycotoxin (inhaled), *Staphylococcus* enterotoxin B (inhaled), plague, tularemia, *Brucella* spp., and influenza (super-flu).**

21. Four protective measures the first responder should take to ensure that no further spread of a disease caused by a biological agent occurs include: **barrier protection, high-efficiency particulate air (HEPA) filter mask (N-95 or better), communication with medical command, communication with the receiving facility to ensure that quarantine can be maintained, and decontamination of the transport vehicle before return to service, depending on the suspected agent involved.**

22. **b**

23. **c**

24. **False:** A standard Geiger counter can be used to determine the presence or absence of radioactivity at a scene.

25. **True**

26. **True**

27. **True**

28. **False**

CHAPTER 40

1. An incident management system is a **coordinated system of procedures that assists in the control, direction, and coordination of emergency response resources.**

2. **Incident management systems provide an orderly method for communicating and decision making at emergency scenes regardless of the size. Incident management systems also make communication and interaction among different agencies more efficient.**

3. **False.** Law enforcement, fire departments, EMS agencies, local hospitals, and support services such as the Red Cross, Salvation Army, health departments, and public works departments use the incident command system.

4. **True**

5. **False:** Usually the incident plan determines who assumes the initial command.

6. **c**

7. During major incidents, several **sectors** are established, each with unique **responsibilities**.

8. The seven recognized EMS sectors are:
   - **Incident command**
   - **Triage**
   - **Extrication**
   - **Treatment**
   - **Staging**
   - **Transportation**
   - **Supply (support)**

9. **a**

10. **d**

11. Priority levels with the correct conditions: **a. highest priority:** airway or breathing difficulties, uncontrolled or severe bleeding, decreased or altered mental status, severe medical problems, signs and symptoms of shock (hypoperfusion), and severe burns with airway compromise; **b. second priority:** burns without airway compromise, multiple or major bone or joint injuries, and back injuries with or without spinal cord damage; **c. lowest priority:** minor bone or joint injuries, minor soft tissue injuries, prolonged respiratory arrest, cardiopulmonary arrest, and death.

12. **True**

CHAPTER 41

1. Tactical Emergency Medical Support (TEMS) **is the area of EMS directly involved with supporting law enforcement operations.**

2. **TEMS provides medical support in unique environments that have a high risk of injury and limited potential for standard "load and go" situations. This allows for the provision of medical treatment when there are limited resources and decreased ability to evacuate the patient.**

3. **True**

4. **b:** The tactical commander has ultimate authority over all members of the tactical team, *including TEMS members*.

5. Tactical environment zones with descriptions: **a. Cold zone:** sometimes referred to as safe zone, area of no threat; **b. Warm zone:** area of potential threat; **c. Hot zone:** sometimes referred to as the kill zone, area of direct or immediate threat.

6. Six responsibilities of TEMS:
   - **Proper health maintenance and medical preparation of all tactical team members.**
   - **Preplanning potential medical responses related to the mission.**
   - **Medical intelligence gathering on perpetrators, hostages, or other involved civilians.**
   - **Providing medical support during the operational phase of the mission.**
   - **Establishing and operating a rest and rehabilitation area.**
   - **Medical and behavior health debriefing as needed at the completion of the operational phase.**

7. **c**

8. **d**

9. The **entry** phase is the most dangerous.

10. Typical TEMS equipment is carried in **black** or **camouflage** bags to limit visibility during operations.

11. **a**

12. **True**